P9-DZZ-947

Cleft Palate Speech

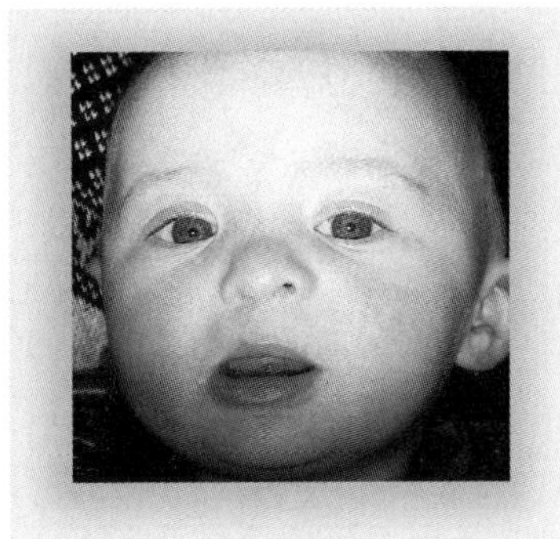

Cleft Palate Speech

THIRD EDITION

Sally J. Peterson-Falzone, PhD

Clinical Professor
Department of Growth and Development
Speech-Language Pathologist
Center for Craniofacial Anomalies
University of California
San Francisco, California

Mary A. Hardin-Jones, PhD

Associate Professor
Division of Communication Disorders
University of Wyoming
Laramie, Wyoming

Michael P. Karnell, PhD

Associate Professor
Department of Otolaryngology—Head and Neck Surgery
Department of Speech Pathology and Audiology
University of Iowa
Iowa City, Iowa

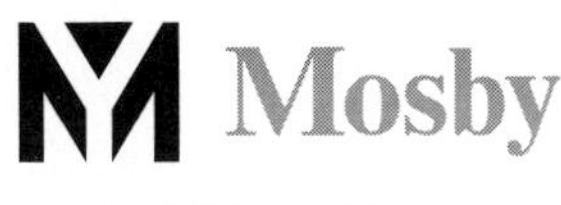

An Affiliate of Elsevier

WB

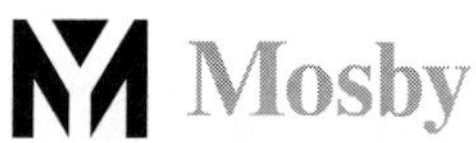

An Affiliate of Elsevier

Editor John A. Schrefer
Developmental Editor Christie M. Hart
Project Manager Carol Sullivan Weis
Production Editor Florence Achenbach
Designer Mark A. Oberkrom

THIRD EDITION

Mosby, Inc.
An Affiliate of Elsevier
11830 Westline Industrial Drive
St. Louis, Missouri 63146

Printed in the United States of America

Library of Congress Cataloging-in-Publication Data

Peterson-Falzone, Sally J.
Cleft palate speech. — 3rd ed. / Sally J. Peterson-Falzone, Mary A. Hardin-Jones, Michael P. Karnell.
p. ; cm.
Includes bibliographical references and index.
ISBN-13: 978-0-8151-3153-3 ISBN-10: 0-8151-3153-4 (hard cover)
1. Cleft palate—Complications. 2. Cleft lip—Complications. 3. Speech disorders. 4. Speech disorders in children. I. Hardin-Jones, Mary A. II. Karnell, Michael P. III. McWilliams, Betty Jane. IV. Title.
[DNLM: 1. Cleft Palate. 2. Speech Disorders. WV 440 P485c 2000]
RD525.M38 2000
617.5'22501—dc21

00-055908

ISBN-13: 978-0-8151-3153-3
ISBN-10: 0-8151-3153-4

06 07 08 09 10 GW/MP 9 8 7 6 5

7/19/07

To

Drs. Betty Jane McWilliams, Hughlett L. Morris,
and **Ralph L. Shelton, Jr.**

the master clinicians, researchers, and teachers
who wrote the first two editions of *Cleft Palate Speech* (1984, 1990).
Their research and scholarship defined many of the questions
asked during the last four decades and continue
to inspire young investigators today.

PREFACE

Betty Jane McWilliams, Hughlett L. Morris, and Ralph L. Shelton, Jr., wrote *Cleft Palate Speech* as both a text and a reference source for upper level undergraduate students and graduate students in speech pathology. They struggled to find the right mix of readable, comprehensive, but also comprehensible material to offer young professionals. When they passed this task along to us for the third edition, we also struggled. To no one's surprise, the amount of material had grown exponentially in the 16 years between the first and third editions of the book. Moreover, access to scientific material had changed from paper and pencil searches of printed material in libraries to instantaneous electronic access to innumerable journals and databases throughout the world. The attempt to update the original book had to begin with hard decisions about what to include, what to omit, and what to cite as additional sources.

There is no doubt that the information contained in these pages will be, to some extent, out of date by the time the ink dries. We have tried to give students and other readers a perspective on how to evaluate both old and new information. Some of the old information still holds value; much of it does not, and we have tried to demonstrate the difference. But the ability to judge new "data" and to differentiate data from opinions will always be critical for clinicians and researchers; otherwise, professionals will make errors that will cause patients unnecessary problems. None of the three of us is a perfect clinician, but we hope the information offered in this book will help new clinicians avoid the mistakes that we and others have made.

Sally J. Peterson-Falzone, PhD
Mary A. Hardin-Jones, PhD
Michael P. Karnell, PhD

Acknowledgments

From Sally Peterson-Falzone

Nick Falzone pushed me to accept the responsibility of spearheading the rewriting of *Cleft Palate Speech* and promised not to complain too much about all the time and attention it would take. He was true to his word. He emitted deep sighs of neglect only occasionally and endured no small number of temper tantrums. (I will always remember that, when we first met, I struggled mightily to explain "craniofacial speech pathology." He listened patiently for a few minutes, then interrupted to say, "That sounds like a nice way to talk about some not-very-nice things." I was struck by his instant empathy for conditions that were previously unknown to him, and I remain stricken 25 years later.)

My coworkers at the Center for Craniofacial Anomalies at the University of California, San Francisco, also endured me while this project was underway, offering any help I needed. Dr. Karin Vargervik helped edit and revise the sections on dental and prosthetic issues. Others (Anne Boekelheide, Alison Winder, Judith Waskow, Bill Hoffman, Ilse Sauerwald) helped locate photographs or obtain new ones and generally tried to keep me sane.

The Mosby editors, Christie Hart and John Schrefer, were more patient than they had ever planned to be and did a perfect job of combining encouragement with prodding. I sincerely hope the quality of this product rewards their endurance.

When I was first given this assignment, I went immediately to Mike Karnell and Mary Hardin-Jones to ask them to accept the other two thirds of the responsibility. They graciously accepted, although each already was overly committed to teaching, clinical duties, research, and writing assignments. They did not flinch; they just kept working. They know I love them. Some of their students and protégés already know how key their contributions are in this field, and others will learn.

Many professionals both in my own field and in other fields have taught me. Apart from our beloved Hugh, the two most important, for me, are long gone. I would never have developed a career in craniofacial anomalies if it had not been for a very complex, difficult, and wonderful man who founded the first center for craniofacial anomalies in the United States, the late Samuel Pruzansky. And I could never have stayed in the field, let alone endured Sam, without Donna Pruzansky, who was one of the first nurses to study feeding problems of infants with clefts and who was, more importantly, the personification of the word "nurturer."

Finally, children and families are the best teachers. Those who come to the UCSF Center for Craniofacial Anomalies seem to give anything they can so that the burden will be a little lighter for those who follow. I am always tempted to think that one day we will know everything we need to know if we will just hush up and listen to the kids.

From Mary Hardin-Jones

Tasks of this kind often are accomplished at someone else's expense. Colleagues who once counted on you to provide that extra bit of support learn to live without you or at least without your full participation. To friends and colleagues who tolerated my absence (and presence!) at times, endured the vacant stares, and continually offered their support—my heartfelt thanks. To kids such as Clarissa, Amanda, and Sheena, who have taught me so much, and to all the others who continually force me to admit that I don't know as much as I like to think I do—a special thank you. You and your lessons will not be forgotten. Finally, to David and Kathryn—my love and gratitude. You both provided more patience and support than I had a right to expect.

From Michael Karnell

The very special role that Hugh Morris has played as mentor and friend to all three authors of *Cleft Palate Speech,* third edition, deserves special acknowledgment. It is impossible to overstate the importance of his influence on the careers of these three authors and on the body of knowledge regarding cleft palate and craniofacial anomalies that exists today. Without his encouragement, this latest edition would not have been initiated, much less completed. A simple "Thank you, Hugh" seems inadequate, but it will have to do.

The work of Hugh, Betty Jane McWilliams, and Ralph Shelton, which made the first two editions of this book successful and which continues to enhance the current edition, provided a target we could only hope to approximate in this edition. Speaking only of my own contribution, I hope what has been done here will meet with their acceptance, if not necessarily their complete approval.

The readers of this third edition should know that the bulk of the careful hard work that went into this project came from Sally Peterson-Falzone. Sally has always been and will continue to be a role model and inspiration to me. My sincere thanks go out to her for so skillfully driving this often difficult-to-manage bus.

Finally, I acknowledge my dear wife, Lucy Hynds Karnell, and loving children, Jessica (age 14) and Cohen (age 9). They are a daily reminder of what a fortunate person I am.

Contents

Chapter 1

Cleft Lip and Palate

Cleft lip and palate and related congenital disorders assume many forms. These structural defects that occur very early in the embryo are present at birth. A cleft of the lip and a cleft of the palate can occur separately, although they are more likely to occur together. Clefts can occur as isolated defects, but on the whole they are more likely to occur with at least one minor or one major associated malformation. In this chapter you will learn about types of clefts, variations in severity of clefts, the incidence of clefts, and the association with other defects or syndromes. We will also discuss how clefts form in the embryo and review what is known about possible causes. As of this writing, the body of knowledge about causes of clefts and other birth defects is burgeoning, practically changing from day to day as we acquire new information from the Human Genome Project.[1] Thus the information presented here will be current only to the date of composition.

AN INTRODUCTORY GLOSSARY

As a background for this material, you will need a basic vocabulary having to do with birth defects:

Association a pattern of anomalies identified in two or more individuals but not yet identified as either a syndrome or a sequence.

Chromosomal caused by abnormalities in the number or structure of chromosomes. Probably the best known example of a chromosomal disorder is Down syndrome. Most individuals with this syndrome have an extra chromosome 21, a condition designated as "trisomy 21." Some individuals, however, have only a partial extra chromosome; others are "mosaics," with only part of their somatic cells carrying the extra chromosome.

Congenital present at birth. This is a term that is often misused, and one that is confusing for several reasons. A congenital disorder is one for which the underlying pathologic mechanism occurred before birth, yet there are some congenital disorders that do not become clinically apparent until many years later (e.g., Huntington's chorea). "Congenital" is not equivalent to "inherited" because many congenital traits or disorders are not inherited from either parent but are the result of a change in the genetic material at the time of formation of the egg or sperm (termed a "spontaneous mutation") or of various factors influencing intrauterine life such as an abnormally shaped uterus or maternal substance abuse.

Deformation abnormal form, shape, or position of a part of the body caused by mechanical forces (Spranger et al., 1982). Examples include abnormal shape of an external ear or even the cranium as a result of inadequate room within the mother's uterus. However, the mechanical force that causes a deformation may also be intrinsic to the fetus itself: The fetus has to move to provide room for itself to grow; if there is inadequate movement because of an inherent neurological or muscular defect, that defect becomes an intrinsic force that causes deformation of a body part.

Disruption a morphologic defect of an organ or a larger region of the body caused by extrinsic breakdown of, or interference with, an originally normal developmental process (Spranger et al., 1982). A classic example is the damage that can be done to a developing fetus by amniotic bands—abnormal fibrous bands that form within the amnion—amputating parts of limbs and even causing atypical orofacial "clefts" if the fetus swallows the bands.

Epidemiology the study of the incidence and distribution of diseases and of their control and prevention.

Etiology the science and study of the causes of disease (commonly shortened simply to "cause").

Genetic determined by properties of the genes. By definition, genetic conditions are congenital (present at

[1]The Human Genome Project is attempting to map and identify all the approximately 100,000 human genes arranged on our 46 chromosomes. This work is progressing so rapidly that on-line computer updates are virtually the only way for clinicians to keep current. In 1995 Sperber stated that 53 genes related to craniofacial disorders had been mapped: 30 related to dental tissue development, 20 related to cleft defects, and 3 related to craniosynostosis. As of this writing (June 1999), there are almost 100 loci identified for clefting, and nine genes have been mapped for craniosynostosis syndromes.

birth), but the opposite is not true because congenital conditions may be genetic, chromosomal, teratogenic, multifactorial, or unknown in etiology.

Malformation a defect in the formation of an organ, part of an organ, or a larger region of the body resulting from an intrinsically abnormal developmental process (Spranger et al., 1982). That is, the formation of the organ was "misprogrammed" from the moment of fertilization.

Pathogenesis the pathologic, physiologic, or biochemical mechanism resulting in the development of a disease or morbid process.

Sequence one anomaly causing a cascade of secondary anomalies. Probably the most familiar example is Pierre Robin sequence, in which it is theorized that the initial anomaly is an abnormally small (either deformed or malformed) mandible that keeps the tongue between the palatal shelves, preventing them from meeting and fusing, thus causing a cleft palate.[2] The anomalies in Robin sequence do not constitute a syndrome, although the sequence often does occur as part of a syndrome, particularly anomalies in which the mandible is inherently defective. The most common examples are mandibulofacial dysostosis (Treacher Collins syndrome) and Stickler syndrome (hereditary arthro-ophthalmopathy).

Syndrome multiple anomalies (multiple defects in one or more tissues) occurring together in an individual but having a single pathogenesis. For example, there are many structural and developmental problems in Down syndrome, but they all stem from the excess chromosome 21.

Teratogenic tending to produce abnormalities of formation. This term is applied to environmental factors. In craniofacial clinics we are currently seeing an increasing number of children with a variety of structural and developmental disorders resulting from maternal drug and alcohol intake.

TYPES OF CLEFTS

The speech-language pathologist working in the public schools or other nonmedical settings may never have the opportunity to see children with unrepaired clefts and thus has little opportunity to appreciate the great variation in types and severity of clefts in infants before surgical intervention. Historically, admirable effort was put into developing categorization systems for clefts, all of which were essentially elaborations on the basic dichotomy of cleft lip with or without (+/−) cleft palate (CL +/− P) versus cleft palate alone (CPO).[3] Clefts of the lip +/− palate may be either unilateral or bilateral and "incomplete" versus "complete." The latter designation speaks only to whether there is any tissue across the line of the cleft, although that tissue may be minimal. It will help to keep in mind that, in addition to unilateral versus bilateral, clefts vary in three other dimensions: anterior to posterior, width, and "depth" or "top to bottom" (nasal mucosa, bone of the hard palate or muscle of the soft palate, oral mucosa). Even the dichotomy of "unilateral" versus "bilateral" is not always helpful in terms of describing severity because some unilateral clefts are very wide. Thus the clinician who has not seen the child from early infancy may be left guessing about the severity of the original defect and the influence of that severity on both the success of surgical reconstruction and the development of communication skills.

Although the terminology may seem confusing if you have not had a course in embryology, your ability to picture or conceptualize types of clefts will be enhanced if you keep in mind that the middle portion of the lip (that portion extending from one lateral incisor to the other lateral incisor) and the anterior portion of the palate are formed from an embryonic structure called the "primary palate." This structure is wedge shaped, the posterior point of the wedge corresponding to the incisive foramen. A cleft of the lip or cleft of the lip and alveolus may be termed a "cleft of the primary palate" by some clinicians. All the rest of the hard palate and the soft palate form from the embryonic "secondary palate." Thus a cleft of the "palate only" is often clinically labeled a "cleft of the secondary palate." This will be explained in greater detail in a following section.

Cleft Lip

Clinically, clefts of the lip vary from a small defect (Fig. 1-1, *A*) to a complete cleft extending up to and through the floor of the nostril (Fig. 1-1, *B*). "Microforms" of cleft lip may include a minimal notch in the vermilion, a minor defect where the mucosa of the lip meets the cutaneous portion (skin), a fibrous band or depressed groove running up to the nostril, and minor deformity of the nose on the same side (Lehman and Artz, 1976). These defects are often associated with a minor alveolar deformity (Cosman and Crikelair, 1966; Ranta, 1988). A minimal defect of the lip with or without a minimal defect of the alveolus may also be called a "forme fruste." Microforms of cleft lip have no clinical significance for the speech-language pathologist but the patient or family may desire surgical repair. In addition, the geneticist studying the family will note all microforms of clefts, as well as other minor defects. When there is a cleft on both sides of the lip, the two defects may be symmetrical or quite asymmetrical (e.g., complete on one side, incomplete on the other) (Fig. 1-2). There may be a partial bridge of soft tissue across a cleft of the lip +/− alveolus, as seen on the right side of the lip in Fig. 1-2. A very thin bridge of soft tissue across a cleft lip may be termed a "Simonart's band" (Fig. 1-3). A cleft of the lip, even if incomplete, is typically associated with deformity of the nose, causing collapse or flattening on the affected side and a flaring of the alar base (Fig. 1-4).

Cleft lip is usually, but not always, accompanied by a cleft of the alveolus or dental arch (Fig. 1-4). The cleft in

---

[2]However, there is dissent about this sequence. Please see the section on embryology.

[3]Many texts recap classic categorization systems for clefts. However, if clinicians do not agree on the details or dimensions that must be present for a cleft to fit a certain category, the categorization system serves no purpose. Rather than repeat the historical systems, we prefer to urge clinicians to describe in detail the cleft in any given patient.

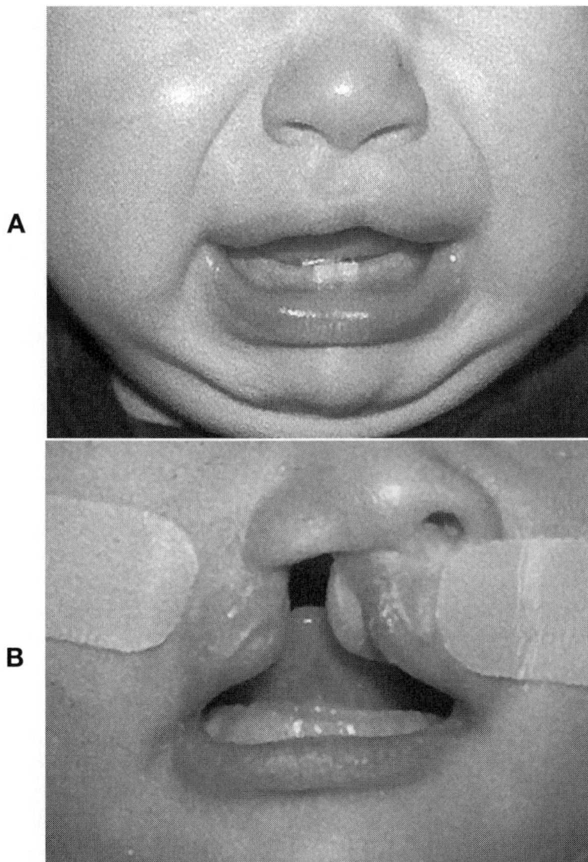

Figure 1-1 Unilateral cleft of the lip may vary from a barely detectable "microform" **(A)** to a complete cleft through the lip and base of the nose **(B).** (The tape on the lateral segments in **B** is there in preparation for a small additional device or tape that will serve to bring the protrusive premaxilla [*baby's left*] into a better position for surgical repair. See Chapters 4 and 5 on dental and surgical management for details on such treatment).

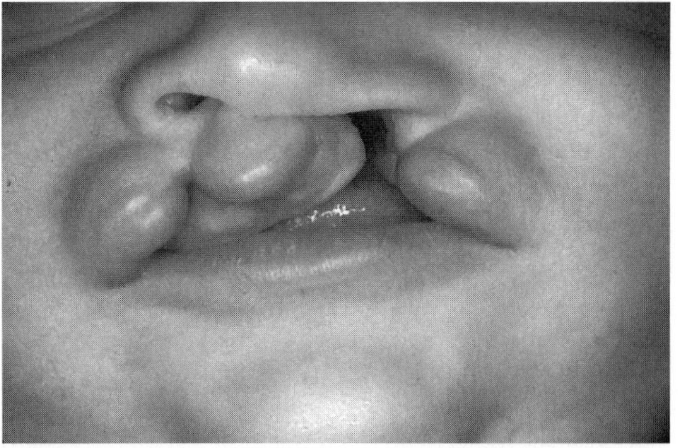

Figure 1-2 Asymmetrical bilateral cleft lip, complete on the baby's left side but incomplete on the right.

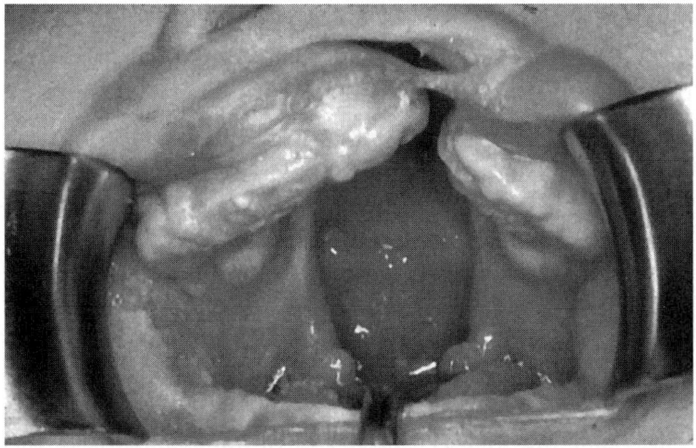

Figure 1-3 Very thin bridge of soft tissue across an otherwise complete cleft of the lip and palate. This bridge of tissue is often called a "Simonart's band." If you look closely, you will see that this baby actually has an "incomplete bilateral cleft" of the primary palate because there is also a small defect of the lip on the baby's right side (not easily seen in this picture) and a more easily seen but small defect of the alveolus. The cleft of the secondary palate is quite wide in this infant.

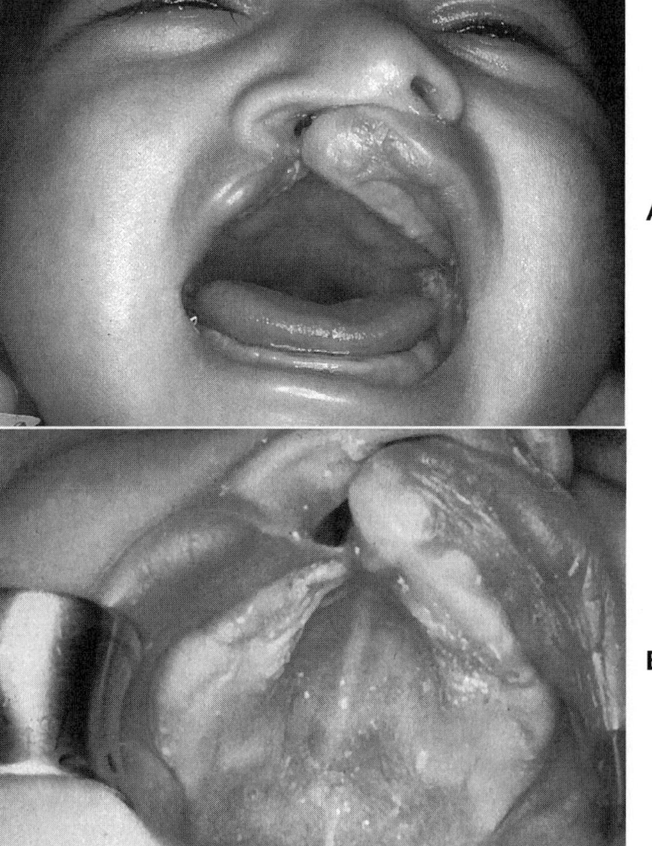

Figure 1-4 **A** and **B,** Incomplete cleft of the lip and alveolus on the right side, but the nostril on this side is still very flattened.

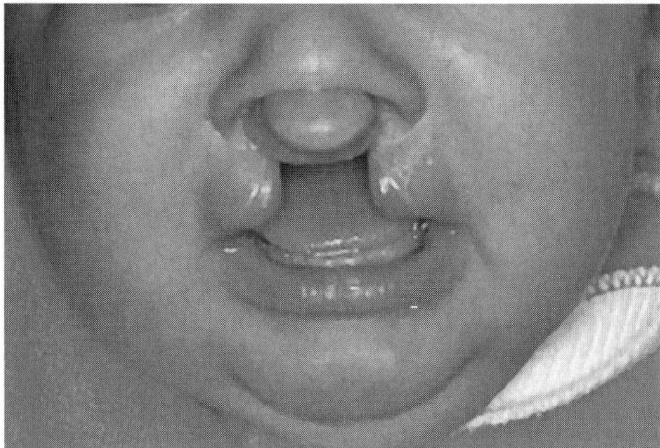

Figure 1-5 Bilateral cleft lip and alveolus with the central portions of the upper lip and alveolus attached to the tip of the nose with little or no columella.

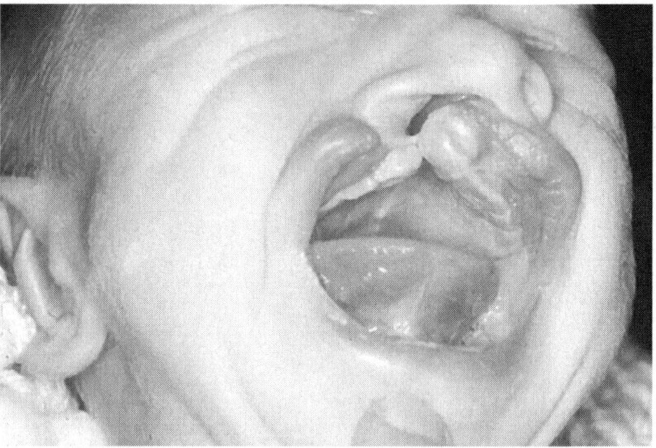

Figure 1-6 As in Fig. 1-4, incomplete cleft of the lip and alveolus on one side (with a microform cleft on the other side) but no involvement of the secondary palate. (Note that the judgment of "no involvement of the secondary palate" is not made on the basis of visual inspection alone but on digital palpation plus lack of early history of feeding difficulties and later evidence of good velopharyngeal closure for speech and corroborating evidence drawn from imaging studies, as deemed necessary.)

the alveolus may be minimal (only a notch or a submucous defect), or it may extend completely through the arch. Although somewhat difficult to explain embryologically, there have been reports of congenital alveolar defects without defects of the lip (Ranta and Rintala, 1989). A complete cleft through the alveolus can extend as far posteriorly as the region of the incisive foramen. If there is a bilateral complete cleft of the lip and alveolus, the central portions of the upper lip and alveolus are attached to the tip of the nose with little or no columella, the strip of tissue between the base and tip of the nose (Fig. 1-5).

Unilateral or bilateral clefts of the lip and alveolus are more often than not associated with clefts of the secondary palate, although there are cases of clefts of the lip and alveolus with no involvement of the secondary palate (Figs. 1-4, 1-6, and 1-7).

Cleft Palate

Clefts of the secondary palate also range from minimal defects to complete clefts extending all the way forward to the region of the incisive foramen. The "minimal defects" may pose more of a conceptual challenge than the overt, complete cleft because of the dimensions along which these defects can vary. Technically, a defect of the secondary palate may be as small as a slight scallop or streak in the uvula (Fig. 1-8). The defect that is visible on the clinician's intraoral examination ranges from these slight variations in the configuration of the uvula to overt clefts of the uvula, clefts extending further forward into the velum itself, and those extending still further forward into the hard palate (Fig. 1-9, *A* to *J*). However, this is just one dimension: There may be submucous defects of the soft and hard palate existing either in conjunction with overt clefts or without any overt cleft. In some submucous clefts the clinician will see one or more "stigmata" or signs on the intraoral examination of the patient, but in many others the physical defect is not detectable, let alone fully delineated, without special observation techniques (see following section).

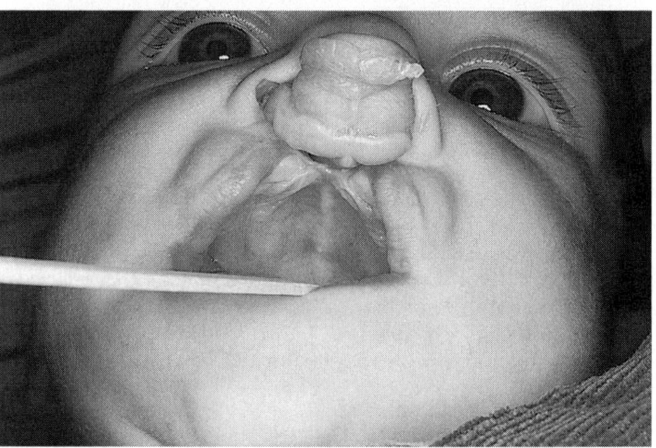

Figure 1-7 A more dramatic illustration of the points made in Figs. 1-4 and 1-6. This baby also has an intact secondary palate but in the presence of a severe bilateral cleft of the primary palate.

An overt cleft of the secondary palate may be complete up to the area of the incisive foramen, and, even if it is not complete, it usually has a submucous extension anterior to the overt portion. Variation in width of clefts of the secondary palate can be quite remarkable, with the extreme case resembling a horseshoe, as seen in Fig. 1-9, *J*. Technically, a complete cleft of the secondary palate is termed "bilateral" when neither palatine shelf has fused with the vomer bone. When clefts of the secondary palate, particularly small ones, occur without clefts of the lip and alveolus (clefts of the primary palate), they are less likely to be detected in the immediate postnatal period unless the baby is having problems feeding.

Given the above information, the clinician should now know that a patient described as having "a complete unilateral cleft lip and palate" has a cleft through the lip,

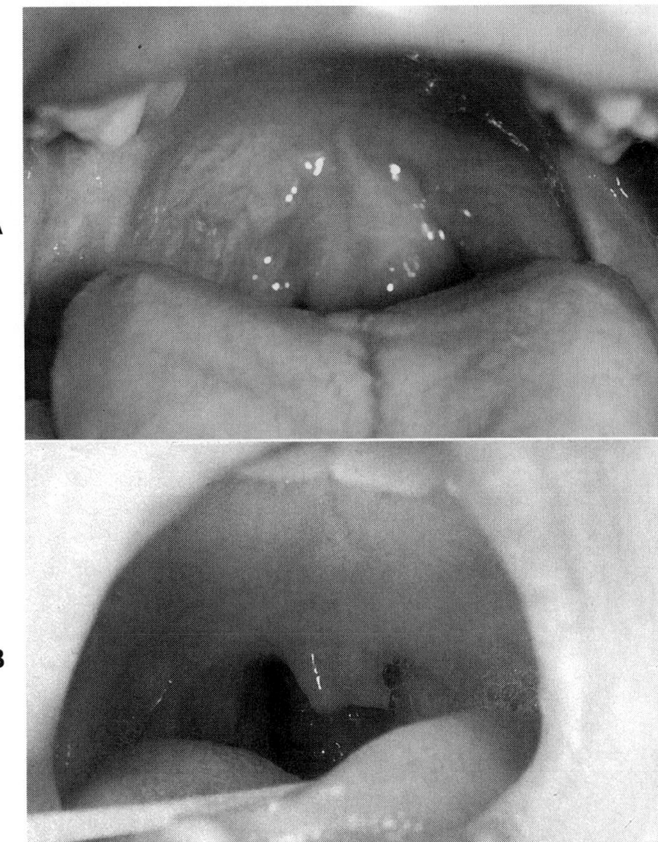

Figure 1-8 A and B, Submucous defects of the secondary palate with a bifid uvula, which may escape detection on a quick or careless intraoral examination. These photographs illustrate what we may consider "microforms" of clefts of the secondary palate, but it is important to remember that the patients may be either asymptomatic in speech or exhibiting significant velopharyngeal inadequacy—the intraoral view alone tells us very little of clinical significance although the presence of the bifid uvula is important for the genetic documentation of each case regardless of whether that person is symptomatic in speech.

alveolus, and anterior section of the hard palate (back to the region of the incisive foramen) combined with a complete cleft of the secondary palate (all the way forward to the region of the incisive foramen). Fig. 1-10 shows the facial and intraoral views of an infant with an incomplete unilateral cleft, in that the lip is only partially cleft but nevertheless there is a quite wide cleft palate. Fig. 1-11 shows two babies with unilateral complete clefts, one substantially wider than the other. In a "complete bilateral cleft of the lip and palate" there is an opening through the lip and alveolus on both sides, with the premaxilla unattached to anything but the columella of the nose, combined with a complete cleft of the secondary palate (Fig. 1-12). The premaxilla in bilateral clefts is often very protrusive, as seen in Fig. 1-12, *C* and *E*). Various configurations of incomplete bilateral clefts are shown in Fig. 1-13.

Submucous Clefts of the Secondary Palate

There may be significant defects of the secondary palate in the absence of an actual opening into the nasal cavity. The three classic "intraorally visible" stigmata of a submucous cleft are a bifid uvula, a midline division or "diastasis" of the musculature of the soft palate (sometimes the lack of normal muscle causes the overlying mucosa to look so thin that the defect is termed a "zona pellucida"), and a notch into the hard palate (all three of these findings are present in the patient pictured in Fig. 1-14).[4] However, for several reasons clinicians historically have been confused in their attempts to describe and categorize submucous clefts:

1. The three classic stigmata do not always appear together, that is, one may be present without the other two, or two without the third. A patient may have only a small defect in the uvula or a bifid uvula and muscular diastasis of the soft palate with an intact hard palate. In fact, although somewhat difficult to explain embryologically, there may be a clinically intact uvula with a defect in the soft palate and/or the hard palate, as seen in Fig. 1-15 (Fara, Hrivnakova, and Sedlackova, 1971; Shprintzen et al., 1985a).[5]
2. Even when none of the three classic stigmata is present, there may be a defect in the muscular bulk of the soft palate that can be seen only on nasal endoscopy. This is sometimes called an "occult submucous cleft." Before the advent of nasal endoscopy, also called nasopharyngoscopy, we had no way to determine if the nasal surface or upper muscular layer of the velum was intact except at the operating table (Kaplan, 1975).
3. Although nasal endoscopy has been a routine clinical examination procedure for at least 15 years, overall only a relatively small percentage of those cases of "submucous cleft palate" reported in the extensive literature on this subject have undergone a nasopharyngoscopic examination. This is one reason

[4]A relatively recent study (Park et al., 1994) revealed that one or more of the palatal rugae in individuals with submucous bony defects of the hard palate curve toward the region of the bony notch, a common finding in overt clefts of the secondary palate as well. Such a finding could prove clinically useful in working with young children in whom complete examination of the posterior palate proves difficult.

[5]The literature dating back to at least 1835 has contained reports of anomalous overt clefts or "congenital palatal fistulae" in the hard palate or anterior soft palate, with reported integrity of the rest of the palate and/or uvula (see Peterson-Falzone, 1985, for historical details). As the student might predict, clinical examination of these cases did not include endoscopic evaluations. Even some more recent reports have been relatively naive in the labeling of the findings. For example, Mitts, Garrett, and Hurwitz (1981) reported "cleft of the hard palate with soft palate integrity" in one case but the velum in their patient actually exhibited abnormal muscle insertion and a bifid uvula. Similarly, in each of the five cases reported by Fara (1971), there was also a submucous cleft. The topic of congenital palatal fistulae or perforations has interested investigators studying theoretical mechanisms of cleft formation in the embryo, as will be discussed in a following section.

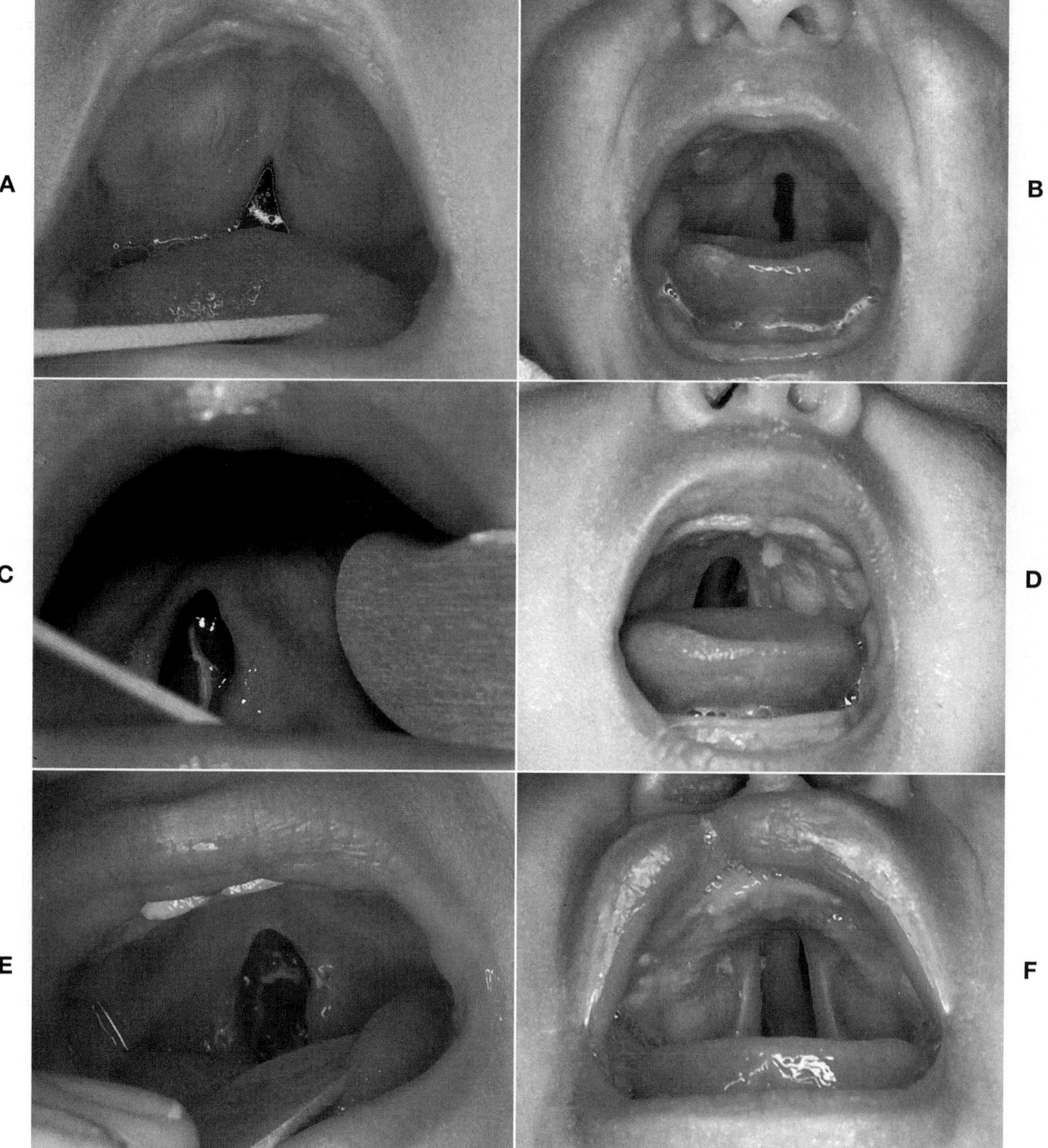

Figure 1-9 **A** to **J**, Wide range in severity of clefts of the secondary palate. Actually, the range also includes, on the lesser end, the clefts shown in Fig. 1-8 and even smaller, less easily detectable (and occult) clefts of the secondary palate. *Continued*

our frequency figures on submucous clefts are highly questionable: without complete examinations, we cannot know how often one clinical finding appears in conjunction with others. Furthermore, because submucous clefts are part of the same gene pool as overt clefts, the fact that we do not have accurate numbers regarding the occurrence of submucous defects means that we do not have fully accurate numbers regarding the frequency of genes for clefting.

4. In older literature, patients were sometimes diagnosed as having "submucous clefts" simply on the basis of hypernasal speech, without evidence of submucous defects on physical examination. In some reports, patients with other anatomical or neurological findings in the velopharyngeal system were grouped with patients with submucous clefts.

At this point, it will help to review the conceptualization of clefts in the three dimensions of space: the front-to-back (anterior-to-posterior extent), the side-to-side (lateral di-

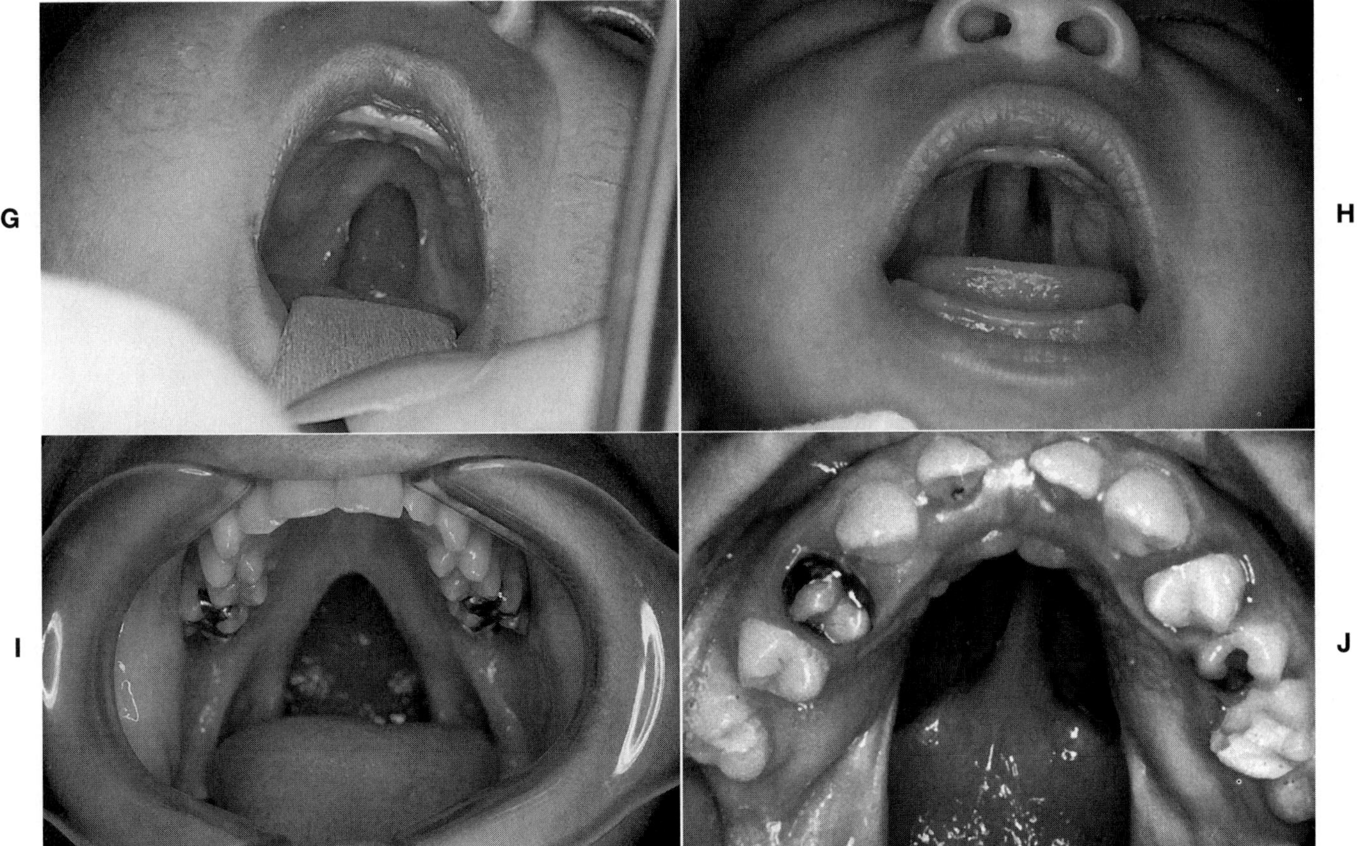

Figure 1-9, cont'd For legend see opposite page.

mension or width), and the vertical dimension. The latter term may be easy to understand in terms of the lip but a mystery in terms of the palate. The "hard palate" is made up of the oral mucosa (the lowermost layer), the bone layers (oral mucoperiosteum, bone, nasal mucoperiosteum), and the nasal mucosa (the uppermost layer). The comparable layers in the soft palate are the oral mucosa, the muscular layer, and the nasal mucosa. Minimal defects can be present on either the upper or lower aspects, or both, without penetrating all the bone or all the muscle. The extent to which the congenital defect is longer, wider, or "deeper" (in the vertical dimension) affects the likelihood of clinical identification and also the likelihood of significant speech problems, although there are speakers with all three of the classical stigmata of a submucous cleft (bifid uvula, muscular diastasis of the soft palate, bony notch in the hard palate) who do not exhibit velopharyngeal inadequacy.

Rare Forms of Clefts

Median clefts. True midline or median clefts of the lip, which may or may not continue through the palate, occur in several different forms and look very different from the clefts just described. Median clefts may be isolated defects or may occur as part of frontonasal dysplasia sequence or holoprosencephaly sequence (DeMyer, 1971). In frontonasal dysplasia (Fig. 1-16) the median cleft will be associated with wide-spaced eyes (hypertelorism), a broad or possibly bifid nose, and sometimes a single central incisor but basically normal development. In holoprosencephaly sequence (Fig. 1-17), there are congenitally absent midline structures, including structures of the central nervous system. The eyes are close set (hypotelorism), and the premaxilla is often absent. Although there is a range of severity in holoprosencephaly, for many affected babies the central nervous system defects are so severe that the life span is very limited (less than one year.) Unfortunately, inexperienced clinicians may see a child such as the youngster pictured in Fig. 1-17 and make the mistaken diagnosis of "unilateral cleft lip and palate."

Oblique facial clefts. A second form of rare facial clefts consists of oblique defects that were categorized by Tessier (1976) according to the scheme shown in Fig. 1-18. These defects may be due to amniotic bands (fibrous bands of amnion that cut through normally developing facial structures when they are swallowed by the embryo) or of failure of normal fusion of the facial prominences in the embryo (discussed in the section "How Clefts Form"). When the cause is amniotic bands, there may be strictures or amputations of parts of the limbs. Although oblique facial clefts occur much less frequently than cleft lip +/– palate or cleft palate alone, the defects constitute difficult habilitative challenges in terms of both appearance and

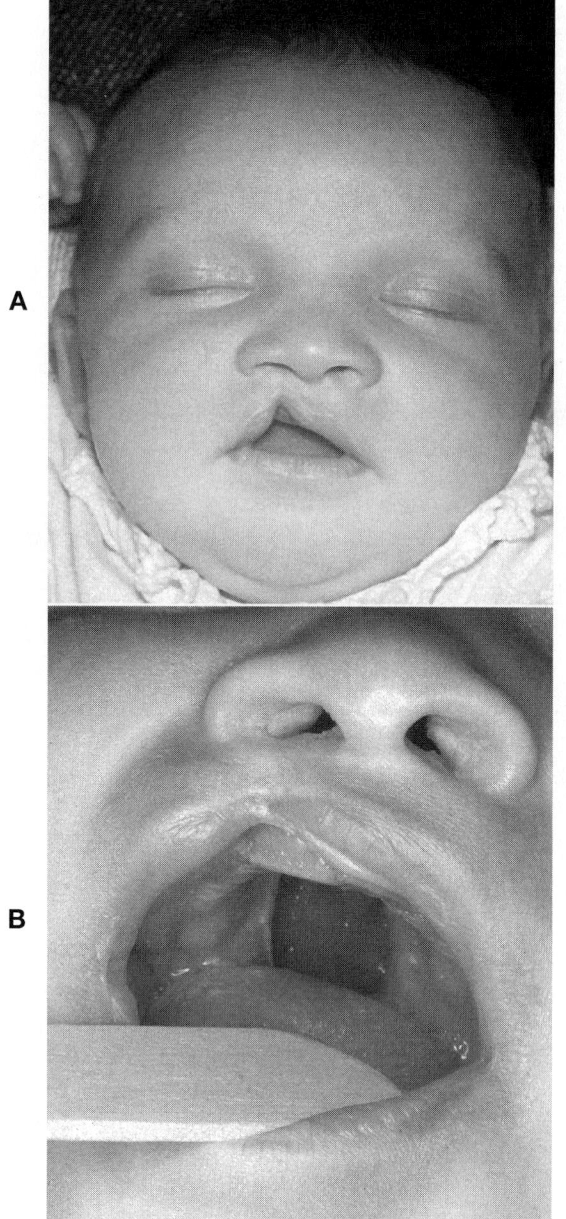

Figure 1-10 **A** and **B**, Facial and intraoral views of an infant with an incomplete unilateral cleft, in that the lip is only partially cleft but there is nevertheless a very wide cleft of the palate **(B)**.

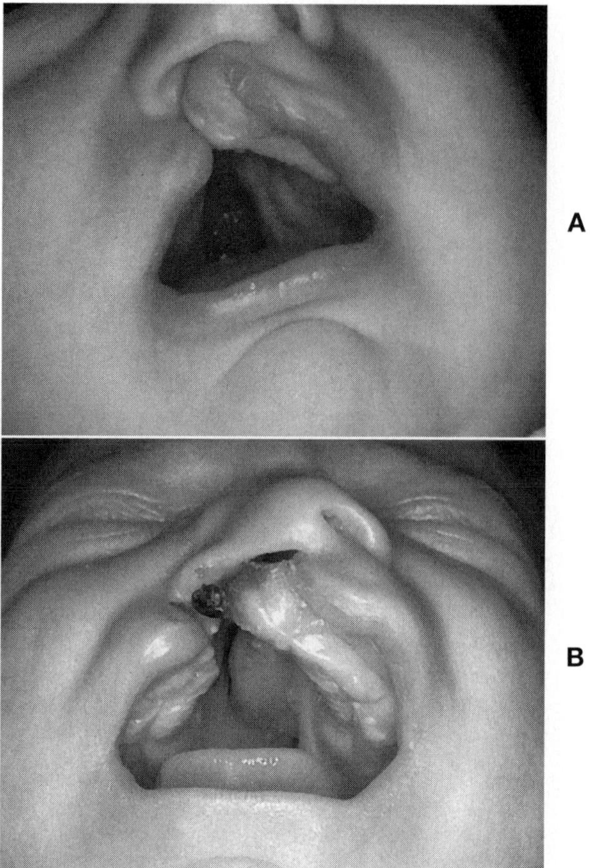

Figure 1-11 Two babies with complete right unilateral cleft lip and palate. In **A**, the cleft is complete although the cleft segment of the lip and alveolus is abutting the noncleft segment. In **B**, notice how the vomer bone is attached to the noncleft segment of the secondary palate on the baby's left side but there is no attachment on the right side. Also notice that the right alar wing (side and roof of the nostril) is severely flattened in both babies.

function. The effects on speech depend on their location and extent. In some babies the clefts extend through the lip and palate, as was the case with the youngsters shown in Figs. 1-19 and 1-20.

Lateral facial clefts. Lateral or transverse facial clefts occur when there is lack of fusion between the maxillary and mandibular prominences in the embryo. Such clefts are often seen as one of the defects in a large family of disorders generically known as "hemifacial microsomia" (see Chapter 2). Clinically, a lateral or transverse cleft is often labeled as "macrostomia" (Fig. 1-21), and corresponds to Tessier's #7 cleft (Fig. 1-18).

Associated Anomalies

It has been shown repeatedly that individuals with clefts of the palate only are far more likely to have associated anomalies than are individuals with clefts of the lip +/− palate (Fogh-Andersen, 1942; Gundlach, 1987; Jones, 1988; Shprintzen et al., 1985b; Womersley and Stone, 1987). Patients with cleft palate only also have a higher percentage of siblings with malformations than do patients with cleft lip +/− palate (Meskin and Pruzansky, 1969). Females have a higher rate of associated anomalies than do males, regardless of the type of cleft (Meskin and Pruzansky, 1969). Two studies (Myrianthopoulos and Chung, 1974; Siegel, 1979) reported a higher incidence of associated anomalies in blacks than in Caucasians. In their study of 1000 patients with clefts, Shprintzen et al. (1985b) reported one or more associated anomalies in 44.6% of the patients with cleft lip only, 50.3% of those with cleft lip and palate, 67.9% of those with cleft of the secondary palate only, and 76.8% of those with submucous clefts, for an overall prevalence of 62.4%. Womersley and Stone (1987)

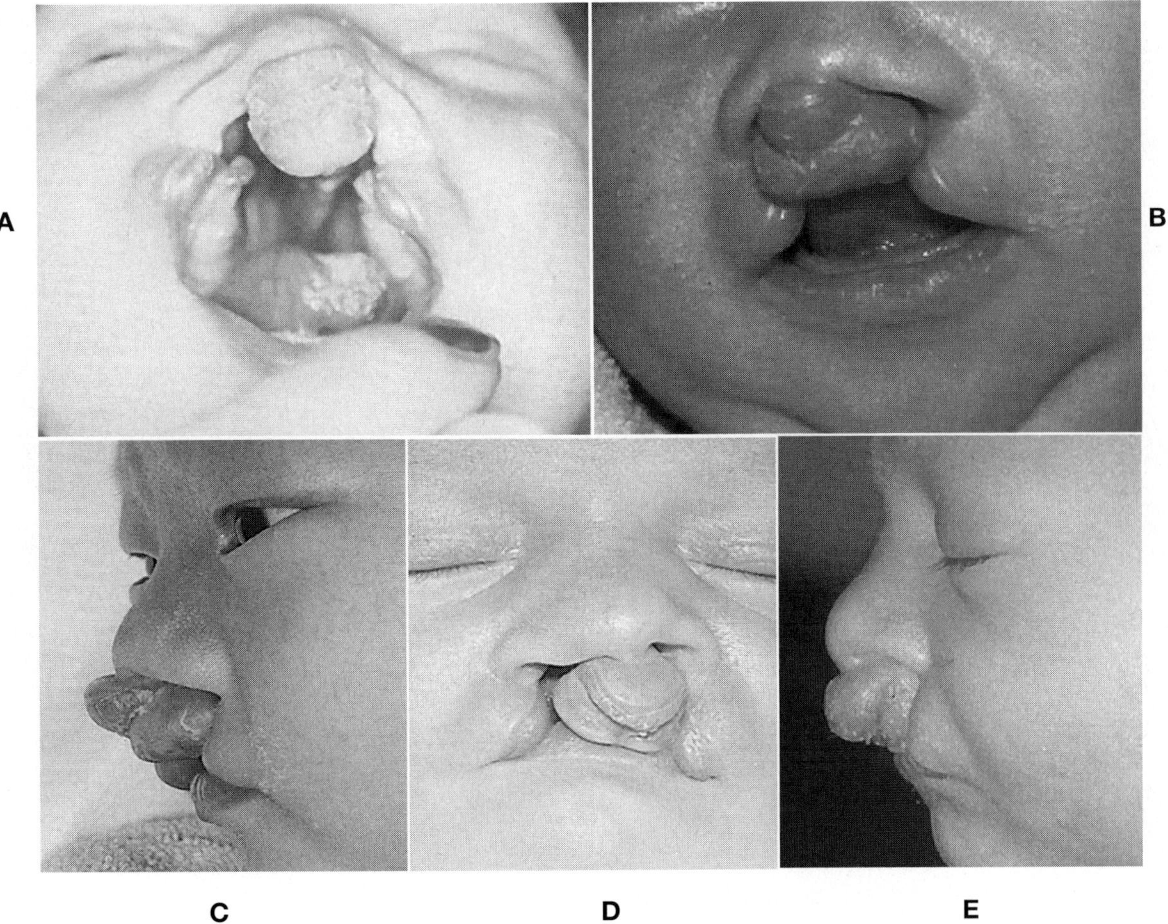

Figure 1-12 **A** to **E**, Prominent, anteriorly displaced premaxilla in infants with complete bilateral cleft lip, with absence of the columella of the nose.

similarly reported that two thirds of their patients with cleft palate only exhibited associated anomalies. Patients with cleft lip +/– cleft of the alveolus have fewer additional defects, and in patients with cleft lip and palate those with bilateral clefts are more likely to have associated anomalies than are those with unilateral clefts (Greene et al., 1964; Gundlach, 1987; Lilius, 1992). In patients with clefts of the secondary palate only, those with more severe clefts are more likely to have associated anomalies than are those with less severe clefts (Gundlach, 1987). In the study of Shprintzen et al. (1985b, 1985c), slightly more than half of those with additional anomalies had a recognizable syndrome, sequence, or association, whereas the remainder had "provisionally unique" sets of findings. The most common identifiable syndromes or associations were velocardiofacial syndrome (Shprintzen et al., 1978), Van der Woude syndrome (Van der Woude, 1954), Stickler syndrome (Stickler et al., 1965), isolated Pierre Robin sequence (Robin, 1923, 1934), and fetal alcohol syndrome (Hanson and Smith, 1975; Jones and Smith, 1975; Jones et al., 1973). These disorders together with other more complex craniofacial disorders will be discussed in Chapter 2. As stated previously, the importance of recognizing associated anomalies in children with clefts is that such anomalies (1) often signal a completely different etiology and (2) usually have dramatic effects on treatment plans.

FREQUENCY OF OCCURRENCE OF CLEFTS

As you review the information both on frequency of occurrence[6] of cleft lip and palate and the possible causes of clefts (next section), there are five major points to keep in mind:

1. The accuracy of any set of numbers on the frequency of occurrence of clefts in a given population depends on how thoroughly each individual was examined. Unfortunately, a large number of studies have relied on information recorded on birth certificates, and all congenital malformations are notoriously underreported on birth records (Green et al., 1979; Gregg, Stanage, and Johnson, 1984; Meskin and Pruzansky,

[6]Epidemiologists make a careful distinction between the terms *incidence* and *prevalence:* "incidence" denotes the number of new cases entering a population in a specified time period and "prevalence" denotes the number of existing cases in the population at some time (Hook, 1988).

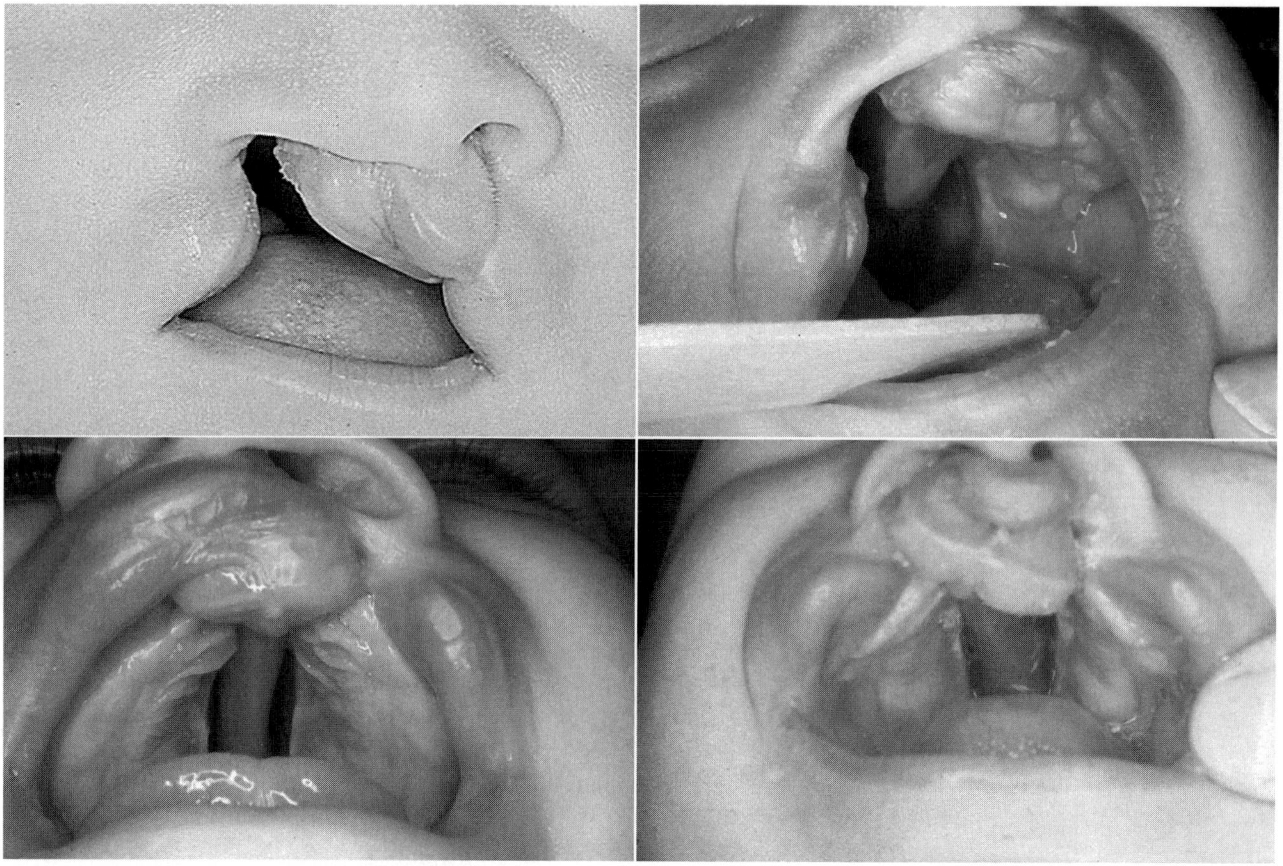

Figure 1-13 A to D, Incomplete bilateral clefts.

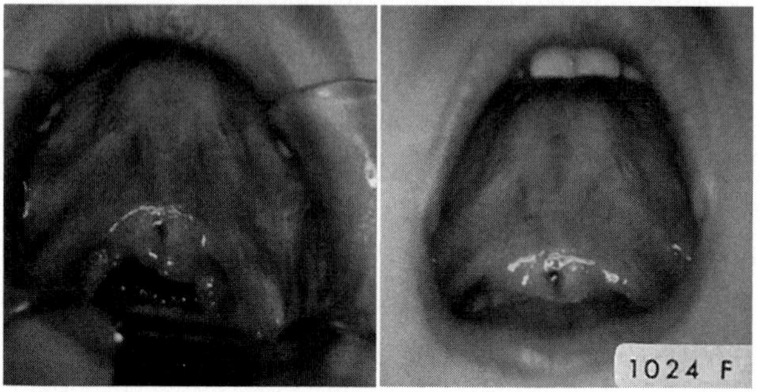

Figure 1-14 Bifid uvula, zona pellucida (transparent area) of the soft palate (difficult to see in a black-and-white photo), and submucous notch in the posterior border of the hard palate.

1967; Rintala and Stegars, 1982). Meskin and Pruzansky (1967) found that birth certificates did not report any type of cleft in 29.4% of their cases and that more than 50% of isolated palatal clefts were not recorded. Green et al. (1979) reported that only 65% of all clefts were noted on birth certificates, and the *accuracy* of reporting (of cleft type) was only 48%.[7]

2. More than half of all clefts are accompanied by at least one minor or one major additional anomaly (Shprintzen et al., 1985b). If the presence of additional anomalies is not recognized, the cleft lip or cleft palate will be erroneously recorded as an isolated defect, a mistake that leads to errors in epidemiologic data and, more important, to errors in determining causation (on a population level) and in planning appropriate treatment for the patient.
3. There is little doubt that cleft lip +/− cleft palate and cleft palate alone are two separate etiologic entities that result from problems at different stages in embryogenesis (Fogh-Andersen, 1942; 1967, 1980; Fraser, 1955; Kaye, 1981; Lynch and Kimberling, 1981; Melnick, 1986; Woolf, Woolf, and Broadbent, 1963a). Geneticists and epidemiologists have found that clefts in families tend to segregate into these two groups, that is, more cases of cleft lip +/− palate than of cleft palate alone in the relatives of a patient with cleft lip +/− palate (Coccia, Bixler, and Conneally, 1969; Curtis, Fraser, and Warburton, 1961; Fogh-Andersen, 1942; Fraser and Baxter, 1954; Fujino, Tanaka, and Sanui, 1963; Woolf et al., 1963a, 1963b, 1969). However, in some historical studies both types of clefts were included in incidence or prevalence figures in ways that are difficult to identify

[7]These data are decades old, and many state cleft palate associations are trying to improve the accuracy of birth records. However, as of this date, we are still awaiting the new data from those efforts.

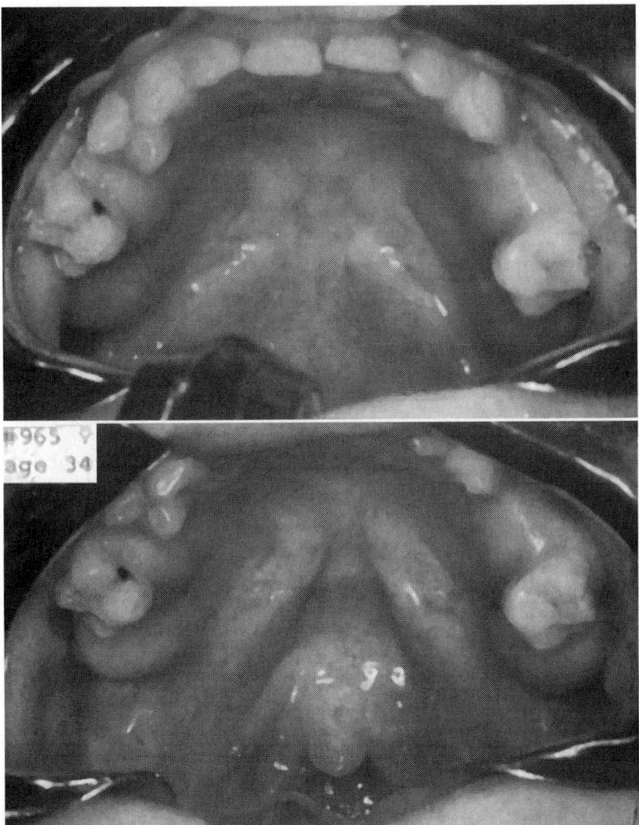

Figure 1-15 The submucous cleft in this patient is not immediately obvious until the patient phonates (*bottom*). Notice that the uvula is not bifid.

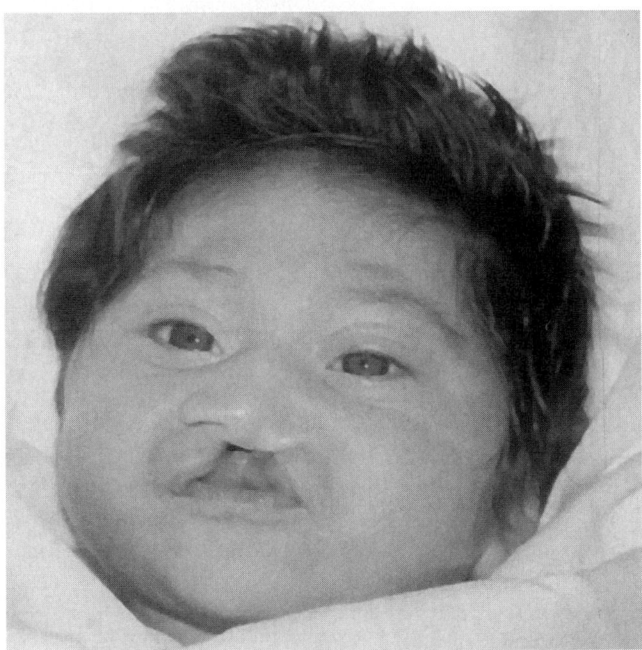

Figure 1-17 Holoprosencephaly sequence, with a midline cleft palate and absent premaxilla, severely hypoplastic nasal structures, closely set eyes, and midline central nervous system defects.

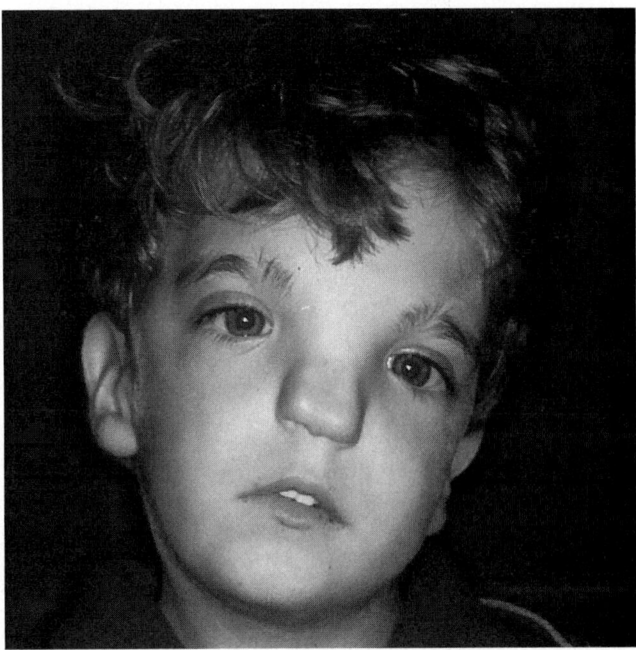

Figure 1-16 A type of median facial clefting known as frontonasal dysplasia. Note the wide-set eyes and the bifid nose. The anomalous eyebrows are consequent to the lateral displacement of the eyes.

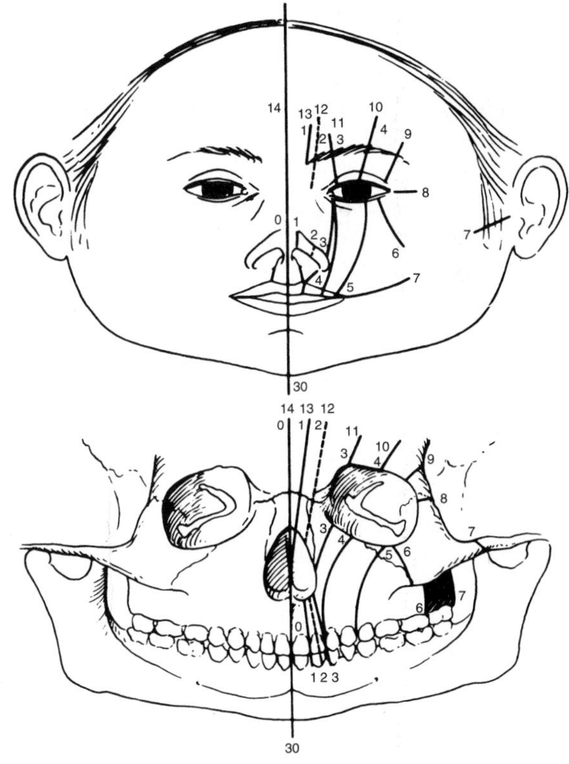

Figure 1-18 Schematic of Tessier's categorization scheme for lateral and oblique facial clefts. *(From Kawamoto HK, Wang MH, McCombes WB: Rare craniofacial clefts. In Converse JM [ed.]:* Reconstructive Plastic Surgery, *vol 4, p. 2129, Philadelphia; WB Saunders, 1977.)*

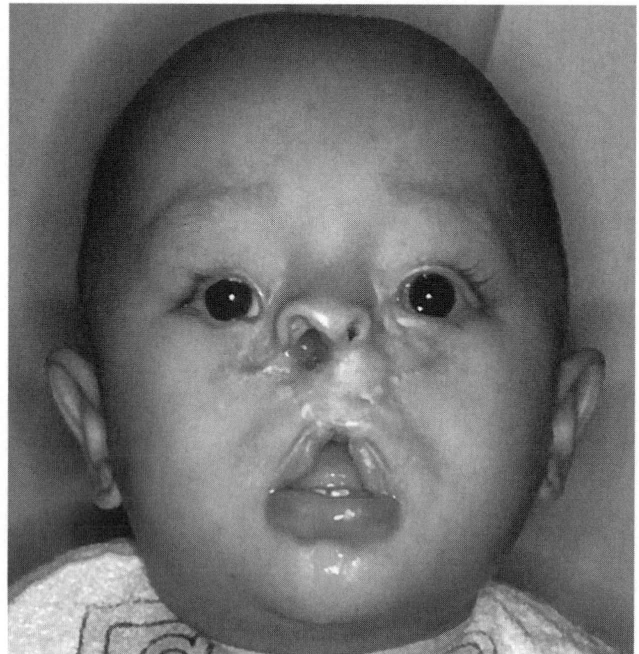

Figure 1-19 This baby initially had bilateral oblique clefts extending upward and outward from the upper lip through the floors of the orbits. There was very little soft tissue available for surgical repair. At the time this photo was taken, he had had two procedures; more surgery will be done as he grows, to provide him with a better nasal airway and a more esthetically acceptable appearance. His development is normal.

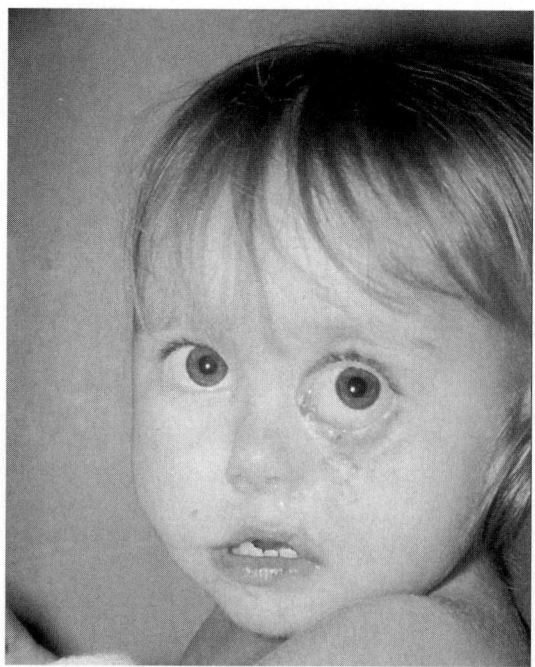

Figure 1-20 This child had an incomplete facial cleft on the left side, not quite as severe as the clefts seen in Fig. 1-19. She will have further reconstruction as she grows. Her development is normal.

on a post-hoc basis. In addition, there are exceptions to the segregation of the two types of clefts in families. For example, both types occur in kindreds with Van der Woude syndrome, an autosomal dominant syndrome combining lower lip pits with clefts that vary from cleft lip alone to cleft lip and alveolus to cleft lip and palate to clefts of the secondary palate only.

4. As already pointed out, because many submucous clefts remain undetected, estimates of the frequency of clefts in any given population are artificially low.
5. In today's (1999) era of profit-driven health care, *not* recognizing birth defects is an economically desirable, conscious decision for the health plan businesses. If a baby is born to a family currently enrolled in such a health plan, the fewer the problems recognized with the baby, the better the financial balance sheets of the health care plan.

General Estimates

New figures on the frequency of clefts are published several times a year, making the tracking of current data a challenging task. Pooling cleft lip +/− palate and cleft palate alone, and ignoring variation according to racial groups,

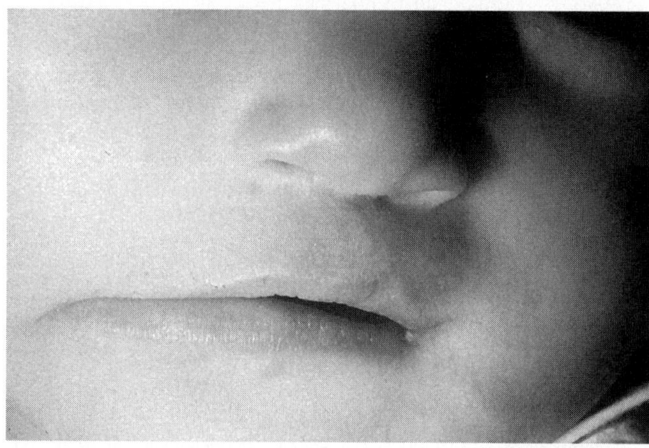

Figure 1-21 Right lateral oral cleft that resulted from incomplete fusion in the embryonic period between the maxillary and mandibular prominences. Clinically, this condition is often labeled as "macrostomia."

current figures on frequency of clefts in live-born babies[8] generally fall between 1:500 and 1:750 (Calzolari et al., 1988; Coupland and Coupland, 1988; Jensen et al., 1988; Myrianthopoulos and Chung, 1974; Natsume and Kawai, 1986; Natsume, Suzuki, and Kawai, 1988; Owens, Jones

[8]The distinction of "live-born babies" is important because frequency of all birth defects is much higher in stillborn babies. For example, cleft palate alone (without cleft lip) occurs nearly seven times as often in stillbirths as in livebirths and cleft lip +/− palate nearly three times as often (Czeizel, 1984).

and Harris, 1985; Pigott, 1992; Tolarova, 1987). Depending on racial group (see section on racial groups), rates for cleft lip +/− palate vary from roughly 1:250 to 1:1000; the rate for cleft palate alone—roughly 1:2500 to 1:3000—is more consistent across racial groups but subject to underestimation because of inadequate ascertainment and also because of inconsistency regarding inclusion of minor defects such as bifid uvula or even complete submucous clefts.

Frequency Data by Type of Cleft and Sex of Individual

Although there are differences according to race and sex, cleft lip and palate occurring together are more common than either defect occurring alone (Fogh-Andersen, 1942; Greene et al., 1964; Jensen et al., 1988; Natsume, Suzuki, and Kawai, 1987, 1988; Oka, 1979; Shaw, Croen, and Curry, 1991; Tolarova, 1987). Proportions vary among racial groups (see section on racial groups), but, as an example, Fogh-Andersen (1942) estimated 25% cleft lip, 50% cleft lip + cleft palate, and 25% cleft palate alone among Danish cases. Later studies have shown somewhat different percentages (Jensen et al., 1988; Natsume, Suzuki, and Kawai, 1988) but the same general findings. Cleft lip with or without cleft palate is at least twice as likely to be unilateral as opposed to bilateral (Czeizel and Tusnadi, 1971; Jensen et al., 1988; Shaw, Croen, and Curry, 1991; Wilson, 1972). Unilateral clefts are much more likely to occur on the left side than the right, regardless of severity or sex of the individual (Fogh-Andersen, 1942; Fraser and Calnan, 1961; Jensen et al., 1988; Tolarova, 1987; Wilson, 1972; Woolf, 1971), although the left > right difference does not hold when the cleft is accompanied by other anomalies. In general, males are more vulnerable to cleft lip +/− cleft palate and females more vulnerable to cleft palate only (Calzolari et al., 1988; Jensen et al., 1988; Owens, Jones, and Harris, 1985; Shaw, Croen, and Curry, 1991; Womersley and Stone, 1987).[9] However, the difference between the sexes varies with the severity of the cleft, with the presence or absence of associated defects, and also to some degree with the racial group (Czeizel and Tusnadi, 1971; Emanuel et al., 1972). In Caucasians the male/female ratio for cleft lip +/− cleft palate increases steadily, proceeding from the mildest form of cleft lip to the most severe bilateral cleft lip and palate (Ross and Johnston, 1978) and for clefts of the secondary palate only the preponderance of females diminishes as the cleft becomes less severe (Fogh-Andersen, 1942; Knox and Braithwaite, 1963; Mazaheri, 1958; Meskin, Pruzansky and Gullen, 1968). There is nearly a 1:1 ratio for bifid uvula (Bagatin, 1985a; Chosack and Eidelman, 1978). For both cleft lip +/− palate and cleft palate only, there is a slight excess of males versus females in blacks (Altemus, 1966) and females versus males in the Chinese (Emanuel et al., 1972).

Historically, the majority of studies on the frequency of clefts were limited to overt clefts and did not include submucous defects. Beginning in the 1960s, a few studies attempted to establish the frequency of one or more of the intraorally visible signs of a submucous defect in nonclinical populations such as groups of schoolchildren, dental or pediatric practices, etc. In the mid-1960s, Meskin, Gorlin, and Isaacson (1964) found bifid uvulas in 1.44% (1 in every 70 people) in individuals drawn from (1) a routine dental practice and (2) incoming freshman students in a large midwestern university. Subsequent studies of the relatives of these individuals led the authors to conclude that defects of the uvula were indeed part of the spectrum of clefts of the secondary palate, with obvious impact on the frequency figures and recurrence risks for such clefts (Meskin, Gorlin, and Isaacson, 1965, 1966). Weatherley-White et al. (1972) reported a frequency of .083% of "submucous cleft palate" in 10,836 school children in Denver (approximately 1 in 1200). However, these authors required that all three of the visible stigmata of bifid uvula, muscular division in the soft palate, and bony defect in the hard palate be present to make the diagnosis of "submucous cleft," and they did not count cases in which they found "only a bifid uvula and a bony notch."[10] Bagatin (1985a, 1985b) also examined a large number of schoolchildren (9720) and reported "cleft uvula" in 2.39% (1/418) and submucous cleft palate in 0.05% (roughly 1 in 10,000), defining the latter only as the presence of a "submucous zone" (Bagatin, 1985b). Shprintzen et al. (1985a) found bifid uvulas in 3.3% of 2500 children (1/303) seen in a pediatric practice. Wharton and Mowrer (1992) found bifid uvulas in 2.26% of more than 700 schoolchildren (or 1 in 442).

Although the numbers vary quite widely in the studies cited above, the point should not be lost that (1) relatively minor defects of the uvula are found in significant numbers of "nonpatients" (people not being seen for speech or other problems), (2) these minor defects are part of the same genetic spectrum as more serious defects of the secondary palate, a fact that changes our perspective regarding the frequency of clefts in given populations, and (3) speech pathologists may well be the first professionals to find these morphologic differences on their routine intraoral examinations. The last point brings up a major dilemma, as pointed out by Cohn (1992): the automatic response should be referral to a geneticist for a complete family workup, but the economics and logistics of such referrals for, say 1 in 70 individuals, are overwhelming.

[9] These sex differences do not hold when clefts occur in association with other defects, for example, when they occur as part of syndromes.

[10] Similarly, the criteria applied by Rintala and Stegars (1982) for the presence of a submucous cleft were abysmally inconsistent. Such inconsistency in criteria continues to plague studies on the frequency of submucous clefts and the proportion of patients who exhibit inadequate velopharyngeal closure (Garcia-Velasco et al., 1985; McWilliams, 1991; Velasco et al., 1988).

Racial Groups

It has long been known that the frequency of clefts varies significantly among racial groups, but obviously the differences become less distinct as people from different racial backgrounds intermarry. Historically, epidemiologists have reported a higher frequency of cleft lip +/– cleft palate among Asian or Mongolian people than among Caucasians, and the lowest frequency in blacks (Altemus, 1966; Altemus and Ferguson, 1965; Chung and Myrianthopoulos, 1968; Chung et al., 1986; Emanuel et al., 1972; Gilmore and Hofman, 1966; Ivy, 1962; Koguchi, 1980; Leck, 1977, 1984; Leck and Lancashire, 1995; Lynch and Kimberling, 1981; Melnick, 1986; Natsume and Kawai, 1986; Oka, 1979; Shaw, Croen, and Curry, 1991; Tyan, 1982; Vanderas, 1987).[11] The differences in these three large groups are generally reported to be on the order of 2 to 1 to 0.5 (twice as many clefts in Asians as Caucasians, twice as many clefts in Caucasians as blacks). The racial background of American Indians is Mongolian, and the occurrence of cleft lip with or without cleft palate is much higher than in Caucasians, with some variation according to the particular group under study (Bardanouve, 1969; Chavez, Cordero, and Becerra, 1989; Erickson, 1976; Jaffe and DeBlanc, 1970; Lowry and Renwick, 1969; Niswander and Adams, 1967; Tretsven, 1963; Vanderas, 1987). Vanderas (1987) reviewed more than 60 studies on this topic and concluded that the highest rates for cleft lip +/– palate occurred in North American Indians (as high as 3.74/1000, or 1 in 267), followed by the Japanese (0.82 to 3.36 per 1000, or 1 in 1219 to 1 in 297), the Chinese (1.45 to 4.04 per 1000, or 1 in 689 to 1 in 247), Caucasians (1 in 1000 to 1 in 372), and blacks (0.18 to 1.67 per 1000, or 1 in 5555 to 1 in 598). The frequency of cleft lip +/– palate is also higher in Mexicans (DeVoss, 1952; Lutz and Moore, 1955).

By contrast, the prevalence of clefts of the secondary palate is approximately the same among Caucasians, African-Americans, American Indians, and Asians (Altemus and Ferguson, 1965; Ching and Chung, 1974; Chung, Rao, and Ching, 1980; Jaffe and DeBlanc, 1970; Myrianthopoulos and Chung, 1974; Niswander and Adams, 1967; Oka, 1979). Lindemann, Riis, and Sewerin (1977) summarized in tabular form the studies on the prevalence of "cleft uvula" that had been published up to that date. Overall, the prevalence figures varied from 0.02% to 18.8%, the highest numbers being found in studies of Chippewa and Navajo Indians and the lowest generally in African-Americans.

Interestingly, there may be a differential effect of maternal versus paternal race on the likelihood of clefts in offspring. Khoury and co-authors (Khoury, Erickson, and James, 1983) reported that offspring of Caucasian mothers had a higher rate of cleft lip +/– palate than did those of black mothers, without a similar effect for cleft palate only, and that race of the father had no effect on likelihood of either type of cleft. In a study of cross-breeding among several different racial groups in Hawaii, Chung, Mi, and Beechert (1987) found a differential effect only for Filipino fathers (not mothers) for the likelihood of producing a child with cleft lip +/– palate. Leck and Lancashire (1995) found that the race of *both* parents influenced the likelihood of cleft lip +/– cleft palate, but not cleft palate alone, and interpreted these findings to mean that genetic influences were more important for cleft lip +/– cleft palate whereas, for cleft palate alone, nongenetic influences could be more important. Other studies on the effect of maternal influences are discussed in a following section.

Is the Frequency of Clefts Changing?

In their 1988 article on the frequency of clefts in Denmark, Jensen et al. noted a significant increase in clefts in that country since 1942: 1.5 per 1000 (1 in 667) live births as recorded by Fogh-Andersen in 1942, increasing to 1.75:1000 in 1971 and 1.89:1000 by 1981. The last figure correlates to 1 in 529 babies. The authors listed the probable or possible factors leading to this increase and did not feel that simple improvement in clinical detection of clefts (e.g., small clefts of the secondary palate) was the sole explanation. Their list included decreased neonatal mortality, environmental factors such as drugs, increased frequencies of intermarriage (among racial groups in Denmark), and "childbirths in cleft patients because of better acceptability and fertility." The last factor is interpreted to mean that, in Denmark as in other parts of the world, an ever-increasing number of men and women who were born with clefts go through successful habilitation (surgery, orthodontics, prosthodontics, speech-language services, psychosocial services, etc.) so that they become normal members of their social community, and as such, find partners and reproduce. Data published since the 1988 report largely verify the findings and interpretation, with some variation depending on types of clefts and racial or ethnic factors. Not surprisingly, rates for cleft palate only are more likely to be affected by thoroughness of examination of the newborn than are rates for the more obvious clefts of lip +/– palate. For example, Lowry, Thunem, and Hong (1989) reported that birth prevalence rates for cleft lip +/– cleft palate in British Columbia showed no increase or decrease over the period from 1952 to 1986, but that rates for cleft palate only showed an increase, which these authors attributed to better clinical ascertainment (more thorough examinations and more accurate recordings of findings).

A Brief Summary

For practical purposes, current information about frequency of clefts is summarized here, but the reader must bear in mind the limitations of the studies cited above:

Overall frequency: Roughly 1 in 500 to 1 in 750; more

[11] In the United States the term "African-Americans" is appropriate, but the same low frequency of cleft lip with or without cleft palate holds true in blacks in other parts of the world.

frequent in some Asian and American Indian populations.

Type of cleft: Depending on racial group, generally more frequent occurrence of cleft lip and palate than cleft lip alone or cleft palate alone.

Sex: Again with some variation in racial groups, CL +/– P is apt to be more frequent in males, CPO in girls. Sex differences in the occurrence of cleft palate only diminish as the severity of the cleft diminishes (e.g., there is a more remarkable predominance of females versus males for complete clefts of the secondary palate but almost no sex difference for small clefts of the soft palate or bifid uvulas).

Racial/ethnic groups: Higher occurrence of CL +/– P in Asians compared with Caucasians and higher in Caucasians compared with blacks. About the same rate of occurrence of CPO across racial groups.

Associated anomalies: Always more likely to be found in individuals with CPO. More likely to occur in patients with bilateral cleft lip and palate than unilateral clefts.

Recurrence Risks

When a baby is born with a cleft or any other birth defect, the family wants to know why it happened and whether there is a chance it can happen again in subsequent children. Clearly, it is not the responsibility of the speech-language pathologist to counsel families about recurrence risks; to do so would in fact be irresponsible because genetic counseling requires highly trained specialists. However, some basic information is provided here to help you understand the process.

When a geneticist sees the family of a child with a cleft, the first step is physical examination of the child or "proband" (index case), together with obtaining a detailed prenatal and birth history. The examination of the child may include laboratory tests, radiographic and nonradiographic imaging studies, various forms of chromosome analysis, and referral to other specialists such as cardiologists, endocrinologists, etc. The purpose is to establish an accurate diagnosis of the proband. Taking a detailed family history and examining available family members is also a part of that process because findings in the proband may be interpreted differently depending on what findings are present in other family members or what the family history indicates.

In addition to the physical findings in the proband and available family members, the geneticist and genetic counselor record racial background in the family, any history of illnesses or exposure to possible teratogens in the parents (particularly in the mother), the reproductive history of the parents plus that of their siblings and the grandparents, and the family history of clefts and related defects. Some of the many factors that may influence recurrence risks for the family are discussed in a following section. The fact that there are so many variables in predicting the possibility of a cleft in future children is the reason no one other than qualified specialists should undertake this task.

Table 1-1 Theoretical Recurrence Risk (%) for Cleft Lip +/– Cleft Palate

Other Relatives	Neither Affected	Parents One Affected	Both Affected
None affected	.08	2.1	26.2
One sibling affected	2.4	7.6	29.0
One sibling affected, one not affected	2.3	7.1	28.1
Two siblings affected	7.7	14.0	31.3
One sibling affected, five not affected	1.9	5.5	24.5

Adapted from Tenconi R, Clementi M, and Turolla L: Theoretical recurrence risks for cleft lip derived from a population of consecutive newborns. *Journal of Medical Genetics* 25:243-246, 1988.

Unless otherwise specified, the following information presented in the tables on recurrence risks is based on the presumption of (1) Caucasian racial background and (2) absence of any associated anomalies in the proband. Table 1-1 shows theoretical recurrence risks for cleft lip +/– palate adapted from Tenconi, Clementi, and Turolla (1988). The figures mean, for example, in a baby born into a family with no affected parents and no previous children with clefts, the likelihood of cleft lip +/– palate is 0.08%, or a little less than 1 in 1000. By contrast, if there is one affected parent and one affected sibling, the risk for affected subsequent children is 7.6, or about 1 in 131. The figures in this table are roughly in agreement with earlier estimates from Melnick (1986): 3% to 5% recurrence risk if there are no other affected first-degree relatives (parents, siblings, offspring) or second-degree relatives (grandparents, uncles, aunts) and 15% to 20% if there is one affected first- or second-degree relative. Tenconi, Clementi, and Turolla (1988) noted that the frequency of clefts in first-degree relatives was significantly dependent on severity of the cleft in the proband, although they defined severity only in terms of the structures involved: 0.5% versus 4.1% for cleft lip versus cleft lip + palate and 1.5% versus 5.8% for unilateral versus bilateral clefts. In second-degree relatives (e.g., grandparents or grandchildren) frequency was independent of severity of cleft in the proband (Tenconi, Clementi, and Turolla, 1988).

An earlier table (Table 1-2) offered by Fraser (1971) is a little more difficult to interpret but is included here because it gives recurrence risks for cleft palate alone as well as for cleft lip +/– cleft palate.

The reader is again urged *not* to use these tables to offer numbers for recurrence risks to families. The speech-language pathologist, as well as other clinicians, can help families find appropriate resources for exploring the etiology of the cleft and for learning as much as possible

Table 1-2 **Risks (%) for Cleft Lip +/– Cleft Palate and Cleft Palate**

Situation	*Proband Has CL +/– CP*	*Proband Has CP*
Frequency of defect in general population	0.1	0.04
My spouse and I are unaffected. We have an affected child. What is the probability that our next baby will have the same condition if:		
• We have no affected relatives?	4	2
• There is an affected relative?	4	7
• Our affected child also has another malformation?	2	—
What is the probability that our next baby will have some other sort of malformation?	Same as general population	
We have two affected children. What is the probability that our next baby will have the same condition?	9	1
I am affected (or my spouse is): We have no affected children. What is the probability that our next baby will be affected?	4	6
We have an affected child. What is the probability that our next baby will be affected?	17	15

From Fraser FC: Etiology of cleft lip and palate. In Grabb WC, Rosenstein SW, Bzoch KR (eds.): Cleft lip and palate: surgical, dental, and speech aspects. Boston: Little, Brown, 1971, pp. 54-65.

about the likelihood of future clefts or other malformations in the family.

HOW CLEFTS FORM

Cleft lip and palate result from developmental variations that occur during the embryonic period (the fourth to eighth weeks) and the very early fetal period (9 weeks and beyond). Understanding how these variations occur requires a basic grasp of normal development of the head and face.[12] Slavkin (1979) saw embryology as a means of simplifying the study of both normal anatomy and congenital anomalies, citing no less a source than Aristotle (384-322 BC) in support: "He who sees things grow from the beginning will have the finest view of them."

Normal Embryological Development

The structures that will form the face and palate begin within layers of different kinds of cells even before the about-to-be baby is officially an embryo.[13] During the first 3 weeks after conception the product of the sperm + ovum progresses from a single cell into a multicellular structure that assumes the shape of a flat disc of one layer *(embryonic endoderm)* on about the seventh day, two layers (embryonic endoderm and *epiblast*) at the beginning of the second week, and then three layers when the epiblast separates into the *embryonic ectoderm* and *mesoderm.* The embryonic ectoderm, mesoderm, and endoderm—the three layers of the trilaminar embryonic disc—give rise to all the tissues and organs of the developing baby. The disc thickens as cells differentiate, with the greater thickening occurring in the cranial end as opposed to the caudal or tail end, giving the disc something of an inverse pear shape.

The outermost of the three primary germ layers—the ectoderm—generally gives rise to those organs and structures that maintain contact with the outside world, including the central and peripheral nervous systems. Differentiated ectodermal cells become *neuroectodermal cells* that form the primitive *neural plate.* About the eighteenth day the neural plate invaginates along its axis to form a longitudinal *neural groove* that is flanked by *neural folds.* These folds move toward each other over the groove (something like crossed swords at a military wedding) and start to fuse to form the *neural tube,* the cephalic or rostral end of which will become the brain. The fusion begins in the region of the neck and proceeds in both directions (cephalic and caudal). Initially, the tube is widely open at both ends, called the *rostral* and *caudal neuropores.* The rostral neuropore (head end) closes on the twenty-fourth to twenty-fifth day, and the caudal neuropore on the twenty-sixth to twenty-seventh day.

As the neural folds are fusing, some of the neuroectodermal cells beneath the peak of each fold fuse into a crest just above the neural tube and just under the cutaneous surface on the dorsal (back) side of the developing embryo. These *neural crest cells* proliferate and migrate at different rates into the developing facial structures to play a crucial role in the formation of those structures.

As all this is happening, the embryo is growing more rapidly at its center than at its periphery and more rapidly along its longitudinal axis than its transverse axis. This

[12]The material presented here is necessarily limited in scope and detail. If at all possible, the student in speech-language pathology should take, or at least audit, a course in human embryology.

[13]The official stages are "zygote" (the initial product of the joining of the ovum and sperm), "morula" (about 3 days after fertilization), "blastocyst" (which embeds in the uterine wall on the 5th or 6th days after conception), "gastrula" (14th day to 20th day), "embryo" (from the beginning of the 4th week through the 8th week), and "fetus." Many authors simply use the term "embryo" when discussing events in the first 8 weeks, and we will do the same.

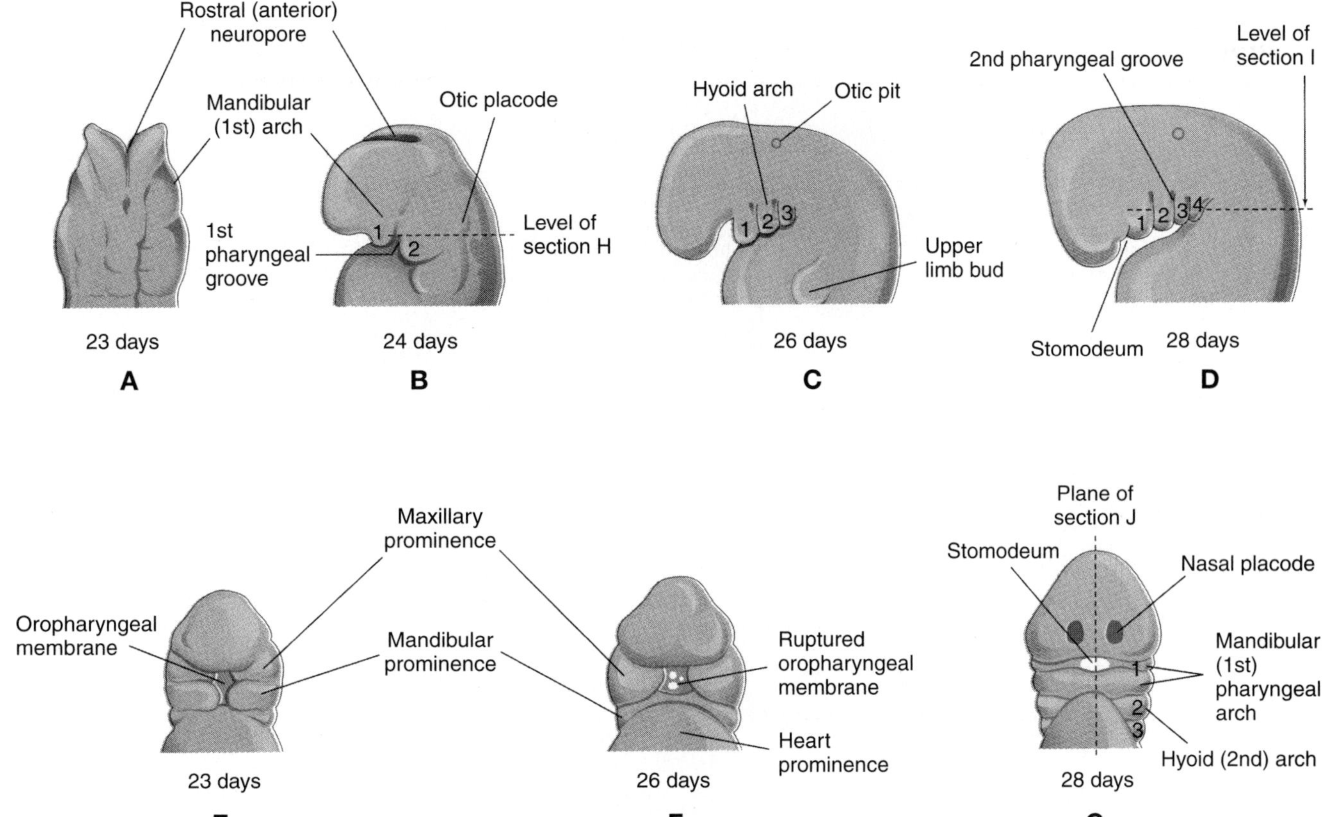

Figure 1-22 Schematic representations of the development of the human branchial or pharyngeal apparatus during the fourth week of embryonic life. **A,** Dorsal view. **B** to **D,** Lateral views. **E** to **G,** Frontal views. *(From Moore KL, and Persaud TVN:* The developing human: clinically oriented embryology, *ed. 6. Philadelphia: WB Saunders, 1998, p. 216.)*

differential growth causes the embryo to fold in on itself in two dimensions. By the twenty-eighth day, it has acquired head and tail folds, giving it something of a "C" shape viewed from the side. It has also acquired a midline fold, as though it were trying to grasp a tightrope by squeezing it with the sides of the developing body. The folding process changes the once disc-like embryo into a more recognizable (if not quite human) form, with a disproportionately large cranial end.

At the beginning of the fourth week, just before the folding process begins, two rounded ridges appear on each side of the future head and neck region. These two pairs of structures are the first signs of development of the *branchial apparatus,* which eventually gives rise to the ears, maxilla, mandible, and anterior portion of the neck. The apparatus consists of paired (one left, one right) *branchial* or *pharyngeal arches* (visible on the external surface of the embryo), *branchial grooves* between the arches (the first branchial groove becomes the external auditory canal), internal *pharyngeal pouches* reaching toward those grooves, and *branchial membranes,* which separate the pouches from the grooves (Fig. 1-22). On the twenty-second day, the paired first branchial arches are separated by a midline depression, as seen in a "frontal" view, called the *stomadeum* or *primitive mouth.*

By the end of the fourth week, four pairs of branchial arches are visible (Fig. 1-23). The first arch is also called the *mandibular arch,* and consists of a lower *mandibular process* and an upper *maxillary process.* The second arch is termed the *hyoid arch;* the third and fourth branchial arches are designated by number only. Sometimes a rudimentary fifth arch is present. Each arch except the fifth contains an artery, a cartilaginous bar, a muscle element, and a nerve growing into it from the brain.[14]

The migrating neural crest cells arrive in the developing facial structures by two routes, one longer than the other. The first cells to reach the area migrate from the forebrain fold, over the top of the cranial end of the embryo, to form the *frontonasal process,* from which the nose and adjacent structures will form. Neural crest cells migrating into branchial arches have a little further to travel, and so arrive

[14]For a detailed discussion of the derivatives of the branchial arteries, cartilage, muscles, and nerves, plus the derivatives of the pharyngeal pouches, please see Slavkin (1979).

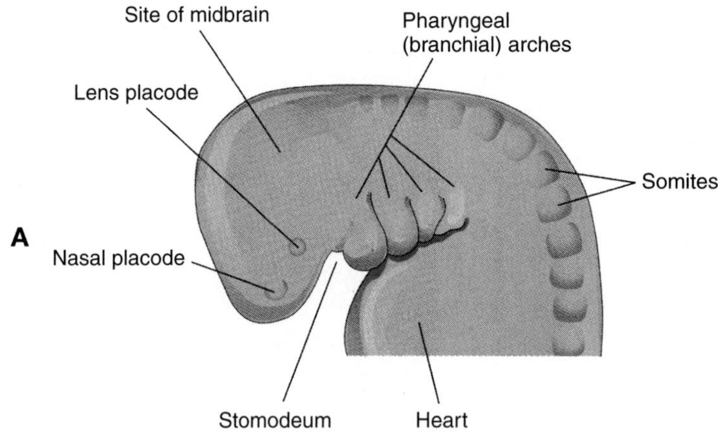

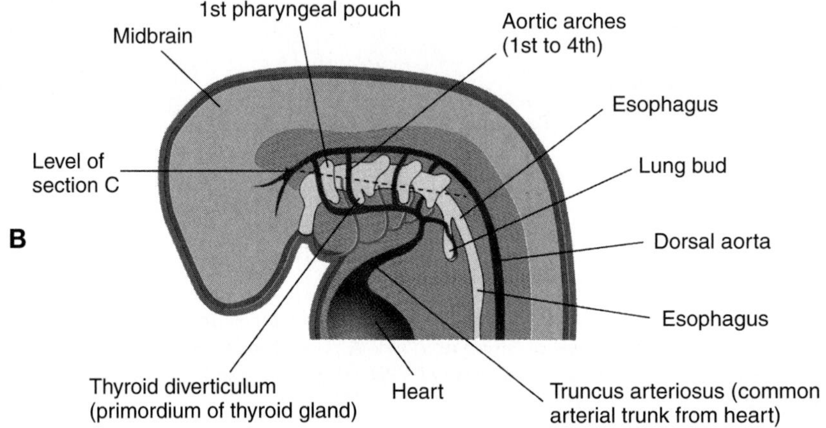

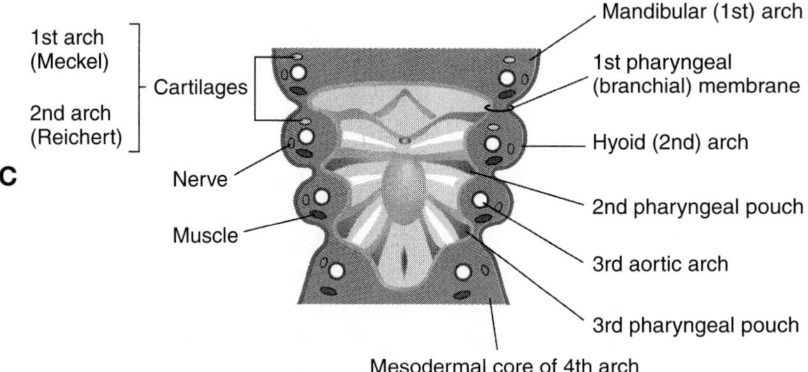

Figure 1-23 Schematic representations of the head and neck regions of the embryo at about 28 days' gestation. **A,** Side view. **B,** Longitudinal section through the midline. **C,** Horizontal section. *(From Moore KL, and Persaud TVN:* The developing human: clinically oriented embryology, *ed. 6. Philadelphia: WB Saunders, 1998, p. 218.)*

a little later. The "job" of the neural crest cells is to surround the mesoderm of the structures in their new environment to form the mesenchyme (loosely organized embryonic connective tissue), which will provide most of the bone and soft tissue of the face. As you already suspect, if the migration of the neural crest cells fails to take place at the critical time or if there is a deficiency of the mesoderm that is the "target" for those cells, clefts and other facial abnormalities may result.

The *frontonasal process* or *frontonasal prominence* forms *two medial nasal processes* between the *nasal pits* and *two lateral nasal processes* lateral to the pits (Fig. 1-24). The median and lateral nasal processes form the upper boundary of the stomodeum. The lateral boundary is formed by the paired maxillary processes of the first branchial arch and the lower boundary by the paired mandibular processes. Development of an intact nose, nasal floor, lip, and palate depends on normal growth and successful joining of the lateral and median nasal processes and the maxillary processes in the correct way and at the correct time.

How processes join to form facial and palatal structures. Two terms are used to denote different modes of the "joining" or blending of the facial and palatal processes to form normal structures: "fusion" and "merging" (Fig. 1-25). Unfortunately, the terms are not consistently differentiated because researchers have argued about which is the most appropriate, particularly with regard to the formation of the soft palate (discussed below). The paired facial and palatal processes, as they grow towards their counterparts, have an epithelial covering that adheres to the covering of the counterpart process. Normal formation of the structure then depends on breakdown of that epithelial "seam" and subsequent mesenchymal consolidation (Ferguson, 1987, 1988). This is the process labeled "fusion." Some anatomists and embryologists have hypothesized that lack of breakdown of the epithelium leads to clefts, as will be discussed below. In contrast, "merging" is defined as the coalescence of growth centers in tissues where there is already a confluence of the mesenchyme that seems to "smooth out" grooves in the epithelium. (See Johnston and Sulik, 1984, for a more complete explanation.)

Formation of the primary palate. Fusion of the median nasal processes, the lateral nasal processes, and the paired maxillary prominences produces the embryonic *primary palate,* which forms most of the upper lip (roughly the middle two thirds), the corresponding portion of the alveolar ridge, and the anterior portion of the maxilla back to the incisive foramen. (These portions of the alveolar ridge and the hard palate are collectively called the *premaxilla,* and the associated portion of the lip is called the *prolabium.*) The nasal septum grows downward and fuses with the palate, completing the separation of the two nostrils. The formation of the primary palate takes place during the sixth week after conception, approximately 2 weeks after fusion of the left and right mandibular prominences or processes has produced the mandible, lower lip, and lower part of the face.

Formation of the secondary palate. The secondary palate is formed by the meeting and fusion (and perhaps merging) of the *palatine processes* or *palatal shelves,* which are medial projections from the right and left maxillary processes. The palatal shelves also fuse with the primary palate along the *premaxillary sutures* and with the nasal septum and vomer bone superiorly (Fig. 1-26). The process by which the palatal shelves develop and create the secondary palate has been the point of a rather interesting controversy in embryology for several decades.

The palatal shelves initially develop as two "vertical floppy flaps" (Sperber, 1992) hanging down on either side of the rapidly growing embryonic tongue. For them to meet and fuse, the shelves must somehow get into a horizontal position above the tongue, adhere to each other, and fuse. Anatomists and embryologists have offered two different sequences of events. The most widely postulated sequence has been that the developing tongue keeps the palatal shelves apart and in a vertical position until there is enough growth or extension of the neck to allow the mandible to get off the chest, letting the mandible grow forward and thus providing room for the tongue to drop down from between the shelves (Diewert, 1974; Zeiler, Weinstein, and Gibson, 1964). The alternative sequence starts with the shelves rotating upward past the tongue to reach an appropriate horizontal position, grow toward each other and fuse, forcing the tongue down into the mandible, which then pushes the mandible forward (Kjaer et al., 1993). This theory was given impetus by findings indicating that the mandibular growth spurt in human embryos *follows* rather than precedes closure of the secondary palate (Burdi and Silvey, 1969; Humphrey, 1969, 1971).

The shelves move upward very quickly in a sort of floppy barn door fashion, with the posterior portions moving upward first. Fusion between the shelves takes place in the opposite direction, that is, front to back. Shelf contact in the region of the soft palate seems to involve a "remodeling of tissues" (Johnston and Millicovsky, 1985) rather than the barn door type of elevation. Whether the soft palate forms by fusion or merging (Burdi and Faist, 1967; Smiley, 1972), formation of the secondary palate is complete somewhere between the tenth and twelfth weeks. The process of shelf elevation and fusion takes place about 1 week later in girls than in boys (Burdi and Silvey, 1969), which may help to explain why girls are more vulnerable than boys to clefts of the secondary palate; that is, the process of formation of the secondary palate takes more time in girls, providing more of a time window for adverse effects from environmental agents.

For a thumbnail summary of the formation of the structures of the primary and secondary palates, these structures form from roughly the end of the fifth week to perhaps the end of the twelfth week (some scientists say the end of the 10th week, others say the 12th week). Clearly the developing embryo is subject to insults of myriad and unknown origins throughout all of this time of "organo-

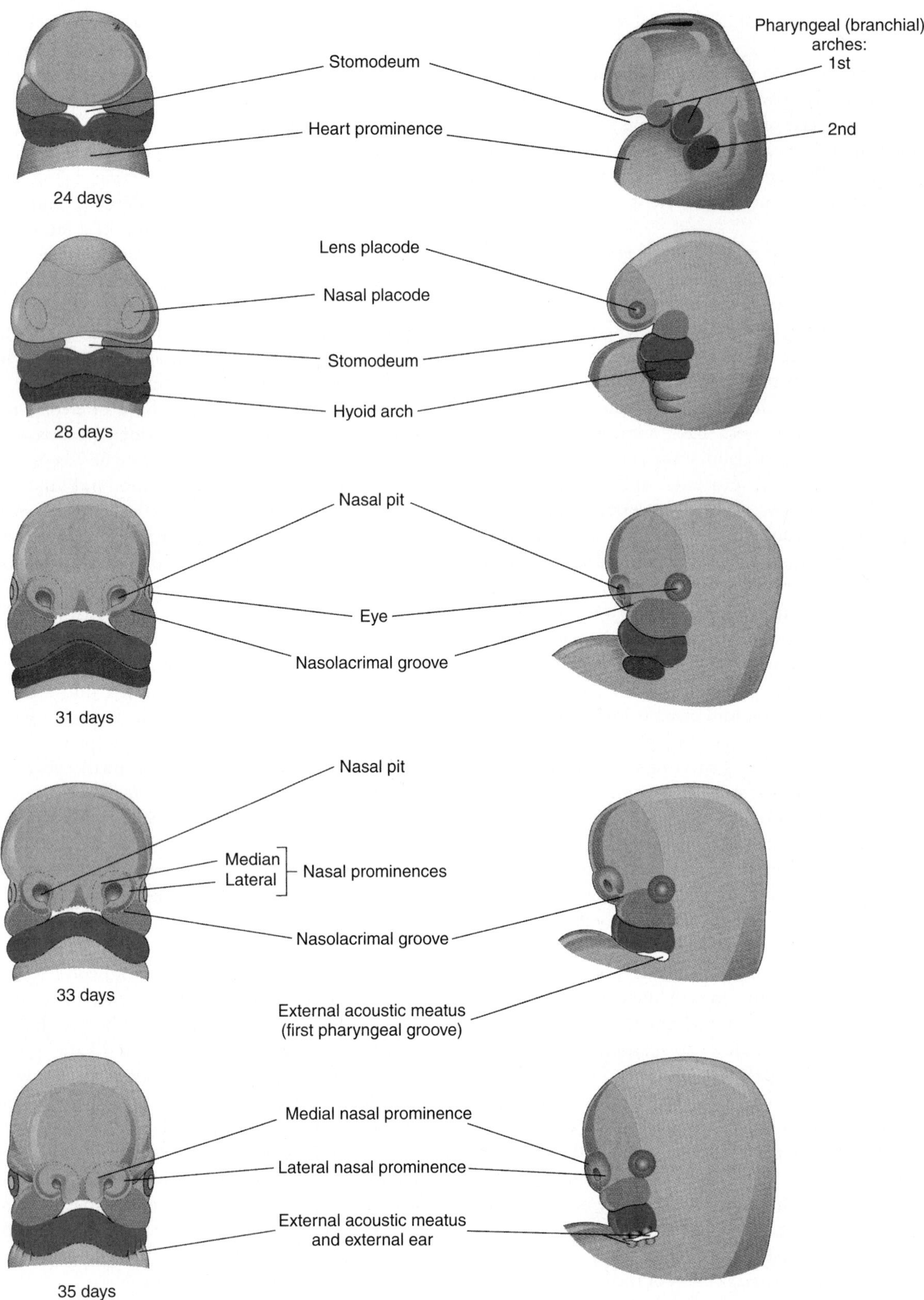

Figure 1-24 Sequential schematic representations of the development of the face in frontal and lateral views of the embryo from about the 24th day of gestation to 14 weeks of gestation. *(From Moore KL, and Persaud TVN:* The developing human: clinically oriented embryology, *ed. 6. Philadelphia: WB Saunders, 1998, pp. 237-238.)*

Continued

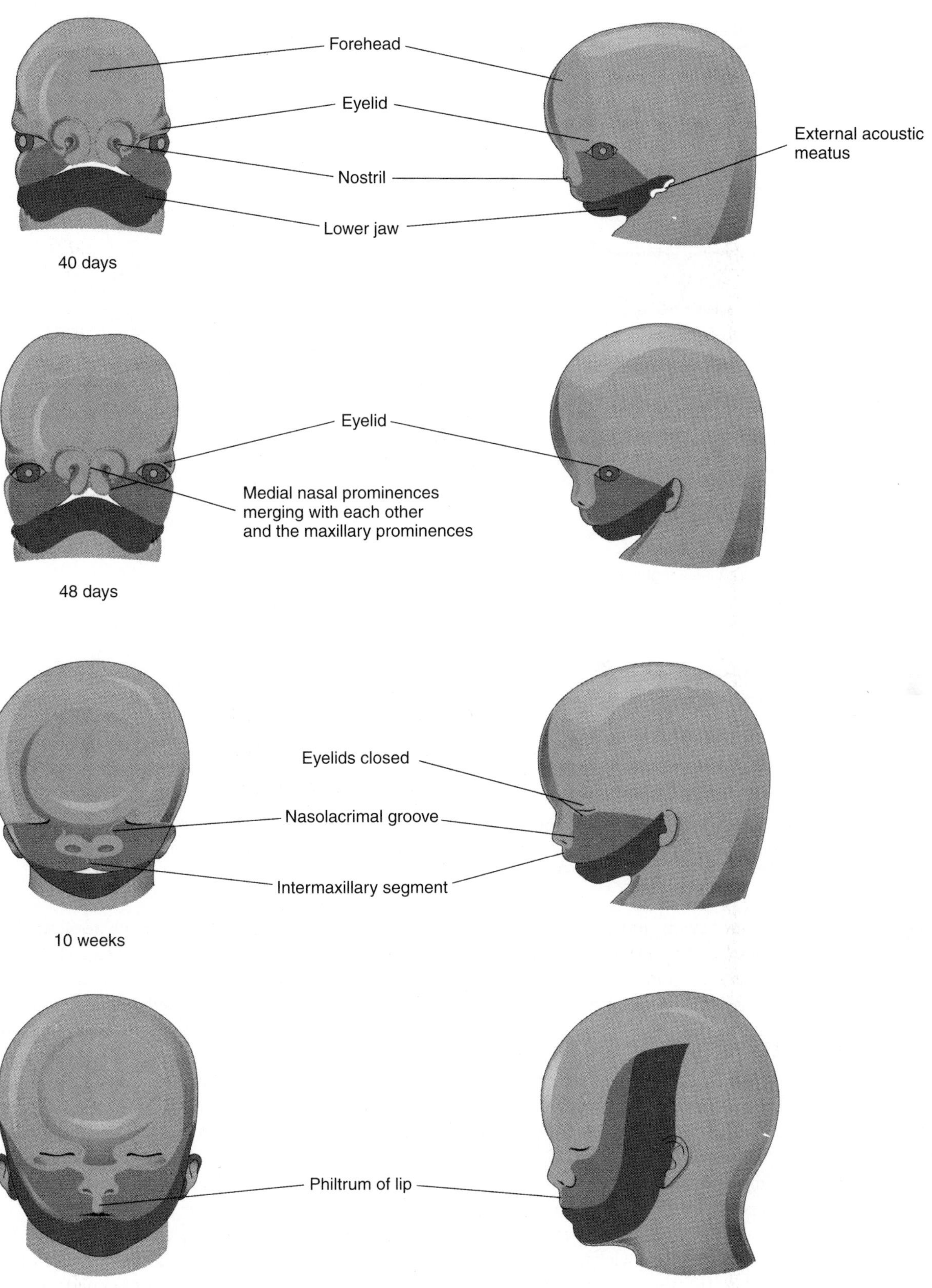

Figure 1-24, cont'd For legend see opposite page.

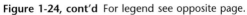

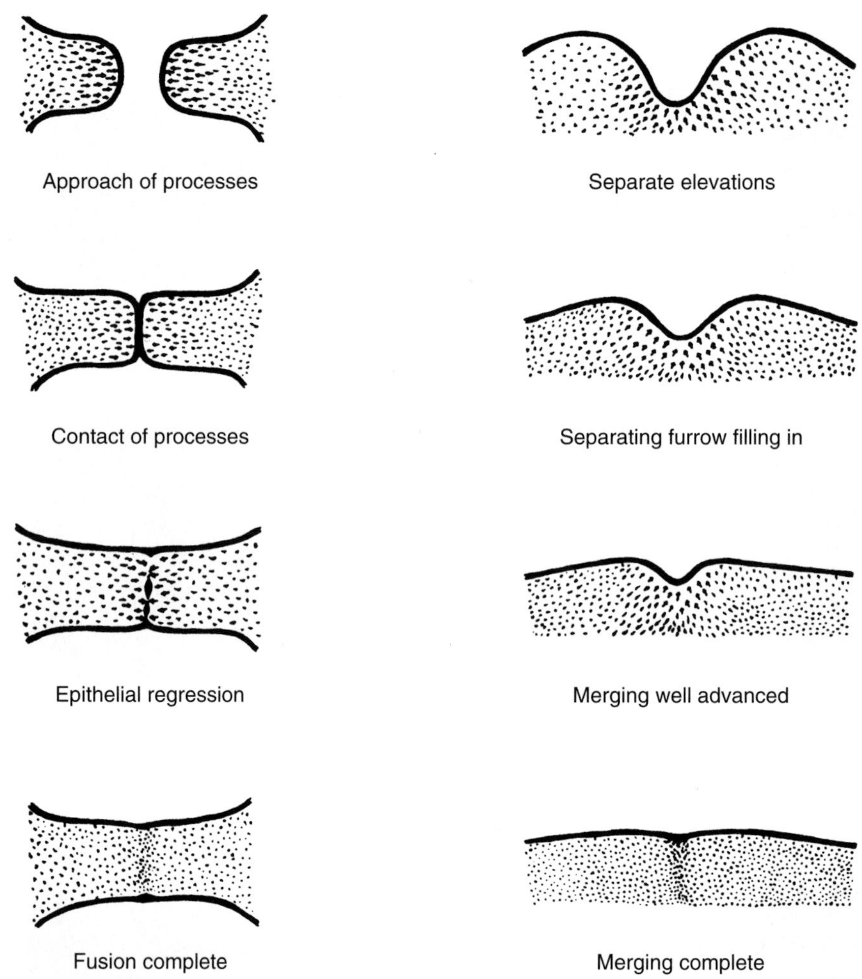

Figure 1-25 Schematic representation of the difference between "merging" and "fusion" in the embryo. *(From Patten BM: Normal development of the facial region. In Purzansky S [ed.].* Congenital anomalies of the face and associated structures. *Springfield, Il: CC Thomas, 1961:35.)*

genesis" (formation of major organs and tissues). Sperber (1992, p. 111) put it this way: "These events of the first few weeks of intrauterine life are the most important occurrences predicting one's entire extrauterine life."

Embryology of Clefts

Clefts of the primary palate appear if the lateral nasal processes, median nasal processes, and maxillary processes do not grow to sufficient size at the right time to meet each other or if the fusion between paired processes and associated structures is impaired. In addition to this "too little or too late" conceptualization, embryologists have considered "postfusion" rupture as the pathogenetic mechanism for the formation of some clefts both of the primary and secondary palate (Kitamura, 1966, 1991). In the latter theory, some interference in the formation of the epithelial seam between the structures or in the subsequent breakdown of that seam and replacement by mesenchyme leads to later ruptures or tears, perhaps as a consequence of continued growth of the embryo. Clinically, both a "Simonart's band" in the primary palate and congenital fistulae of the secondary palate have been cited as evidence of postfusion rupture (Bagatin and Zajc, 1985; Fara, 1971; Kitamura, 1991; Mitts, Garrett, and Hurwitz, 1981). Researchers who have explored this theory at the cellular level have cited various abnormal histologic findings in embryonic tissues (animal and human) after cleft formation. However, others have reported that similar cellular changes were present even before contact of the palatal shelves (Mato, Aikawa, and Smiley, 1972). Johnston (1991) cited problems in several aspects of the "postfusion rupture" theory, and currently this theory is not as widely accepted an explanation for cleft formation as is the more classic "prefusion" interference with growth, positioning, and adherence of structures. However, post-fusion rupture is still considered a *possible* pathogenetic mechanism for some clefts (Ferguson, 1987).

Because combined clefts of the primary and secondary palate are more common than either defect alone, anatomists and embryologists have theorized that the cleft of the lip and alveolus (forming first) somehow predisposes toward a cleft of the secondary palate. One theory about

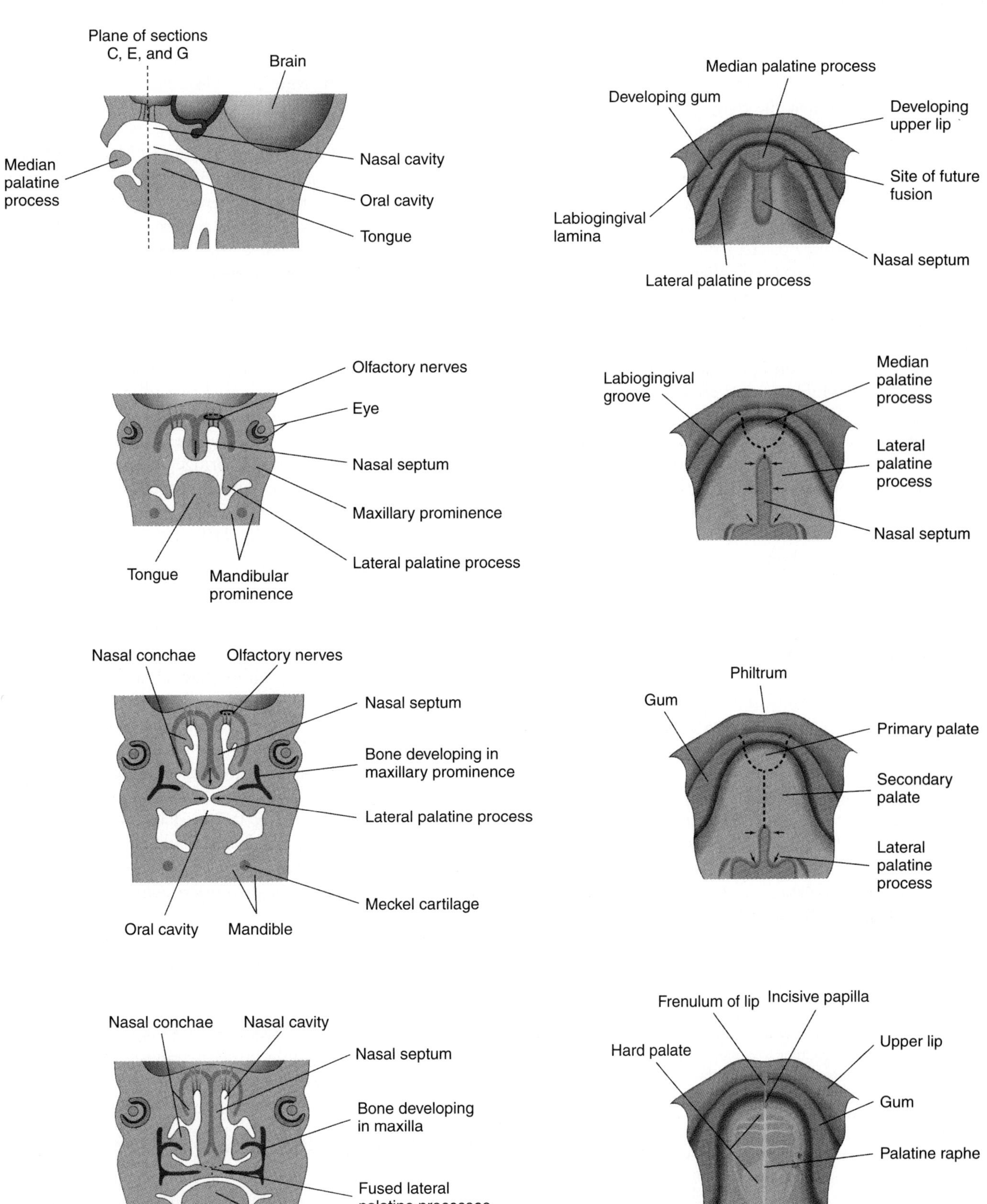

Figure 1-26 Schematic representations of the formation of the structures of the mouth from the ages of about 6 weeks to 12 weeks of gestation. *(From Moore KL, and Persaud TVN:* The developing human: clinically oriented embryology, *ed. 6. Philadelphia: WB Saunders, 1998, p. 246.)*

this link is that lack of lip closure leads to "overgrowth" of the prolabial tissues, diverting the tongue up into the nasal cavity in such a way that the tongue delays movement of one or both palatal shelves to the point that the optimal time for fusion is lost (Trasler, 1968). However, normal formation of the secondary palate in the presence of a cleft of the primary palate certainly does occur because there are many individuals with cleft lip (or cleft lip and alveolus) but no cleft of the secondary palate.

Clefts of the secondary palate obviously do not all form in the same way or for the same reason. Various authors have discussed factors that can interfere with growth of the palatal shelves, shelf elevation, adherence, and fusion (Ferguson, 1987; Johnston and Millicovsky, 1985; Johnston, Bronsky, and Millicovsky, 1990; Poswillo, 1988; Ross and Johnston, 1978). A frequently mentioned "culprit" in terms of shelf elevation is interference by the tongue, but, as discussed in the brief review of normal embryologic development the lowering of the tongue into the mandible and the subsequent growth spurt of the mandible reportedly *follows* shelf elevation in human embryos (Burdi and Silvey, 1969; Humphrey, 1969, 1971).[15] Nevertheless, most major tutorials on cleft formation continue to include discussion of the possible role of tongue position.

Clearly, normal formation of the lip and palate is a finely tuned, intricately timed process. The embryonic structures must be the right size and in the right place at the right time for normal development to occur. If, for example, palatal shelf elevation is delayed beyond a critical threshold in time, fusion may no longer be possible (Fraser, 1971), perhaps because the head is continuing to grow and the shelves can no longer meet even when elevated. Johnston, Bronsky, and Millicovsky (1990) discussed the "threshold" concept in a slightly different context in their perspective on the possible role of environmental factors in predisposing toward cleft lip +/− palate: ". . . the facial prominences of individuals with CL(P) [may] have barely missed making contact, and slight improvements in the conditions affecting the pregnancy . . . could substantially improve the chances of contact and prevent an appreciable number of clefts from occurring. The fact that so many clefts are incomplete (when contact is insufficient for complete fusion) indicates that a large number of embryos are sitting squarely on the threshold" (p. 2539).

This "threshold" conceptualization[16] blends with the concept of a *continuum* of the effects or consequences of factors interfering with normal growth, positional changes, and consolidation of the facial processes: The earlier the interruption or interference, the greater the effect and, conversely, the later the interference the milder the effect. Johnston, Bronsky, and Millicovsky (1990) cited the "many degrees of severity of CL(P), from lip scarring or notching to complete bilateral CL(P)" as evidence that "the process of contact and fusion may cease at any point" (p. 2526). Poswillo (1988) stated that submucous clefts of the secondary palate and bifid uvulas "are probably the result of disturbances in the local mesenchyme at the time of ossification of the palatal bridge and merging of the margins of the soft palate. These phenomena occur late in morphogenesis, between the seventh and tenth weeks of human development . . ." (p. 210). The intriguing cases of submucous defects of the hard and/or soft palate with integrity of tissue *posterior* to the defect (Shprintzen et al., 1985a) suggests that mesenchymal consolidation may be interrupted very briefly and then resume.

A special note should be made here about the formation of the rare median (or midline), lateral, and oblique clefts mentioned earlier. Midline clefts result when there is interference with neural crest cell flow into the developing frontonasal process (Poswillo, 1988). Lateral clefts may result from lack of normal fusion between the maxillary and mandibular processes. Oblique clefts may result from lack of normal fusion between the median and lateral nasal processes, or between the lateral nasal processes and the maxillary processes. Oblique clefts and other atypical facial clefts can be the result of disruption, which can be vascular (interruption in the blood supply to the developing processes) or "mechanical" such as the amniotic rupture sequence in which the embryo swallows amniotic bands, tearing developing tissues (Poswillo, 1988).

WHY CLEFTS OCCUR (ETIOLOGY OF CLEFTS)

We will discuss this topic in two sections: current theories about the genetic bases of clefts and current knowledge about factors that may predispose families to clefts.

Theories About the Etiology of Clefts

Both cleft lip +/− palate and cleft palate alone are etiologically heterogeneous. There is not a single cause nor any single etiological model that explains the occurrence of either type of cleft. Clefts may be caused by single genes,

[15]The theoretical role of the tongue in preventing normal shelf elevation and contact has been most emphasized in the literature on Pierre Robin sequence, the classic features of which are a small mandible, cleft of the secondary palate (frequent but not obligatory), glossoptosis (retraction of the tongue), and consequent respiratory problems. The traditional explanation for the "sequence" of defects in Robin babies has been that something has prevented the mandible from growing normally, which has kept the tongue between the palatal shelves, which has led to a cleft. The cleft is often described as "U shaped," presumably mimicking the shape of the interfering tongue. However, Rintala, Ranta, and Stegars (1984) reported both "V-shaped" and "U-shaped" clefts in Robin patients and in non-Robin patients with clefts of the secondary palate, and two Robin patients with submucous clefts. They also reported unexpected findings of "conical elevations" on the lower lip and hypodontia in high percentages of their Robin patients and concluded that the defects in Robins sequence were more likely due to "a genetically influenced growth disturbance in the maxilla and mandible" rather than "foetal malposition with the tongue between the palatal shelves."

[16]In the next section we will discuss the "multifactorial threshold" or "MFT" theory of the etiology of clefts; the use of the word "threshold" in these two different contexts is not merely coincidental because the "MFT" theory addresses what factors may play a role in pushing the embryo over the threshold for clefting.

chromosomal disorders, or environmental factors. Some of the 300+ syndromes in which a cleft is a feature are known to be caused by an abnormal gene. Examples of single-gene disorders that include clefts are Treacher Collins syndrome, velocardiofacial syndrome, Stickler syndrome, EEC syndrome (ectrodactyly-ectodermal dysplasia-cleft syndrome), and van der Woude syndrome, all of which are autosomal dominant.[17] There are some chromosomal disorders in which a cleft is often present, but many individuals with chromosomal disorders are not reproductively fit and others have a short life span. For example, the chromosomal disorder in which clefts are most common is trisomy 13 (Patau syndrome), but the mean life expectancy is 130 days (Gorlin, Cohen, and Levin, 1990). For the clefts that are not clearly part of a known-genesis syndrome or a chromosomal disorder, geneticists and epidemiologists have struggled to derive models that could help to predict recurrence within families. For the past several decades the most popular theory has been the "polygenic, multifactorial threshold" model of inheritance (Carter, 1970; Ferguson, 1987; Fraser, 1970, 1971, 1977, 1978; Fraser and Pashayan, 1970). However, many scientists believe a better explanation for clefts lies in some "single mutant gene" model.

The "multifactorial threshold" model. Most human traits are multifactorial in origin—height, weight, hair color, eye color, and so on. This means that there are probably several genes, possibly combined with environmental factors, that determine the expression of the trait. The frequency with which the trait is found in the family, and the extent to which it is expressed will depend on sex, degree of relationship (first degree versus second degree or beyond), and possibly environmental factors (e.g., diet). When a birth defect such as CL +/− P follows a multifactorial pattern of inheritance, (1) the affected relatives, if there are any at all, will more likely be first-degree rather than second-degree relatives, (2) the more severe the defect in the proband, the more likely there will be affected relatives, (3) the affected relatives will more likely be of the same sex as the proband, and (4) the more affected relatives there are in the family history, the higher the likelihood of recurrence in future babies.

The multifactorial model postulates a "threshold" as illustrated in Fig. 1-27. Most embryos theoretically fall to the left of the threshold and will not have clefts. But if enough of the predisposing factors (genetic factors plus possible environmental factors) are present, the embryo is pushed over the threshold. The "MFT" model has been widely accepted as a model for the majority of cases of nonsyndromic cleft lip +/− palate (Chung et al., 1986; Czeizel and Nagy, 1986; Ferguson, 1987; Fraser, 1970, 1971, 1977, 1978; Fraser and Pashayan, 1970; Johnston and Millicovsky, 1985; Johnston, Bronsky, and Millicovsky, 1990), but the data for cleft palate only do not fit the model so well, leaving scientists to emphasize the diversity of causes for cleft palate only (Czeizel and Nagy, 1986).[18] Some studies have reported "microforms" of cleft lip +/− palate (e.g., deformities of the nose, notches of the lip, hypoplasia of the premaxilla, anomalies of the lateral incisors) in relatives of affected individuals, providing support for this model (Schubert et al., 1988).[19]

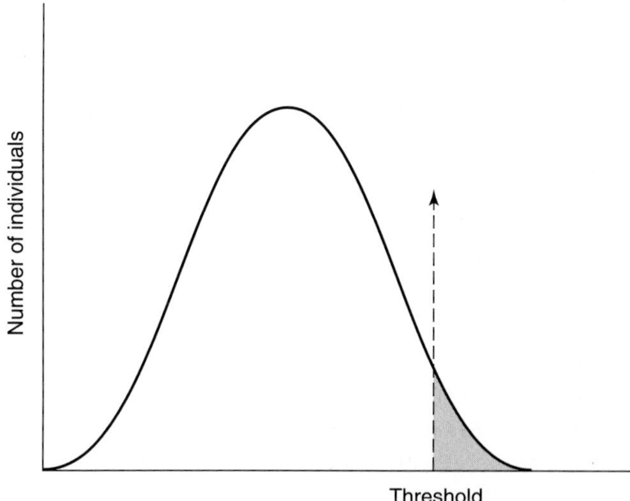

Figure 1-27 Schematic portrayal of the multifactorial model. The threshold for expression of a trait is determined by many genetic factors and possibly some environmental factors. With regard to clefts, most embryos fall to the left of the threshold and will not have clefts. This model does not apply to syndromic clefts.

The "major gene" hypothesis. For the past three decades there has been increasing interest in the possibility that many nonsyndromic clefts may actually be caused by a single mutant (abnormal) gene, rather than by many unidentified genes acting together (Bixler, 1981; Chabora and Horowitz, 1974; Coccia, Bixler, and Conneally, 1969; Fukuhara, 1965; Melnick, 1986; Marazita et al., 1986; Marazita, Spence, and Melnick, 1984; Melnick and Shields, 1976; Melnick et al., 1980; Mitchell and Risch, 1992; Ray, Field, and Marazita, 1993). Some investigators have felt that the patterns occurrence of cleft lip +/− palate in families best fit the model of an autosomal recessive gene with reduced penetrance and variable expressivity (Chung et al., 1986; Melnick, 1986; Melnick et al., 1980).[20]

[17]An individual with an autosomal dominant disorder has a 50% risk for transmitting the disorder to offspring (50% risk with *each* pregnancy).

[18]Remember that clefts of the secondary palate are far more likely to occur with associated anomalies, including multi-anomaly syndromes.

[19]Schubert et al. (1988) also reported "microforms" of clefts of the palate only in relatives of individuals with such clefts, leading the authors to support the MFT model for both types of clefts.

[20]An "autosomal recessive" trait is transmitted to offspring if each parent contributes one mutant gene, that is, both genes of the pair present in baby must be abnormal for the trait to be present. In autosomal dominant inheritance, only one must be abnormal. "Penetrance" is expressed as the percentage of time that a trait for which the gene is present (or genes are present) that the offspring will actually have the trait. "Expressivity" refers to the severity of the trait in a given affected individual.

However, some clinicians have reported evidence of autosomal dominant inheritance (Fukuhara, 1965; Jenkins and Stady, 1980; Temple et al., 1989). Current gene linkage studies are uncovering more possibilities of major gene loci (Christensen and Mitchell, 1996; Stein et al., 1995).

Epidemiologists and geneticists have not found that a single model (MFT vs. major gene) fits all available population data. For example, Chung et al. (1986) found that the population data for cleft lip +/– palate in Japan fit the multifactorial model, without evidence for a major gene; but the same authors reported evidence of a combination of major gene action and multifactorial inheritance in Danish population data. In 1986, Melnick asked, "Is there a major gene for CL +/– P?" and answered his own question with "an unqualified 'probably.' " At the same time, however, he felt that in utero exposure to environmental teratogens played a role in whether the theoretical gene actually produced a cleft. The advantage to finding a major gene (or genes) for nonsyndromic clefts is that the occurrence of clefts could be predicted more accurately, both for families and within given populations. Some current researchers view the multifactorial inheritance model for clefts as something that was useful when geneticists had no other way to predict recurrence of clefts and feel that the need for such a model will gradually diminish as more genes are mapped and identified. As of this writing, however, the multifactorial threshold model is still used in the counseling of the majority of families.

Factors Related to the Etiology of Clefts

Because scientists have not had a clear, simple model to explain the occurrence of most clefts, they have looked at physical findings in families and possible environmental influences.

Characteristics within families. The factors that have received the most attention are parental age and a variety of radiographic and anthropometric findings in parents and other relatives. In the latter case, the findings have inevitably been intertwined with racial influences.

Researchers looking for a possible link between paternal or maternal age on the occurrence of clefts have been careful to control for age of the other parent and have looked at consecutive brackets of age groups. This search dates back to at least 1953, and the findings have often been contradictory (Fraser and Calnan, 1961; Loretz, Westmoreland, and Richards, 1961; MacMahon and McKeown, 1953; Shaw, Croen, and Curry, 1991; Womersley and Stone, 1987; Woolf, 1963; Woolf, Woolf, and Broadbent, 1963b). Recent studies have shown no maternal age effect for either cleft lip +/– palate or cleft palate only (Baird, Sadovnick, and Yee, 1994) but a slight increased risk for cleft lip +/– palate when fathers are less than 20 or more than 40 years old (McIntosh, Olshan, and Baird, 1995).

The search for a link between clefts and various radiographic or anthropometric measurements in the relatives of affected individuals has generally yielded positive, potentially helpful information (Chung and Kau, 1985; Coccaro, D'Amico, and Chavoor, 1972; Fraser and Pashayan, 1970; Kurisu et al., 1974; Nakasima and Ichinose, 1983; Prochazkova and Tolarova, 1986; Prochazkova and Vinsova, 1995; Raghavan, Sidhu, and Kharbanda, 1994; Sato, 1989). In general, this research has shown that there may indeed be physical markers, such as wider heads, in families of individuals with clefts. The practicality of such information on a prospective basis remains somewhat elusive, but the search continues because, as stated by Ward, Bixler, and Jamison in 1994, "The ability to identify minimally affected gene carriers within families would provide critical information needed in the search for molecular markers that segregate with the genetic risk for clefting" (p. 57).

Environmental influences. The most intriguing focus of study in terms of the influence of environmental factors has been the effects of possible teratogens, but scientists have also looked at seasonal variations in the occurrence of clefts on the theory that some environmental factors such as pesticides will vary with the time of year (Coupland and Coupland, 1988; Gordon and Shy, 1981; Owens, Jones, and Harris, 1985), maternal epilepsy, and maternal diet and vitamin intake.

One study (Tyan, 1982) reported that the frequency of CL +/– P among Japanese and other Asians born in California and New York was significantly lower than the frequency in the same groups born in Japan and Hawaii; these authors postulated that the effect could be due to better diet. In the early 1980s Tolarova (1982) found evidence that the occurrence of CL +/– P, as well as other neural tube defects, might be reduced by maternal intake of folic acid. The investigation of folic acid as a factor for reducing occurrence of clefts continues (Tolarova, 1987) and remains one of the few "proactive" areas of research for helping to eliminate birth defects.

In the early 1960s maternal epilepsy was linked to an increased risk for clefts (Friis, 1989), but scientists had a difficult time segregating the effects of the disease from the effects of drugs used to treat the disease. More recent studies have demonstrated the effects of various anticonvulsant drugs as teratogens linked to an increased risk for clefts (Czeizel and Nagy, 1986; Friis, 1989; Hanson, 1989; Hanson et al., 1976; Meadow, 1968; Owens, Jones, and Harris, 1985).

Our body of knowledge regarding environmental agents that predispose toward birth defects continues to grow. The student must understand that research in this area is necessarily limited when it comes to birth defects in humans because humans cannot be experimentally "dosed" with suspected teratogens as can laboratory animals. Nevertheless, as humans "dose" themselves with possibly harmful agents, the incidence of birth defects grows.[21] In

[21] An embryo (actually, the "blastocyst") becomes vulnerable to possible teratogens only after it embeds in the uterine wall. However, the prenatal environment may be influenced by diet and vitamins even before pregnancy.

addition to anticonvulsant medications, the drugs or other environmental agents that have been linked to an increased risk for clefts in offspring include alcohol (Clarren and Smith, 1978; Hanson and Smith, 1975; Jones et al., 1973); retinoids, which are members of the vitamin A family (Fernhoff and Lammer, 1984; Lammer et al., 1985); nitrate compounds (Dorsch et al., 1984); organic solvents (Holmberg et al., 1982); and cigarettes (Ericson, Kallen, and Westerholm, 1979; Khoury, Gomez-Farias, and Mulinare, 1989; Khoury et al., 1977; Werler et al., 1990).[22] As of this writing, the evidence of cigarette smoking as a significant influence on the likelihood of clefts continues to grow, to the extent that the California Birth Defects Monitoring Program warns potential parents as strongly against the use of tobacco as against the use of alcohol and illegal drugs.

Finally, the influence of various illegal drugs on the incidence of birth defects has been under investigation for several years, but the current clinical reality is that many babies seen for a variety of structural and neurologic deficits have parents with a history of multiple substance abuse (alcohol, tobacco, marijuana, cocaine, crack cocaine, heroin, etc.). Segregation of the effects of these various agents is nearly impossible under such circumstances.

REFERENCES

Altemus LA: The incidence of cleft lip and cleft palate among North American Negroes. *Cleft Palate Journal* 3:357-361, 1966.

Altemus LA, and Ferguson AD: Comparative incidence of birth defects in Negro and white children. *Pediatrics* 36:56-61, 1965.

Bagatin M: Cleft uvula. *Acta Chirurgiae Plasticae* 37:202-206, 1985a.

Bagatin M: Submucous cleft palate. *Journal of Maxillofacial Surgery* 13:37-38, 1985b.

Bagatin M, and Zajc I: Perforation of submucous cleft palate. *Chirurgiae Maxillofacial Plasticae* 15:65-67, 1985.

Baird PA, Sadovnick AD, and Yee IMI: Maternal age and oral cleft malformations: data from a population-based series of 576,815 consecutive livebirths. *Teratology* 49:448-451, 1994.

Bardanouve V: Cleft palate in Montana: a 10-year report. *Cleft Palate Journal* 6:213-220, 1969.

Bixler D: Genetics and clefting. *Cleft Palate Journal* 18:10-18, 1981.

Burdi AR, and Faist K: Morphogenesis of the palate in normal human embryos with special emphasis on the mechanisms involved. *American Journal of Anatomy* 120:149-159, 1967.

Burdi AR, and Silvey RG: Sexual differences in closure of the human palatal shelves. *Cleft Palate Journal* 6:1-7, 1969.

Calzolari E, Milan M, Cavazzuti GB, Cocchi G, Gandini E, Magnani C, Moretti M, Garani GP, Salvioli GB, and Volpato S: Epidemiological and genetic study of 200 cases of oral cleft in the Emilia Romagna region of Northern Italy. *Teratology* 38:559-564, 1988.

Carter CO: Multifactorial inheritance revisited. In Fraser FC, and McKusick VA (eds.): *Congenital malformations.* Amsterdam: Excepta Medica, 1970, pp. 227-232.

Chabora AJ, and Horowitz SL: Cleft lip and cleft palate: one genetic system. A new hypothesis. *Oral Surgery, Oral Diagnosis, Oral Pathology* 38:181-186, 1974.

[22]In the mid-1970s, a link was suspected between Valium (diazepam) and clefts (Safra and Oakley, 1976) but later research failed to verify this drug as a possible teratogen (Shiono and Mills, 1984).

Chavez GF, Cordero JF, Becerra JE: Leading major congenital malformations among minority groups in the United States, 1981-1986. *Journal of the American Medical Association* 261:205-209, 1989.

Ching GHS, and Chung CS: A genetic study of cleft lip and palate in Hawaii. I. Interracial crosses. *American Journal of Human Genetics* 26:162-176, 1974.

Chosack A, and Eidelman E: Cleft uvula: Prevalence and genetics. *Cleft Palate Journal* 5:63-67, 1978.

Christensen K, and Mitchell LE: Familial recurrence-pattern analysis of nonsyndromic isolated cleft palate—a Danish registry study. *American Journal of Human Genetics* 58:182-190, 1996.

Chung CS, and Kau MCW: Racial differences in cephalometric measurements and incidence of cleft lip with or without cleft palate. *Journal of Craniofacial Genetics and Developmental Biology* 5:341-349, 1985.

Chung CS, and Myrianthopoulos NC: Racial and prenatal factors in major congenital malformations. *American Journal of Human Genetics* 20:44-60, 1968.

Chung CS, Mi MP, and Beechert AM: Genetic epidemiology of cleft lip with or without cleft palate in the population of Hawaii. *Genetic Epidemiology* 4:415-423, 1987.

Chung CS, Rao DC, and Ching GHS: Population and family studies of cleft lip ana palate. In Melnick M, Bixler D, and Shields ED (eds.): *Etiology of cleft lip and cleft palate.* New York: Alan R. Liss, 1980, pp. 325-352.

Chung CS, Bixler D, Watanabe T, Koguchi H, and Fogh-Andersen P: Segregation analysis of cleft lip with or without cleft palate: a comparison of Danish and Japanese data. *American Journal of Human Genetics* 39:603-611, 1986.

Clarren SK, and Smith DW: The fetal alcohol syndrome. *New England Journal of Medicine* 298:1063-1067, 1978.

Coccaro PJ, D'Amico R, and Chavoor A: Craniofacial morphology of parents with and without cleft lip and palate children. *Cleft Palate Journal* 9:28-38, 1972.

Coccia CT, Bixler D, and Conneally PM: Cleft lip and cleft palate: a genetic study. *Cleft Palate Journal* 6:323-336, 1969.

Cohn ER: Commentary on prevalence of cleft uvula among school children in kindergarten through grade five. *Cleft Palate-Craniofacial Journal* 29:13-14, 1992.

Cosman B, and Crikelair GF. The minimal cleft lip. *Plastic and Reconstructive Surgery* 37:334-340, 1966.

Coupland MA, and Coupland AI: Seasonality, incidence, and sex distribution of cleft lip and palate births in Trent region, 1973-1982. *Cleft Palate Journal* 25:33-37, 1988.

Curtis E, Fraser FC, and Warburton D: Congenital cleft lip and palate: risk figures for counseling. *Archives of Pediatric and Adolescent Medicine* 102:853-857, 1961.

Czeizel A, and Nagy E: A recent aetiological study on facial clefting in Hungary. *Acta Paediatrica Hungarica* 27:145-160, 1986.

Czeizel A, and Tusnadi G: An epidemiologic study of cleft lip with or without cleft palate in Hungary. *Human Heredity* 21:17-38, 1971.

Czeizel A: Re: "Incidence and prevalence as measures of the frequency of birth defects" [letter]. *American Journal of Epidemiology* 119:141-142, 1984.

DeMyer W: Median cleft lip. In Grabb WC, Rosenstein SW, Bzoch KR (eds): *Cleft lip and palate: surgical, dental, and speech aspects.* Boston: Little, Brown, 1971, pp. 359-369.

DeVoss H: A study of the factors relative to the incidence of cleft palate births from 1945 through 1949 in San Bernadino County. *Speech Monographs* 19:303-308, 1952.

Diewert V: A cephalometric study of orofacial structures during secondary palate closure in the rat. *Archives of Oral Biology* 19:303-315, 1974.

Dorsch MM, Scragg RKR, McMichael AJ, Baghurst APA, and Dyer KF: Congenital malformations and maternal drinking water supply in rural South Australia: a case-control study. *American Journal of Epidemiology* 119:473-486, 1984.

Emanuel I, Huang S-W, Gutman L, Yu F-C, and Ling C-C: The incidence of congenital malformations in a Chinese population: the Taipei collaborative study. *Teratology* 5:159-169, 1972.

Erickson JD: Racial variations in the incidence of congenital malformations. *Annals of Human Genetics* 39:315-320, 1976.

Ericson A, Kallen B, and Westerholm P: Cigarette smoking as an etiologic factor in cleft lip and palate. *American Journal of Obstetrics and Gynecology* 135:348-351, 1979.

Fara M: Congenital defects in the hard palate. *Plastic and Reconstructive Surgery* 48:44-47, 1971.

Fara M, Hrivnakova J, and Sedlackova E: Submucous cleft palates. *Acta Chirurgiae Plasticae* 13:221-234, 1971.

Ferguson MWJ: Palate development: mechanisms and malformations. *Irish Journal of Medical Science* 156:309-315, 1987.

Ferguson MWJ: Palate development. *Development* 103(Supplement):41-60, 1988.

Fernhoff PM, and Lammer EJ: Craniofacial features of isotretonoin embryopathy. *Pediatrics* 105:595-597, 1984.

Fogh-Andersen P: *Inheritance of harelip and cleft palate.* Copenhagen: Munksgaard, 1942.

Fogh-Andersen P: Genetic and non-genetic factors in the etiology of facial clefts. *Scandinavian Journal of Plastic and Reconstructive Surgery* 1:22-29, 1967.

Fogh-Andersen P: Incidence and aetiology. In Edwards J, and Watson A (eds.): *Advances in the management of cleft palate.* Edinburgh: Churchill Livingstone, 1980, pp. 43-48.

Fraser FC: Thoughts on the etiology of clefts of the palate and lip. *Acta Geneticae* (Basel) 5:358-369, 1955.

Fraser FC: The genetics of cleft lip and palate. *American Journal of Human Genetics* 22:336-352, 1970.

Fraser FC: Etiology of cleft lip and palate. In Grabb WC, Rosenstein SW, Bzoch KR (eds.): *Cleft lip and palate: surgical, dental, and speech aspects.* Boston: Little, Brown, 1971, pp. 54-65.

Fraser FC: Interactions and multiple causes. In Wilson JC, and Fraser FC (eds.): *Handbook of teratology: general principles and etiology.* Volume 1. New York: Plenum Press, 1977, pp. 445-463.

Fraser FC: The multifactorial threshold concept—uses and misuses. *Teratology* 14:267-280, 1978.

Fraser FC, and Baxter H: The familial distribution of congenital clefts of the lip and palate. *American Journal of Surgery* 87:656-659, 1954.

Fraser FC, and Calnan J: Cleft lip and palate: Seasonal incidence, birth weight, birth rank, sex, site, associated malformations, and parental age. A statistical survey. *Archives of Diseases of Children* 36:420-423, 1961.

Fraser FC, and Pashayan H: Relation of face shape to susceptibility to congenital cleft lip: a preliminary report. *Journal of Medical Genetics* 7:112-117, 1970.

Friis ML: Facial clefts and congenital heart defects in children of parents with epilepsy: Genetic and environmental etiologic factors. *Acta Neurologica Scandinavia* 79:433-459, 1989.

Fujino H, Tanaka K, and Sanui Y: Genetic study of cleft lips and cleft palates based on 2828 Japanese cases. *Kyushu Journal of Medical Science* 14:317-331, 1963.

Fukuhara T: New method and approach to the genetics of cleft lip and palate. *Journal of Dental Research* 44:259-268, 1965.

Garcia-Velasco M, Galvez-Perez F, Ysunza-Rivera A, and Ortiz-Monasterio F: Conceptos actuales sobre el paladar hendido submucoso. *Boletin Medicina Hospital de Infant de Mexico* 42:657-661, 1985.

Gilmore SI, and Hofman SM: Clefts in Wisconsin: incidence and related factors. *Cleft Palate Journal* 3:186-199, 1966.

Gordon JE, and Shy CM: Agricultural chemical use and congenital cleft lip and/or palate. *Archives of Environmental Health* 36:213-221, 1981.

Gorlin RJ, Cohen MM Jr., and Levin LS: *Syndromes of the head and neck,* 3rd ed. New York: Oxford University Press, 1990.

Green HG, Nelson CJ, Gaylor DW, and Holson JF: Accuracy of birth certificate data for detecting facial cleft defects in Arkansas children. *Cleft Palate Journal* 16:167-170, 1979.

Greene JC, Vermillion JR, Hay S, Gibbens SF, and Kerschbaum S. Epidemiologic study of cleft lip and cleft palate in four states. *Journal of the American Dental Association* 68:387-404, 1964.

Gregg JH, Stanage WF, and Johnson W: Birth certificate data: how reliable? [letter]. *South Dakota Journal of Medicine* 37:20-21, 1984.

Gundlach KKH: Concomitant developmental anomalies of the face in patients with clefts of lip (alveolus, and palate) or cleft palates. *Scandinavian Journal of Plastic and Reconstructive Surgery* 21:27-30, 1987.

Hanson JW, and Smith DW: Fetal alcohol syndrome: experience with 41 cases. *Journal of Pediatrics* 87:285-290, 1975.

Hanson JW, Myrianthopoulos NC, Harvey MAS, and Smith DW: Risks to the offspring of women treated with hydantoin anticonvulsants with emphasis on the fetal hydantoin syndrome. *Journal of Pediatrics* 89:662-668, 1976.

Holmberg PC, Hernberg S, Kruppa K, Rantala K, and Riala R: Oral clefts and organic solvent exposure during pregnancy. *International Archives of Occupational and Environmental Health* 50:371-376, 1982.

Hook EB: "Incidence" and "prevalence" as measures of the frequency of congenital malformations and genetic outcomes: application to oral clefts. *Cleft Palate Journal* 25:97-102, 1988.

Humphrey T: The relation between human fetal mouth opening reflexes and closure of the palate. *American Journal of Anatomy* 125:317-344, 1969.

Humphrey T: Development of oral and facial motor mechanisms in human fetuses and their relation to human craniofacial growth. *Journal of Dental Research* 50:1428-1441, 1971.

Ivy RH: The influence of race on the incidence of certain congenital anomalies, notably cleft lip-palate. *Plastic and Reconstructive Surgery* 30:581-585, 1962.

Jaffe B, and DeBlanc G: Cleft palate, cleft lip, and cleft uvula in Navajo Indians: incidence and otorhinolaryngolic problems. *Cleft Palate Journal* 7:300-305, 1970.

Jenkins J, and Stady C: Dominant inheritance of cleft of the soft palate. *Human Genetics* 53:341-342, 1980.

Jensen BL, Kreiborg S, Dahl E, and Fogh-Andersen P: Cleft lip and palate in Denmark, 1976-1981: epidemiology, variability, and early somatic development. *Cleft Palate Journal* 25:258-269, 1988.

Johnston MC: Commentary on evidence for cleft palate as a postfusion phenomenon. *Cleft Palate-Craniofacial Journal* 28:210-211, 1991.

Johnston MC, and Millicovsky G: Normal and abnormal development of the lip and palate. *Clinics in Plastic Surgery* 12:521-532, 1985.

Johnston MC, and Sulik KK: Embryology of the head and neck. In Serafin D, and Georgiade NG (eds.): *Pediatric plastic surgery.* St. Louis: CV Mosby, 1984, pp. 184-215.

Johnston MC, Bronsky PT, and Millicovsky G: Embryogenesis of cleft lip and palate. In McCarthy J (ed.): *Plastic surgery.* Volume 4: *Cleft lip and palate and craniofacial deformities.* Philadelphia: WB Saunders, 1990, pp. 2515-2552.

Jones MC: Etiology of facial clefts: Prospective evaluation of 428 patients. *Cleft Palate Journal* 25:16-20, 1988.

Jones KL, and Smith DW: The fetal alcohol syndrome. *Teratology* 12:1-10, 1975.

Jones KL, Smith DW, Ulleland CN, and Streissguth AP: Pattern of malformation in offspring of chronic alcoholic mothers. *Lancet* 1:1267-1271, 1973.

Kaplan EN: The occult submucous cleft palate. *Cleft Palate Journal* 12:356-368, 1975.

Kaye CI: Classification, etiology and genetic aspects of craniofacial anomalies. In Caldarelli D (ed.): *Otolaryngologic Clinics of North America* 14: *Symposium on Craniofacial Anomalies,* 1981, pp. 827-864.

Khoury MJ, Erickson JD, and James LM: Maternal factors in cleft lip with or without palate: evidence from interracial crosses in the United States. *Teratology* 27:351-357, 1983.

Khoury MJ, Gomez-Farias J, and Mulinare J: Does maternal cigarette smoking during pregnancy cause cleft lip and palate in offspring? *American Journal of Diseases in Children* 143:333-337, 1989.

Khoury MJ, Weinstein A, Panny S, Holtzman NA, Lindsay PK, Farrel K, and Eisenberg M: Maternal cigarette smoking and oral clefts: a population-based study. *American Journal of Public Health* 77:623-625, 1977.

Kitamura H: Epithelial remnants and pearls in the secondary palate in the human abortus: a contribution to the study of the mechanism of cleft palate formation. *Cleft Palate Journal* 3:240-257, 1966.

Kitamura H: Evidence for cleft palate as a postfusion phenomenon. *Cleft Palate-Craniofacial Journal* 28:195-210, 1991.

Kjaer I, Bach-Petersen S, Graem N, and Kjaer T: Changes in human palatine bone location and tongue position during prenatal palatal closure. *Journal of Craniofacial Genetics and Developmental Biology* 13:18-23, 1993.

Knox G, and Braithwaite F: Cleft lips and palates in Northumberland and Durham. *Archives of Diseases of Children* 38:66-70, 1963.

Koguchi H: Population data on cleft lip and cleft palate in the Japanese. In Melnick M, Bixler D, and Shields E (eds.): *Progress in Clinical and Biological Research,* Volume 46: *Etiology of cleft lip and cleft palate.* New York: Alan R Liss, 1980, pp. 297-323.

Kurisu K, Nishwander JD, Johnston MC, and Mazaheri M: Facial morphology as an indicator of genetic predisposition to cleft lip and palate. *American Journal of Human Genetics* 26:702-714, 1974.

Lammer EJ, Chen DT, Hoar RM, Agnish ND, Benke PJ, Braun JT, Curry CJ, Fernhoff PM, Grix AW, Lott IT, Richard JM, and Sun SC: Retinoic acid embryopathy. *New England Journal of Medicine* 313:837-841, 1985.

Leck I: Correlations of malformation frequency with environmental and genetic attributes in man. In Wilson JG, Fraser FC (eds.): *Handbook of teratology: comparative, maternal, and epidemiologic aspects.* Volume 3. New York: Plenum Press, 1977, pp. 243-324.

Leck I: The geographical distribution of neural tube defects and oral clefts. *British Medical Bulletin* 40:390-395, 1984.

Leck I, and Lancashire RJ: Birth prevalence of malformations in members of different ethnic groups and in the offspring of matings between them, in Birmingham, England. *Journal of Epidemiology and Community Health* 49:171-179, 1995.

Lehman JA, and Artz JS: The minimal cleft lip. *Plastic and Reconstructive Surgery* 58:306-309, 1976.

Lilius GP: Clefts with associated anomalies and syndromes in Finland. *Scandinavian Journal of Plastic and Reconstructive and Hand Surgery* 26:185-196, 1992.

Lindemann G, Riis B, and Sewerin I: Prevalence of cleft uvula among 2,732 Danes. *Cleft Palate Journal* 14:226-229, 1977.

Loretz W, Westmoreland WW, and Richards LF: A study of cleft lip and cleft palate births in California, 1955. *American Journal of Public Health* 51:873-877, 1961.

Lowry RB, and Renwick D: Incidence of cleft lip and palate in British Columbia Indians. *Journal of Medical Genetics* 6:67-69, 1969.

Lowry RB, Thunem HY, and Hong S: Birth prevalence of cleft lip and palate in British Columbia between 1952 and 1986: stability of rates. *Canadian Medical Association Journal* 140:1167-1170, 1989.

Lutz K, and Moore F: A study of factors in the occurrence of cleft palate. *Journal of Speech and Hearing Disorders* 20:271-276, 1955.

Lynch HT, and Kimberling WJ: Genetic counseling in cleft lip and cleft palate. *Plastic and Reconstructive Surgery* 38:800-815, 1981.

MacMahon B, and McKeown T: The incidence of harelip and cleft palate related to birth rank and maternal age. *American Journal of Human Genetics* 5:176-183, 1953.

Marazita ML, Spence MA, and Melnick M: Genetic analysis of cleft lip with or without cleft palate in Danish kindreds. *American Journal of Medical Genetics* 19:9-18, 1984.

Marazita ML, Goldstein AM, Smalley SL, and Spence MA: Cleft lip with or without cleft palate: reanalysis of a three-generation family study from England. *Genetic Epidemiology* 3:335-342, 1986.

Mato M, Aikawa E, and Smiley GR: Invagination of human palatal epithelium prior to contact. *Cleft Palate Journal* 9:335-340, 1972.

Mazaheri M: Statistical analysis of patients with congenital cleft lip and/or palate at the Lancaster Cleft Palate Clinic. *Plastic and Reconstructive Surgery* 21:193-203, 1958.

McIntosh GC, Olshan AF, and Baird PA: Paternal age and the risk of birth defects in offspring. *Epidemiology* 6:282-288, 1995.

McWilliams BJ: Submucous clefts of the palate: how likely are they to be symptomatic? *Cleft Palate Craniofacial Journal* 28:247-249, 1991.

Meadow SF: Anticonvulsant drugs and congenital abnormalities. *Lancet* 2:1269, 1968.

Melnick M: Cleft lip with or without cleft palate: etiology and pathogenesis. *Canadian Dental Association Journal* 14:92-96, 1986.

Melnick M, and Shields ED: Allelic restriction: a biologic alternative to multifactorial threshold inheritance. *Lancet* 1:176-179, 1976.

Melnick M, Bixler D, Fogh-Andersen P, and Conneally PM: Cleft lip +/− cleft palate: an overview of the literature and an analysis of Danish cases born between 1941 and 1968. *American Journal of Medical Genetics* 6:83-97, 1980.

Meskin L, and Pruzansky S: Validity of the birth certificate in the epidemiologic assessment of facial clefts. *Journal of Dental Research* 46:1456-1459, 1967.

Meskin L, and Pruzansky S: A malformation profile of facial cleft patients and their siblings. *Cleft Palate Journal* 6:309-315, 1969.

Meskin L, Gorlin R, and Isaacson R: Abnormal morphology of the soft palate: I. The prevalence of cleft uvula. *Cleft Palate Journal* 1:342-346, 1964.

Meskin L, Gorlin R, and Isaacson R: Abnormal morphology of the soft palate: II. The genetics of cleft uvula. *Cleft Palate Journal* 1:40-45, 1965.

Meskin L, Gorlin R, and Isaacson R: Cleft uvula—a microform of cleft palate. *Acta Chirurgiae Plasticae* 8:91-96, 1966.

Meskin L, Pruzansky S, and Gullen W: An epidemiologic investigation of factors related to the extent of facial clefts: I. Sex of patient. *Cleft Palate Journal* 5:23-29, 1968.

Mitchell LE, and Risch H: Mode of inheritance of nonsyndromic cleft lip with or without cleft palate: a reanalysis. *American Journal of Human Genetics* 51:323-332, 1992.

Mitts T, Garrett W, and Hurwitz D: Cleft of the hard palate with soft palate integrity. *Cleft Palate Journal* 18:204-206, 1981.

Myrianthopoulos N, and Chung C: Congenital malformations in singletons: epidemiologic survey. *Birth Defects: Original Article Series X* 11:1-54, 1974.

Nakasima A, and Ichinose M: Characteristics of craniofacial structures of parents of children with cleft lip and/or palate. *American Journal of Orthodontics* 84:140-146, 1983.

Natsume N, and Kawai T: Incidence of cleft lip and cleft palate in 39,696 Japanese babies born during 1983. *International Journal of Oral and Maxillofacial Surgery* 15:565-586, 1986.

Natsume H, Suzuki T, and Kawai T: The prevalence of cleft lip and palate in the Japanese: their birth prevalence in 40,304 infants born during 1982. *Oral Surgery, Oral Medicine, and Oral Pathology* 63:421-423, 1987.

Natsume N, Suzuki T, and Kawai T: The prevalence of cleft lip and palate in Japanese. *British Journal of Oral and Maxillofacial Surgery* 26:232-236, 1988.

Niswander J, and Adams M: Oral clefts in the American Indians. *Public Health Reports* 82:807-812, 1967.

Oka SW: Epidemiology and genetics of clefting: with implications for etiology. In Cooper HK, Harding RL, Krogman WM, Mazaheri M, Millard RT (eds.): *Cleft palate and cleft lip: a team approach to clinical management and rehabilitation of the patient.* Philadelphia: WB Saunders, 1979, pp. 108-143.

Owens JR, Jones JW, and Harris F: Epidemiology of facial clefting. *Archives of Disease in Childhood* 60:521-524, 1985.

Park S, Eguti T, Kato K, Nitta H, and Kitano I: The pattern of palatal rugae in submucous clefts palates and isolated cleft palate. *British Journal of Plastic Surgery* 47:395-399, 1994.

Peterson-Falzone SJ: Velopharyngeal inadequacy in the absence of overt cleft palate. *Journal of Craniofacial Genetics and Developmental Biology* 1(Supplement):97-124, 1985.

Pigott RW: Organisation of cleft lip and palate services. *British Journal of Plastic Surgery* 45:385-387, 1992.

Poswillo D: The aetiology and pathogenesis of craniofacial deformity. *Development* 103(Supplement):207-212, 1988.

Prochazkova J, and Tolarova M: Craniofacial morphological features in parents of children with isolated cleft palate. *Acta Chirurgiae Plasticae* 28:194-204, 1986.

Prochazkova J, and Vinsova J: Craniofacial morphology as a marker of predisposition to isolated cleft palate. *Journal of Craniofacial Genetics and Developmental Biology* 15:162-168, 1995.

Raghavan R, Sidhu SS, and Kharbanda OP: Craniofacial pattern of parents of children having cleft lip and/or cleft palate anomaly. *The Angle Orthodontist* 64:137-144, 1994.

Ranta R: Minimal cleft lip: Comparison of associated abnormalities. *International Journal of Oral and Maxillofacial Surgery* 17:183-185, 1988.

Ranta R, and Rintala A: Unusual alveolar clefts: report of cases. *Journal of Dentistry for Children* 56:363-365, 1989.

Ray AK, Field LL, and Marazita ML: Nonsyndromic cleft lip with or without cleft palate in West Bengal, India: evidence for an autosomal major locus. *American Journal of Human Genetics* 52:1006-1011, 1993.

Rintala A, and Stegars T: Increasing incidence of clefts in Finland: reliability of hospital records and central register of congenital malformations. *Scandinavian Journal of Plastic and Reconstructive Surgery* 16:35-40, 1982.

Rintala A, Ranta R, and Stegars T: On the pathogenesis of cleft palate in the Pierre Robin syndrome. *Scandinavian Journal of Plastic and Reconstructive Surgery* 18:237-240, 1984.

Robin P: La chute de la base de la langue consideree comme und velle cause de gene dans la respiration naso-pharyngienne. *Bulletin de l'Academie Nationale de Medecine* (Paris) 89:37-44, 1923.

Robin P: Glossoptosis due to atresia and hypotrophy of the mandible. *Archives of Pediatric and Adolescent Medicine* 48:541-547, 1934.

Ross RB, and Johnston MC: *Cleft lip and palate.* Huntington, NY: Robert E. Kreiger, 1978.

Safra MJ, and Oakley GP: Valium: an oral cleft teratogen? *Cleft Palate Journal* 13:198-200, 1976.

Sato T: Craniofacial morphology of parents with cleft lip and palate children. *Shikwa Gakuho* 89:1479-1506, 1989.

Schubert J, Metzke H, Bittroff H, Hintz J, and Lindner H: The significance of microforms of CLP for anomalies and malformations of the jaw and face. *Acta Chirurgiae Plasticae* 30:14-20, 1988.

Shaw GM, Croen LA, and Curry CJ: Isolated oral cleft malformations: associations with maternal and infant characteristics in a California population. *Teratology* 43:225-228, 1991.

Shprintzen RJ, Goldberg RB, Lewin M, Sidoti E, Berkman M, Argamaso R, and Young D: A new syndrome involving cleft palate, cardiac anomalies, typical facies, and learning disabilities: velo-cardio-facial syndrome. *Cleft Palate Journal* 15:56-62, 1978.

Shprintzen RJ, Schwartz RH, Daniller A, and Hoch L: Morphologic significance of bifid uvula. *Pediatrics* 75:553-561, 1985.

Shprintzen RJ, Siegel-Sadewitz VL, Amato J, and Goldberg RB: Anomalies associated with cleft lip, cleft palate, or both. *American Journal of Medical Genetics* 20:585-595, 1985a.

Shprintzen RJ, Siegel-Sadewitz VL, Amato J, and Goldberg RB: Retrospective diagnoses of previously missed syndromic disorders among 1000 patients with cleft lip, cleft palate, or both. *Birth Defects: Original Article Series* 21:85-92, 1985b.

Siegel B: A racial comparison of cleft patients in a clinic population: associated anomalies and recurrence rates. *Cleft Palate Journal* 16:193-197, 1979.

Slavkin H: *Developmental craniofacial biology.* Philadelphia: Lea & Febiger, 1979.

Smiley GR: A possible genesis for cleft palate formation. *Plastic and Reconstructive Surgery* 50:390-393, 1972.

Sperber GH: First year of life: prenatal craniofacial development. *Cleft Palate-Craniofacial Journal* 29:109-111, 1992.

Sperber GH: Commentary: confluence of clinical, theoretical, and laboratory research in syndromology. *Cleft Palate-Craniofacial Journal* 32:527-528, 1995.

Spranger J, Benirschke K, Hall JG, Lenz W, Lowry RB, Opitz JM, Pinsky L, Schwarzacher HG, and Smith DW: Errors of morphogenesis: concepts and terms. *Journal of Pediatrics* 100:160-165, 1982.

Stein J, Mulliken JB, Stal S, Gasser DL, Malcolm S, Winter R, Blanton SH, Amos C, Seemanova E, and Hecht JT: Nonsyndromic cleft lip with or without cleft palate: evidence of linkage to BCLE in 17 multigenerational families. *American Journal of Human Genetics* 57:257-272, 1995.

Temple K, Calvert M, Plint D, Thompson D, and Pembrey M: Dominantly inherited cleft lip and palate in two families. *Journal of Medical Genetics* 26:386-389, 1989.

Tenconi R, Clementi M, and Turolla L: Theoretical recurrence risks for cleft lip derived from a population of consecutive newborns. *Journal of Medical Genetics* 25:243-246, 1988.

Tessier P: Anatomical classification of facial, cranio-facial and latero-facial clefts. *Journal of Maxillofacial Surgery* 4:69-92, 1976.

Tolarova M: Periconceptional supplementation with vitamins and folic acid to prevent recurrence of cleft lip. *Lancet* 2:217, 1982.

Tolarova M: A study of the incidence sex-ratio, laterality, and clinical severity in 3,660 probands with facial clefts in Czechoslovakia. *Acta Chirurgiae Plasticae* 19:77-87, 1987.

Trasler DG: Pathogenesis of cleft lip and its relation to embryonic face shape in A/J and CC57BL mice. *Teratology* 1:33-43, 1968.

Tretsven VS: Incidence of cleft lip and palate in Montana Indians. *Journal of Speech Disorders* 28:52-57, 1963.

Tyan ML: Differences in the reported frequencies of cleft lip plus cleft lip and palate in Asians born in Hawaii and the continental United States. *Proceedings of the Society for Experimental Biology and Medicine* 171:41-45, 1982.

Van der Woude A: Fistula labii inferioris congenita and its association with cleft lip and palate. *American Journal of Human Genetics* 6:244-256, 1954.

Vanderas AP: Incidence of cleft lip, cleft palate, and cleft lip and palate among races: a review. *Cleft Palate Journal* 24:216-225, 1987.

Velasco MG, Ysunza A, Hernandez X, and Marquez C: Diagnosis and treatment of submucous cleft palate: a review of 108 cases. *Cleft Palate Journal* 25:171-173, 1988.

Ward RE, Bixler D, and Jamison PL: Cephalometric evidence for a dominantly inherited predisposition to cleft lip-cleft palate in a single large kindred. *American Journal of Medical Genetics* 50:57-63, 1994.

Weatherley-White RCA, Sakura C, Brenner L, Stewart J, and Ott J: Submucous cleft palate: its incidence, natural history, and indications for treatment. *Plastic and Reconstructive Surgery* 49:297-304, 1972.

Werler MM, Lammer EJ, Rosenberg L, and Mitchell AA: Maternal cigarette smoking during pregnancy in relation to oral clefts. *American Journal of Epidemiology* 132:926-932, 1990.

Wharton P, and Mowrer DE: Prevalence of cleft uvula among school children in kindergarten through grade five. *Cleft Palate-Craniofacial Journal* 29:10-12, 1992.

Wilson M: A ten-year survey of cleft lip and cleft palate in the south west region. *British Journal of Plastic Surgery* 25:224-228, 1972.

Womersley J, and Stone DH: Epidemiology of facial clefts. *Archives of Disease in Childhood* 62:717-720, 1987.

Woolf, CM: Paternal age effect for cleft lip and palate. *American Journal of Human Genetics* 15:389-393, 1963.

Woolf CM: Congenital cleft lip: a genetic study of 496 propositi. *Journal of Medical Genetics* 8:65-83, 1971.

Woolf CM, Woolf RM, and Broadbent TR: A genetic study of cleft lip and palate in Utah. *American Journal of Human Genetics* 15:209-215, 1963a.

Woolf CM, Woolf RM, and Broadbent TR: Genetics and non-genetic variables related to cleft lip and palate. *Plastic and Reconstructive Surgery* 32:65-74, 1963b.

Woolf CM, Woolf RM, and Broadbent TR: Cleft lip and palate in parent and child. *Plastic and Reconstructive Surgery* 44:436-440, 1969.

Zeiler K, Weinstein S, and Gibson S: A study of the morphology and the time of closure of the palate in the albino rat. *Archives of Oral Biology* 9:545-554, 1964.

Chapter 2

Multi-Anomaly Cleft Disorders

In Chapter 1 you learned about the high probability that additional anomalies will be present in a child with a cleft, even if the child is functioning at a relatively normal level and the associated anomalies are quite mild. In 1991 Cohen and Bankier estimated that there were more than 340 known syndromes involving orofacial clefting. That number is currently estimated to be close to 350. The rate of identification of multi-anomaly disorders involving various types of orofacial clefts has accelerated as a result of technological advances at three levels: imaging (e.g., magnetic resonance imaging, three-dimensional computed tomography scans), laboratory studies (e.g., gene mapping), and computer networks linking the geneticists and dysmorphologists as they recognize and sort these conditions.[1]

Clearly there are far too many syndromes, sequences, and associations involving clefting to allow a comprehensive discussion in a single chapter. This chapter will be limited to some of the more "common" multi-anomaly conditions likely to include cleft palate or other problems of velopharyngeal function.

GUIDELINES FOR LEARNING ABOUT MULTI-ANOMALY DISORDERS

As you study material about patients with multi-anomaly conditions, you will need to bear in mind the following points:

1. For many conditions there is no universal agreement among dysmorphologists regarding what features must be present for a given diagnosis to be made. A classic example is Robin sequence, discussed on page 32.
2. Most multi-anomaly conditions vary significantly in expressivity, that is, in the severity of expression of physical findings from patient to patient with the same disorder. Many mild cases are likely to be missed or erroneously diagnosed (Shprintzen et al., 1985a, 1985b). In addition, as more individuals with a given condition are recognized, dysmorphologists expand the description of likely, probable, or associated findings in that condition.
3. It is very confusing to new clinicians, and sometimes to experienced clinicians as well, that patients can have overlapping signs or stigmata of two or more sequences, associations, or syndromes. Often this overlap is later sorted out into a "new" multi-anomaly condition, or the geneticists and dysmorphologists learn that what were formerly thought of as two separate conditions actually represent variable expressions of the same disorder.
4. Frequently there is a poor correlation between the severity of expression of the physical manifestations of a disorder and various aspects of developmental, cognitive, communicative, and psychosocial function. Patients who appear to have minimal physical involvement may exhibit severe functional difficulties; conversely, some individuals with relatively severe physical findings exhibit cognitive, social, and communicative skills within normal limits.
5. In dealing with patients who have structural abnormalities of the craniofacial complex, the clinician may focus too readily on the visible problems and not pay sufficient attention to less obvious factors such as hearing loss (a highly probable finding in virtually all of the conditions discussed here) and psychosocial adjustment.

VAN DER WOUDE SYNDROME

Perhaps the least complex of the congenital disorders discussed in this chapter is van der Woude syndrome, to which you were introduced in Chapter 1. This syndrome

[1]There are several on-line systems and CD-ROM resources available to assist clinicians in accurate diagnosis. However, each requires the clinical experience to know what dysmorphologic findings to look for in a given patient. In other words, a basic background in dysmorphology is requisite to being able to use such programs or networks. Because computer-based resources change and expand on such a rapid basis, you are advised to consult with a local medical library about updated systems.

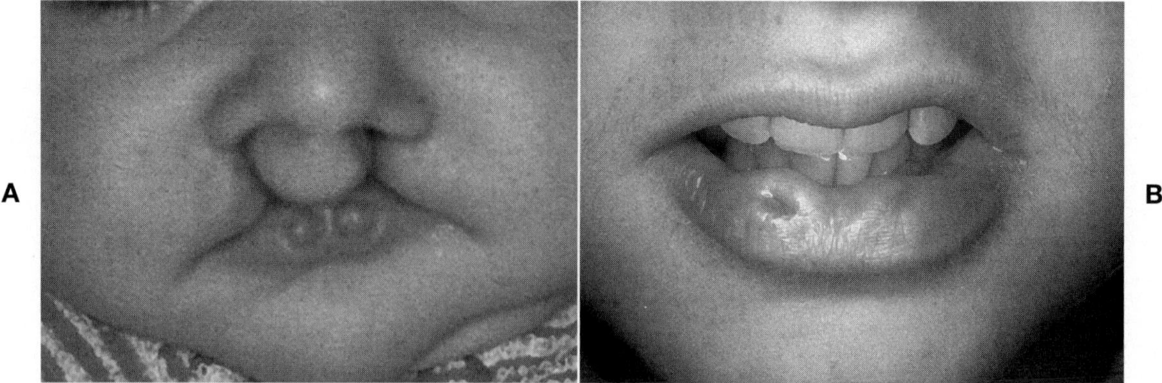

Figure 2-1 **A** and **B**, Two youngsters with van der Woude syndrome. In the first baby the paramedian lip mounds are quite prominent. In the second child, there are less prominent mounds, with a pit in each one (more easily seen in the mound on the child's right).

combines paramedian pits or conical elevations on the lower lip (Fig. 2-1) with various forms of clefting (Fogh-Andersen, 1943; van der Woude, 1954). [2] Although the syndrome carries the name of the pediatrician who described a set of patients in 1954 (van der Woude, 1954), it was actually first described by Demarquay more than 100 years earlier (Demarquay, 1845). Expression of the syndrome varies significantly from one affected individual to another: (1) the clefts can be unilateral or bilateral cleft lip and palate, clefts of the primary palate only, or clefts of the secondary palate only, including submucous clefts and less obvious defects such as a bifid uvula or occult submucous cleft; (2) the lip defects may be found on the inner or gingival surface of the lip rather than on the vermilion, or they may be asymmetrically placed; (3) some individuals may have only the lip defects, without any type of cleft; and, in contrast, (4) some members of an affected family may have a cleft but no lip pits (Cervenka, Gorlin, and Anderson, 1967; Janku et al., 1980; Rintala and Ranta, 1981; Shprintzen, Goldberg, and Sidoti, 1980).

There have been several studies of large kindreds with Van der Woude syndrome establishing the fact that the gene is present in an individual family member with a cleft even if he or she does not have lip defects (Burdick, Bixler, and Puckett, 1985; Janku et al., 1980; Shprintzen et al., 1980; Wienker et al., 1987). Hypodontia (lack of the normal number of teeth) is an associated finding, and some authors have proposed that it may be a "forme fruste," that is, a signpost for the syndrome even when other expected findings are not present (Ranta and Rintala, 1983; Wienker et al., 1987). You will recall from Chapter 1 that Van der Woude syndrome is an autosomal dominant syndrome, carrying a 50% recurrence risk. The gene has been mapped to chromosome 1 (Bocian and Walker, 1987; Murray et al., 1990; Sander, Schmelzle, and Murray, 1994). Cytogenetic studies can now be used to identify individuals who may carry the gene but in whom no clinical findings are visible. Also, in large kindreds there may be clinically normal individuals who are identified as carrying the gene because, although the individuals have no clefts or lip pits, clinical findings were present in one of their parents and also in one or more of their own children (Shprintzen et al., 1980).

For the speech-language pathologist, the importance of this syndrome may be summarized as follows. (1) In your routine oral examination of a patient, be sure to note abnormalities of the lower lip, and to evert the lip (examine the inner or gingival surface) as you do so. (2) As you would for any child or adult with a cleft, even in the absence of lip abnormalities, help your patient and the family locate appropriate genetic counseling if such counseling has not already been given. In terms of effects on communication skills, the bulk of the information on this syndrome leads us to expect only those problems that concern us about any child with a cleft. However, a few cases reported in the literature have exhibited cognitive delay together with some other craniofacial and skeletal findings (Bocian and Walker, 1987; Lacombe et al., 1995). One of the cases described by Lacombe et al. (1995) had midline brain abnormalities on magnetic resonance imaging, which the authors proposed as "part of the clinical spectrum of VWS" (p. 221). Future detailed descriptions of patients, including imaging studies of the central nervous system, may uncover additional cases of anomalies with potential significance for development.

ROBIN SEQUENCE

In 1923, a French stomatologist, Pierre Robin, described a combination of micrognathia, glossoptosis (retracted and elevated tongue), and respiratory distress in a series of babies. Robin later reported infants with these findings who also had cleft palate (Robin, 1934). This group of findings came to be associated with Robin's name, although there had been several earlier reports of infants with similar problems in the 1800s and early 1900s (see Gorlin, Cohen, and Levin, 1990, for historical references).

[2] Lip pits are also inconsistently found in other syndromes: oral-facial-digital syndrome, type I (OFD I), popliteal pterygium syndrome (LaCombe et al., 1995), and Kabuki syndrome (Franceschini et al., 1993; McDonald-McGinn et al., 2000).

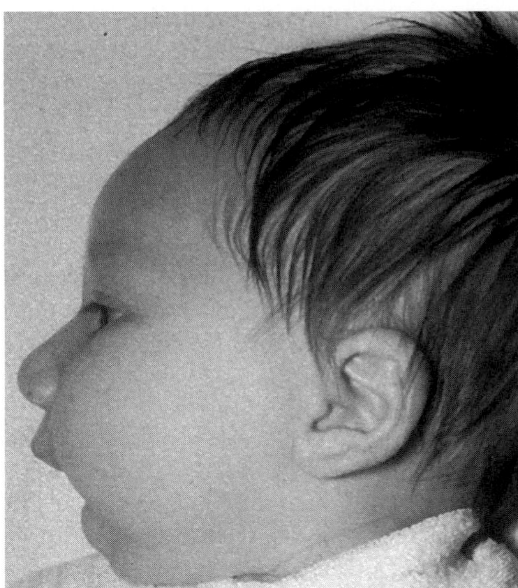

Figure 2-2 Severe micrognathia in an infant with Pierre Robin sequence.

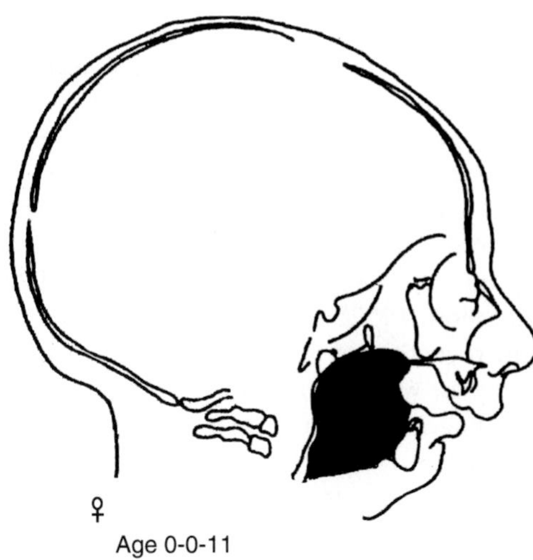

Figure 2-3 Tracing of lateral x-ray film of 11-day-old infant with Robin sequence. The tongue has been blacked in to more clearly illustrate the glossoptosis.

The literature on Robin sequence is characterized by three problems:

1. *Disagreement about what features constitute the disorder:* Some articles specify micrognathia (Fig. 2-2) and glossoptosis (Fig. 2-3) with or without cleft palate (Fig. 2-4); others specify micrognathia, glossoptosis, and respiratory distress; and still others list micrognathia, glossoptosis, and cleft palate (Caouette-Laberge, Bayet, and Larocque, 1994; Elliott, Studen-Pavlovich, and Ranalli, 1995; Sheffield et al., 1987; Tomaski, Zalzal, and Saal, 1995). Gorlin, Cohen, and Levin (1990), in one of the comprehensive resources for dysmorphologists, listed micrognathia, glossoptosis, and cleft palate as the obligatory features. Obviously, lack of consistency in defining the disorder leads to problems in estimating frequency of occurrence: Gorlin, Cohen, and Levin (1990) cited estimates ranging from 1:2000 to 1:30,000. However, because many of these babies have life-threatening problems in early infancy, estimates of frequency of occurrence also depend on the ages of the patients in any epidemiologic study.
2. *Change in nomenclature:* Until approximately 20 years ago, the eponym "syndrome" was consistently used for this disorder (notwithstanding the fact that sources did not agree on what the pathognomonic features should be). When it was later realized that this was a nonspecific association of findings without a single etiology, "syndrome" was discarded, first for "anomalad" (Cohen, 1976), then "complex" (Cohen, 1978), and then "sequence" as the emphasis was placed upon the cascade of effects from a poorly developing mandible in the embryo (Shprintzen and Singer, 1992).

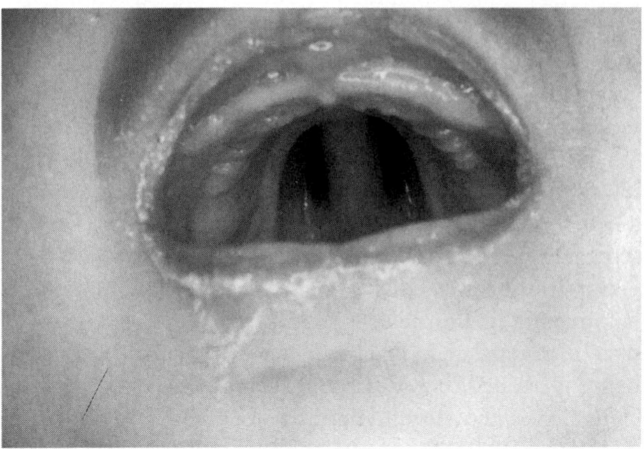

Figure 2-4 The wide, U-shaped cleft of the secondary palate seen in most, but not all, infants with Robin sequence.

3. *Incomplete diagnosis:* Because clinical reports on patients with Robin sequence have been published over several decades, the accuracy of diagnosis of associated abnormalities and syndromes has obviously increased. Findings that were considered only as coincidental in older articles were later found to be part of syndromes. According to Gorlin, Cohen, and Levin (1990), Robin sequence occurs in more than 30 syndromes or associations. In a series of 100 cases of Robin sequence, Shprintzen (1992) reported that 34% had Stickler syndrome, 11% had velocardiofacial syndrome, 10% had fetal alcohol syndrome, 10% had provisionally unique pattern syndromes, and 5% had Treacher Collins syndrome. Thirteen cases had other syndromes, meaning that only 17% had

nonsyndromic Robin sequence. A more recent report (Elliott, Studen-Pavlovich, and Ranalli, 1995) indicated a much lower prevalence of multi-anomaly syndromes among Robin cases (9.1%). However, the latter report was based on retrospective chart review rather than on actual examination of patients by a dysmorphologist or geneticist. An additional point is that many of the syndromes in which Robin sequence is likely to occur may not be easily detected or diagnosed in the first weeks of life (Sadewitz and Shprintzen, 1986; Shprintzen, 1988, 1992; Singer and Sidoti, 1992).

The micrognathia in Robin sequence can have many different causes, which illustrates the heterogeneous etiology and pathogenesis of the sequence (Cohen 1976, 1982; Shprintzen, 1988, 1992). Shprintzen (1992) grouped these causes as genetic syndromes, chromosomal syndromes, teratogenic influences, mechanically induced factors, and "multifactorial contributions." The mandible may be small as a result of fetal constraint, that is, inadequate room for the head to move off the chest as the embryo is growing. Fetal constraint itself has many different causes, two of which are an abnormally small or misshapen uterus and inadequate amniotic fluid. The embryo may also not move enough to allow normal growth for some inherent reason such as hypotonicity or other neuromuscular problems. When the mandible is mechanically constrained, it is technically "deformed" (see definition of deformation in Chapter 1) rather than "malformed" (the result of a primary error in morphogenesis), and the sequence itself is a "deformation sequence" rather than "malformation sequence." In such cases the mandible often shows catch-up growth postnatally. This is not the case when the mandible is inherently malformed.[3]

The cleft palate in Robin sequence is usually described as being U shaped, but V-shaped clefts as well as submucous clefts have also been described (LeBlanc and Golding-Kushner, 1992; Poradowska, Reszke, and Lenkiewica, 1981; Ranta, Laatikainen, and Laitinen, 1985; Rintala, Ranta, and Stegars, 1984; Shprintzen, 1988). In many infants, the tongue continues to be positioned between the palatal shelves until surgical or prosthetic intervention. Surgical closure of the cleft may be delayed in infants who have significant early respiratory problems (Lehman, Fishman, and Neiman, 1995), although Shprintzen (personal communication, 1993) has advocated consideration of earlier-than-normal palatal surgery when imaging studies show the velar halves to be hanging low in the oropharynx and adding to obstruction of the airway (discussed in the following paragraph). In fact, in 1956 Champion advocated surgical closure of the cleft palate in Robin sequence infants within the first 2 days of life in an effort to improve the airway.

The early weeks of life are often hazardous for infants with Robin sequence, with significant problems occurring in respiration and feeding (Benjamin and Walker, 1991; Pashayan and Lewis, 1984; Sheffied et al., 1987; Shprintzen, 1992; Shprintzen and Singer, 1992; Singer and Sidoti, 1992; Tomaski, Zalzal, and Saal, 1995; Williams et al., 1981). Even in contemporary reports, the mortality rate in the first few months of life is often high. In some infants significant obstruction is not present at birth but develops within the first month (Bull et al., 1990). In most of the historical literature, and even in many current reports, the cause of the respiratory distress is presumed to be the retraction of the tongue into the upper pharynx. Several decades ago observations of this tongue position motivated the development of a surgical procedure for anchoring the tongue tip to the lower lip (Douglas, 1946, 1950), a procedure that has undergone various modifications in the ensuing years (Argamaso, 1992; Parsons and Smith, 1980; Routledge, 1960; Smith, 1981) and that is generally known under the rubric of "glossopexy." Other surgical procedures that have been used in the effort to bring the tongue forward include fixation to the anterior portion of the mandible with a wire (Hadley and Johnson, 1963) or sling of fascia lata (Lewis, Lynch, and Blocker, 1968), fixation to the cheeks (Minervini, 1973), resection and repositioning of sublingual musculature (Delorme, Larocque, and Caouette-Laberge, 1989), and suspension (elevation) of the hyoid bone (Bergoin, Giraud, and Chaix, 1971). Palatal plates (obturators) with posterior extensions have also been used in infants in the effort to push the tongue downward and forward (Hotz and Gnoinski, 1982).

In the 1980s and 1990s endoscopic studies revealed other mechanisms and sites of airway obstruction in children with Robin sequence, specifically (1) posterior positioning of the tongue "sandwiching" the soft palate (when there is no cleft palate) or the palatal tags against the posterior pharyngeal wall, (2) medial constriction of the lateral pharyngeal walls to the extent that they touch in the midline, and (3) sphincteric pharyngeal constriction (Sadewitz and Shprintzen, 1986; Sher, 1992; Sher, Shprintzen, and Thorpy, 1986; Shprintzen, 1988). In either of the latter two types of obstruction it is unlikely that simple forward anchoring of the tongue tip would alleviate the problem. Different strategies of management are necessary for different babies. The options range from simple changes in positioning for sleep and feeding to nasopharyngeal intubation, surgical repositioning of the tongue, and tracheotomy (Benjamin and Walker, 1991; Pashayan and Lewis, 1984; Sadewitz and Shprintzen, 1986; Sher, 1992; Sher et al., 1986; Shprintzen 1988; Singer and

[3]Pruzansky and Richmond (1954) described catch-up growth of the mandible in children with Pierre Robin "syndrome." Although their work has been widely cited over the last four decades, several of the syndromes that include Robin sequence were not widely recognized at that time (e.g., Stickler syndrome, velocardiofacial syndrome). A later cephalometric study of nonsyndromic Robin children demonstrated "partial mandibular catch-up growth" (Figueroa et al., 1991). In the latter study Robin infants showed mandibular growth approximately 10% greater than that of normal infants during the first year of life, although their measurements still did not equal those of the normal children by age 2 years.

Sidoti, 1992). As you would expect, clinicians prefer to try simpler, less invasive approaches first unless the infant is so compromised that the need for aggressive intervention is obvious on initial examination. The effects of chronic respiratory problems caused by intermittent airway obstruction can be catastrophic (Singer and Sidoti, 1992).[4]

The feeding difficulties in Robin infants are often reported to be proportional to the severity of the airway problems (Benjamin and Walker, 1991; Pashayan and Lewis, 1984; Sadewitz and Shprintzen, 1986; Sher, 1992; Sher, Shprintzen, and Thorpy, 1986; Shprintzen 1988; Singer and Sidoti, 1992), and again are managed by a variety of approaches ranging from conservative (positioning, use of modified nipples and bottles) to aggressive (nasogastric tube or gastrostomy). Singer and Sidoti (1992) noted that gastrostomy is rarely used, the exceptions being in infants with severe neurologic problems. Long-term use of nonoral feedings through a nasogastric tube or a gastrostomy is a threat to development of normal suckling patterns and feeding skills and may lead to oral defensiveness, adding to the complex clinical problems for these babies.

If you are attempting to gather information from the literature regarding expectations of speech and language development in children with Robin sequence, you will have some difficulty deciding which reports are relevant because of the likelihood of associated anomalies or syndromes, particularly in clinical reports before the 1980s. If your patient truly has nonsyndromic Robin sequence with a cleft of the secondary palate, expectations for speech problems should be generally equivalent to the expectations in other individuals with clefts of the secondary palate, depending to some extent on how complicated the early medical problems were and what interventions were necessary. One complication may be a delay in palatal surgery in the infant with significant early medical problems. Late closure of the palate can result in delayed acquisition of normal phonology and persistence of compensatory articulations (Trost, 1981; Trost-Cardamone, 1987; Trost-Cardamone and Bernthal, 1993) as the child's language development places phonetic demands on a physical system not yet capable of oral productions. Prolonged presence of a tracheotomy can lead to delays in speech development, especially if the child is unable to produce any phonation at all while the tube is open. If normal oral feeding cannot be successfully established in early infancy, there may be subsequent effects on the control and coordination of oral motor activity for speech. If glossopexy is used to improve the airway, there may be temporary effects on early speech sound production: LeBlanc and Golding-Kushner (1992) observed such effects in infants whose glossopexies were released between 9 and 15 months but found that the effects had disappeared within 12 months of the glossopexy release. Gould (1989) reported the prevalence of ear disease and hearing loss to be essentially the same as in other cases of cleft palate. However, in a more recent report (Handzic et al., 1995), the prevalence of hearing loss in 18 patients with Robin sequence was 83.33% (in 36 ears) as opposed to 59.67% in 243 patients with cleft lip and palate or cleft palate. The authors of the latter report suggested that early problems with upper airway obstruction in these infants may produce more frequent problems of middle ear effusion. Earlier reports of ossicular malformations actually included data from patients with additional malformations (Bergstrom, Hemenway, and Sando, 1972; Igarashi, Filippone, and Alford, 1976), making the accuracy of diagnosis suspect. As pointed out by Shprintzen (1988, 1992), accuracy of diagnosis is the crucial and time-sensitive basis for optimal care and management.

STICKLER SYNDROME

Before the case descriptions that appeared in the 1960s and 1970s, there is little doubt that patients with Stickler syndrome were recorded as having Pierre Robin "syndrome" (or perhaps simply "cleft palate") with clusters of associated findings (e.g., Smith and Stowe, 1961). This syndrome, also called hereditary arthroophthalmopathy, was described in 1965 (Stickler et al., 1965), with subsequent case descriptions by Stickler and Pugh (1967), Spranger (1968), Herrmann et al. (1975), and Hall (1974). Stickler syndrome was estimated to be the most common connective tissue disorder (Herrmann et al., 1975) prior to the identification of velocardiofacial syndrome (discussed in a following section). It is an autosomal dominant syndrome (50% recurrence risk for offspring of affected individuals) with high penetrance and variable expression. In about 50% of patients the syndrome is due to abnormalities of the type II collagen gene located on chromosome 12 (Brown et al., 1992; Francomano et al., 1987). However, another Stickler syndrome gene has been mapped to chromosome 6 (Brunner et al., 1994). Many authors have recorded the variability in findings from patient to patient. Affected members of one family are more likely to have similar findings than are patients from different families (intrafamilial similarities versus interfamilial dissimilarities), lending support to the hypothesis that Stickler syndrome is not a single genetic entity (Zlotogora et al., 1992).

Because many of the physical findings are progressive in nature, the likelihood of detecting the presence of the syndrome increases with age (Gorlin, Cohen, and Levin, 1990). Thus the diagnosis will be missed in many young children.[5]

The major features of Stickler syndrome include high myopia in early childhood, retinal detachment and

[4]The converse point, equally as important, is that central nervous system problems in these infants, which might have been presumed to be caused by hypoxia in older reports, could well have been the result of unrecognized syndromes (Shprintzen, 1988, 1992).

[5]If a child with a cleft palate is referred only to a plastic surgeon on the presumption that all that is required is surgical closure of the cleft, the probability of accurate detection of Stickler syndrome is minimal, with potentially dire consequences.

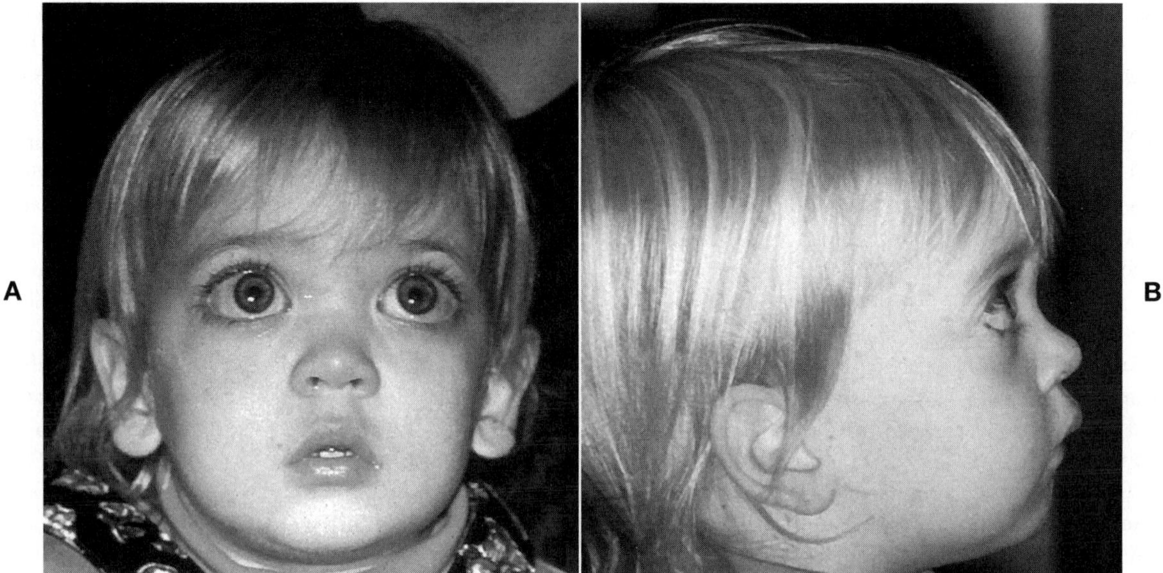

Figure 2-5 **A** and **B**, Frontal and profile views of a child with Stickler syndrome, demonstrating the prominent eyes, rather flat midface, depressed nasal bridge with epicanthal folds, and long philtrum. Mandibular hypoplasia is not as clearly demonstrated in this youngster as it is in many other children with this syndrome.

cataracts, hearing loss, cleft palate, and progressive arthropathy. Although cleft palate or other abnormalities of velopharyngeal function may be the main focus for the speech-language pathologist, for the patient and family the ophthalmologic, orthopedic, and hearing problems are often far more threatening. Forty percent of patients have myopia by age 10 years and 75% by age 20 years; in some patients it does not develop until after age 50 years (Jones, 1997). Retinal detachment can occur in childhood but usually does not occur until after the age of 20 years. The threat of blindness is reduced if the likelihood of retinal detachment is recognized and treated early (Jones, 1997). The orthopedic findings are extensive, mainly affecting the long bones and epiphyses (Gorlin, Cohen, and Levin, 1990; Jones, 1997). Although the specific bone and joint problems are highly variable, they become more severe as the affected individual matures. Progressive sensorineural hearing loss occurs in 80% of cases (Gorlin, Cohen, and Levin, 1990).[6]

The craniofacial features of Stickler syndrome are highly variable. Some affected individuals have a relatively normal face. More typical, however, is a flat midface resulting from maxillary hypoplasia, prominent eyes, depressed nasal bridge with epicanthal folds, long philtrum, and mandibular hypoplasia (Fig. 2-5). The palatal anomalies range from overt clefts to submucous clefts to inadequate velopharyngeal motion in the absence of either overt or submucous clefts. Earlier estimates of the prevalence of palatal problems were roughly 20% (Hall, 1974; Hall and Herrod, 1975). Lucarini, Liberfarb, and Eavey (1987) reported a prevalence of 57% for overt or submucous cleft palate among 14 patients with Stickler syndrome ages 4 to 17 years who were identified when they were admitted to a hospital because of retinal detachment. The prevalence of palatal problems is difficult to determine: estimates are bound to vary depending on how the condition is first ascertained (e.g., through cleft palate clinics, ophthalmologic clinics, or orthopedic clinics).

The impact of Stickler syndrome on communication skills depends on the severity of expression of the syndrome in a given patient. In early childhood the major concern may be velopharyngeal function if a cleft or other palatal anomaly is present. However, hearing loss (mixed or sensorineural) is a factor of equal or greater concern, particularly in view of the progressive nature of the loss. Although the loss may not be of sufficient magnitude in early childhood to affect development of speech and language, the potential effects in later life are significant, especially when combined with the likelihood of concurrent progressive loss of vision.

VELOCARDIOFACIAL SYNDROME

In 1955 Sedlackova described an association of facial findings and velopharyngeal problems together with cupped ears and digital abnormalities in what was later to become recognized as the most frequently occurring syndrome of clefting.[7] Subsequent reports in the 1960s and

[6]A significant associated finding is mitral valve prolapse in 50% of Stickler cases (Liberfarb and Goldblatt, 1986).

[7]Some of the patients in the 1955 Sedlackova report also had manifestations of ectodermal dysplasia, but ectodermal dysplasia was not included as a sign of "Sedlackova syndrome" in subsequent reports.

1970s described inadequate velopharyngeal function for speech together with mildly dysmorphic facies and reduced facial expression (Calnan, 1971; Fara, Hrivnakova, and Sedlackova, 1971; Kruk and Tronczynska, 1978; Pitt and Ingram, 1975; Sedlackova, 1967; Sedlackova, Lastovka, and Sram 1973; Vrticka and Sedlackova, 1962; Winters, 1975). This group of findings was commonly referred to as "Sedlackova syndrome" until a 1978 report by Shprintzen and colleagues described "velocardiofacial syndrome" as a purportedly newly identified syndrome (Shprintzen et al., 1978).

The report of Shprintzen et al. (1978) did not in fact describe a new entity but did lead to (1) the recognition of additional findings, (2) subsequent worldwide recognition of this entity as the most common syndrome involving clefts, and (3) eventual identification of what may be the most "mutable" (changeable) portion of the human genome. The syndrome is an autosomal dominant condition, with about 75% of the cases showing a microdeletion of genetic material on the long arm of chromosome 22 (locus 22q11) (Driscoll et al., 1992; Kelly et al., 1993; Lindsay et al., 1995; Morrow et al., 1995; Scambler et al., 1992). There is both a genetic overlap and an overlap of clinical features between velocardiofacial syndrome and DiGeorge sequence, a condition that includes variable defects of the thymus gland, parathyroids, and cardiovascular vessels (Driscoll et al., 1992; Goldberg et al., 1985; Jones, 1997; Scambler et al., 1992; Stevens, Carey, and Shigeoka, 1990). That is, the microdeletions on chromosome 22 found in patients with velocardiofacial syndrome encompass the region where deletions are found in DiGeorge syndrome, and many patients carry the signs of both disorders, to the extent that Driscoll et al. (1992) suggested that the two disorders are etiologically the same.[8]

In the nearly 22 years since the 1978 report, clinicians have documented an increasingly wider range of findings. The phenotypic spectrum has broadened as both more mildly affected and more severely affected individuals are identified (Goldberg et al., 1993). As you read the catalog of physical and functional findings in the following paragraphs, keep in mind the high variability in features of the syndrome from patient to patient.

According to Shprintzen et al. (1978), the facial features of velocardiofacial syndrome include a vertically long face with a broad nasal root, narrow alar base, flattened malar region, narrow and downward-slanted palpebral fissures, abundant scalp hair, and retruded mandible[9] (Fig. 2-6). This report emanated from a large cleft palate–craniofacial program, so it is not surprising that all 12 of the patients had clefts: seven submucous clefts, five overt clefts. The two additional common findings in this group of patients were ventricular septal defects (nine patients) and specific learning disabilities (11 patients).[10] In a subsequent report 100% of 39 individuals had clefts of the secondary palate and learning disabilities (Shprintzen et al., 1981). Goldberg et al. (1993) further documented the extensive list of findings in 120 patients: learning disabilities (99%), cleft palate (98%), pharyngeal hypotonia (90%), lymphoid tissue hypoplasia (83%), cardiac anomalies (82%), retrognathia (80%), obtuse cranial base (75%), malar flatness (70%), minor ear anomalies (70%), slender hands and digits (Fig. 2-7) (63%), microcephaly (40%), mental retardation (40%), tortuous retinal vessels (33%), small stature (33%), inguinal hernia (30%), medial displacement of internal carotid arteries (25%), umbilical hernia (23%), Robin sequence (17%), scoliosis (13%), hypospadias in 10% of males, and ocular coloboma (3%). Unilateral facial palsy has been reported in a few cases (Beemer et al., 1968).

As more cases of this syndrome have been documented in various centers, occult submucous clefts of palate (see Chapter 1 for description) have proved to account for a significant percentage of the palatal anomalies (Croft et al., 1978; Finkelstein et al., 1992; Finkelstein et al., 1993). Finkelstein et al. (1993) reported 67% occult submucous cleft, 24% submucous cleft, and 9.5% overt cleft in a series of 21 patients. There have also been a few cases of cleft lip (Fig. 2-8) (Lipson et al., 1991). Velopharyngeal function in these patients can be compromised by pharyngeal hypotonia and adenoid hypoplasia (Williams, Shprintzen, and Rakoff, 1987). An additional complication in terms of treating velopharyngeal inadequacy is abnormal medial placement and tortuosity of the internal carotids, posing a problem if pharyngeal flap surgery is planned (D'Antonio and Marsh, 1987; MacKenzie-Stepner et al., 1987).

The threats to overall development, communication skills, educational progress, and life competency in this syndrome are myriad and complex. In addition to the speech problems resulting from cleft palate or inadequate velopharyngeal function, children with velocardiofacial syndrome are apt to exhibit language and learning difficulties. More than a decade ago, Golding-Kushner and colleagues (Golding-Kushner, Weller, and Shprintzen, 1985) described specific problems in motor coordination and development of numerical concepts, which, together with bland affect, seemed to be a better predictor of later school problems than intelligence tests before age 6 years. Mental retardation is reportedly present in 40% of patients (Goldberg et al., 1993). A recent report on the psychoedu-

[8]Overlap with CHARGE association (Hall, 1979; Pagon et al., 1981) has also been noted in some patients, and Shprintzen (1987) commented that CHARGE may be a part of the phenotypic spectrum of velocardiofacial syndrome. Association with holoprosencephaly has also been described (Wraith et al., 1985).

[9]The mandible is actual relatively normal in size and shape but is retruded because of posterior displacement of the temporomandibular joint as a result of flattening of the cranial base (Arvystas and Shprintzen, 1984; Glander and Cisneros, 1992).

[10]Other findings that were variable from patient to patient in the 1978 report included minor ear anomalies, conductive hearing loss (and one case of sensorineural loss), hypotonia in infancy, reduced fine motor coordination, pyloric stenosis, hypospadias, inguinal hernia, undescended testes, joint hyperextensibility, and laryngeal web.

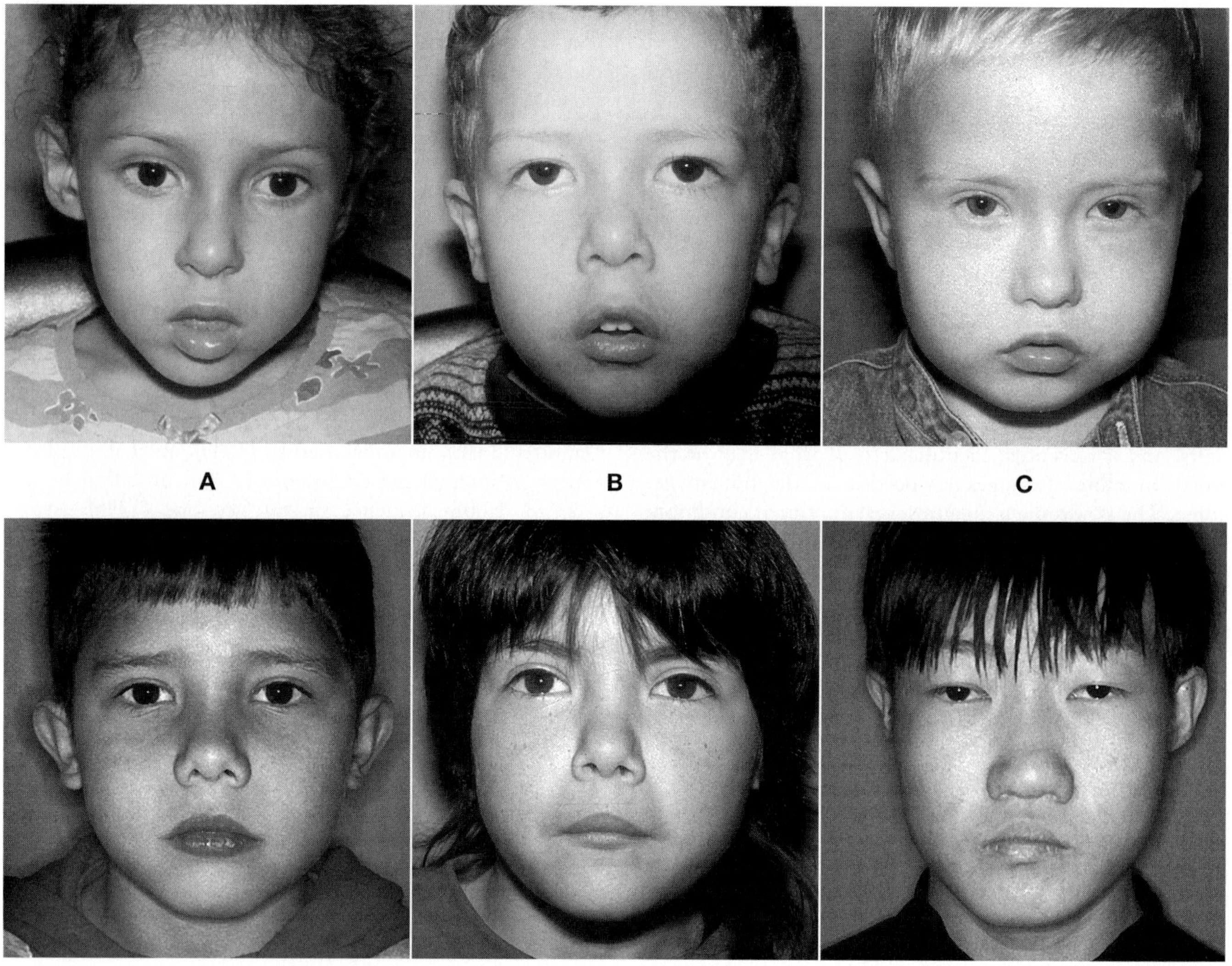

A B C

D E F

Figure 2-6 **A** to **F,** Six youngsters with velocardiofacial syndrome. The children in **D** and **E** are brother and sister. The expression of the syndrome is more severe in the boy than in the girl: his facial features are more remarkable and his intellectual development is more impaired.

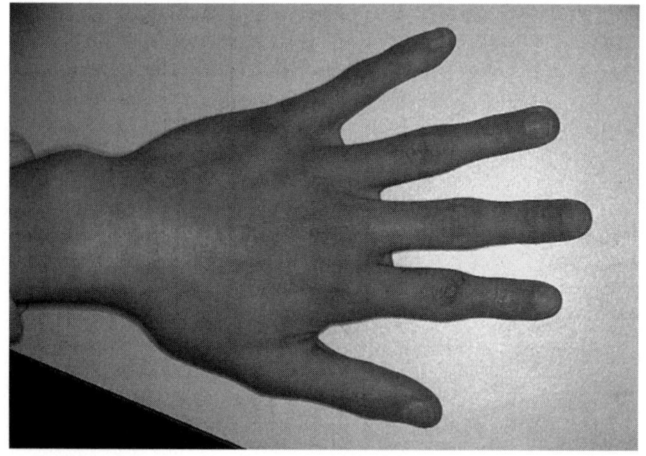

Figure 2-7 The slender, tapered fingers of the young man shown in Fig. 2-6, *F.*

cational profile in this syndrome documented full-scale intelligence quotients (IQ) ranging from normal to moderately retarded in 33 patients and, interestingly, a significantly higher mean verbal IQ than performance IQ (Moss et al., 1999). In addition, many children in this study showed clinically significant language impairments, with mean language scores lower than mean verbal IQ. They felt that the IQ and academic profiles were reminiscent of a "nonverbal" learning disability but urged that educational programming for children with velocardiofacial syndrome address both verbal and nonverbal deficits. Structural brain anomalies have been documented by magnetic resonance imaging in enough patients to suggest that such anomalies are probably common in this syndrome (Altman et al., 1995; Mitnick, Bello, and Shprintzen, 1994). The catalog of functional problems also unfortunately includes a significant threat of onset of psychosis as the patient

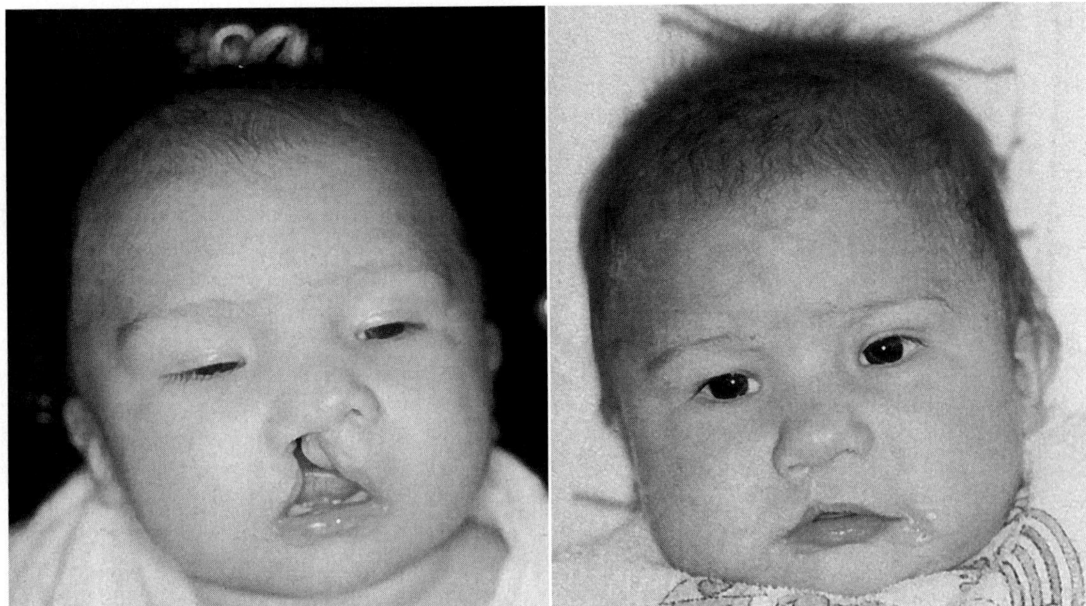

Figure 2-8 Preoperative and postoperative photos of a child with velocardiofacial syndrome who also had a cleft lip, a relatively rare but not unknown finding in this syndrome.

matures. The original alert to the possibility of mental illness appeared in a letter to the editor of a genetic journal in 1992 (Shprintzen et al., 1992). At that time it was thought that the prevalence might be on the order of 10%; subsequent investigations have shown an alarming association with psychotic illness and a genetic overlap between schizophrenia and velocardiofacial syndrome (Chow, Bassett, and Weksberg, 1994; Karayiorgou et al., 1995; Pulver et al., 1994).

Every child or adult with a cleft or other type of dysfunction of the velopharyngeal mechanism should be evaluated and followed by an interdisciplinary team of specialists, and the patient with velocardiofacial syndrome, whether exhibiting a mild or severe expression of the syndrome, illustrates the pitfalls in diagnosis and care if this model for care is not followed. Many of the potential problems for children with this syndrome will not become apparent until later years, to the point that the diagnosis may not even be made until the child has encountered difficulties in school and social experiences, to say nothing of medical complications. An additional problem with delays in diagnosis is family planning, because any individual showing clinical signs of the syndrome or the microdeletion on chromosome 22 has a 50% risk of passing the syndrome on to his or her children.

HEMIFACIAL MICROSOMIA OR OCULOAURICULOVERTEBRAL SPECTRUM

There is a large, heterogeneous family of disorders in which there is asymmetric development of the facial structures, primarily those arising from the first and second branchial arches. The most popular umbrella terms used for these disorders are "hemifacial microsomia" and "oculoauriculovertebral spectrum" (Cohen, Rollnick, and Kaye, 1989; Gorlin, Cohen, Levin, 1990). Although the term "hemifacial" denotes problems on just one side of the face, the majority of patients actually have abnormalities of both sides of the face, with one side more severely involved than the other. In the many clinical descriptions that appeared in the 1960s, 1970s, and 1980s, there was confusion about what constituted "obligatory" findings, and the addition of new or associated findings often led to new labels. In 1989 Cohen, Rollnick, and Kaye offered a list of the names that had been applied to these disorders; that list is repeated here (in alphabetical rather than chronological order) to assist you in identifying pertinent articles in the literature:

- Auriculo-branchiogenic dysplasia
- Facio-auriculo-vertebral (FAV) malformation spectrum
- Familial facial dysplasia
- First arch syndrome
- First and second arch syndrome
- Goldenhar syndrome
- Goldenhar-Gorlin syndrome
- Hemifacial microsomia
- Hemicraniofacial microsomia (not included in the list of Cohen, Rollnick, and Levin [1989])
- Lateral facial dysplasia
- Microtia syndrome (not included in the list of Cohen, Rollnick, and Levin [1989])
- Oculoauriculovertebral dysplasia
- Oral-mandibular-auricular syndrome
- Otomandibular dysostosis
- Unilateral craniofacial microsomia
- Unilateral intrauterine facial necrosis
- Unilateral mandibulofacial dysostosis

Hemifacial microsomia is not a syndrome but a spectrum of disorders, the core of which consists of deformities of the ear, maxilla, and mandible. The deformities can occur alone or as part of complex malformation syndromes (e.g., branchio-oto-renal syndrome, Klippel-Feil syndrome, Klinefelter syndrome, cri-du-chat syndrome, Saethre-Chotzen syndrome, Seckel syndrome, and others). The overall frequency of occurrence of hemifacial microsomia has been estimated to range from 1:3000 to 1:5000 (Jones, 1997). Most authors have described it as a sporadic disorder, but some have reported evidence of autosomal dominant inheritance with reduced penetrance (Gorlin, Cohen, and Levin, 1990; Kaye et al., 1992; Tsai and Tsai, 1993). In a recent survey of 121 patients with hemifacial microsomia, more than half were found to have at least one additional anomaly *outside* the craniofacial complex, and more than 40% had anomalies of multiple organ systems (Horgan et al., 1995). Cohen, Rollnick, and Kaye (1989) and Gorlin, Cohen, and Levin (1990) offered extensive reviews of this disorder, emphasizing the heterogeneity in etiology, pathogenesis, and clinical findings, and also tried to lead clinicians through the maze of differential diagnosis. Each individual identified as having hemifacial microsomia should have a full spectrum of evaluations because so many systems may be affected: ears (a full audiologic exam should be carried out as soon as an ear anomaly is suspected), eyes, heart, spine, and kidneys.[11]

Dysmorphologists do not agree on what constitutes the minimal criteria for a diagnosis of hemifacial microsomia. As stated by Gorlin, Cohen, and Levin (1990, p. 641), "Extreme variability of expression is characteristic." Some consider microtia (deformity of the auricle) alone to be a microform, whereas others insist on deformity of the jaw as a pathognomonic feature. Smith (1981) estimated that about 70% of cases are unilateral and 30% bilateral. When one side is rather severely affected, it is easy for clinicians to miss microforms on the opposite side, although such microforms may be indicative of significant deformities that are not visible (e.g., ossicular chain malformations).

The ear deformities in hemifacial microsomia range from mild differences in the auricle (Fig. 2-9) to complete absence of the external ear and auditory canal (Fig. 2-10). The deformities of the middle ear and ossicles also range from mild to severe. There may be malformations of the temporal bone, together with incomplete pneumatization of the mastoid. There is typically a conductive hearing loss, again ranging from mild to severe, with a maximum conductive loss in many cases. There have been some reported cases of cochlear involvement and sensorineural hearing loss (Bassila and Goldberg, 1989). Hearing loss may be bilateral even if the clinically obvious deformities are only unilateral.

The jaw deformity also ranges from mild to severe (Fig. 2-11), at its mildest producing an open bite on the affected side, at its worst characterized by a rudimentary mandible incapable of opening-closing movements and unable to articulate with the maxilla. Although the mandible, external ear, and middle ear all develop from the first and second branchial arches (thus the term "first and second arch syndrome"), there is no strong correlation among the deformities of these structures. More severely affected mandibles *tend* to be associated with more severely affected external ears, but there are exceptions (Figueroa and Pruzansky, 1982). There may be partial ankylosis of the tongue, and severe cases may exhibit a combination of a poorly developed, anchored tongue sitting in a retruded, ankylosed mandible. A deformed, retruded mandible, combined with retrusion of the tongue, may contribute to upper airway obstruction, a problem exacerbated by hypotonic pharyngeal musculature on the affected side (Shprintzen et al., 1980).

Asymmetry of the bulk and strength of facial muscles is common in hemifacial microsomia (Fig. 2-12). Because the facial nerve courses through the middle ear cavity, it may be damaged when that cavity is not normally developed (Caldarelli et al., 1980; Sedee, 1973). Other cranial nerves may also be abnormal in development and function, but the most common is the facial nerve (Converse et al., 1979). The facial muscular asymmetry in hemifacial microsomia may have several bases: primary hypoplasia of muscle itself, abnormality of the bones to which the muscle is attached, deficiency in innervation, and secondary overdevelopment of the musculature on the normal or lesser affected side.

Unilateral or bilateral cleft lip and/or cleft palate occurs in an estimated 7% to 15% of patients with hemifacial microsomia, with cleft palate alone occurring about twice as often as cleft lip +/– cleft palate (Rollnick et al., 1987). In

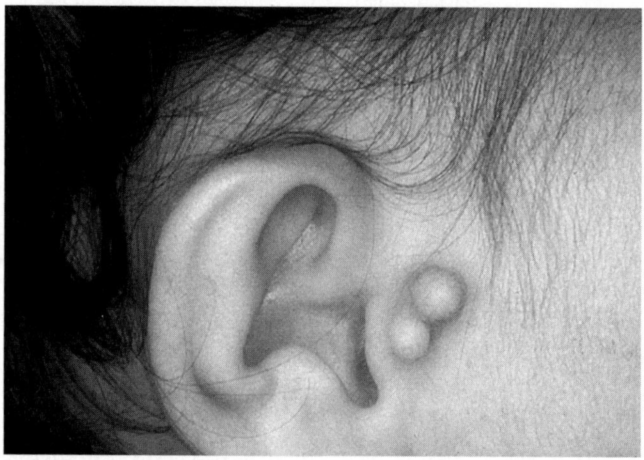

Figure 2-9 Preauricular tags in a baby born with hemifacial microsomia.

[11]Because the ears and the kidneys form at the same time in the embryo, any individual with an ear deformity should have a renal sonogram as a minimal diagnostic step, even in the absence of clinically recognizable renal problems.

addition, these patients may exhibit noncleft velopharyngeal incompetency resulting from asymmetric movement of the velum and/or pharyngeal musculature (Luce, McGibbon, and Hoopes, 1977; Shprintzen et al., 1980).

When vertebral anomalies are present together with anomalies of the eye and ear, the label "oculoauriculovertebral" spectrum or Goldenhar syndrome is applied (Fig. 2-13). The vertebral anomalies carry several potential threats to health and development (Gibson, Sillence, and Taylor, 1996) including various forms of neurologic compromise (Gosain, McCarthy, and Pinto, 1994). In addition, individuals with Goldenhar syndrome show a

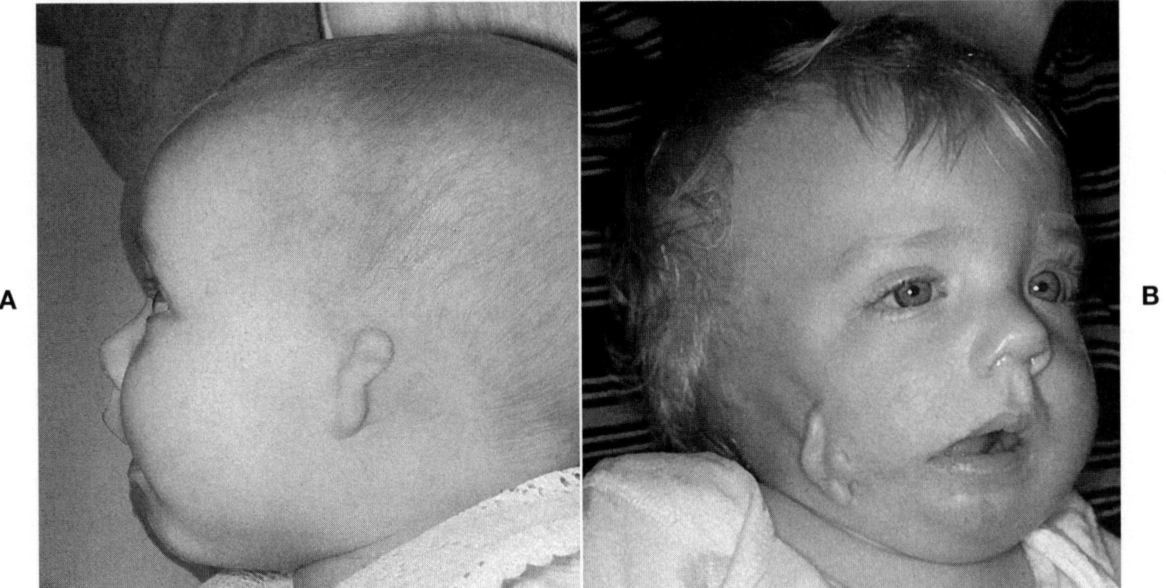

Figure 2-10 A and **B,** Deformity of the auricle in two children with hemifacial microsomia. Note the displacement of the auricle down onto the cheek and the preauricular pits in the second child.

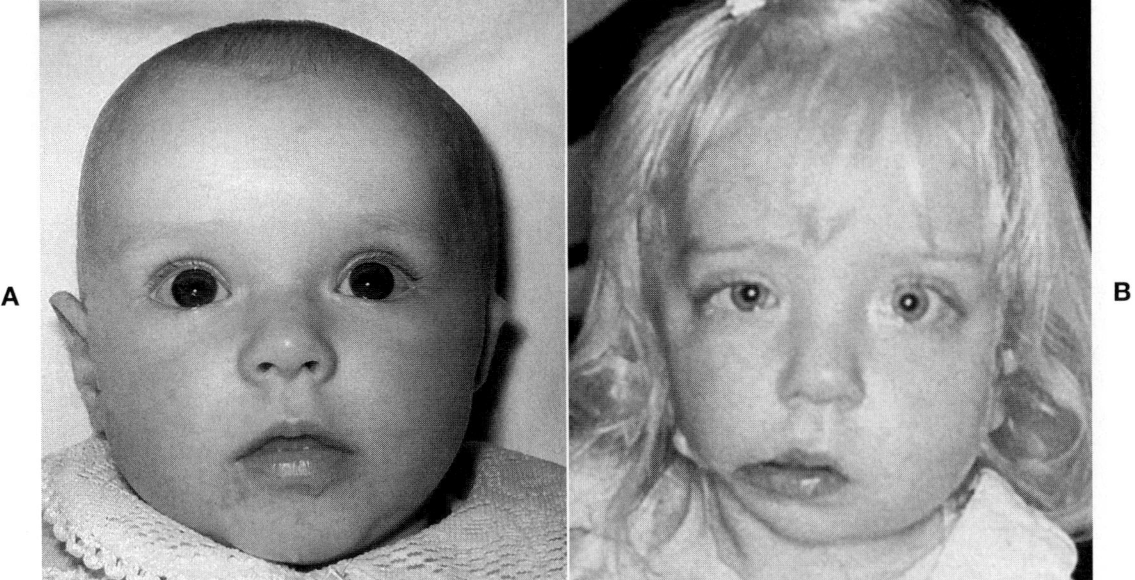

Figure 2-11 A and **B,** Frontal views of the same two children in Fig. 2-10. In the first child, note that there is good symmetry of the facial structures despite the relatively severe deformity of the left auricle. The second child actually has bilateral, asymmetric hemifacial microsomia, with less severe deformities on her left side than on her right. Note the right macrostomia, also seen in her earlier photo (Fig. 2-10, *B*).

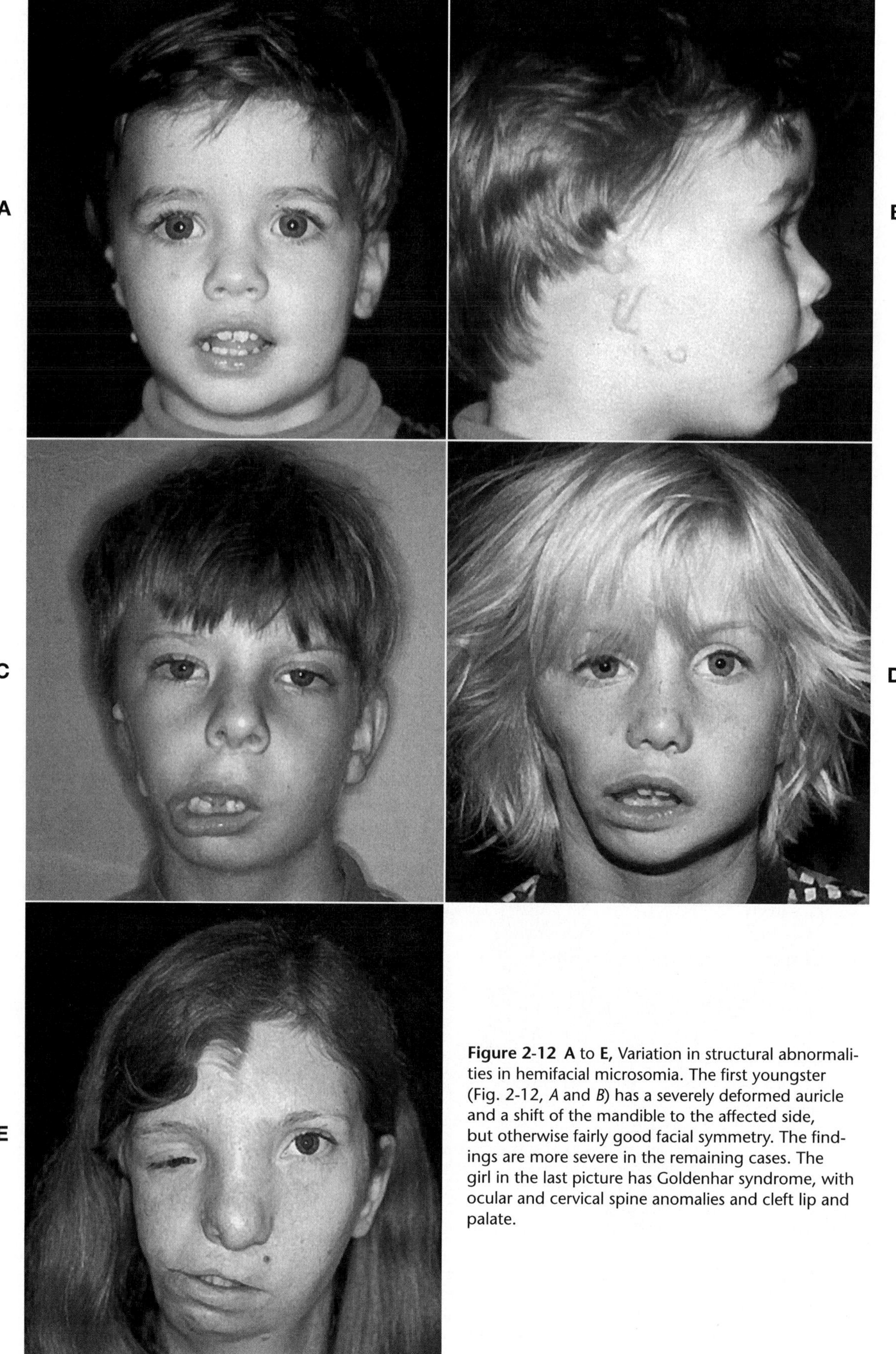

Figure 2-12 A to **E,** Variation in structural abnormalities in hemifacial microsomia. The first youngster (Fig. 2-12, *A* and *B*) has a severely deformed auricle and a shift of the mandible to the affected side, but otherwise fairly good facial symmetry. The findings are more severe in the remaining cases. The girl in the last picture has Goldenhar syndrome, with ocular and cervical spine anomalies and cleft lip and palate.

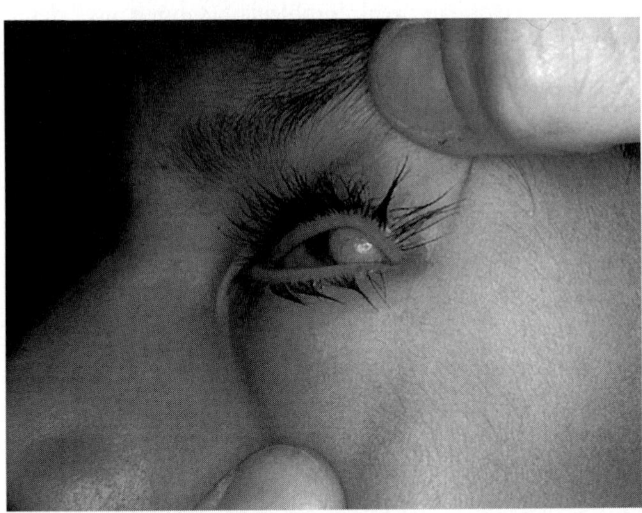

Figure 2-13 An epibulbar dermoid, one of the characteristics of Goldenhar syndrome.

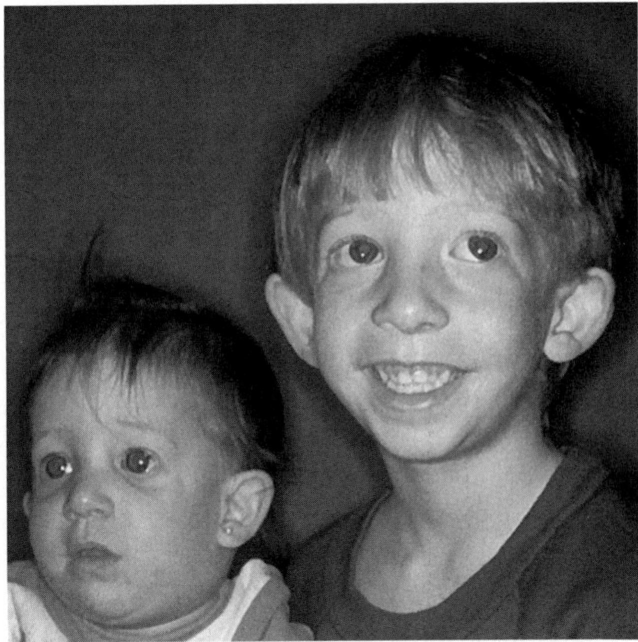

Figure 2-14 A baby girl with mild expression of mandibulofacial dysostosis, pictured with her older brother, who is also mildly affected.

high frequency of cardiac anomalies (Abe, Ishikawa, and Murakami, 1965; Friedman and Saraclar, 1974; Greenwood et al., 1974; Kumar et al., 1993).

There is no coherent body of literature regarding speech problems in hemifacial microsomia, partly because there is such a range in severity of physical findings among patients and partly because patients exhibit different capabilities to adapt to or compensate for their physical differences. The possible threats to normal development of communication skills include hearing loss, malocclusion, ankyloglossia, velopharyngeal inadequacy, and even secondary delay if the threats—especially the hearing loss—are not recognized and treated early. Given all the possible hazards, it is amazing that so many individuals with hemifacial microsomia exhibit normal speech or speech characterized only by mild articulation problems. Speech problems may be temporarily exacerbated by physical treatment, such as orthodontic or surgical repositioning of the jaws. As of this writing, such treatment is taking a new direction for children and adults with unilateral or bilateral micrognathia (small jaw), namely, distraction osteogenesis (Chin and Toth, 1996; Molina and Ortiz Monasterio, 1995).

In summary, communication skills in patients with hemifacial microsomia may be quite normal or may be threatened by multiple physical abnormalities. Any speech pathologist involved in the evaluation and care of such patients should first be certain that appropriate assessments have been completed, most notably a hearing evaluation and a genetics-dysmorphology examination. Finally, the communication skills of any individual with hemifacial microsomia may change over time as he or she goes through stages of physical management, meaning that the responsibilities of the speech-language pathologist do not end with a one-time assessment.

MANDIBULOFACIAL DYSOSTOSIS

Mandibulofacial dysostosis is a multi-anomaly disorder primarily affecting the eyes, ears, maxilla, and mandible. The first cases were probably the patients with ear deformities and hearing loss described by Thomson in 1846. In 1889 Berry described the lower eyelid defects in a mother and daughter. The syndrome came to be associated with the name of Treacher Collins, an English ophthalmologist who described the malar hypoplasia (poor development of the cheekbones) that is one of key features (Treacher Collins, 1900). Franceschetti and Klein (1949) coined the term "mandibulofacial dysostosis" for what they erroneously thought was a newly identified craniofacial syndrome. The syndrome is autosomal dominant, and the gene has been mapped to the long arm of chromosome 5 (Dixon et al., 1991; Edery et al., 1994; Jabs et al., 1991; Marres et al., 1995).

Mandibulofacial dysostosis is relatively rare (approximately 1 in 50,000 live births) but is so variable in expressivity that many minimally involved cases are undoubtedly missed. Affected members of the same family often vary markedly in severity of findings (Fig. 2-14) (Dixon et al., 1994; Fazen, Elmore, and Nadler, 1967; Hansen et al., 1996).

The facial features of mandibulofacial dysostosis include malar hypoplasia, downward slant of the palpebral fissures (outer corners of the eyes), lower eyelid defects including colobomata (notches) and partial to total absence of lower eyelashes, colobomata of the iris, and hypoplasia of the mandible and maxilla (Fig. 2-15). About 25% of cases have a tongue-shaped projection of scalp hair onto the cheek (Gorlin, Cohen, and Levin, 1990; Jones, 1997). A few cases with cleft lip have been reported (Gorlin, Cohen, and Levin, 1990). The facial deformities are usually described as symmetric on clinical examination, but there are exceptions, particularly in the ear malformations.

The oral and pharyngeal deformities in mandibulofacial dysostosis are complex. The mandible is both small (micrognathic) and deformed, with antegonial notching that creates a sort of "S curve" of the inferior border (Fig. 2-16) and contributes to an open bite. The mandibular deformity tends to become worse with time (Goldberg et al., 1981; Roberts, Pruzansky, and Aduss, 1975). The maxilla is also small. About 30% to 35% of cases have overt clefts (Fig. 2-17), and another 30% to 40% exhibit other types of velopharyngeal problems (submucous clefts, inadequate velopharyngeal motion) (Peterson-Falzone and Pruzansky, 1976). The pharynx is small in diameter (Peterson-Falzone and Pruzansky, 1976; Shprintzen et al., 1979), partly as a result of posterior displacement of the

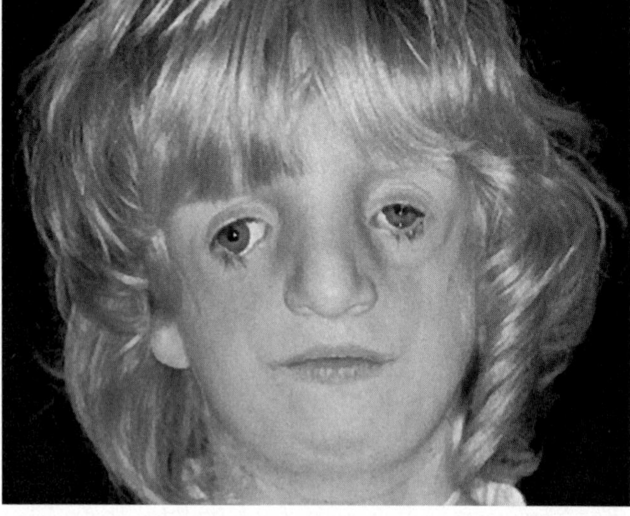

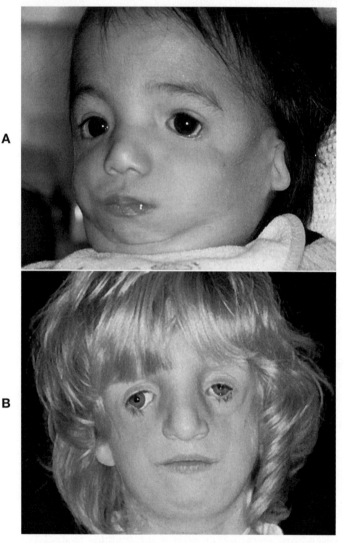

Figure 2-15 A and **B,** These youngsters (unrelated) have more severe cases of mandibulofacial dysostosis than the children pictured in Fig. 2-14. Note the auricular deformities and the drooped position of the lower lateral portions of the eyes (caused by deformities of the malar bones). In the child in **A** the mandibular hypoplasia is also easily seen.

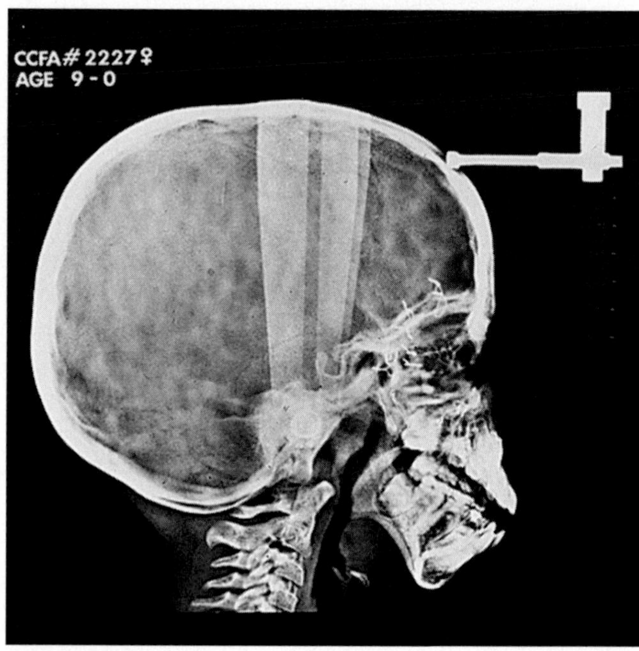

Figure 2-16 Lateral cephalometric film of 9-year-old child with mandibulofacial dysostosis, demonstrating the curvature of the lower border of the mandible, which tends to become worse over time.

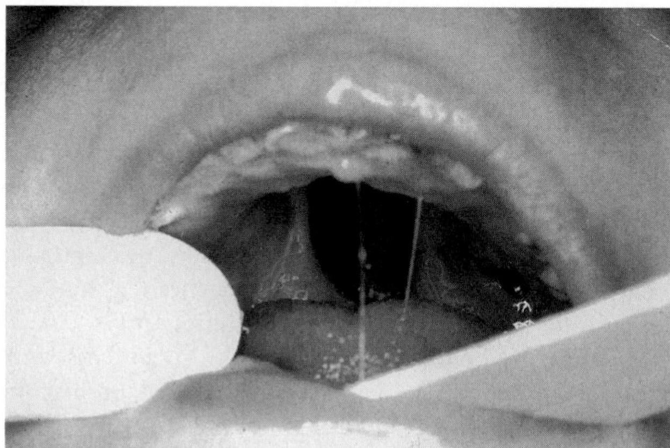

Figure 2-17 Palatal cleft in a patient with mandibulofacial dysostosis.

tongue (a consequence of the small and retrognathic mandible), and maxillary deficiency with reduced forward projection (Figueroa, 1991). Other factors adding to crowding of the airway include medial displacement of the pterygoid plates (Shprintzen, 1982), and a progressive bending of the cranial base, bringing the posterior pharyngeal wall forward into an already crowded airway (Figueroa, 1991; Kreiborg and Dahl, 1993; Peterson-Falzone and Figueroa, 1986) (Fig. 2-18).

Children with mandibulofacial dysostosis are subject to significant respiratory problems as infants (see the preceding section on Robin sequence, p. 32), and tracheotomies are frequently required. The literature contains multiple reports of neonatal deaths (Book and Fraccaro, 1955; Fazen, Elmore, and Nadler, 1967; Franceschetti and Klein, 1949; Rogers, 1964). Airway problems may persist or, in fact, recur as the child grows because of the progressive deformities of the mandible and cranial base (Kreiborg and Dahl, 1993). Obstructive sleep apnea and apnea during wakefulness are serious concerns in both children and adults (Arvystas and Shprintzen, 1991; Colmenero et al., 1991; Fazen, Elmore, and Nadler, 1967; Johnston et al., 1981; Schafer, 1982; Sher, Shprintzen, and Thorpy, 1986; Shprintzen, 1982; Shprintzen et al., 1979). Sometimes, surgical closure of a cleft in an infant may be contraindicated because of the airway complications (Crysdale, 1981), and later surgery such as a pharyngeal flap for velopharyngeal inadequacy may be similarly contraindicated because of the already hypoplastic airway. Kreiborg and Dahl (1993), focusing on the progressive changes in mandible and cranial base with the consequent effect upon the airway, urged monitoring of these patients from infancy through adolescence. However, the deleterious changes in the cranial base may go on into early adulthood (Peterson-Falzone and Figueroa, 1986).

There are extensive reports on the variation in structural deformities of the outer and middle ears, temporal bones, and the hearing loss in patients with mandibulofacial dysostosis (Cremers and Teunissen, 1991; Jahrsdoefer, Aguilar, Yeakley, and Cole, 1989; Jahrsdoefer and Jacobson, 1995; Kay and Kay, 1989; Marsh et al., 1986; Phelps, Poswillo, and Lloyd, 1981; Pron et al., 1993; Sando, Suehiro, and Wood, 1983). The ear deformities are usually, but not always, limited to the structures from the first and second branchial arches. The outer ear deformities range from minimal abnormality to complete agenesis ("anotia"), and the external auditory canal ranges from normal to stenotic to atretic to absent. The major threat to hearing, however, is found in the deformities of the middle ear: hypoplastic tympanic and epitympanic cavities and ossicular malformations ranging from minor to complete absence. The temporal bone often lacks normal pneumatization. In some cases the deformities of the external ears, middle ear cavities, and temporal bones are asymmetric (Marsh et al., 1986; Phelps, Poswillo, and Lloyd, 1981; van Vierzen et al., 1995). The typical hearing loss is a bilateral conductive loss, often of maximum degree in both ears, the contour of the loss being flat or rising. A few cases with a mixed conductive-sensorineural loss have been reported (Jahrsdoefer and Jacobson, 1995; Sando, Suehiro, and Wood, 1983).

The hazards to normal early childhood development in mandibulofacial dysostoses are multiple and potentially severe, with obvious specific threats to communication development. Although the audiologist and the speech-language pathologist know instantly that a child with ear deformities needs neonatal audiologic testing and often the

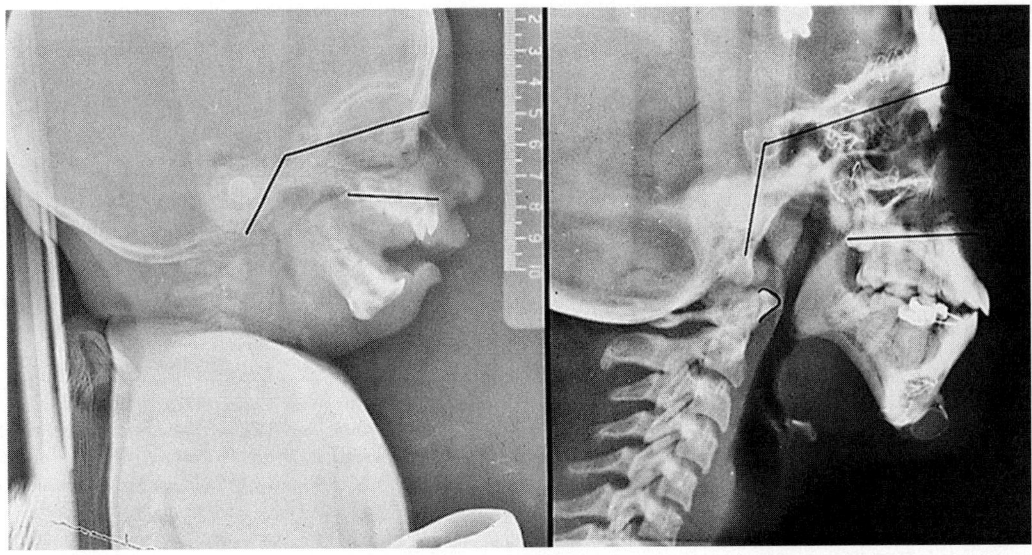

Figure 2-18 The change in the cranial base in a patient with mandibulofacial dysostosis. Note how the cranial base angle becomes more acute from the age of 5 months to the age of 17 years.

fitting of amplification, that knowledge is not always shared by parents or even other caregivers.[12] Some of the early reports on individuals with this syndrome listed "mental retardation" as an associated finding, but as you would expect, this finding has gradually dropped out of most clinical reports as more children diagnosed in the early weeks and months of life have had appropriate audiologic assessment and habilitation for hearing problems. Note the statement of geneticist Kenneth L. Jones (1997, p. 250): "As the great majority of these patients are of normal intelligence, the early recognition of deafness and its correction with hearing aids or surgery (when possible) are of great importance to development."

Although many individuals with mandibulofacial dysostosis have clefts or other problems in the function of the velopharyngeal system, the treatment decisions are not straightforward. Even surgical closure of an overt cleft may be contraindicated in the presence of severe crowding of the airway (Crysdale, 1981; Peterson-Falzone and Pruzansky, 1976). A pharyngeal flap for inadequate velopharyngeal function may be impossible, even in older children, for the same reason. Conversely, there are patients who have a submucous cleft or other potential threats to velopharyngeal closure (e.g., minimal movement of the velum) for whom surgery is actually not necessary because of the small size of the pharyngeal space. Even when velopharyngeal function is adequate, the abnormal size and shape of the oral and pharyngeal cavities in this syndrome can produce an abnormal resonance that has been variously labeled as "muffled," "hot potato," and "cul-de-sac" resonance.

RARER SYNDROMES THAT RESEMBLE MANDIBULOFACIAL DYSOSTOSIS

There are several disorders in which the facial and oral anomalies are often confused with mandibulofacial dysostosis. As a group, they are known as syndromes of acrofacial dysostosis. The term "acrofacial" was coined by Nager and de Reynier in 1948 when they described patients with facial deformities similar to mandibulofacial dysostosis but also exhibiting limb abnormalities. At least eight types of acrofacial dysostosis have been described to date (Opitz et al., 1993); "new" types are often challenged as simply being variants of previously described disorders (Gorlin, Cohen, and Levin, 1990). Each of the acrofacial syndromes occurs less frequently than mandibulofacial dysostosis does. Nager syndrome occurs more often than any other type, and it is the only one to be discussed here in detail. The likelihood of your encountering a child or adult with any of these disorders is very low. However, if you do, your input will be crucial, especially if the patient is a child.

[12]In California there was a case in 1996 in which the third-party payer for a family of a child with bilateral severe deformities of the auricles refused authorization for audiologic testing because "he doesn't have any ears."

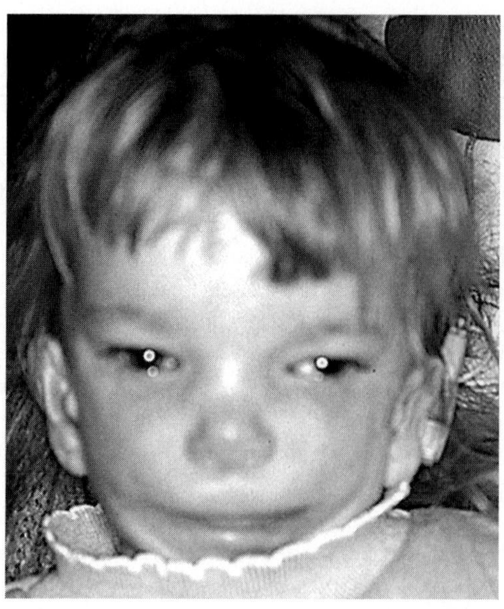

Figure 2-19 Facial features of a child with Nager syndrome.

Nager Syndrome (Preaxial Acrofacial Dysotosis)[13]

This syndrome was probably first described by Slingenberg in 1908 (Gorlin, Cohen, and Levin, 1990). As of 1993, 76 cases had been reported in the literature (McDonald and Gorski, 1993). The facial features (Fig. 2-19) are very similar to those of mandibulofacial dysostosis. Although there is variation in expressivity from patient to patient (Fig. 2-20), the craniofacial abnormalities are multiple and frequently of sufficient severity to preclude intelligible speech. A particularly devastating complication is the fact that the syndrome includes anomalies of the arms and hands (Fig. 2-21), often so severe that signing as an alternative or adjunctive mode of communication is significantly impaired. There is evidence for both autosomal recessive and autosomal dominant transmission of Nager syndrome (Chemke et al., 1988; Hecht et al., 1987; Kawira, Weaver, and Bender, 1984; Opitz et al., 1993), but many cases are sporadic (Opitz et al., 1993).

The craniofacial features include hypoplasia of the zygomas and downward slanting of the palpebral fissures, cheek extensions of scalp hair, malformations of the external and middle ears, lower eyelid defects, and mandibular and maxillary hypoplasia—all as listed in mandibulofacial dysostosis. The lower jaw is typically even

[13]In the arm, "preaxial" means side of the thumb (the side of the radius). In the lower limb, preaxial means the medial side, or side of the tibia. In the upper extremity, "postaxial" means the side of the little finger (side of the ulnar bone), whereas in the lower limb it means the outer or lateral aspect. Although this may seem unnecessarily confusing, if you have had a course in anatomy you know that in the "anatomical position" the human figure is positioned with the palms facing forward. Thus the thumbs of the hands in this position are actually "lateral" to the long axis of the arm.

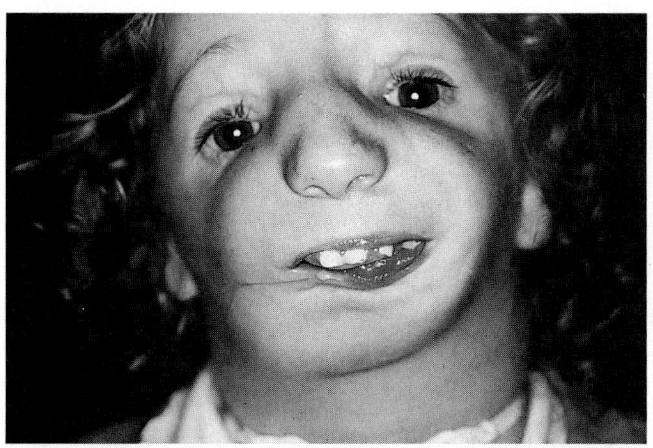

Figure 2-20 Facial features in another child with Nager syndrome. Children with this syndrome have normal intellectual function but have severe orofacial structural hazards to oral communication skills.

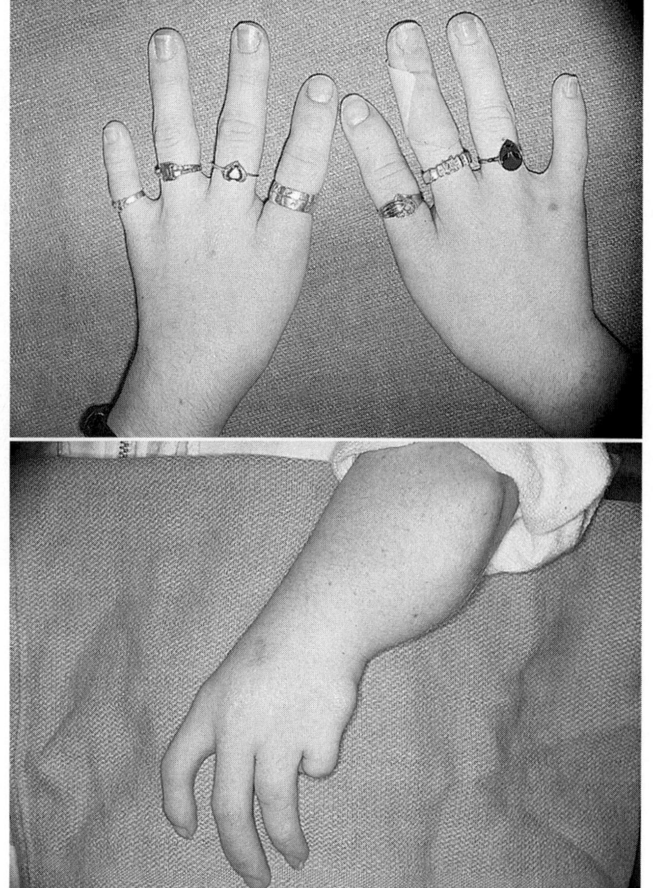

Figure 2-21 The digital anomalies in Nager syndrome. **A,** The fingers of a young adult, who likes to wear rings on her fingers despite the absence of thumbs. **B,** The absence of the thumb, plus anomalies of the other digits, in another child with this syndrome.

smaller and more deformed than in mandibulofacial dysostosis (Fig. 2-22) (Gorlin, Cohen, and Levin, 1990); the mandibular deformities include the ramus and condyle, causing problems in jaw opening that may be progressive. The inability to open the mouth produces, in turn, problems in oral hygiene and dental care and may prohibit surgical or prosthetic treatment of velopharyngeal abnormalities. The velopharyngeal abnormalities are also more severe than in mandibulofacial dysostosis, because patients with Nager syndrome often exhibit agenesis (virtual lack of) the soft palate (Jackson et al., 1989).

The limb deformities vary from patient to patient, but some form of upper limb malformation is always present. The thumbs may be hypoplastic, triphalangeal (looking more like fingers than thumbs), or missing (aplastic), as seen in Fig. 2-21. About half the cases exhibit hypoplasia or aplasia of the radii or synostosis of the radial and ulnar bones of the arm, either unilateral or bilateral. In practical terms, this means that many of these children have rudimentary or absent forearms, and attached to the arms are hands without thumbs. The lower limb problems are variable but tend to be less devastating than those of the upper limbs (Halal et al., 1983). These children often exhibit short stature and poor growth (Gellis, Feingold, and Miller, 1978; Goodman and Gorlin, 1983; Halal et al., 1983; Temtamy and McKusick, 1978).

Occasional associated craniofacial anomalies in Nager syndrome include cleft lip (Kawira, Weaver, and Bender, 1984; Le Merrer et al., 1989; Verloes, Foret, and Lambotte, 1987), lateral facial clefts (Goldstein and Mirkin, 1988; Kawira, Weaver, and Bender, 1984), and laryngeal hypoplasia (Krauss, Hassell, and Gang, 1985).

As in mandibulofacial dysostosis, some cases of Nager syndrome are so mild that they are misdiagnosed or never recognized. The likelihood of an individual being misdiagnosed as having mandibulofacial dysostosis is high if the limb abnormalities are not recognized.

The threats to survival for neonates with Nager syndrome are severe. The hypoplasia of the maxilla and mandible and associated retrodisplacement of the tongue, together with the limitations in jaw opening, predispose toward airway obstruction that is often progressive (Danziger et al., 1990; Friedman et al., 1996). In reviewing the cases reported in the literature, Friedman et al. (1996) concluded that tracheotomy is necessary in 37% of these infants.

In early childhood the opportunity to explore the environment is limited by limb deformities and the multiple necessary medical interventions. Similarly, the opportunity for normal interaction between baby and parent or between baby and other aspects of the environment is often impaired. Stimulation for the infant is limited by the hearing loss until the loss is assessed and appropriate amplification provided, and also by the inability of adults to recognize and reinforce early speech attempts. Some authors have reported mild mental retardation (Klein, Konig, and Tobler, 1970; Walker, 1974), and there have been sporadic reports of severe retardation (Halal et al., 1983; Verloes, Foret, and Lambotte, 1987). However, such

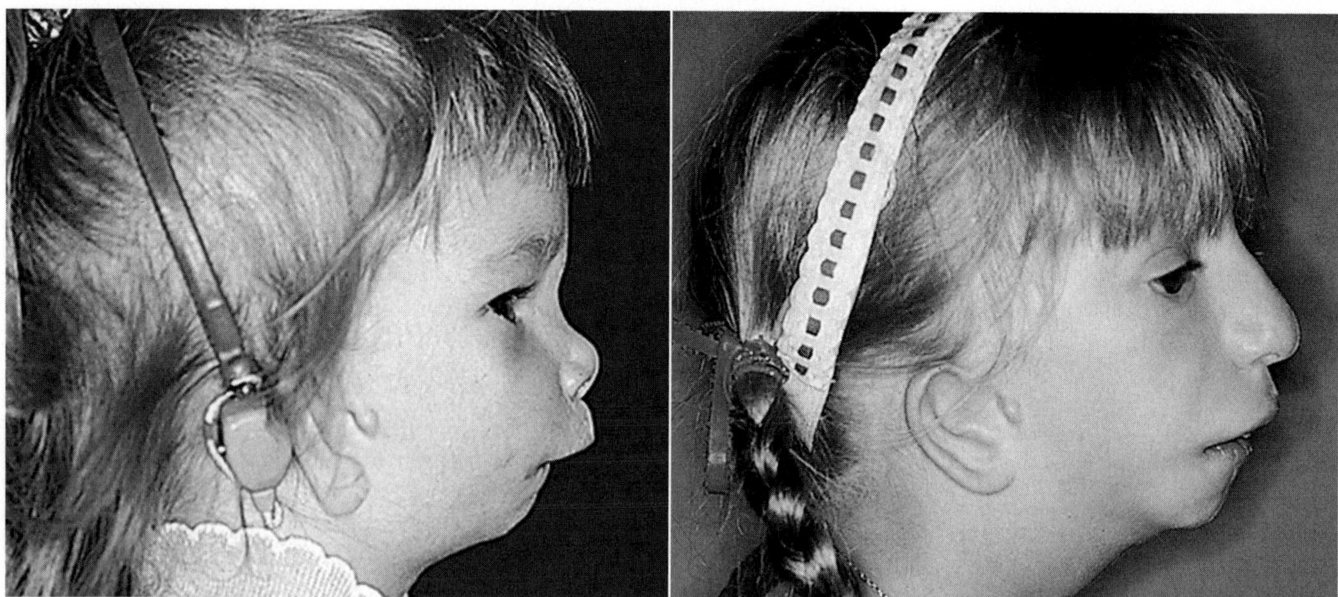

Figure 2-22 Profiles of two children with Nager syndrome, particularly demonstrating the mandibular hypoplasia.

reports should be viewed with caution unless care has been taken to discriminate primary limitations in intellectual development from the secondary effects of hearing loss. Each child with Nager syndrome requires early assessment and continuing individualized habilitative and educational planning to maximize communication skills (Meyerson and Nisbet, 1987; Meyerson et al., 1977).

Other Syndromes of Acrofacial Dysostosis

As of this writing, seven additional syndromes of acrofacial dysostosis have been described (Opitz et al., 1993). In terms of estimated frequency of occurrence, Miller syndrome probably ranks just after Nager syndrome, with about half the known number of cases (Donnai, Hughes, and Winter, 1987; Genee, 1969; Miller, Fineman, and Smith, 1979; Opitz et al., 1993). This syndrome consists of acrofacial dysostosis plus postaxial limb abnormalities. Cleft lip and palate are frequent (Chrzanowska et al., 1989; Fryns and Van den Berghe, 1988; Hauss-Albert and Passarge, 1988; Meinecke and Wiedemann, 1987; Miller, Fineman, and Smith, 1979), and one of the patients with "Nager" syndrome in the 1989 report by Jackson et al. actually had Miller syndrome. Other types of acrofacial dysostosis syndromes are discussed by Gorlin, Cohen, and Levin (1990) and Opitz et al. (1993). You are advised to check current computer updates for more extensive listings of newly described variants.

ECTRODACTYLY–ECTODERMAL DYSPLASIA–CLEFT SYNDROME

Although the ectrodactyly–ectodermal dysplasia–cleft syndrome occurs infrequently, it is another autosomal dominant syndrome in which cleft lip and cleft palate are integral features (Fig. 2-23). Ectrodactyly is the medical term for "claw-like" hands and feet, meaning that there may be only a thumb and little finger or ring finger and little finger on each hand and similar deformities of the feet (Fig. 2-24). Ectodermal dysplasia means that the structures derived from the embryonic ectoderm (skin, hair, teeth, nails) are poorly developed. There are many forms of ectodermal dysplasia. The most common form is hypohydrotic, meaning that the skin is dry with little to no formation of sweat glands. Affected individuals must be very careful in high heat because there is serious danger of hyperthermia. The hair is usually blond, coarse, and sparse. The eyelashes and eyebrows are also sparse. The cleft lip and palate in this syndrome is often bilateral. An additional cardinal feature is obstruction of the nasolacrimal duct. There is strong evidence of autosomal dominant transmission of this syndrome with penetrance between 93% and 98% (Roelfsema and Cobben, 1996), although there is marked variability in findings even among members of the same family (Anneren et al., 1991; Majewski and Kuster, 1988). No single symptom is obligatory; the most constant feature is some degree of ectodermal dysplasia, but even that is not 100% consistent (Rodini, Freitas, and Richieri-Costa, 1991).

In very mild cases with incomplete expression of the syndrome, there may be no significant problems affecting speech or hearing. However, there are several sources of problems in more fully affected cases. Hypodontia (Fig. 2-25) can contribute to articulation problems until the dentition is replaced through dentures, bridges, or implants. The ectodermal dysplasia, particularly the hypohydrotic type, may result in lack of normal lubrication of the vocal folds with an incomplete seal between the folds in the

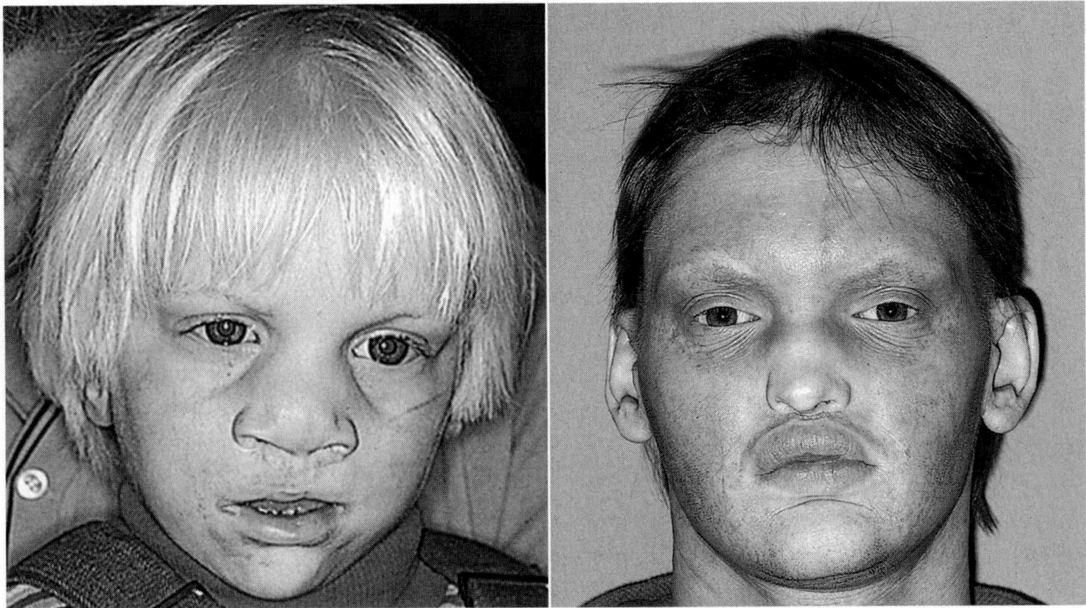

Figure 2-23 The typical facial features in patients with ectodermal dysplasia–ectrodactyly–cleft syndrome in a little boy and his father.

adduction phase of phonation, producing a breathy voice (Peterson-Falzone, Caldarelli, and Landahl, 1981).[14] The cleft palate is an obvious threat to communication development. Conductive hearing loss has been reported repeatedly (Buss, Hughes, and Clarke, 1995; Bystrom, Snager, and Stewart, 1975; Chiang and Robinson, 1974; Kaiser-Kupfer, 1973; Pashayan, Pruzansky, and Solomon, 1974), which is not surprising in view of the cleft.

Although ectrodactyly–ectodermal dysplasia–cleft is a relatively rare syndrome (about 260 cases published to date), the above description and accompanying pictures should alert you to the additional anomalies when you are seeing a child or adult with a cleft, particularly if there has not been a prior full evaluation by a dysmorphologist or geneticist.

SYNDROMES OF PREMATURE CRANIOFACIAL SYNOSTOSIS

The normal shape of the human skull is dependent on a number of interactive factors both inside the head and in the skull bones themselves, and both early and late in the formation of the baby, including during the postnatal period.[15] There are many syndromes in which the shape of the skull is abnormal. Most of these involve a generalized dysplasia, meaning that other parts of the body are affected as well. The situation typically becomes worse as the child grows, that is, it may seem benign or mild in infancy but become more disfiguring and more injurious to function with time. Although the syndromes of premature craniofacial synostosis occur only once in several thousand births, they usually entail significant hazards to the development of communication skills. There are many more syndromes than can be presented here. We have chosen to discuss four of these syndromes, the selection based on the relative frequency with which affected individuals are seen in craniofacial treatment centers. These four syndromes—Apert, Crouzon, Pfeiffer, and Saethre-Chotzen—are closely related in structural anomalies, symptoms, and to some extent etiology. In fact, Cohen (1986, p. 435) noted, "On occasion, some of these entities appear to overlap within the same family."[16]

Defining Premature Craniofacial Synostosis

You will remember from your course work in anatomy and embryology that the sutures between the skull bones and between the bones of the facial skeleton are growth sites. That is, increase in size of the skull or facial skeleton is dependent on new bone being gradually added along the "edges" of each bone. Eventually, there is fusion between adjacent bones, but this fusion is programed to occur at specific times. If it occurs too early, deformity and deficient craniofacial growth will result. In fact, complete fusion of the craniofacial skeleton does not occur until late in adulthood.

[14]In any individual with ectodermal dysplasia and a breathy voice, be careful not to encourage use of an increased loudness level in the effort to reduce the breathiness: use of increased vocal effort will only result in increased trauma to the vocal folds, which are not protected by a normal mucosal covering.

[15]Currently there is a very vocal controversy in the United States regarding the effect of placing babies on their backs to avoid SIDS (sudden infant death syndrome), a positioning that can cause flattening of the back of the head.

[16]Cohen's remark also included Carpenter syndrome, which will not be discussed here.

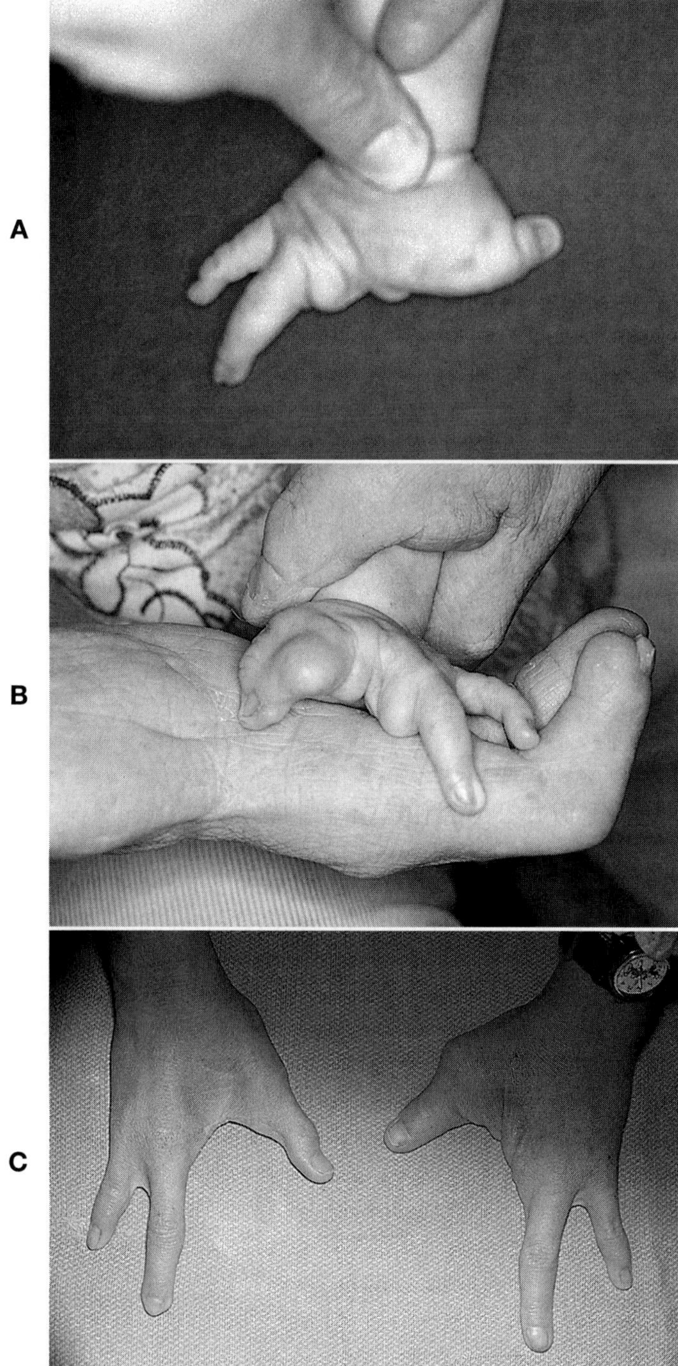

Figure 2-24 Digital anomalies in an infant (A and B) and adult (C) with ectrodactyly.

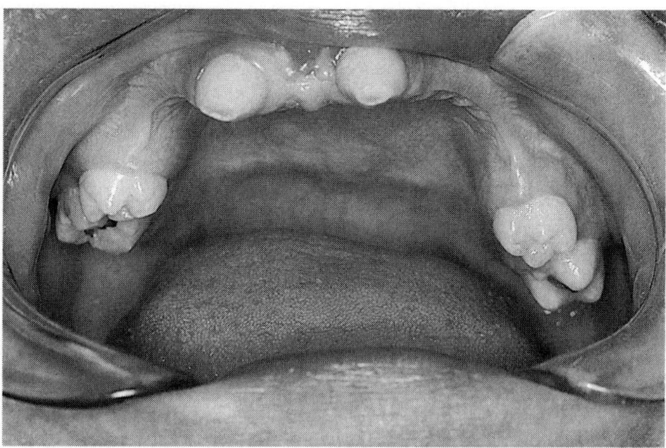

Figure 2-25 Missing teeth in a patient with ectodermal dysplasia–ectrodactyly–cleft syndrome.

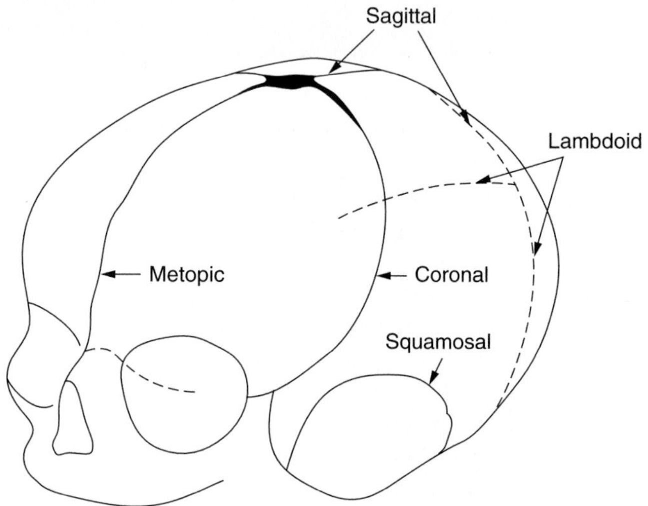

Figure 2-26 Locations of the major sutures of the skull.

In premature craniofacial synostosis, the shape of the skull will depend on what sutures fuse and at what time. When a suture has closed, growth is restricted at right angles to the suture and there is compensatory overgrowth in the same direction as the fused suture. Fig. 2-26 shows the location of the major sutures of the skull, and Fig. 2-27 is a schematic diagram demonstrating the effect on skull growth of premature closure of a suture. Isolated (nonsyndromic) premature fusion of a single suture or just one side (left or right) of a suture produces a misshapen skull but usually not the serious functional problems such as we will discuss below. When craniofacial synostosis occurs as part of a syndrome, there is also premature fusion of the bones of the cranial base, meaning that there is distortion and restriction of growth of the bony "foundation" of the skull and facial skeleton. This fusion contributes to the outward deformities and complicates attempts at surgical reconstruction.

Apert Syndrome (Acrocephalosyndactyly, Type I)

Apert syndrome is characterized by multiple deformities of the skull, face, maxilla, mandible, hands, feet, and joints (Fig. 2-28). This syndrome, which is autosomal dominant, is caused by mutation of a gene located on chromosome 10 (Jones, 1997). In 1967, Tunte and Lenz estimated the frequency of occurrence at 1 in 100,000 live births, but Cohen (1986) felt this estimate to be low. There are very

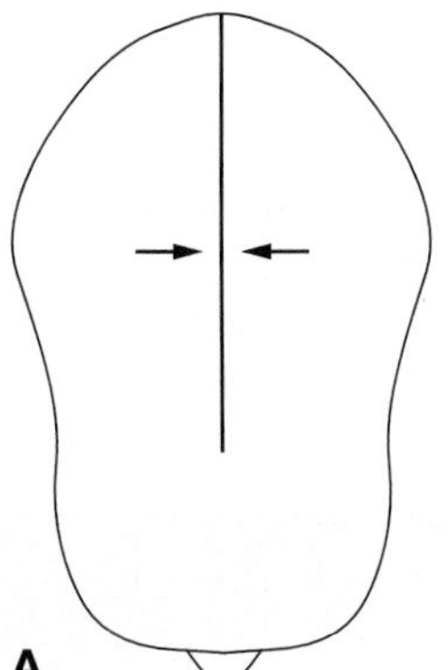

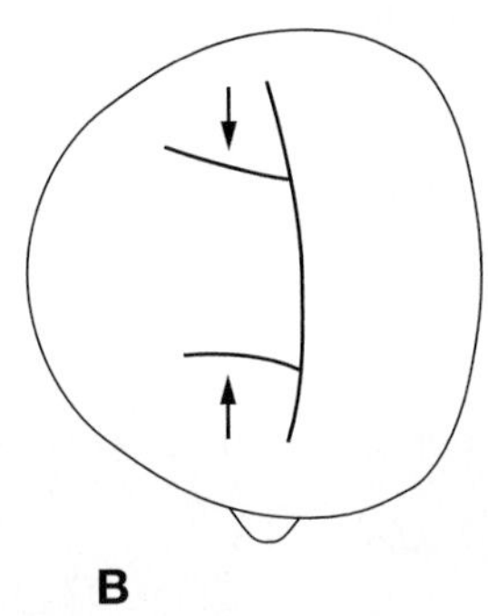

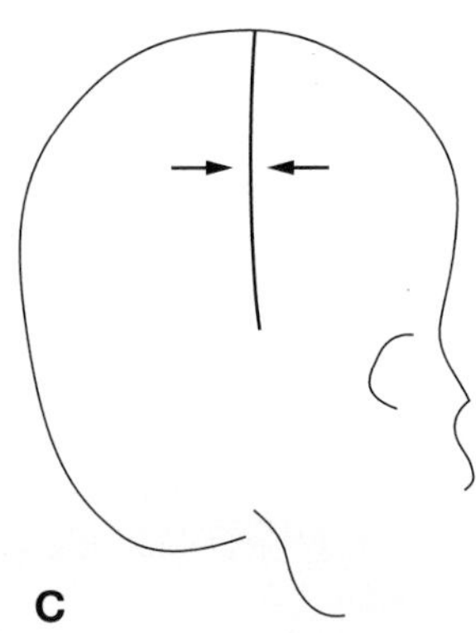

Figure 2-27 Schematic representations of the restriction of skull growth at right angles to a prematurely closed skull suture and the compensatory overgrowth that takes place in the same direction as the prematurely closed suture. In **A,** premature closure of the sagittal suture has kept the skull from expanding laterally, so it has overgrown from front to back. In **B,** premature closure of the lambdoid and coronal suture *just on one side* has shortened the skull from front to back (on the child's *right* side) and caused some outward bulging that is not seen on the side with the open sutures *(left).* In **C,** premature closure of the entire coronal suture has shortened the skull from front to back and lengthened it in the vertical dimension.

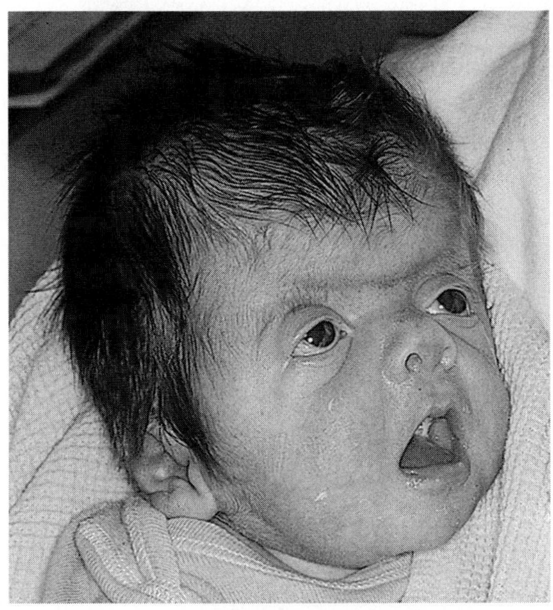

Figure 2-28 The severe facial and cranial deformities in an infant with Apert syndrome.

few reported cases of transmission of the syndrome from parent to child, which Gorlin, Cohen, and Levin (1990) attributed to reduced fitness of affected individuals to reproduce. In practical terms, the physical deformities in Apert syndrome are so striking that the opportunity for mating and reproduction is low. Thus most cases are sporadic, that is, attributable to a new mutation occurring in a family.

In Apert syndrome there is synostosis of the coronal suture, with variable involvement of other sutures as well. Premature synostosis of the coronal suture produces a skull that is vertically long but foreshortened in the anterior-to-posterior dimension. Usually there is early surgery to advance the forehead and help protect the eyes, but the midface remains retruded (Fig. 2-29). There is also synostosis and malformation of the cranial base, contributing to the distortion of the skull and face (Matras, Watsek and Perneczky, 1977; Ousterhout and Melsen, 1982). The midface, including the maxilla, is poorly formed and retruded (Fig. 2-30), providing little bony support for the eyes inferiorly and contributing to exophthalmus (abnormally prominent eyes). The primary cause of the exophthalmus is malformation of the bony orbits: instead of being cup shaped they are flat plates. The small, retruded upper jaw causes the more normally formed lower jaw to appear overly large (Fig. 2-31), a condition called "relative prognathism."[17] The nose is beak shaped, with a depressed nasal bridge (Fig. 2-32).

The maxilla is particularly deformed, compressed into a V shape with ectopic eruption of teeth (Fig. 2-33). The result is a severe Class III malocclusion (underbite) and open bite (Fig. 2-34). In addition, the palatal vault is characterized by progressive accumulation of soft tissue[18] along the palatine shelves (Fig. 2-35). The early stages of these accumulations are often visible in the infant's mouth within the first few months of life (Fig. 2-36), and they progress to the point that only a narrow slit of 1 or 2 mm remains between them, effectively flattening the palatal vault (Peterson and Pruzansky, 1974). Sometimes the palatal configuration, such as those pictured in Figs. 2-33, 2-35, and 2-36, is mistaken for a palatal cleft. Actual palatal

---

[17]However, the mandible itself is actually smaller than normal (Costaras-Volarich and Pruzansky, 1984.)

[18]Caused by accumulation of acid mucopolysaccharides (Solomon et al., 1973).

clefts (Fig. 2-37) and submucous clefts do occur in Apert syndrome in about 30% of cases (Gorlin, Cohen, and Levin, 1990). The pharynx is reduced in height and depth, and the soft palate is abnormally long and thick, crowding and sometimes virtually obliterating the nasopharyngeal airway, a problem that is apt to become more severe with age (Fig. 2-38) (Peterson and Pruzansky, 1974; Peterson-Falzone et al., 1981).

There is syndactyly of both the hands and feet, meaning that the digits (fingers and toes) appear to be melted together (Figs. 2-39 and 2-40). The syndactyly particularly involves digits 2, 3, and 4. A portion of the syndactyly may

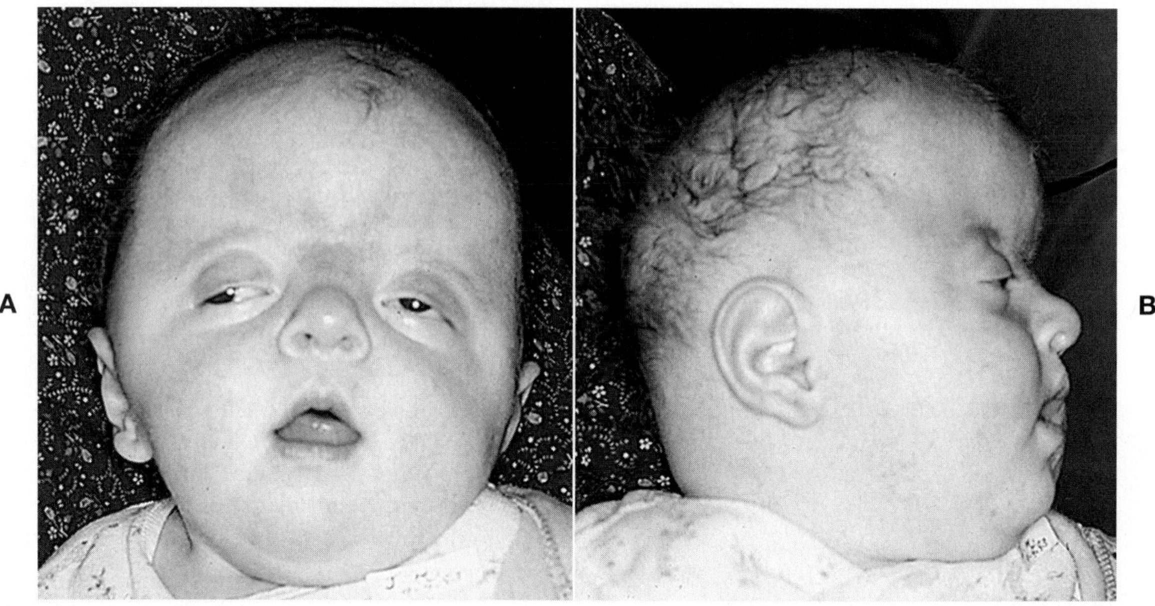

Figure 2-29 **A** and **B**, An infant with Apert syndrome who has had an early surgical advancement of the forehead (also known as "canthal advancement"), but the midface remains retruded.

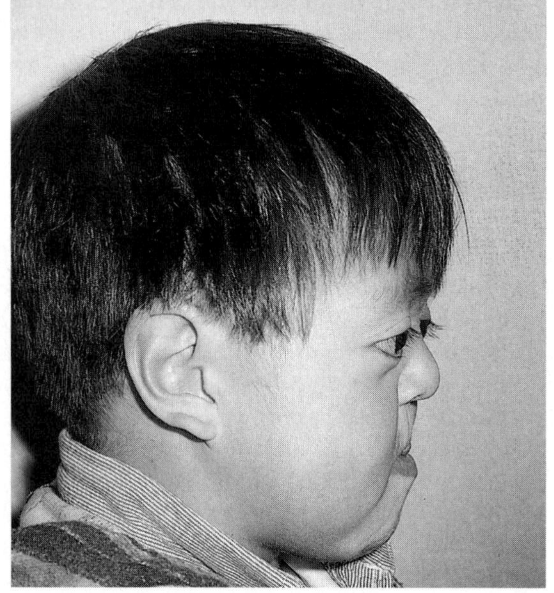

Figure 2-30 A preschooler with Apert syndrome who has good skull shape (subsequent to cranial remodeling in infancy) but persistent midface retrusion and exophthalmus (also called proptosis).

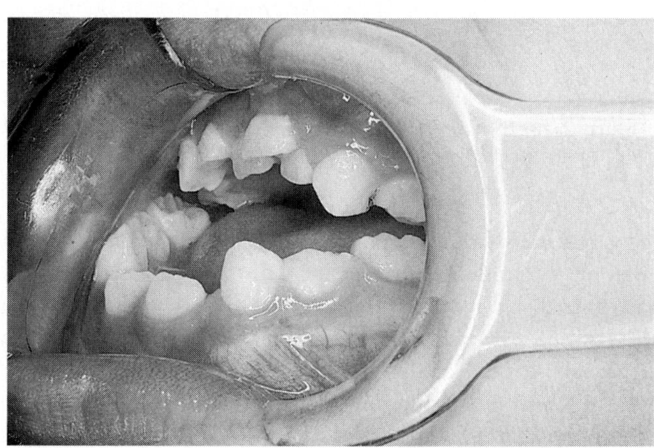

Figure 2-31 The dentition of the child shown in Fig. 2-30. The small, retruded upper jaw with a more normal-sized lower jaw contributes to "relative prognathism," meaning that the lower jaw looks abnormally large but actually is not.

be only soft tissue, although the bones underneath are not normal. The limbs are short, contributing to reduced linear growth (Cohen and Kreiborg, 1993b). There are restrictions in movement of the elbows, shoulders, hips, and knees that tend to become worse with time, another indication that Apert syndrome involves a progressive dysostosis (Cohen and Kreiborg, 1993c; Harris, Beligere, and Pruzansky, 1977; Wood, Sauser, and O'Hara, 1995). Calcification and fusion of the bones of the hands and feet are also progressive (Schuarte and St. Aubin, 1966).

Abnormalities of soft tissue and bony structures are found in other parts of the body as well. Fusions and other anomalies of the cervical spine occur in more than 65% to 70% of patients with Apert syndrome, and the fusions are typically progressive (Hemmer, McAlister, and Marsh, 1987; Kreiborg, 1987; Sherk, Whitaker, and Pasquariello, 1982).

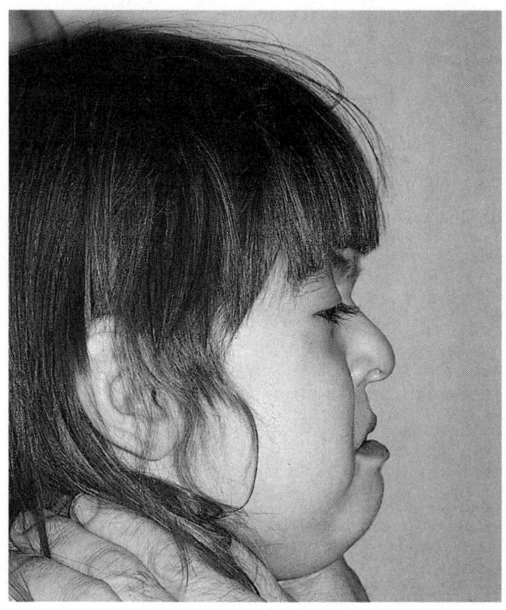

Figure 2-32 The "beak-shaped" nose in Apert syndrome, also seen in Fig. 2-29, *B*.

Two areas of chronic problems, sometimes very serious, are the airway and the ears. The upper airway is severely crowded as a result of bony and soft tissue abnormalities (see Fig. 2-37). Some individuals with Apert syndrome have stenosis of the posterior part of the nose, called "choanal atresia" (Perkins et al., 1997). The trachea may be a solid cartilaginous tube (Cohen and Kreiborg, 1993d). Infants and children with Apert syndrome are at risk for life-threatening respiratory problems (Crysdale, 1981: Perkins et al., 1997). Interestingly, surgery to position the midface further forward does not consistently produce a larger airway (Jarund and Lauritzen, 1996; McCarthy et al., 1995). The dysmorphic, crowded nasopharyngeal space also leads to inadequate aeration of the middle ear. Many patients have nearly unrelenting middle ear disease. In addition, some have malformations of the structures of the middle ear (Crysdale, 1981; Gould and Caldarelli, 1982; Phillips and Miyamoto, 1986). Both the airway problems

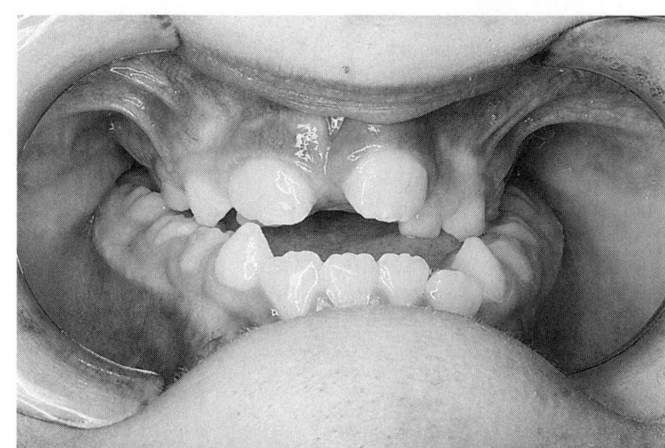

Figure 2-34 Class III malocclusion (underbite) and open bite in Apert syndrome.

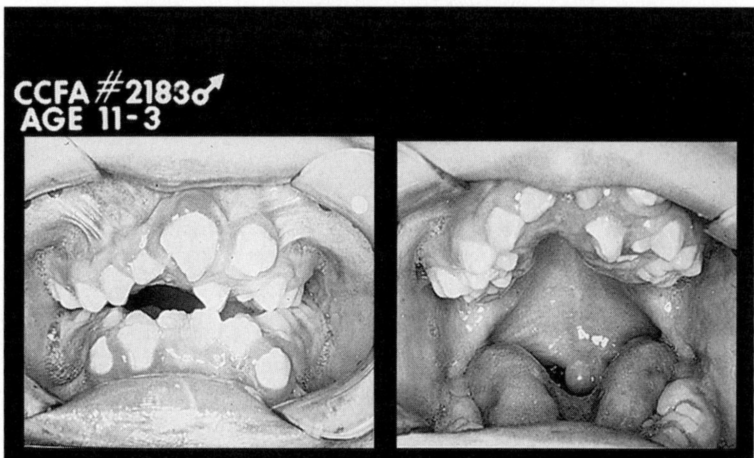

Figure 2-33 The malformed maxilla in Apert syndrome, compressed into a V shape with ectopic eruption of teeth.

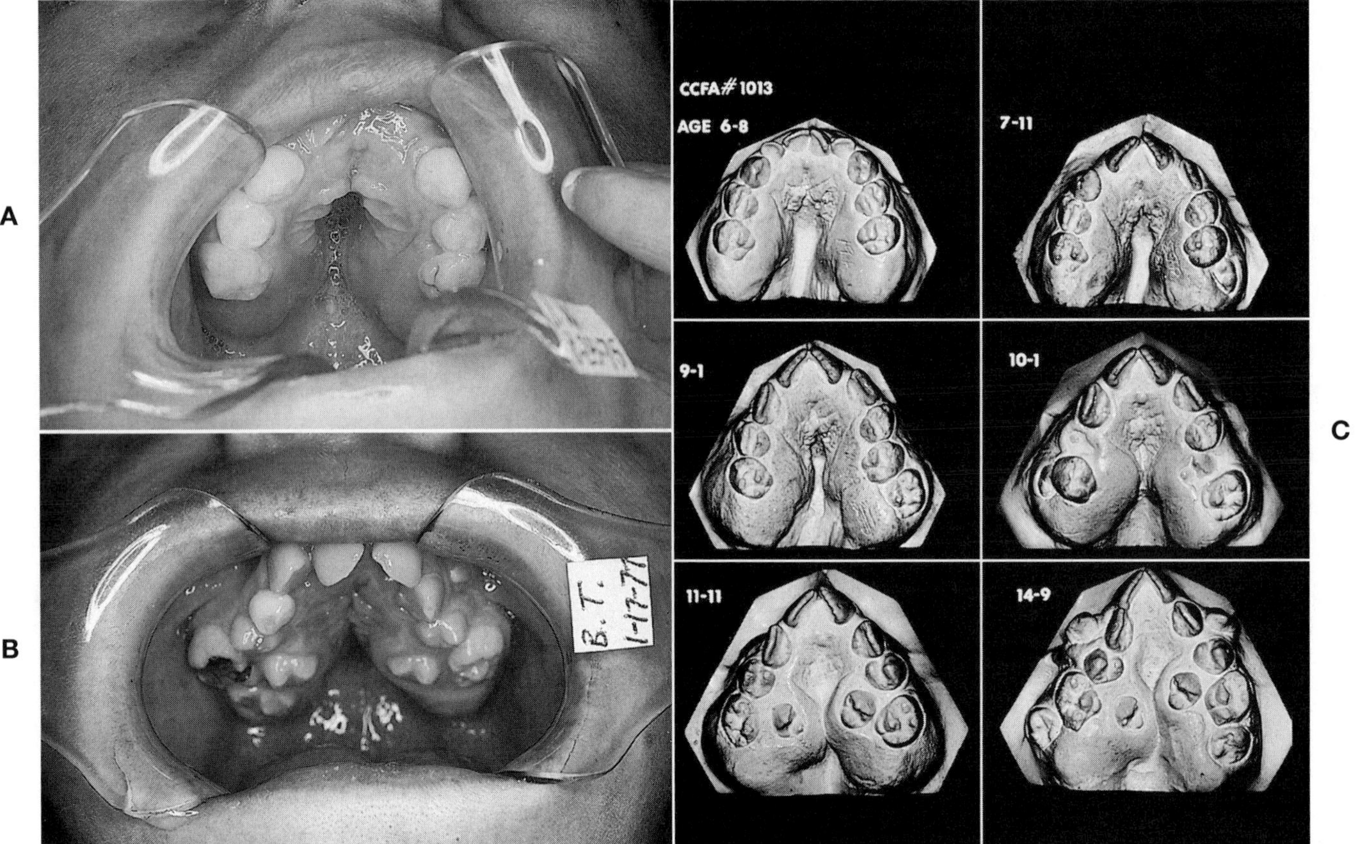

Figure 2-35 **A** to **C,** The accumulations of soft tissue along the palatine shelves in Apert syndrome. **C,** The progressive nature of this problem in serial dental casts of a youngster from ages 6 years 8 months through 14 years 9 months. This configuration often leads to a misdiagnosis of cleft palate.

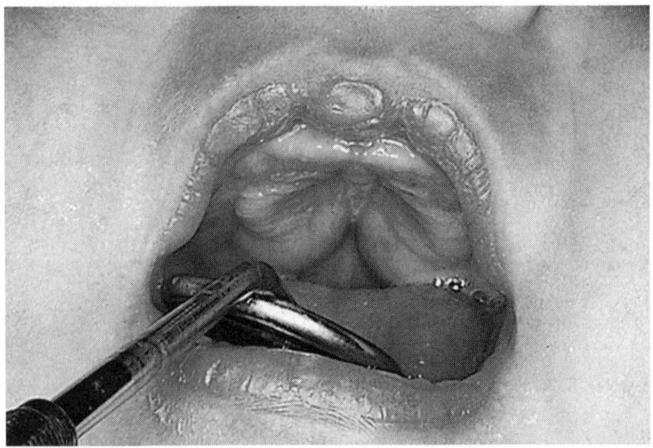

Figure 2-36 The soft tissue accumulations in Apert syndrome are usually visible in the infant's mouth in the early weeks of life.

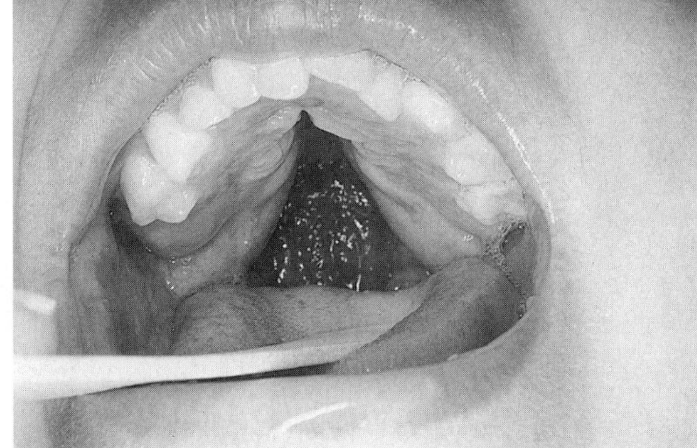

Figure 2-37 An actual palatal cleft in a patient with Apert syndrome.

and the ear problems are in fact common in all the craniofacial synostosis syndromes discussed here.

Not surprisingly, Apert syndrome also includes malformations of the central nervous system (Cohen and Kreiborg, 1990, 1993a; Gupta and Popli, 1995; Renier et al., 1996; Tokumaru et al., 1996). It is difficult to specify a percentage of patients in which these findings are present because not all patients receive evaluations of sufficient rigor or thoroughness to identify such malformations (Gorlin, Cohen, and Levin, 1990). Abnormally high

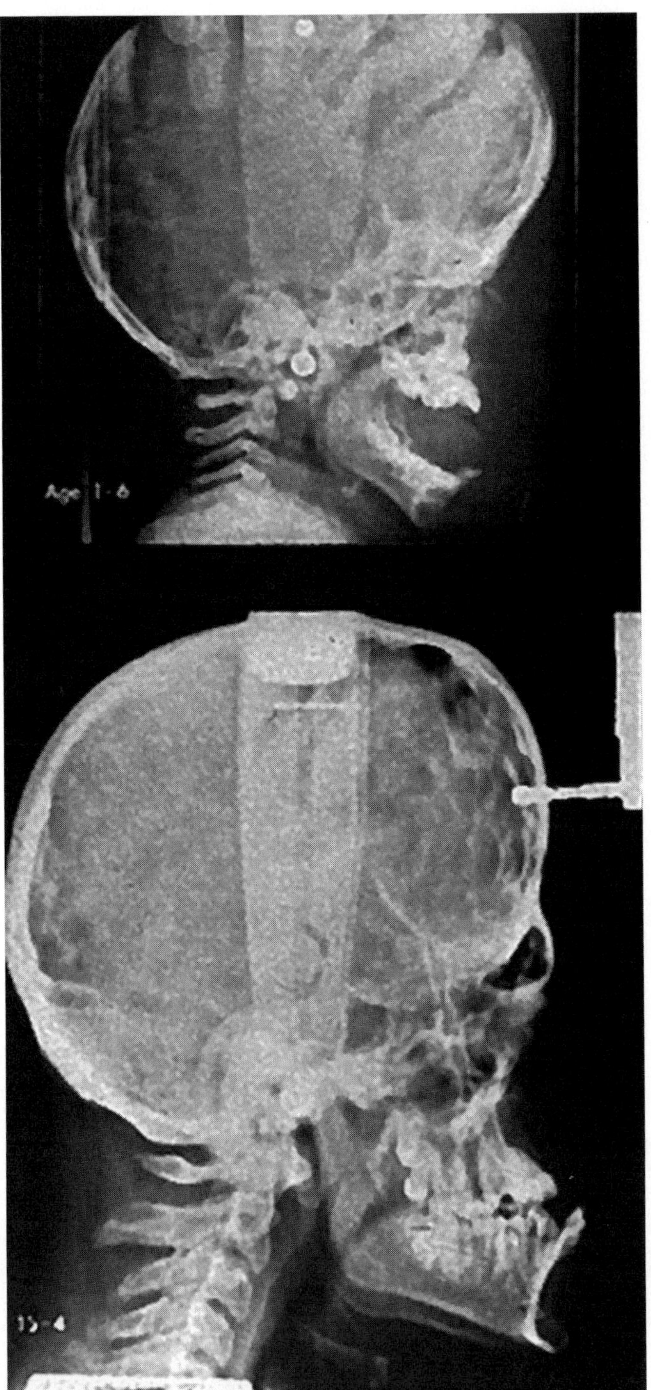

Figure 2-38 Lateral cephalometric films on a patient with Apert syndrome at ages 1 year 6 months and 15 years 4 months. Note the long, thick soft palate already in evidence in the early film and the extreme crowding of the nasopharyngeal airway in the later film.

intracranial pressure and hydrocephalus are frequent problems that are not always eliminated by surgery to release the sutures (Gosain, McCarthy, and Wisoff, 1996; Gosain et al., 1995). Ventriculoperitoneal shunts to reduce the intracranial pressure are often necessary. Cohen and Kreiborg (1990) pointed out that malformations of the

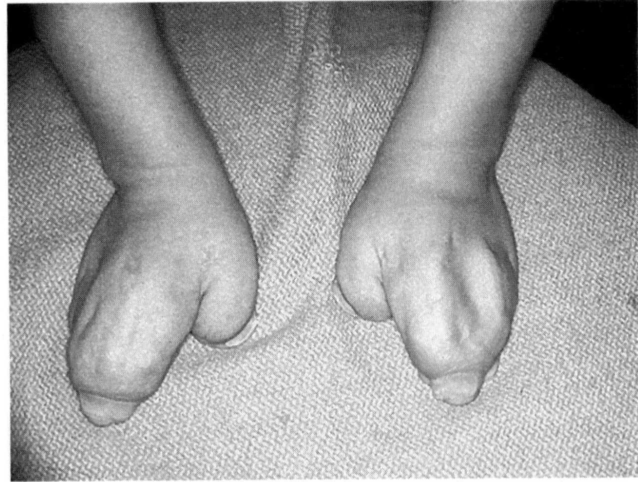

Figure 2-39 Syndactyly of the hands in Apert syndrome.

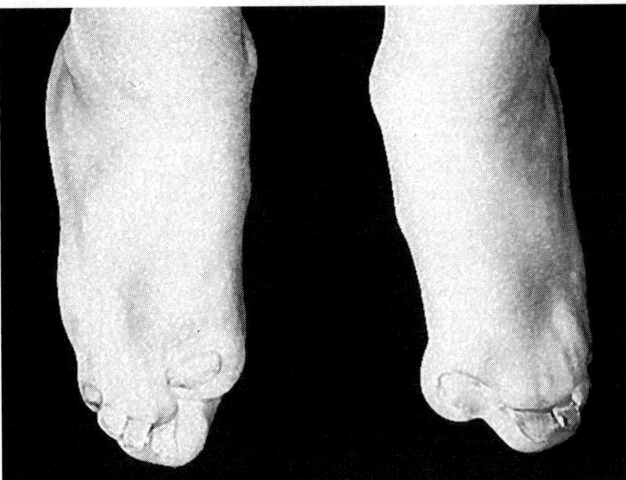

Figure 2-40 Syndactyly of the feet in Apert syndrome.

central nervous system may be responsible for the mental retardation frequently reported in this syndrome.

Mental retardation has long been listed as a common, although not universal, finding in Apert syndrome. In recent years craniofacial teams have attempted to study the relationship between intellectual function and craniofacial surgery and/or neurosurgery.[19] Renier et al. (1996) reported that age at operation for release of craniofacial sutures had a significant effect on later measurements of intelligence: 32% of patients operated on before 1 year of

[19]Craniofacial surgery is basically of four types: surgery to release the stenosis of sutures, surgery to advance the forehead, surgery to advance the midface, and surgery to remodel specific parts of the skull or face, such as the orbits, nose, etc. Within each of these general categories there are subtypes or special modifications. In craniofacial synostosis it is common for the child to undergo release of one or more sutures and advancement of the forehead in the first few months of life. Timing of the remaining surgeries is controversial, especially since results are not consistent.

age had IQs higher than 70 versus only 7.1% of those operated on after 1 year of age. Comparison to other studies is difficult because investigators used different cutoff points. Patton et al. (1988) reported no relationship between IQ testing results and early craniectomies: approximately half of their 29 patients (aged 8 to 35 years) had IQs higher than 70, but none had an IQ more than 100. In a study of 20 children, all of whom had undergone early neurosurgical intervention, LeFebvre and coworkers (LeFebvre et al., 1986) reported a mean full-scale IQ of 73.6, with a range from 52 to 89. Murovic et al. (1993) reported an average IQ of 72.5 on the Wechlser Intelligence Scale for 15 patients with Apert syndrome who had undergone surgery to relieve hydrocephalus within the first year of life. In general, IQ scores clustering around 70 seem to be commonly reported even when the patients have undergone early neurosurgery. However, a few individuals with IQs in the normal range have been reported (Cohen and Kreiborg, 1990).

Clearly there are many threats to overall development and specifically to communication development in Apert syndrome: airway compromise, malocclusion not easily treated by orthodontics alone, probable limitation in mental development, negative psychosocial input because of the severe facial and limb deformities,[20] likelihood of conductive hearing loss, and the effect of multiple hospitalizations and resultant isolation from family and other "normal" sources of stimulation. We have very little data on communication skills in Apert syndrome, perhaps because clinicians who see these patients are aware of the multiple and complex variables affecting each child and adult with Apert syndrome. Articulation and resonance problems presumably attributable to the malocclusion and nasopharyngeal dysmorphologic features have been reported in a few cases (Elfenbein, Waziri, and Morris, 1981; Peterson, 1973). Midface advancement had no effect on articulation or articulation in six cases reported by McCarthy, Coccaro, and Schwartz (1977). Such surgery has been reported to benefit articulation in some patients without congenital anomalies and also in some patients with cleft palate; lack of this improvement may reflect other complications (e.g., anomalous configuration of the palatal vault). In general, clinicians are advised to be alert for all the possible sources of speech and language problems in this population and to follow each patient on a longitudinal basis until maximum habilitation has been attained.

[20]In addition to the other physical problems, approximately 70% of patients have severe, atypical acne that extends onto the forearms (Solomon, Fretzin, and Pruzansky, 1970). This can be one of the most debilitating and disturbing problems for the patient.

Crouzon Syndrome (Craniofacial Dysostosis)

Crouzon syndrome shares many of the deformities and functional problems seen in Apert syndrome, but there is a much wider range of severity. Patients with this disease have malformations of the skull and face (Fig. 2-41) but not the limb deformities found in Apert syndrome. Like Apert syndrome, Crouzon syndrome is caused by mutation of a gene mapped to chromosome 10. The estimated frequency of occurrence is 1:25,000 births (Cohen, 1986). Although the physical and functional problems can be debilitating, many patients function well enough to be active members of society and to mate and reproduce. In Kreiborg's study of 61 patients (1981), 44% were familial and 56% were sporadic. The higher percentage of cases transmitted from parent to child, in comparison to Apert syndrome, is evidence of the relative fitness of Crouzon patients.

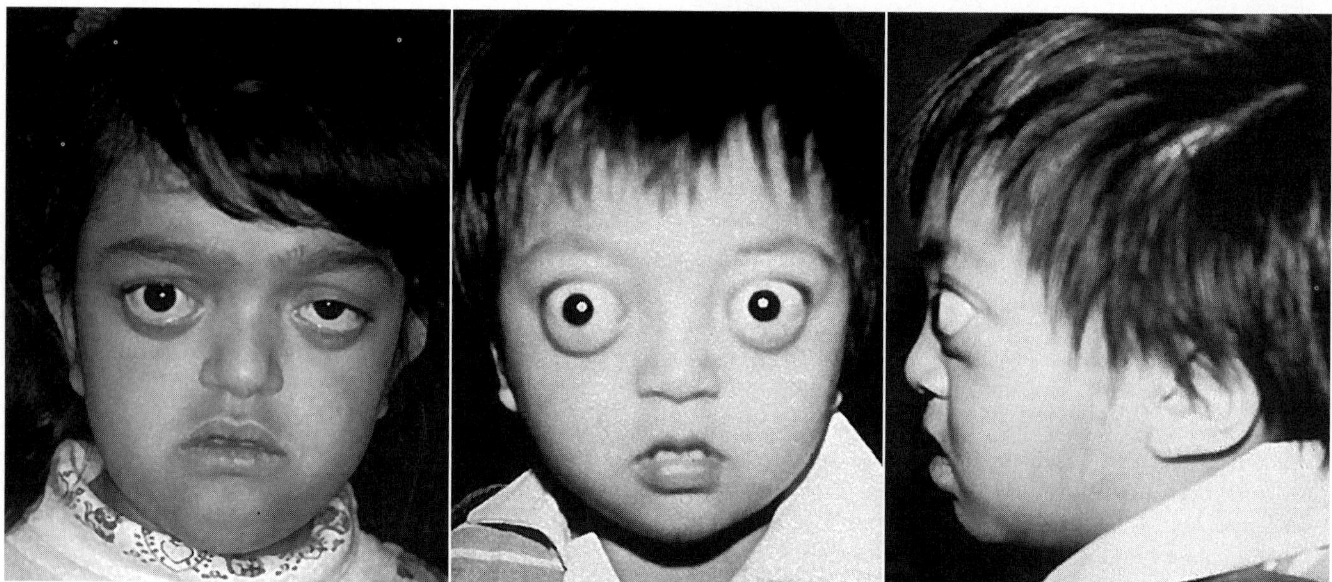

Figure 2-41 Two youngsters with Crouzon syndrome. Exophthalmus is present in both children but is particularly severe in the second child.

Crouzon syndrome entails synostosis of the coronal suture, with a high probability of involvement of the sagittal and lambdoidal sutures as well. Kreiborg (1981) found coronal synostosis in 100% of his cases and combined coronal-sagittal-lambdoidal synostosis in 75%. The synostosis may not be present at birth but usually begins within the first year of life and is complete by 2 to 3 years of age (Cohen, 1986). As in Apert syndrome, the facial features include hypoplasia and retrusion of the midface, shallow orbits, and exophthalmus (also called "ocular proptosis") (Fig. 2-41, *B* and *C*). The proptosis may be so severe that the globes of the eyes pop out in front of the orbital rims. There are many eye problems in patients with Crouzon syndrome (Miller, 1986), including possible atrophy of the optic nerve (Kreiborg, 1981).

The maxillary hypoplasia typically leads to a class III malocclusion; dental crowding and ectopic eruption of teeth are common (Fig. 2-42). Lateral accumulations of soft tissue in the palatal vault occur in an estimated 50% of cases, but usually not to the severe degree seen in Apert syndrome (Kreiborg, 1981; Peterson and Pruzansky, 1974). Cleft palate occurs in some cases (Gorlin, Cohen, and Levin, 1990; Selle and Jacobs, 1977).

As in Apert syndrome, patients with Crouzon syndrome are subject to nasopharyngeal crowding (Fig. 2-43) and chronic respiratory problems, often necessitating tracheotomy (Fig. 2-44) (Chandra-Sekhar, 1979; Crysdale, 1981; Jarund and Lauritzen, 1996; Moore, 1993; Schafer, 1982; Sirotnak, Brodsky, and Pizzuto, 1995). There have also been several reports of anomalous tracheal struc-

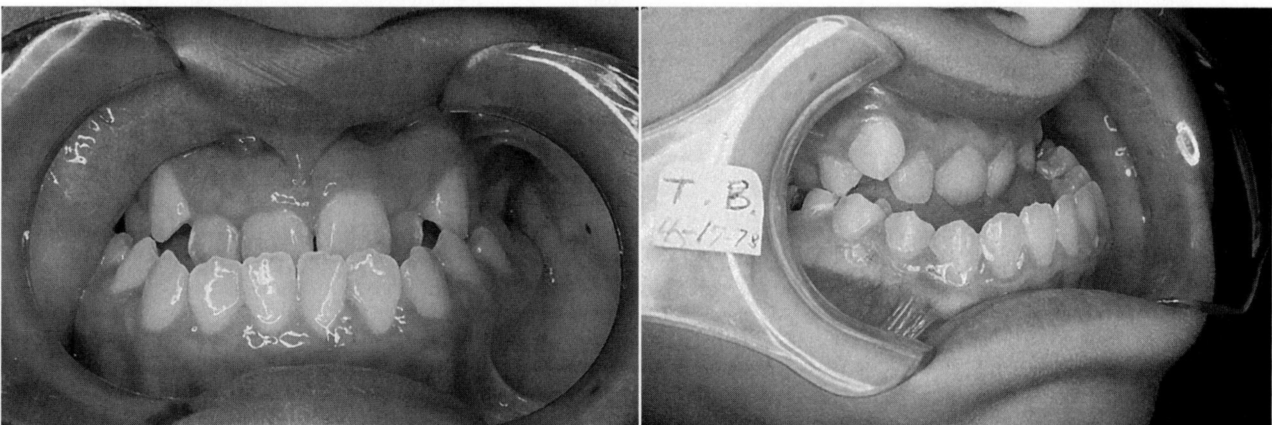

Figure 2-42 Class III malocclusions in Crouzon syndrome.

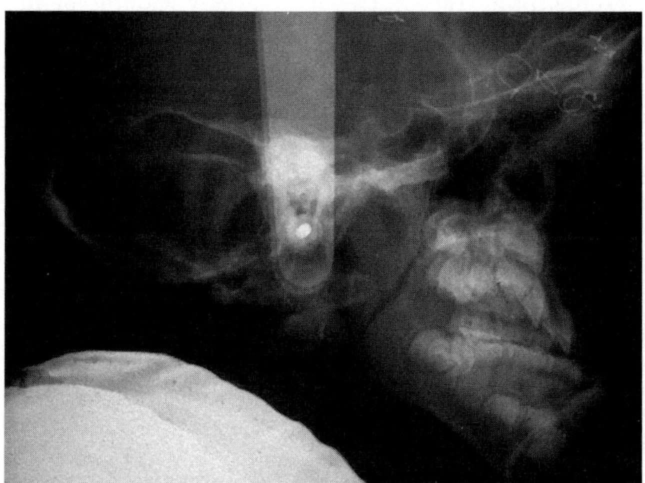

Figure 2-43 Lateral cephalometric film of a patient with Crouzon syndrome demonstrating the extreme crowding of the airway (seen only as a very narrow slit in this patient).

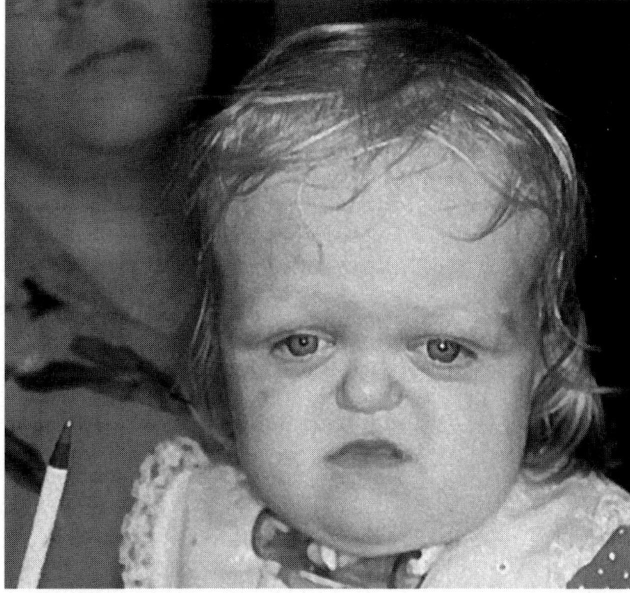

Figure 2-44 Tracheotomy in a toddler with Crouzon syndrome.

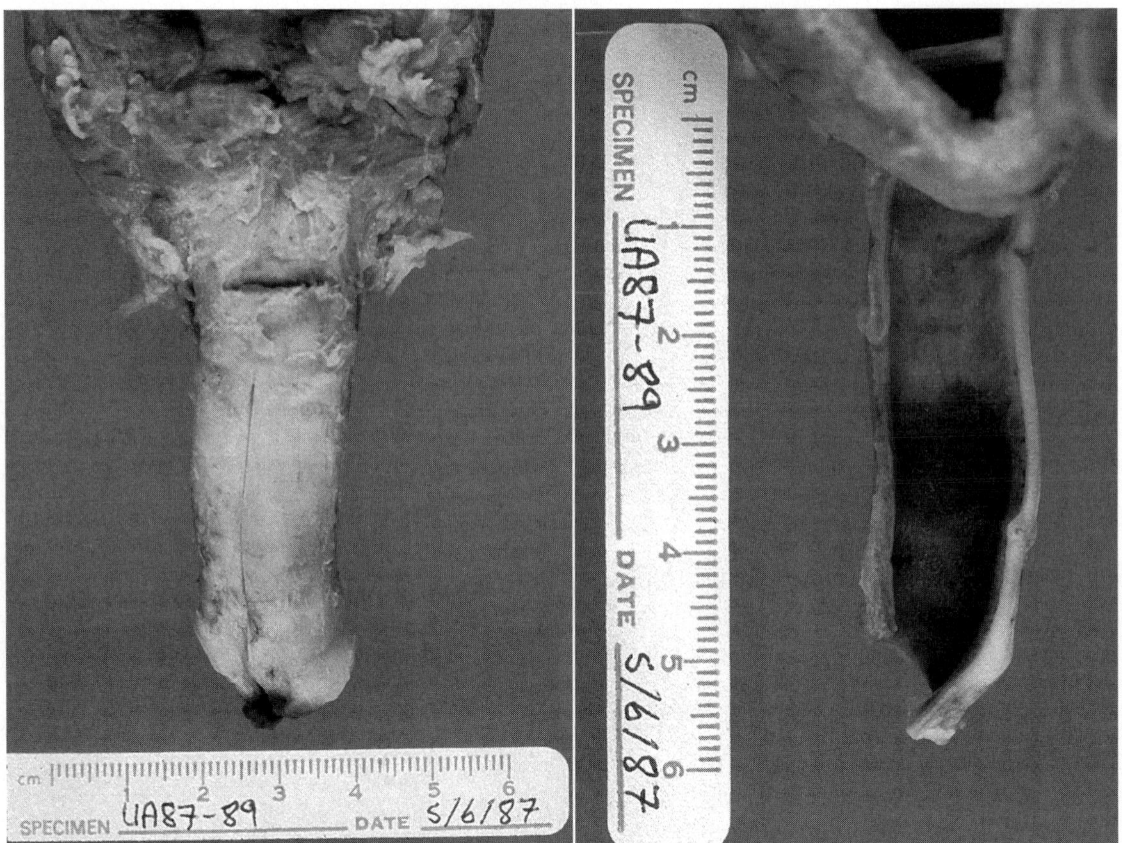

Figure 2-45 Anomalous trachea of a child with Crouzon syndrome who died of extreme respiratory complications. The trachea is essentially one smooth piece of cartilage, without the support of tracheal rings.

ture (Fig. 2-45) (Devine et al., 1984; Sagehashi, 1992; Schmid, 1971).

Cervical spine anomalies are common (Hemmer, McAlister, and Marsh, 1987; Kreiborg, 1981). Malformations of the central nervous system have been reported but not with the high frequency found in Apert syndrome (Proudman et al., 1995; Tokumaru et al., 1996). In the report of Proudman et al. (1995), 51% of 59 patients had enlarged cerebral ventricles and 14% had other central nervous system anomalies.

Although marked mental retardation may be found in some patients with Crouzon syndrome, the range also includes many patients with unimpaired intellectual function. Kreiborg (1981) reported mental deficiency in only 3% of his 61 cases and Proudman et al. (1995) only 12%. (The criteria used for decreased mental function in either of these studies were not specified.)

Otologic disease is common in this syndrome, and it does not necessarily improve as the patient matures. In addition, some patients have malformations of the external and/or middle ear. Kreiborg (1981) reported conductive hearing loss in 55% of his cases and atresia of the external auditory canals in 13%. Corey, Caldarelli, and Gould (1987) found otopathologic conditions in 37% of infants and 62% of older patients with Crouzon syndrome. Cremers and Teunissen (1991) reported one case with ossicular malformations and hypoplasia of the mastoid.

Threats to communication skills in Crouzon syndrome depend to a large extent on the severity of expression of the syndrome in the individual, although even an apparently mildly affected individual may have specific problems such as unrelenting ear disease. In the early months of life, problems with respiration and feeding may preoccupy parents and other caregivers, making it difficult to focus on adequate language stimulation for the child. Later in life the threats to communication may diminish. Many patients with midface retrusion and resultant Class III malocclusion manage to make amazing articulatory adjustments. McCarthy, Coccaro, and Schwartz (1977) reported that hyponasality was eliminated by maxillary advancement in five patients and that some showed improvement in articulation as well. To date, there have been no published reports of onset of velopharyngeal inadequacy in patients with Crouzon syndrome after such advancement.

Pfeiffer Syndrome

Pfeiffer syndrome is a third craniosynostosis syndrome that has been mapped to chromosome 10. Like Apert and Crouzon syndromes, it is autosomal dominant. In this syndrome there is progressive synostosis of both sides (left

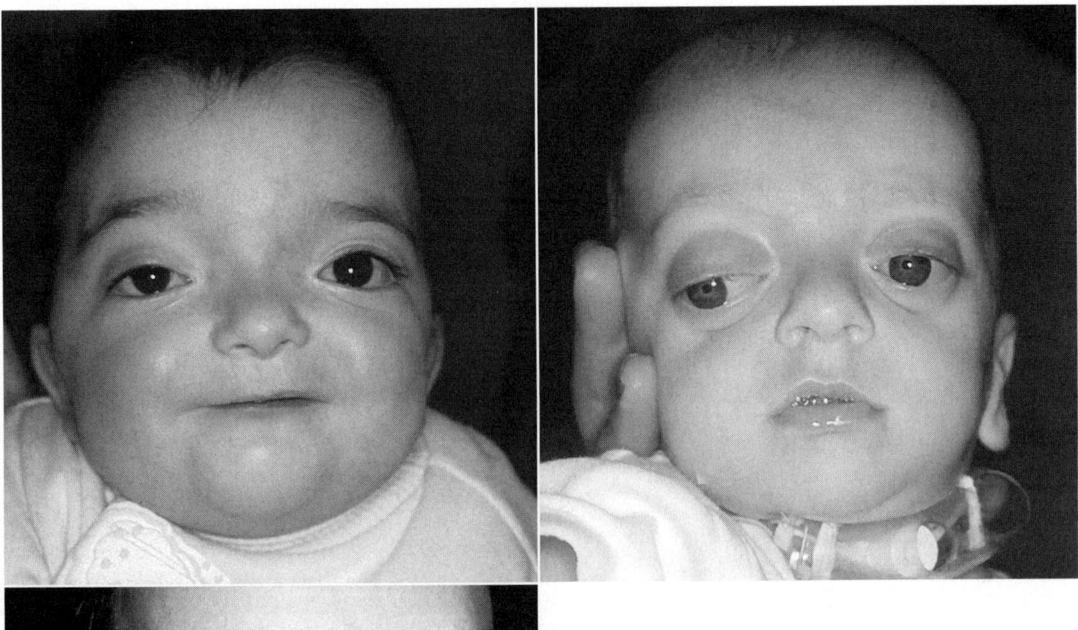

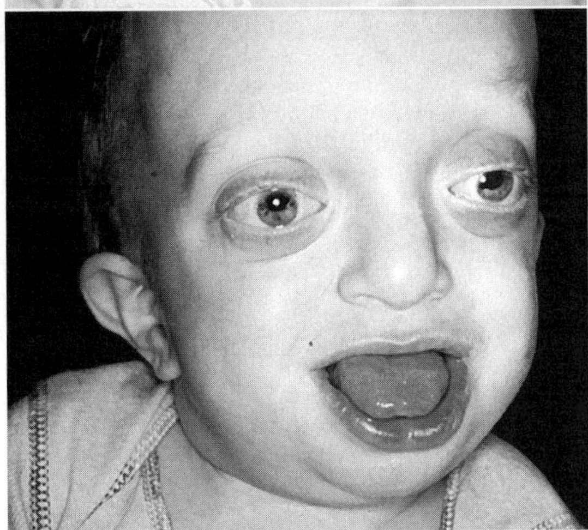

Figure 2-46 Facial features in three babies with Pfeiffer syndrome.

and right) of the coronal suture. Cohen (1993) categorized Pfeiffer syndrome patients into three clinical subtypes, with the classic form as type 1 (Fig. 2-46). In Pfeiffer type 2, there is a cloverleaf-shaped skull resulting from synostosis of virtually all of the cranial sutures,[21] severe ocular proptosis, severe involvement of the central nervous system, ankylosis or synostosis of the elbows, and a cluster of variable low-frequency anomalies. These patients usually do poorly and die early in life (Cohen, 1993; Moore et al., 1995). Cohen (1993) added a suspected type 3 of Pfeiffer syndrome, in which there is no cloverleaf skull but there is ocular proptosis, shallow orbits, marked shortness of the anterior cranial base, and a poor prognosis. All known cases of types 2 and 3 have been sporadic, as would be expected given the poor prognosis. However, Pfeiffer type 1 is compatible with life and these patients may reproduce.

[21]Cloverleaf or "kleeblatschadl" skull can occur in other craniosynostosis syndromes as well.

In classic cases, the facial features are similar to those of Apert syndrome: depressed nasal bridge with a prominent nasal dome, maxillary hypoplasia with resultant malocclusion; and dental crowding. The facial features are even more exaggerated in Pfeiffer type 2 (Fig. 2-47). Patients have broad thumbs and great toes (Fig. 2-48) and partial soft tissue syndactyly of the hands (Cohen, 1993; Moore, Lodge, and Clark, 1995b). Depending on the severity of the deformities in individual cases, these patients are subject to the same nasopharyngeal crowding (Fig. 2-49) and respiratory problems described in Apert and Crouzon syndromes (Jarund and Lauritzen, 1996; Moore, 1993; Perkins et al., 1997). In addition, there may be congenital anomalies of the trachea (Stone et al., 1990). The bony abnormalities include vertebral fusion, particularly in the cervical spine (Anderson et al., 1996; Hemmer, McAlister, and Marsh, 1987; Moore, Lodge, and Clark, 1995a).

Vallino-Napoli (1996) reported a high prevalence of stenosis or atresia of the auditory canal, middle ear hypoplasia, and ossicular hypoplasia in nine patients with

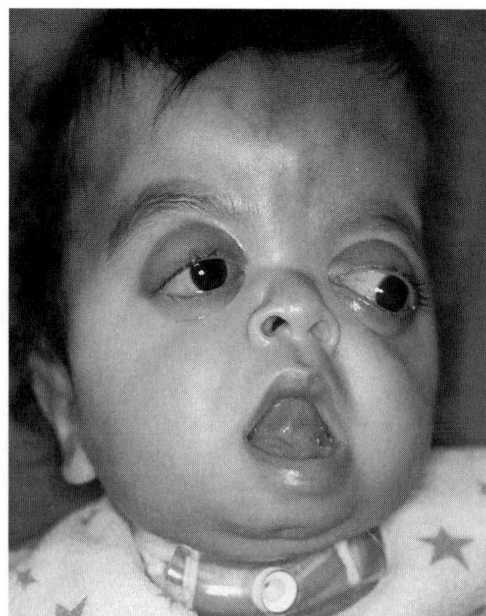

Figure 2-47 Facial deformities in an infant with Pfeiffer type 2.

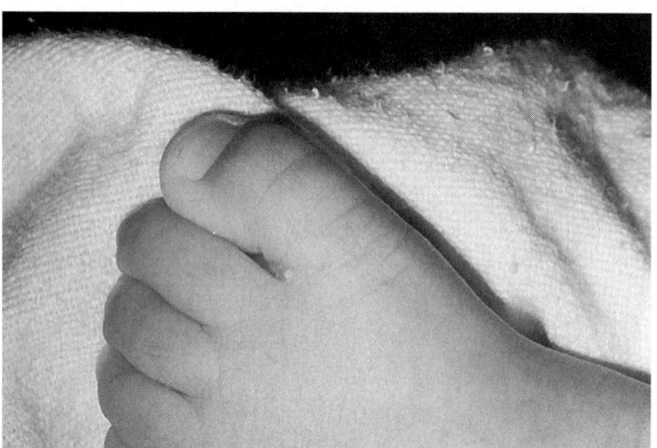

Figure 2-48 Broad great toe in Pfeiffer syndrome.

Pfeiffer syndrome. These conditions, together with recurrent middle ear disease, predispose patients to conductive hearing loss (Cremers, 1981; Martsolf et al., 1971; Vallino-Napoli, 1996).

Speech-language pathologists are more likely to become involved with the habilitation of patients with type 1 Pfeiffer syndrome than with types 2 or 3, although if children with types 2 or 3 live long enough to make communication attempts the speech-language pathologist may be called on to help implement alternative means of communication (e.g., rudimentary sign language, communication boards, etc.). In type I Pfeiffer syndrome the hazards to communication skills are primarily the malocclusion and the hearing loss. Some patients exhibit mild to moderate deficiency in intellectual function, but most exhibit normal intelligence (Cohen, 1993). Many are

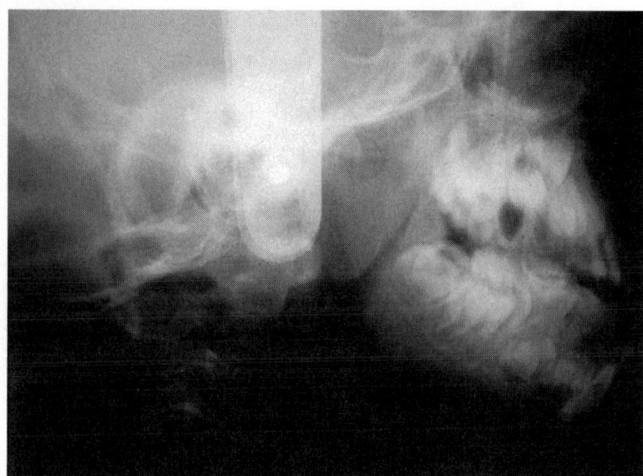

Figure 2-49 Extreme crowding of the airway in Pfeiffer syndrome. This boy (seen as an infant in Fig. 2-46, C) is now a teenager and continues to require a tracheotomy despite midface advancement (which had not been done at time this film was taken).

hyponasal because of the crowding of the nasopharyngeal airway. Tracheotomies are sometimes necessary, even in later childhood, especially if midface advancement does not provide a larger pharyngeal airway.

Saethre-Chotzen Syndrome

Saethre-Chotzen syndrome was first described in the 1930s (Chotzen, 1932; Saethre, 1932). It is characterized by a variable pattern of malformations that includes craniosynostosis, low frontal hairline, facial asymmetry, ptosis (drooping) of the eyelids (Fig. 2-50), deviated nasal septum, various skeletal anomalies, and digital findings including brachydactyly (short fingers) and partial soft tissue syndactyly (Gorlin, Cohen, and Levin, 1990). This is yet another autosomal dominant condition); it has been mapped to a genetic mutation on chromosome 7 (Brueton et al., 1992; Reardon et al., 1993).

Craniosynostosis is not an obligatory finding in Saethre-Chotzen syndrome, but it is usually present and usually involves the coronal suture (Cohen, 1986). The timing of onset of the synostosis and the ultimate degree of involvement is quite variable (Gorlin, Cohen, and Levin, 1990). The forehead is high and may be either sloping or protuberant. The eyes are usually wide set ("hypertelorie").

The maxilla may be hypoplastic, with a narrow dental arch and resultant malocclusion. There have been sporadic reports of cleft palate, extra teeth, and other dental defects (Bartsocas, Weber, and Crawford, 1970; Cohen, 1986; Friedman et al., 1977; Gorlin, Cohen, and Levin, 1990; Pantke et al., 1975). The ears may be low set and posteriorly rotated or may exhibit other minor anomalies. Conductive

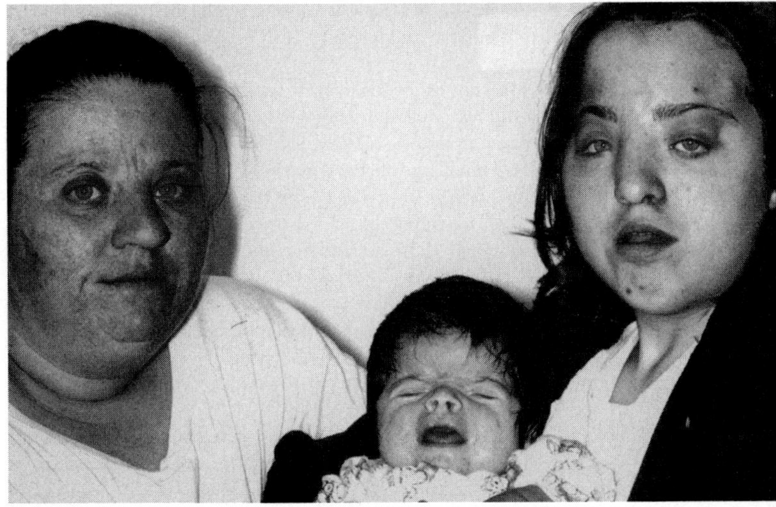

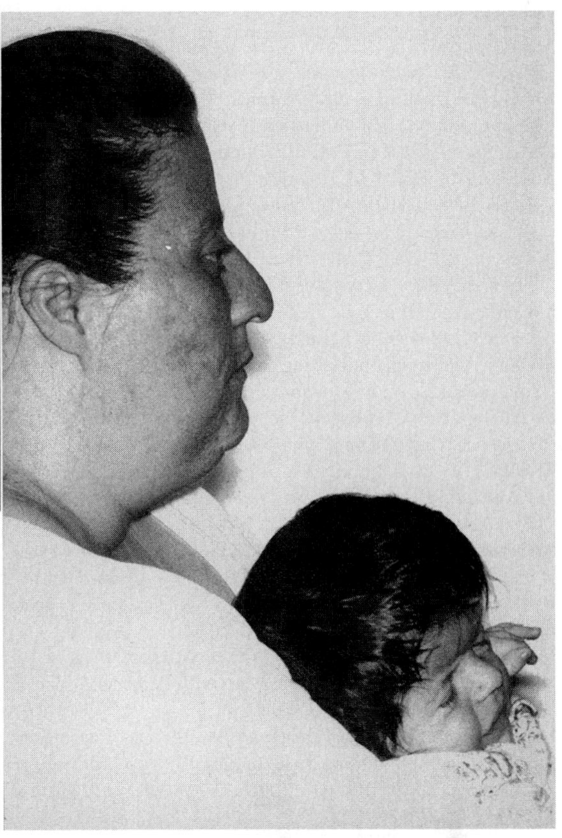

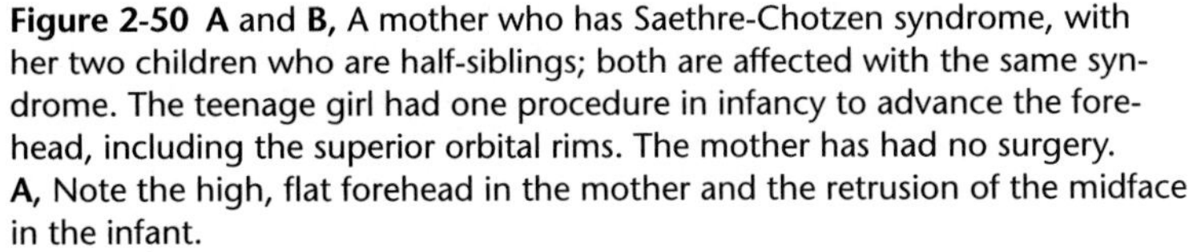
Figure 2-50 **A** and **B,** A mother who has Saethre-Chotzen syndrome, with her two children who are half-siblings; both are affected with the same syndrome. The teenage girl had one procedure in infancy to advance the forehead, including the superior orbital rims. The mother has had no surgery. **A,** Note the high, flat forehead in the mother and the retrusion of the midface in the infant.

hearing loss is common (Ensink et al., 1996; Konigsmark and Gorlin, 1976, Pantke et al., 1975).

Recent studies have revealed cervical spine fusions in approximately 50% of examined cases (Anderson et al., 1997) and various types of involvement of the central nervous system (Elia et al., 1996).

There is a wide range of expression of this syndrome, and many individuals are so mildly affected that they are asymptomatic and go undiagnosed. The danger for undiagnosed individuals is, of course, that they will not be aware that they carry a 50% chance of transmitting the syndrome to their children. In more severely involved cases the concerns are likely to be airway problems, malocclusion, and hearing loss, as well as variable speech problems.

A POSTSCRIPT REGARDING SURGICAL HABILITATION OF MULTI-ANOMALY CLEFT DISORDERS

By now you realize that both the nonsurgical and surgical habilitation for most of the patients described in this chapter are likely to be long term, complex, and mutually interrelated or interdependent over several years of the child's life. There are multiple sources both in the print media and in on-line computer sources for you to learn about current treatment as you deal with any of these patients. It may provide you with a useful perspective to know that, before the early 1970s, the only "reconstructive" surgical procedures available for many of these patients, at least in the United States, consisted of more or less compartmentalized, palliative treatments (e.g., advancements or set-backs of the mandible). With the advent of Tessier's revolutionary craniofacial surgery (Tessier 1967, 1971), the entire approach to habilitation of patients with mandibulofacial dysostosis, the premature craniosynostosis syndromes, and other disorders changed dramatically. Faces began to be "re-made" rather than simply remodeled. Some patients experienced such drastic changes in their own appearance that psychological problems ensued, especially if they were not adequately prepared for the changes about to take place. Craniofacial teams depend on the expertise of professionals in the psychosocial fields to assess the status of patients and their families and to help prepare them for both surgery and the postsurgical outcome. Patients and families are often misled either by their own hopes or the optimistic predictions of caregivers. For example, when parents of a child with microtia are told that the outer ear will be "reconstructed," they may expect that such surgery will provide their youngster with normal hearing on the affected side plus a normal appearance of the ear itself. The opportunities for confusion, heartbreak, and anger increase nearly in proportion to the complexity of the craniofacial deformity. Each professional on the craniofacial team, including the speech-language pathologist, must be sufficiently prepared to assist families as they face surgery and other physical interventions and to avoid misleading them into unrealistic expectations.

REFERENCES

Abe K, Ishikawa N, and Murakami Y: Goldenhar's syndrome associated with cardiac malformations. *Helvetica Paediatria Acta* 30:57-60, 1975.

Altman DH, Altman NR, Mitnick RJ, and Shprintzen RJ: Further delineation of brain anomalies in velo-cardio-facial syndrome [letter]. *American Journal of Medical Genetics* 60:174-175, 1995.

Anderson PJ, Hall CM, Evans RD, Hayward RD, Harkness WJ, and Jones BM: The cervical spine in Saethre-Chotzen syndrome. *Cleft Palate–Craniofacial Journal* 34:79-82, 1997.

Anderson PJ, Hall CM, Evans RD, Jones BM, Harkness W, and Hayward RD: Cervical spine in Pfeiffer's syndrome. *Journal of Craniofacial Surgery* 7:275-279, 1996.

Anneren G, Andersson T, Lindgren PG, and Kjartansson S: Ectrodactyly-ectodermal dysplasia-clefting syndrome (EEC): the clinical variation and prenatal diagnosis. *Clinical Genetics* 40:257-262, 1991.

Argamaso RV: Glossopexy for upper airway obstruction in Robin sequence. *Cleft Palate–Craniofacial Journal* 29:232-238, 1992.

Arvystas M, and Shprintzen RJ: Craniofacial morphology in the velo-cardio-facial syndrome. *Journal of Craniofacial Genetics and Developmental Biology* 4:39-45, 1984.

Arvystas M, and Shprintzen RJ: Craniofacial morphology in Treacher Collins syndrome. *Cleft Palate-Craniofacial Journal* 26:14-22, 1991.

Bartsocas CS, Weber AL, and Crawford JD: Chotzen's syndrome. *Journal of Pediatrics* 77:267-272, 1970.

Bassila MK, and Goldberg RB: The association of facial palsy and/or sensorineural hearing loss in patients with hemifacial microsomia. *Cleft Palate Journal* 26:287-291, 1989.

Beemer FA, de Nef JJEM, Delleman JW, Bleeker-Wagemakers EM, and Shprintzen RJ: Additional eye findings in a girl with the velo-cardio-facial syndrome [letter]. *American Journal of Medical Genetics* 24:541-542, 1986.

Benjamin B, and Walker P: Management of airway obstruction in the Pierre Robin sequence. *International Journal of Pediatric Otorhinolaryngology* 22:29-37, 1991.

Bergoin M, Giraud J-P, and Chaix C: L'hyomandibulopexie dans le traitment des formes graves du syndrome de Pierre Robin. *Annales Chirugie Infant* 2:85-90, 1971.

Bergstrom L, Hemenway W, and Sando I: Pathological changes in congenital deafness. *Laryngoscope* 82:1777-1792, 1972.

Berry GA: Note on a congenital defect (?coloboma) of the lower lid. *Royal London Ophthalmologic Hospital* Report 12:255-257, 1889.

Bocian M, and Walker AP: Lip pits and deletion 1q32-41. *American Journal of Medical Genetics* 26:437-443, 1987.

Book JA, and Fraccaro J: Genetical investigations in a North-Swedish population mandibulofacial dysostosis. *Acta Genetica et Statistica Medica* 5:327-333, 1955.

Brown DM, Nichols BE, Weingeist TA, Sheffield VC, Kimura AE, and Stone EM: Procollagen II gene mutation in Stickler syndrome. *Archives of Ophthalmology* 110:1589-1593, 1992.

Brueton LA, van Herwerden I, Chotai KA, and Winter RM: The mapping of a gene for craniosynostosis: evidence for linkage of the Saethre-Chotzen syndrome to distal chromosome 7p. *Journal of Medical Genetics* 29:681-685, 1992.

Brunner HG, van Beersum SE, Warman ML, Olsen BR, Ropers HH, and Mariman EC: A Stickler syndrome gene is linked to chromosome 6 near the COL11A2 gene. *Human Molecular Genetics* 3:1561-1564, 1994.

Bull MJ, Given DC, Sadove M, Bixler D, and Hearn D: Improved outcome in Pierre Robin sequence: effect of multidisciplinary evaluation and management. *Pediatrics* 86:294-301, 1990.

Burdick AB, Bixler D, and Puckett CL: Genetic analysis in families with van der Woude syndrome. *Journal of Craniofacial Genetics and Developmental Biology* 5:181-208, 1985.

Buss PW, Hughes HE, and Clarke A: Twenty-four cases of the EEC syndrome: clinical presentation and management. *Journal of Medical Genetics* 32:716-723, 1995.

Bystrom E, Snager R, and Stewart R: The syndrome of ectrodactyly, ectodermal dysplasia and clefting (EEC). *Journal of Oral Surgery* 33:192-198, 1975.

Caldarelli D, Hutchinson J, Pruzansky S, and Valvassori G: A comparison of microtia and temporal bone anomalies in hemifacial microsomia and mandibulofacial dysostosis. *Cleft Palate Journal* 17:103-110, 1980.

Calnan JS: Congenital large pharynx: a new syndrome with a report of 41 personal cases. *British Journal of Plastic Surgery* 24:263-271, 1971.

Caouette-Laberge L, Bayet B, and Larocque Y: The Pierre Robin sequence: review of 125 cases and evolution of treatment modalities. *Plastic and Reconstructive Surgery* 93:934-942, 1994.

Cervenka J, Gorlin RJ, and Anderson VE: The syndrome of pits of the lower lip and cleft lip and/or palate: genetic considerations. *American Journal of Human Genetics* 19:416-432, 1967.

Champion R: Treatment of cleft palate associated with micrognathia. *British Journal of Plastic Surgery* 8:283-290, 1956.

Chandra-Sekhar H: Airway problems in craniofacial dysostosis. In Converse J, McCarthy JG, and Wood-Smith D (eds.): *Symposium on Diagnosis and Treatment of Craniofacial Anomalies.* St. Louis: CV Mosby, 1979, pp. 274-276.

Chemke J, Mogilner BM, Ben-Litzhak I, Zurkowski L, and Ophir D: Autosomal recessive inheritance of Nager acrofacial dysostosis. *Journal of Medical Genetics* 25:230-232, 1988.

Chiang TP, and Robinson GC: Ectrodactyly, ectodermal dysplasia, and cleft lip/palate syndrome: the importance of dental anomalies. *Journal of Dentistry for Children* 41:38-42, 1974.

Chin M, and Toth BA: Distraction osteogenesis in maxillofacial surgery using internal devices: review of five cases. *Journal of Oral and Maxillofacial Surgery* 54:45-53, 1996.

Chotzen F: Eine eigenqrtige familiare Entwicklungwsstorung. (Akrocephalosyndaktylie, Dysostosis craniofacialis und Hypertelorismus. *Monatsschrift Kinderheilkunde* 55:97-122, 1932.

Chow EWC, Bassett AS, and Weksberg R: Velo-cardio-facial syndrome and psychotic disorders: implications for psychiatric genetics. *American Journal of Medical Genetics* 54:107-112, 1994.

Chrzanowska KH, Fryns JP, Krajewska-Walasek M, Wisniewski L, and Van den Berghe J: Phenotype variability in the Miller acrofacial dysostosis syndrome. Report of two further patients. *Clinical Genetics* 35:157-160, 1989.

Cohen MM Jr: The Robin anomalad—its nonspecificity and associated syndromes. *Journal of Oral Surgery* 34:587-593, 1976.

Cohen MM Jr: Syndromes with cleft lip and palate. *Cleft Palate Journal* 15:306-328, 1978.

Cohen MM Jr: *The child with multiple birth defects.* New York: Raven Press, 1982.

Cohen MM Jr: *Craniosynotosis: diagnosis, evaluation, and management.* New York: Raven Press, 1986.

Cohen MM Jr: Pfeiffer syndrome update, clinical subtypes, and guidelines for differential diagnosis. *American Journal of Medical Genetics* 45:300-307, 1993.

Cohen MM Jr, and Bankier A: Syndrome delineation involving orofacial clefting. *Cleft Palate–Craniofacial Journal* 28:119-120, 1991.

Cohen MM Jr, and Kreiborg S: The central nervous system in the Apert syndrome. *American Journal of Medical Genetics* 35:36-45, 1990.

Cohen MM Jr, and Kreiborg S: An updated pediatric perspective on the Apert syndrome. *American Journal of Diseases of Children* 147:989-993, 1993a.

Cohen MM Jr, and Kreiborg S: Growth pattern in the Apert syndrome. *American Journal of Medical Genetics* 47:617-623, 1993b.

Cohen MM Jr, and Kreiborg S: Skeletal abnormalities in the Apert syndrome. *American Journal of Medical Genetics* 47:624-632, 1993c.

Cohen MM Jr, and Kreiborg S: Visceral anomalies in the Apert syndrome [see comments]. *American Journal of Medical Genetics* 45:758-760, 1993d.

Cohen MM Jr, Rollnick BR, and Kaye CI: Oculoauriculovertebral spectrum: an updated critique. *Cleft Palate Journal* 26:276-286, 1989.

Colmenero C, Esteban R, Albarino AR, and Colmenero B: Sleep apnoea syndrome associated with maxillofacial abnormalities. *The Journal of Laryngology and Otology* 105:94-100, 1991.

Converse JM, McCarthy J, Coccaro P, and Wood-Smith D: *Clinical aspects of craniofacial microsomia.* In Converse JM, McCarthy J, and Wood-Smith D (eds.): St. Louis: CV Mosby, 1979, pp. 461-475.

Corey JP, Caldarelli DD, and Gould HJ: Otopathology in cranial facial dysostosis. *American Journal of Otology* 8:14-17, 1987.

Costaras-Volarich M, and Pruzansky S: Is the mandible intrinsically different in Apert and Crouzon syndromes? *American Journal of Orthodontics* 85:475-487, 1984.

Cremers CWRJ: Hearing loss in Pfeiffer's syndrome. *International Journal of Pediatric Otorhinolaryngology* 8:343-353, 1981.

Cremers CWRJ, and Teunissen E: The impact of a syndrome diagnosis on surgery for congenital minor ear anomalies. *International Journal of Pediatric Otorhinolaryngology* 22:59-74, 1991.

Croft C, Shprintzen RJ, Daniller A, and Lewin M: The occult submucous cleft palate and the musculus uvulae. *Cleft Palate Journal* 15:150-154, 1978.

Crysdale W: Otorhinolaryngologic problems in patients with craniofacial anomalies. *Otolaryngologic Clinics of North America* 14:145-155, 1981.

D'Antonio LL, and Marsh JL: Abnormal carotid arteries in the velocardiofacial syndrome. *Plastic and Reconstructive Surgery* 80:471-472, 1987.

Danziger I, Brodsky L, Perry R, Nusbaum S, Bernat F, and Robinson L: Nager acrofacial dysostosis: case report and review of the literature. *International Journal of Pediatric Otorhinolaryngology* 20:225-240, 1990.

Delorme R-P, Larocque Y, and Caouette-Laberge L: Innovative surgical approach for the Pierre Robin anomalad: subperiosteal release of the floor of the mouth musculature. *Plastic and Reconstructive Surgery* 83:960-964, 1989.

Demarquay JN: Quelques considerations sur le bec-de-lievre. *Gazette Medicale de Paris* 13:52-53, 1845.

Devine P, Bhan I, Feingold M, Leonidas JC, and Wolpert SM: Completely cartilaginous trachea in a child with Crouzon syndrome. *American Journal of Diseases of Childhood* 138:40-43, 1984.

Dixon MJ, Marres HA, Edwards SJ, Dixon J, and Cremers CW: Treacher Collins syndrome: correlation between clinical and genetic linkage studies. *Clinical Dysmorphology* 3:96-103, 1994.

Dixon MJ, Read AP, Donnai D, Colley A, Dixon J, and Williamson R: The gene for Treacher Collins syndrome maps to the long arm of chromosome 5. *American Journal of Human Genetics* 49:17-22, 1991.

Donnai D, Hughes E, and Winter RM: Syndromes of the month: postaxial acrofacial dysostosis (Miller) syndrome. *Journal of Medical Genetics* 29:422-425, 1987.

Douglas B: The treatment of micrognathia associated with obstruction by a plastic operation. *Plastic and Reconstructive Surgery* 1:300-308, 1946.

Douglas B: A further report on the treatment of micrognathia with obstruction by a plastic procedure. *Plastic and Reconstructive Surgery* 5:113-122, 1950.

Driscoll DA, Spinner NB, Budarf ML, McDonald-McGinn DM, Zackal EH, Goldberg RB, Shprintzen RJ, Saal RM, Zonana J, Jones MC, Mascarello JT, and Emanuel BS: Deletions and microdeletions of 22q11.2 in velo-cardio-facial syndrome. *American Journal of Medical Genetics* 44:261-268, 1992.

Edery P, Manach Y, Le Merrer J, Till M, Vignal A, Lyonnet S, and Munnich A: Apparent genetic homogeneity of the Treacher Collins–Franceschetti syndrome. *American Journal of Medical Genetics* 52:174-177, 1994.

Elfenbein J, Waziri M, and Morris HL: Verbal communication skills of six children with craniofacial anomalies. *Cleft Palate Journal* 18:59-64, 1981.

Elia M, Musumeci SA, Ferri R, Greco D, Romano C, Del Gracco S, and Stefanini MC: Saethre-Chotzen syndrome: a clinical, EEG and neuroradiological study. *Child's Nervous System* 12:699-704, 1996.

Elliott MA, Studen-Pavlovich DA, and Ranalli DN: Prevalence of selected pediatric conditions in children with Pierre Robin sequence. *Pediatric Dentistry* 17:106-111, 1995.

Ensink RJ, Marres HA, Brunner HG, and Cremers CW: Hearing loss in the Saethre-Chotzen syndrome. *Journal of Laryngology and Otology* 110:952-957, 1996.

Fara M, Hrivnakova J, and Sedlackova E: Submucous cleft palates. *Acta Chirurgiae Plasticae* (Prague) 13:221-234, 1971.

Fazen LE, Elmore J, and Nadler HL: Mandibulo-facial dysostosis. *American Journal of Diseases of Children* 113:405-410, 1967.

Figueroa AA: Commentary on craniofacial morphology in Treacher Collins syndrome. *Cleft Palate-Craniofacial Journal* 18:230-231, 1991.

Figueroa AA, and Pruzansky S: The external ear, mandible and other components of hemifacial microsomia. *Journal of Maxillofacial Surgery* 4:200-211, 1982.

Figueroa AA, Glupker TJ, Fitz MG, and BeGole EA: Mandible, tongue, and airway in Pierre Robin sequence: a longitudinal cephalometric study. *Cleft Palate–Craniofacial Journal* 28:425-434, 1991.

Finkelstein Y, Hauben DJ, Talmi YP, Nachmani A, and Zohar Y: Occult and overt submucous cleft palate from peroral examination to nasoendoscopy and back again. *International Journal of Pediatric Otorhinolaryngology* 23:25-34, 1992.

Finkelstein Y, Zohar Y, Nachmani A, Talmi YP, Lerner MA, Hauben DB, and Frydman M: The otolaryngologist and the patient with velocardiofacial syndrome. *Archives of Otolaryngology–Head and Neck Surgery* 119:563-569, 1993.

Fogh-Andersen P: Fistula labii inferioris congenita. *Tandlaegebladet* 1943:411-417.

Franceschetti A, and Klein D: Mandibulo-facial dysostosis: new hereditary syndrome. *Acta Ophthalmologica* (Copenhagen) 27:143-224, 1949.

Franceschini P, Vardeau MP, Guala A, Franceschini D, Testa A, Corrias A, and Chiabotto P: Lower lip pits and complete idiopathic prococious puberty in a patient with Kabuki make-up (Kabuki Kuroki) syndrome. *American Journal of Medical Genetics* 47:423-425, 1993.

Francomano CA, Liberfarb RM, Hirose T, Maumenee H, Streeten EA, Meyers DA, and Pyeritz RE: The Stickler syndrome: evidence for close linkage to the structural gene for type II collagen. *Genomics* 1:293-296, 1987.

Friedman JM, Hanson JW, Graham CB, and Smith DW: Saethre-Chotzen syndrome: a broad and variable pattern of skeletal malformations. *Journal of Pediatrics* 91:929-933, 1977.

Friedman RA, Wood E, Pransky SM, Seid AM, and Kearns DB: Nager acrofacial dysostosis: management of a difficult airway. *International Journal of Pediatric Otorhinolaryngology* 35:69-72, 1996.

Friedman S, and Saraclar M: The high frequency of congenita heart disease in oculo-auriculo-vertebral dysplasia (Goldenhar's syndrome) [letter]. *Journal of Pediatrics* 85:874, 1974.

Fryns JP, and Van den Berghe H: Brief clinical report: acrofacial dysostosis with postaxial limb deficiency. *American Journal of Medical Genetics* 29:205-208, 1988.

Gellis SR, Feingold M, and Miller D: Picture of the month: Nager's syndrome (Nager's acrofacial dysostosis). *Archives of Pediatric and Adolescent Medicine* 132:519-520, 1978.

Genee E: Une forme extensive de dysostose mandibulo-facial. *Journal Genetique Humaine* 17:45-52, 1969.

Gibson JM, Sillence DO, and Taylor TK: Abnormalities of the spine in Goldenhar's syndrome. *Journal of Pediatric Orthopedics* 16:344-349, 1996.

Glander K, and Cisneros GJ: Comparison of the craniofacial characteristics of two syndromes associated with Pierre Robin sequence. *Cleft Palate–Craniofacial Journal* 29:210-219, 1992.

Goldberg J, Enlow D, Whitaker L, Zins J, and Kurihara S: Some anatomical characteristics in several craniofacial syndromes. *Journal of Oral Surgery* 39:489-498, 1981.

Goldberg RB, Marion R, Borderon M, Wiznia A, and Shprintzen RJ: Phenotypic overlap between velo-cardio-facial syndrome and the Di George sequence [abstract]. *American Journal of Human Genetics* 37(Supplement):54, 1985.

Goldberg RB, Motzkin B, Marion R, Scambler PJ, and Shprintzen RJ: Velo-cardio-facial syndrome: a review of 120 patients. *American Journal of Medical Genetics* 45:313-319, 1993.

Golding-Kushner KJ, Weller G, and Shprintzen RJ: Velo-cardio-facial syndrome: language and psychological profiles. *Journal of Craniofacial Genetics and Developmental Biology* 51:259-266, 1985.

Goldstein DJ, and Mirkin LD: Nager acrofacial dysostosis: evidence for apparent heterogeneity. *American Journal of Medical Genetics* 30:741-746, 1988.

Goodman RM, and Gorlin RJ: *The malformed infant and child.* New York: Oxford University Press, 1983, p. 280.

Gorlin RJ, Cohen MM Jr, and Levin LS: *Syndromes of the head and neck.* New York: Oxford University Press, 1990.

Gosain AK, McCarthy JG, and Pinto RS: Cervicovertebral anomalies and basilar impression in Goldenhar syndrome. *Plastic and Reconstructive Surgery* 93:498-506, 1994.

Gosain AK, McCarthy JG, and Wisoff JH: Morbidity associated with increased intracranial pressure in Apert and Pfeiffer syndromes: the need for long-term evaluation. *Plastic and Reconstructive Surgery* 97:292-301, 1996.

Gosain AK, McCarthy JG, Glatt P, Staffenberg D, and Hoffmann RG: A study of intracranial volume in Apert syndrome. *Plastic and Reconstructive Surgery* 95:284-295, 1995.

Gould HJ: Audiologic findings in Pierre Robin sequence. *Ear and Hearing* 10:211-213, 1989.

Gould HJ, and Caldarelli D: Hearing and otopathology in Apert syndrome. *Archives of Otolaryngology* 108:347-349, 1982.

Greenwood R, Rosenthal A, Sommer A, Wolff G, and Craenen J: Cardiovascular malformations in oculoauriculovertebral dysplasia (Goldenhar syndrome). *Journal of Pediatrics* 85:816-818, 1974.

Gupta S, and Popli A: Psychosis in Apert's syndrome with partial agenesis of the corpus callosum. *Journal of Psychiatry and Neuroscience* 20:307-309, 1995.

Hadley RC, and Johnson JB: Utilization of the Kirschner wire in Pierre Robin syndrome with case report. *Plastic and Reconstructive Surgery* 31:587-596, 1963.

Halal H, Herrmann J, Pallister PD, Opitz JM, Desgrandes M-F, and Grenier G: Differential diagnosis of Nager acrofacial dysostosis syndrome: report of four patients with Nager syndrome and discussion of other related syndromes. *American Journal of Medical Genetics* 14:209-224, 1983.

Hall BD: Choanal atresia and associated multiple anomalies. *Journal of Pediatrics* 95:395-398, 1979.

Hall JC: Stickler syndrome. In Bergsma D (ed.): *Clinical cytogenetics and genetics, birth defects: Original articles series* 10:157-171, 1974.

Hall JC, and Herrod H: The Stickler syndrome presenting as a dominantly inherited cleft palate and blindness. *Journal of Medical Genetics* 12:397-404, 1975.

Handzic J, Bagatin M, Subotic R, and Cuk V: Hearing levels in Pierre Robin syndrome. *Cleft Palate–Craniofacial Journal* 32:30-36, 1995.

Hansen M, Lucarelli MJ, Whiteman DA, and Mulliden JB: Treacher Collins syndrome: phenotypic variability in a family including an infant with arhinia and uveal colobomas. *American Journal of Medical Genetics* 61:71-74, 1996.

Harris V, Beligere N, and Pruzansky S: Progressive generalized bony dysplasia in Apert syndrome. *Birth Defects: Original Article Series* 14:175, 1977.

Hauss-Albert H, and Passarge E: Postaxial acrofacial dysostosis syndrome with microcephaly, seizures and profound mental retardation [letter]. *American Journal of Medical Genetics* 31:701-703, 1988.

Hecht JT, Immken LL, Harris LF, Malini S, and Scott CI Jr: Brief clinical report: the Nager syndrome. *American Journal of Medical Genetics* 27:965-969, 1987.

Hemmer KM, McAlister WH, and Marsh JL: Cervical spine anomalies in the craniosynostosis syndromes. *Cleft Palate Journal* 24:328-333, 1987.

Herrmann J, France T, Spranger J, Opitz J, and Wiffler C: The Stickler syndrome (hereditary arthoophthalmopathy). *Birth Defects: Original Article Series* 11:76-103, 1975.

Horgan JE, Padwa BL, LaBrie RA, and Mulliken JB: OMENS-Plus: analysis of craniofacial and extracraniofacial anomalies in hemifacial microsomia. *Cleft Palate–Craniofacial Journal* 32:405-412, 1995.

Hotz M, and Gnoinski W: Clefts of the secondary palate associated with the "Pierre Robin syndrome." *Swedish Dental Journal* 15(Supplement): 89-98, 1982.

Igarashi M, Filippone M, and Alford B: Temporal bone findings in Pierre Robin syndrome. *Laryngoscope* 86:1679-1687, 1976.

Jabs EW, Li X, Coss CA, Taylor EW, Meyers DA, and Weber JL: Mapping the Treacher Collins syndrome locus to 5q31.3-q33.3. *Genomics* 11:193-198, 1991.

Jackson IT, Bauer B, Saleh J, Sullivan C, and Argenta LC: A significant feature of Nager's syndrome: palatal agenesis. *Plastic and Reconstructive Surgery* 84:219-226, 1989.

Jahrsdoerfer RA, and Jacobson JT: Treacher Collins syndrome: otologic and auditory management. *Journal of the American Academy of Audiology* 6:93-102, 1995.

Jahrsdoerfer RA, Aguilar EA, Yeakley JW, and Cole RR: Treacher Collins syndrome: an otologic challenge. *Annals of Otology, Rhinology, and Laryngology* 98:807-812, 1989.

Janku P, Robinow M, Kelly T, Bralley R, Baynes A, and Edgerton MT: The van der Woude syndrome in a large kindred: variability, penetrance, genetic risks. *American Journal of Medical Genetics* 5:117-123, 1980.

Jarund M, and Lauritzen C: Craniofacial dysostosis: airway obstruction and craniofacial surgery. *Scandinavian Journal of Plastic and Reconstructive Surgery and Hand Surgery* 30:275-279, 1996.

Johnston C, Taussig LM, Koopmann C, Smith P, and Bjelland J: Obstructive sleep apnea in Treacher-Collins syndrome. *Cleft Palate Journal* 18:39-44, 1981.

Jones KL: *Smith's recognizeable patterns of human malformation,* 5th edition. Philadelphia: WB Saunders, 1997.

Kaiser-Kupfer M: Ectrodactyly, ectodermal dysplasia and clefting syndrome. *American Journal of Ophthalmology* 76:992-998, 1973.

Karayiorgou M, Morris MA, Morrow B, Shprintzen RJ, Goldberg RB, Borrow J, Gos A, Nestadt G, Wolyniec PS, Lasseter VK, Eisen H, Childs B, Kazazian HH, Kucherlapati R, Antonarakis SE, Pulver AE, and Housman DE: Schizophrenia susceptibility associated with interstitial deletions of chromosome 22q11. *Proceedings of the National Academy of Sciences of the United States of America* 92:7612-7616, 1995.

Kawira EL, Weaver DD, and Bender HA: Acrofacial dysostosis with severe facial clefting and limb reduction. *American Journal of Medical Genetics* 17:641-647, 1984.

Kay ED, and Kay CN: Dysmorphogenesis of the mandible, zygoma, and middle ear ossicles in hemifacial microsomia and mandibulofacial dysostosis. *American Journal of Medical Genetics* 32:27-31, 1989.

Kaye CI, Martin AO, Rollnick BR, Nagatoshi K, Israel J, Hermanoff M, Tropea B, Richtsmeier JT, and Morton NE: Oculoauriculovertebral anomaly: segregation analysis. *American Journal of Medical Genetics* 43:913-917, 1992.

Kelly D, Goldberg R, Wilson D, Lindsay E, Carey A, Goodship J, Burn J, Cross I, Shprintzen RJ, and Scambler PJ: Confirmation that the velo-cardio-facial syndrome is associated with haplo-insufficiency of genes at chromosome 22q11. *American Journal of Medical Genetics* 45:308-312, 1993.

Klein D, Konig H, and Tobler R: Sue une forme extensive de dysostose mandibulo-faciale (Franceschetti) accompagnee de malformations des extremites et d'autres anomalies congenitales chez une fille dont le frere ne presente qu'une forme fruste du syndrome (fistula auris congenita retrotragica.) *Revue d'Oto-Neuro-Ophthalmologie* 42:432-440, 1970.

Konigsmark BW, and Gorlin RJ: *Genetic and metabolic deafness.* Philadelphia: WB Saunders, 1976.

Krauss CM, Hassell LA, and Gang DL: Brief clinical reports: anomalies in an infant with Nager acrofacial dysostosis. *American Journal of Medical Genetics* 21:761-764, 1985.

Kreiborg S: Apert's and Crouzon's syndromes contrasted: qualitative craniofacial x-ray findings. In Marchac D (ed.): *Proceedings of the First International Congress of the International Society of Cranio-Maxillo-Facial Surgery.* Berlin: Springer-Verlag, 1987, pp. 91-95.

Kreiborg S: Crouzon syndrome: a clinical and roentgencephalometric study. *Scandinavian Journal of Plastic and Reconstructive Surgery* Supplement:118, 1981.

Kreiborg S, and Dahl E: Cranial base and face in mandibulofacial dysostosis. *American Journal of Medical Genetics* 47:753-760, 1993.

Kruk J, and Tronczynska J: Velopharyngeal insufficiency in children with Sedlackova's syndrome. *Acta Chirurgiae Plasticae* (Prague) 20:13-17, 1978.

Kumar A, Friedman JM, Taylor GP, and Patterson MW: Pattern of cardiac malformation in oculoauriculovertebral spectrum. *American Journal of Medical Genetics* 46:423-426, 1993.

LaCombe D, Pedespan JM, Fortan D, Chateil JF, and Verloes A: Phenotypic variability in van der Woude syndrome. *Genetic Counseling* 6:221-226, 1995.

LeBlanc SM, and Golding-Kushner KJ: Effect of glossopexy on speech sound production in Robin sequence. *Cleft Palate–Craniofacial Journal* 29:239-235, 1992.

LeFebvre A, Travis F, Arndt A, and Munro IR: A psychiatric profile after reconstructive surgery in children with Apert syndrome. *British Journal of Plastic Surgery* 39:510-513, 1986.

Lehman JA, Fishman JRA, and Neiman GS: Treatment of cleft palate associated with Robin sequence: appraisal of risk factors. *Cleft Palate–Craniofacial Journal* 32:25-29, 1995.

Le Merrer M, Cikuli M, Ribier J, and Briard ML: Acrofacial dysostoses. *American Journal of Medical Genetics* 33:318-322, 1989.

Lewis SR, Lynch JB, and Blocker TG Jr: Facial slings for tongue stabilization in the Pierre Robin syndrome. *Plastic and Reconstructive Surgery* 42:237-241, 1968.

Liberfarb RM, and Goldblatt A: Prevalence of mitral valve prolapse in the Stickler syndrome. *American Journal of Medical Genetics* 24:387-392, 1986.

Lindsay EA, Goldberg R, Jurecic V, Morrow B, Carlson C, Kucherlapati RS, Shprintzen RJ, and Baldini A: Velo-cardio-facial syndrome: frequency and extent of 22q11 deletions. *American Journal of Medical Genetics* 57:514-522, 1995.

Lipson AH, Yuille D, Angel M, Thompson PG, Vandervoord JG, and Beckenham EJ: Velocardiofacial (Shprintzen) syndrome: an important syndrome for the dysmorphologist to recognise. *Journal of Medical Genetics* 28:596-604, 1991.

Lucarini JW, Liberfarb RM, and Eavey RD: Otolaryngological manifestations of the Stickler syndrome. *International Journal of Pediatric Otorhinolaryngology* 14:215-222, 1987.

Luce E, McGibbon B, and Hoopes J: Velopharyngeal insufficiency in hemifacial microsomia. *Plastic and Reconstructive Surgery* 60:602-606, 1977.

MacKenzie-Stepner K, Witzel MA, Stringer DA, Lindsay WK, Munro IR, and Hughes H: Abnormal carotid arteries in the velocardiofacial syndrome: a report of three cases. *Plastic and Reconstructive Surgery* 80:347-351, 1987.

Majewski F, and Kuster W: EEC syndrome sine sine? *Clinical Genetics* 33:69-72, 1988.

Marres HAM, Cremers WRJ, Dixon MJ, Huygen PLM, and Joosten FBM: The Treacher Collins syndrome. *Archives of Otolaryngology–Head and Neck Surgery* 121:509-514, 1995.

Marsh JL, Celin SE, Vannier MW, and Gado M: The skeletal anatomy of mandibulofacial dysostosis (Treacher Collins syndrome). *Plastic and Reconstructive Surgery* 78:460-468, 1986.

Martsolf JT, Cracco JB, Carpenter GG, and O'Hara E: Pfeiffer syndrome: an unusual type of acrocephalosyndactyly with broad thumbs and great toes. *Archives of Pediatric and Adolescent Medicine* 121:257-262, 1971.

Matras H, Watzek G, and Perneczky A: Cephalometric observations in premature craniosynostosis. *Journal of Maxillofacial Surgery* 5:298-303, 1977.

McCarthy JG, Coccaro PJ, and Schwartz MD: Velopharyngeal function following maxillary advancement. *Plastic and Reconstructive Surgery* 64:180-188, 1977.

McCarthy JG, Glasberg JB, Cutting CB, Epstein FJ, Grayson BH, Ruff G, Thorne CH, Wisoff J, and Zide BM: Twenty-year experience with early surgery for craniosynostosis: II. The craniofacial synostosis syndromes and pansynostosis—results and unsolved problems. *Plastic and Reconstructive Surgery* 96:284-295, 1995.

McDonald-McGinn DM, LaRossa D, Randall P, Russell MS, Zackai MD: Cleft palate and lip pits in Kabuki syndrome. Presented before the 57th annual meeting of the American Cleft Palate-Craniofacial Association, Atlanta, Georgia, April 14, 2000.

McDonald MT, and Gorski J: Nager acrofacial dysostosis. *Journal of Medical Genetics* 30:779-782, 1993.

Meinecke P, and Wiedemann H-R: Robin sequence and oligodactyly in mother and son—probably a further example of the postaxial acrofacial dysostosis syndrome [letter]. *American Journal of Medical Genetics* 27:953-956, 1987.

Meyerson MD, and Nisbet JG: Nager syndrome: an update of speech and hearing characteristics. *Cleft Palate Journal* 24:142-151, 1987.

Meyerson MD, Jensen KM, Meyers JM, and Hall BD: Nager acrofacial dysostosis: early intervention and long-term planning. *Cleft Palate Journal* 14:35-40, 1977.

Miller M, Fineman R, and Smith DW: Postaxial acrofacial dysostosis syndrome. *Journal of Pediatrics* 95:970-975, 1979.

Miller MT: Ocular findings in craniosynostosis. In Cohen MM Jr (ed.): *Craniosynostosis: diagnosis, evaluation, and management.* New York: Raven Press, 1986, pp. 227-248.

Minervini F: The Duhamel procedure for the treatment of Pierre Robin syndrome [letter]. *Plastic and Reconstructive Surgery* 51:686, 1973.

Mitnick RJ, Bello JA, and Shprintzen RJ: Brain anomalies in velo-cardio-facial syndrome. *American Journal of Medical Genetics* 54:100-106, 1994.

Molina F, and Ortiz Monasterio F: Mandibular elongation and remodeling by distraction: a farewell to major osteotomies. *Plastic and Reconstructive Surgery* 96:825-840, 1995.

Moore MH: Upper airway obstruction in the syndromal craniosynostoses. *British Journal of Plastic Surgery* 46:355-362, 1993.

Moore MH, Lodge ML, and Clark BE: Spinal anomalies in Pfeiffer syndrome. *Cleft Palate–Craniofacial Journal* 32:251-254, 1995a.

Moore MH, Lodge ML, and Clark BE: The infant skull in Pfeiffer's syndrome. *Journal of Craniofacial Surgery* 6:483-486, 1995b.

Moore MH, Cantrell SB, Trott JA, and David DJ: Pfeiffer syndrome: a clinical review. *Cleft Palate–Craniofacial Journal* 32:62-70, 1995.

Morrow B, Goldberg R, Carlson C, Das Gupta R, Sirotkin H, Collins J, Dunham I, O'Donnell H, Scambler P, Shprintzen R, and Kucherlapati R: Molecular definition of the 22q11 deletions in velo-cardio-facial syndrome. *American Journal of Human Genetics* 56:1391-1403, 1995.

Moss EM, Batshaw ML, Solot CB, Gerdes M, McDonald-McGinn DM, Driscoll DA, Emanuel BS, Zackai EH, and Wang PP: Psychoeducational profile of the 22q11.2 microdeletion: qa complex pattern. *Journal of Pediatrics* 134:193-198, 1999.

Murovic JA, Posnick JC, Drake JM, Humphreys RP, Hoffman HJ, and Hendricks ER: Hydrocephalus in Apert syndrome: a retrospective review. *Pediatric Neurosurgery* 19:151-155, 1993.

Murray JC, Nishimura DY, Buetow KH, Ardinger HH, Spence MA, Sparker RS, Falk RE, Falk PM, Gardner RJM, Harkness EM, Glinski LP, Pauli RM, Nakamura Y, Green PP, and Schinzel A: Linkage of an autosomal dominant clefting syndrome (van der Woude) to loci on chromosome 1q. *American Journal of Human Genetics* 46:486-491, 1990.

Nager FR, and de Reynier JP: Das Gehorogan bei den angeborenen Kopf-missbildungen. *Practica Oto-Rhino-Laryngologica* (Basel) 10(Supplement 2):1-128, 1948.

Opitz JM, Mollica F, Sorge G, Milana G, Cimino G, and Caltabiano M: Acrofacial dysostoses: review and report of a previously undescribed condition: the autosomal or X-linked dominant Catania form of acrofacial dysostosis. *American Journal of Medical Genetics* 47:660-678, 1993.

Ousterhout DK, and Melsen B: Cranial base deformity in Apert's syndrome. *Plastic and Reconstructive Surgery* 69:254-263, 1982.

Pagon RA, Graham JM Jr, Zonana J, and Yong SL: Coloboma, congenital heart disease, and choanal atresia with multiple anomalies: CHARGE association. *Journal of Pediatrics* 99:223-227, 1981.

Pantke OA, Cohen MM Jr, Witkop CJ, Feingold M, Schaumann B, Pantke HC, and Gorlin RJ: The Saethre-Chotzen syndrome. *Birth Defects: Original Article Series* 11:190-225, 1975.

Parsons RW, and Smith DJ: A modified tongue-lip adhesion for Pierre Robin anomalad. *Cleft Palate Journal* 17:144-147, 1980.

Pashayan HM, and Lewis MB: Clinical experience with the Robin sequence. *Cleft Palate Journal* 21:270-276, 1984.

Pashayan HM, Pruzansky S, and Solomon L: The EEC syndrome: report of six patients. *Birth Defects: Original Article Series* 10:105-120, 1974.

Patton MA, Goodship J, Hayward R, and Lansdown R: Intellectual development in Apert's syndrome: a long term follow up of 29 patients. *Journal of Medical Genetics* 25:164-167, 1988.

Perkins JA, Sie KC, Milczuk H, and Richardson MA: Airway management in children with craniofacial anomalies. *Cleft Palate–Craniofacial Journal* 34:135-140, 1997.

Peterson SJ: Speech pathology in craniofacial malformations other than cleft lip and palate. ASHA Report 8: *Orofacial Anomalies: Clinical and Research Implications.* Washington DC: American Speech and Hearing Association, 1973, pp. 111-131.

Peterson SJ, and Pruzansky S: Palatal anomalies in the syndromes of Apert and Crouzon. *Cleft Palate Journal* 11:394-403, 1974.

Peterson-Falzone SJ, and Figueroa AA: Longitudinal changes in cranial base angulation in mandibulofacial dysostosis. *Cleft Palate Journal* 26:14-22, 1986.

Peterson-Falzone SJ, and Pruzansky S: Cleft palate and congenital palatopharyngeal incompetency in mandibulofacial dysostosis: frequency and problems in treatment. *Cleft Palate Journal* 13:354-360, 1976.

Peterson-Falzone SJ, Caldarelli DD, and Landahl KL: Abnormal laryngeal vocal quality in ectodermal dysplasia. *Archives of Otolaryngology* 107:300-304, 1981.

Peterson-Falzone SJ, Pruzansky S, Parris PJ, and Laffer JL: Nasopharyngeal dysmorphology in the syndromes of Apert and Crouzon. *Cleft Palate Journal* 18:237-250, 1981.

Phelps PD, Poswillo D, and Lloyd GAS: The ear deformities in mandibulofacial dysostosis (Treacher Collins syndrome). *Clinics in Otolaryngology* 6:15-28, 1981.

Phillips SG, and Miyamoto RT: Congenital conductive hearing loss in Apert syndrome. *Otolaryngology–Head and Neck Surgery* 95:429-433, 1986.

Pitt M, and Ingram TTS: The radiology of speech disorders in childhood. I: Disorders and their study. *Radiography* 41:53-59, 1975.

Poradowska W, Reszke S, and Lenkiewica T: Pierre Robin syndrome. *Pediatria Polska* 56:607-611, 1981.

Pron G, Galloway C, Armstrong D, and Posnick J: Ear malformation and hearing loss in patients with Treacher Collins syndrome. *Cleft Palate–Craniofacial Journal* 30:97-103, 1993.

Proudman TX, Clark BE, Moore MH, Abbott AH, and David DJ: Central nervous system imaging in Crouzon's syndrome. *Journal of Craniofacial Surgery* 6:401-405, 1995.

Pruzansky S, and Richmond JB: Growth of the mandible in infants with micrognathia. *American Journal of Diseases of Children* 88:29-42, 1954.

Pulver AE, Nestadt G, Goldberg R, Shprintzen RJ, Lamacz J, Wolyniec PS, Morrow B, Karayiorgou M, Antonarakis SE, Housman D, and Kucherlapati R: Psychotic illness in patients diagnosed with velo-cardio-facial syndrome and their relatives. *Journal of Nervous and Mental Disease* 182:476-478, 1994.

Ranta R, Laaikainen T, and Laitinen S: Cephalometric comparisons of the cranial base and face in children with Pierre Robin anomalad and isolated cleft palate. *Proceedings of the Finnish Dental Society* 81:82-90, 1985.

Ranta R, and Rintala AE: Correlations between microforms of the van der Woude syndrome and cleft palate. *Cleft Palate Journal* 20:158-162, 1983.

Reardon W, McManus SP, Summers D, and Winter RM: Cytogenetic evidence that the Saethre-Chotzen gene maps to 7p21.2. *American Journal of Medical Genetics* 47:633-636, 1993.

Renier D, Arnaud E, Cinalli G, Sebaq G, Zerah M, and Marchac D: Prognosis for mental function in Apert's syndrome. *Journal of Neurosurgery* 81:66-72, 1996.

Rintala AE, and Ranta R: Lower lip sinuses: I. Epidemiology, microforms and transverse sulci. *British Journal of Plastic Surgery* 34:26-30, 1981.

Rintala AE, Ranta R, and Stegars T: On the pathogenesis of the Pierre Robin syndrome. *Scandinavian Journal of Plastic and Reconstructive Surgery* 18:237-240, 1984.

Roberts F, Pruzansky S, and Aduss H: An x-radiogcephalometric study of mandibulofacial dysostosis in man. *Archives of Oral Biology* 20:265-281, 1975.

Robin P: Glossoptosis due to atresia and hypotrophy of the mandible. *Archives of Pediatric and Adolescent Medicine* 48:541-547, 1934.

Robin P: La chute de la base de la langue consideree comme und veile cause de gene dans la respiration naso-pharyngienne. *Bulletin de l'Academie Nationale de Medecine* (Paris) 89:37-41, 1923.

Rodini ESO, Freitas JAS, and Richieri-Costa A: Ectrodactyly, cleft lip/palate syndrome. *American Journal of Medical Genetics* 38:539-541, 1991.

Roelfsema NM, and Cobben JM: The EEC syndrome: a literature study. *Clinical Dysmorphology* 5:115-127, 1996.

Rogers BO: Berry-Treacher Collins syndrome: a review of 200 cases. *British Journal of Plastic Surgery* 17:109-137, 1964.

Rollnick BR, Kaye CI, Nagatoshi K, Hauck W, and Martin A: Oculoauriculovertebral dysplasia and variants: phenotypic characteristics of 294 patients. *American Journal of Medical Genetics* 26:361-375, 1987.

Routledge RT: The Pierre Robin syndrome: a surgical emergency in the neonatal period. *British Journal of Plastic Surgery* 13:204-218, 1960.

Sadewitz VL, and Shprintzen RJ: *Pierre Robin: a new look at an old disorder.* Videotape. White Plains, NY: March of Dimes Birth Defects Foundation, 1986.

Saethre H: Ein Beitrag zum Turmschadelproblem. (Pathogenese, Erblichkeit und Symptomologie). *Deutsche Zeitschrift fur Nervenheilkunde* (Berlin) 117:533-555, 1931.

Sagehashi N: An infant with Crouzon's syndrome with a cartilaginous trachea and a human tail. *Journal of Cranio-Maxillo-Facial Surgery* 20:21-23, 1992.

Sander A, Schmelzle R, and Murray J: Evidence for a microdeletion in 1q32-41 involving the gene responsible for van der Woude syndrome. *Human Molecular Genetics* 3:575-578, 1994.

Sando I, Suehiro S, and Wood RP: Congenital anomalies of the external and middle ear. In Bluestone C, and Stool S (eds.): *Pediatric otolaryngology,* Volume 1. Philadelphia: WB Saunders, 1983, pp. 309-346.

Scambler PJ, Kelly D, Lindsay E, Williamson R, Goldberg RB, Shprintzen RJ, Wilson DI, Goodship JA, Cross I, and Burn J: The velo-cardio-facial syndrome is associated with chromosome 22 deletions encompassing the DiGeorge locus. *Lancet* 333:1138-1139, 1992.

Schafer ME: Upper airway obstruction and sleep disorders in children with craniofacial anomalies. *Clinics in Plastic Surgery* 9:555-567, 1982.

Schmid H: Synchondrosen des Laryngotrachealskeletts und Trachesotenose beim Apert-Crouzon-Syndrom. *Zentralblatt fur Allgemeine Pathologie und Pathologische Anatomie* 114:326-337, 1971.

Schuarte ES, and St. Aubin PW: Progressive synostosis in Apert's syndrome (acrocephalosyndactyly) with a description of roentgenographic changes in the feet. *American Journal of Roentgenology* 97:67-73, 1966.

Sedee G: Facial nerve and dysplasia of the temporal one. *Journal of Otology, Rhinology, and Laryngology* 35:222-228, 1973.

Sedlackova E: Insuficience patrohitanoveho zaveru jako vyvojova porucha (Insufficiency of the palatolaryngeal passage disorder). *Casopis Lekaru Ceskvch* (Prague) 94:1304-1307, 1955.

Sedlackova E: The syndrome of the congenitally shortened velum. The dual innervation of the soft palate. *Folia Phoniatrica* 19:441-443, 1967.

Sedlackova E, Lastovka M, and Sram F: Contribution to knowledge of soft palate innervation. *Folia Phoniatrica* 12:434-441, 1973.

Selle G, and Jacobs H: Cleft palate in two syndromes. *Cleft Palate Journal* 14:230-233, 1977.

Sheffield LJ, Reiss JA, Strohm K, and Gilding M: A genetic follow-up study of 64 patients with the Pierre Robin complex. *American Journal of Medical Genetics* 28:25-36, 1987.

Sher A: Mechanisms of airway obstruction in Robin sequence: implications for treatment. *Cleft Palate–Craniofacial Journal* 29:224-213, 1992.

Sher A, Shprintzen RJ, and Thorpy MJ: Endoscopic observations of obstructive sleep apnea in children with anomalous upper airways: predictive and therapeutic value. *International Journal of Pediatric Otorhinolaryngology* 11:135-146, 1986.

Sherk H, Whitaker L, and Pasquariello P: Facial malformations and spinal anomalies: a predictable relationship. *Spine* 7:526-531, 1982.

Shprintzen RJ: Palatal and pharyngeal anomalies in craniofacial syndromes. *Birth Defects: Original Article Series* 18:52-78, 1982.

Shprintzen RJ: Reply from Dr. Shprintzen [letter]. *American Journal of Medical Genetics* 28:753-755, 1987.

Shprintzen RJ: Pierre Robin, micrognathia, and airway obstruction: the dependency of treatment on accurate diagnosis. *International Anesthesiology Clinics* 26:84-91, 1988.

Shprintzen RJ: The implications of the diagnosis of Robin sequence. *Cleft Palate–Craniofacial Journal* 29:205-209, 1992.

Shprintzen RJ, and Singer L: Upper airway obstruction and the Robin sequence. *International Anesthesiology Clinics* 30:109-114, 1992.

Shprintzen RJ, Goldberg RB, and Sidoti EJ: The penetrance and variable expression of the Van der Woude syndrome: implications for genetic counseling. *Cleft Palate Journal* 17:52-57, 1980.

Shprintzen RJ, Croft C, Berkman MD, and Rakoff S: Pharyngeal hypoplasia in Treacher Collins syndrome. *Archives of Otolaryngology* 105:127-131, 1979.

Shprintzen RJ, Croft C, Berkman MD, and Rakoff S: Velopharyngeal insufficiency in the facio-auriculo-vertebral malformation complex. *Cleft Palate Journal* 17:132-143, 1980.

Shprintzen RJ, Goldberg RB, Golding-Kushner KJ, and Marion R: Late-onset psychosis in velo-cardio-facial syndrome [letter]. *American Journal of Medical Genetics* 42:141-142, 1992.

Shprintzen RJ, Goldberg RB, Lewin M, Sidoti E, Berkman M, Argamaso R, and Young D: A new syndrome involving cleft palate, cardiac anomalies, typical facies, and learning disabilities: velo-cardio-facial syndrome. *Cleft Palate Journal* 15:56-62, 1978.

Shprintzen RJ, Goldberg RB, Young D, and Wolford L: The velo-cardio-facial syndrome: a clinical and genetic analysis. *Pediatrics* 67:167-172, 1981.

Shprintzen RJ, Siegel Sadewitz V, Amato J, and Goldberg R: Anomalies associated with cleft lip, cleft palate, or both. *American Journal of Medical Genetics* 20:585-595, 1985a.

Shprintzen RJ, Siegel Sadewitz V, Amato J, and Goldberg R: Retrospective diagnoses of previously missed syndromic disorders among 1000 patients with cleft lip, cleft palate, or both. *Birth Defects: Original Article Series* 21:85-92, 1985b.

Singer L, and Sidoti EJ: Pediatric management of Robin sequence. *Cleft Palate–Craniofacial Journal* 29:220-223, 1992.

Sirotnak J, Brodsky L, and Pizzuto M: Airway obstruction in the Crouzon syndrome: case report and review of the literature. *International Journal of Pediatric Otolaryngology* 31:235-246, 1995.

Slingenberg B: Missbildungen von Extremitaten. In *Virchows Archives A. Pathological Anatomy and Histopathology* 193:1-91, 1908.

Smith JD: Treatment of airway obstruction in Pierre Robin syndrome. *Archives of Otolaryngology* 107:419-421, 1981.

Smith JL, and Stowe F: The Pierre Robin syndrome (glossoptosis, micrognathia, cleft palate): a review of 39 cases with emphasis on associated ocular lesions. *Pediatrics* 27:128-133, 1961.

Solomon LM, Fretzin D, and Pruzansky S: Pilosebaceous abnormalities in Apert's syndrome. *Archives of Dermatology* 102:381-385, 1970.

Solomon LM, Medenica M, Pruzansky S, and Kreiborg S: Apert syndrome and palatal mucopolysaccharides. *Teratology* 8:287-292, 1973.

Spranger J: Artho-ophthalmopathia hereditaria. *Annales de Radiologie* (Paris) 11:359-364, 1968.

Stevens CA, Carey JC, and Shigeoka AO: Di George anomaly and velocardiofacial syndrome. *Pediatrics* 85:526-530, 1990.

Stickler G, and Pugh D: Hereditary progressive arthro-ophthalmopathy. II. Additional observations on vertebral abnormalities, a hearing defect, and a report of a similar case. *Mayo Clinic Proceedings* 42:495-500, 1967.

Stickler G, Belau P, Farrell F, Jones J, Pugh D, Steinberg A, and Ward L: Hereditary progressive arthroophthalmopathy. *Mayo Clinic Proceedings* 40:433-455, 1965.

Stone P, Trevenen CL, Mitchell I, and Rudd N: Congenital tracheal stenosis in Pfeiffer syndrome. *Clinical Genetics* 39:145-148, 1990.

Strong WB: Familial syndrome of right-sided aortic arch, mental deficiency, and facial dysmorphism. *Journal of Pediatrics* 73:882-888, 1968.

Temtamy SA, and McKusick VA: The genetics of hand malformations. *Birth Defects: Original Article Series* 14:92-95, 149, 1978.

Tessier P: Osteotomies totales de la face. Syndrome de Crouzon. Syndrome de Apert. Oxycephalies. Scaphocephalies. Turricephalies. *Annales Chirurgie Plasticae* 12:273-286, 1967.

Tessier P: The definitive plastic surgical treatment of the severe facial deformities of craniofacial dysostosis: Crouzon's and Apert's diseases. *Plastic and Reconstructive Surgery* 48:419-442, 1971.

Thomson A: Notice of several cases of malformation of the external ear, together with experiments on the state of hearing in such persons. *Monthly Journal of Medical Science* 7:420-425, 729-738, 1846.

Tokumaru AM, Barkovich AJ, Ciricillo SF, and Edwards MS: Skull base and calvarial deformities: association with intracranial changes in craniofacial syndromes. *American Journal of Neuroradiology* 17:619-630, 1996.

Tomaski SM, Zalzal GH, and Saal HM: Airway obstruction in the Pierre Robin sequence. *Laryngoscope* 105:111-114, 1995.

Treacher Collins E: Case with symmetrical congenital notches in the outer part of each lower lid and defective development of the malar bone. *Transactions of the Ophthalmological Society of the United Kingdom* 20:190-192, 1900.

Trost JE: Articulatory additions to the classical description of the speech of persons with cleft palate. *Cleft Palate Journal* 18:193-203, 1981.

Trost-Cardamone JE: *Cleft palate misarticulations: a teaching tape.* Videotape. Northridge, CA: Instructional Media Center, California State University, 1987.

Trost-Cardamone JE, and Bernthal JE: Articulation assessment and procedures and treatment decisions. In Moller KT, and Starr CD (eds.): *Cleft palate: interdisciplinary issues and treatment.* Austin: Pro-Ed, 1993, pp. 307-336.

Tsai FJ, and Tsai CH: Autosomal dominant inherited oculo-auriculo-vertebral spectrum: report of one family. *Acta Paediatrica Sinica* 34:27-31, 1993.

Tunte W, and Lenz W: Zur Haufigkeit und mutationsrates des Apert-Syndroms. *Human Genetics* (Berlin) 4:104-111, 1967.

Vallino-Napoli LD: Audiologic and otologic characteristics of Pfeiffer syndrome. *Cleft Palate–Craniofacial Journal* 33:524-529, 1996.

Van der Woude A: Fistula labii inferioris congenita and its association with cleft lip and palate. *American Journal of Human Genetics* 6:244-256, 1954.

van Vierzen PBJ, Joosten FBM, Marres HAM, Cremers CWRJ, and Ruijs JHJ: Mandibulofacial dysostosis: CT findings of the temporal bones. *European Journal of Radiology* 21:53-57, 1995.

Verloes A, Foret C, and Lambotte C: Nager acrofacial dysostosis with cleft lip. *Journal Genetique Humaine* 35:415-420, 1987.

Vrticka K, and Sedlackova E: Congenitally shortened velum—investigation of its function. *Proceedings of the 12th Congress of the International Association of Logopedics and Phoniatrics,* Padova, 1962.

Walker F: Apparent autosomal recessive inheritance of the Treacher Collins syndrome. *Birth Defects: Original Article Series* 10:135-139, 1974.

Wienker TF, Hudek G, Bissbort S, Mayerova A, Mauff G, and Bender K: Linkage studies in a pedigree with Van der Woude syndrome. *Journal of Medical Genetics* 24:160-162, 1987.

Williams MA, Shprintzen RJ, and Rakoff SJ: Adenoid hypoplasia in the velo-cardio-facial syndrome. *Journal of Craniofacial Genetics and Developmental Biology* 7:23-26, 1987.

Williams AJ, Williams MA, Walker CA, and Bush PG: The Robin anomalad (Pierre Robin syndrome)—a follow-up study. *Archives of Disease in Childhood* 56:663-668, 1981.

Winters H: *Congenital short palate* [monograph]. Lochem: Kerkard, 1975.

Wood VE, Sauser DD, and O'Hara RC: The shoulder and elbow in Apert's syndrome. *Journal of Pediatric Orthopedics* 15:648-651, 1995.

Wraith J, Super M, Watson G, and Phillips M: Velo-cardio-facial syndrome presenting as holoprosencephaly. *Clinical Genetics* 27:408-410, 1985.

Zlotogora J, Sagi M, Schuper A, Leiba H, and Merin S: Variability of Stickler syndrome. *American Journal of Medical Genetics* 42:337-339, 1992.

Chapter 3

Anatomy and Physiology of the Velopharyngeal System

Normal speech production depends, in part, on the ability to rapidly disconnect (or decouple) and connect (or couple) the nasal cavity from the oral cavity. Nasal speech sounds require oral-nasal coupling. Oral speech sounds require oral-nasal decoupling. The process of coupling and decoupling the oral and nasal cavities is called velopharyngeal valving.

Some individuals who have palatal clefts have inadequate velopharyngeal valving for speech, resulting in abnormal qualities such as hypernasality, audible nasal emission of air, and/or abnormal articulation. Severity of velopharyngeal inadequacy (VPI) is variable across affected individuals. In mild cases the effects on speech may be minimal and not noticeable to most listeners. However, in severe cases problems with speech intelligibility, voice quality, and even nonspeech activities such as blowing, sucking, and swallowing may occur.

It is critical that you understand the structure and function of the normal velopharyngeal valve in order to fully appreciate and appropriately treat speech problems of patients with VPI. In this chapter we will present the anatomy and physiology of the normal velopharyngeal valving mechanism.

ANATOMY OF THE VELOPHARYNGEAL VALVING MECHANISM

The palate is made up of hard and soft portions. The anterior two thirds of the palate is hard because of the underlying bony structures. The skeleton that comprises the *hard palate* includes the premaxilla[1], the paired palatine processes of the maxilla, and the paired palatine bones (Fig. 3-1). Foramina through the hard palate allow for the passage of nerves and blood vessels. The hard palate is covered with mucoperiosteum, a layered combination of mucous membrane, the lining of the passages and cavities which communicate with air, and periosteum, a fibrous membrane which covers bone.

The posterior one third of the palate is soft because it is composed primarily of muscle, adipose tissue, connective tissue, glandular tissue, and overlying mucous membrane. Some of the muscles of the soft palate attach to the sphenoid bone with its lateral and medial pterygoid plates and hamulus (Fig. 3-2). The correct anatomical name for the soft palate is *velum.* The terms *velopharyngeal mechanism* or *velopharyngeal system* refer to the velum along with the lateral and posterior pharyngeal walls at the level of the velum. The space surrounded by the velum, the lateral pharyngeal walls, and the posterior pharyngeal wall is the *velopharyngeal port.*

The histologic makeup of the normal velum is variable along its length. Kuehn and Kahane (1990) and Ettema and Kuehn (1994) reported that tendinous, muscular, and adipose tissue is more prominent in the anterior aspect of the soft palate than in the posterior aspect, whereas glandular and connective tissue is relatively uniform along the length of the soft palate. Epithelium and vascular tissue is more prevalent posteriorly than anteriorly.

The anatomical information in this chapter is intended as a summary or review of information needed for consideration of velopharyngeal function during speech. Additional detailed consideration of this anatomy is provided in anatomy texts such as that by Zemlin (1997). In this chapter muscles are listed, briefly described, diagrammed, and categorized relative to function. Consideration is then given to innervation.

Muscles of the Soft Palate and Pharynx

The muscles of the soft palate and pharynx include the levator veli palatini, the tensor veli palatini, the musculus uvulae, the salpingopharyngeus, the superior pharyngeal

[1]Ross (personal communication) clarified that the premaxilla is not a separate bone. He wrote, "in humans the bone in the anterior of the maxilla arises as centers of ossification which fuse with the maxillary centers and thus do not form a separate bone. . . . When a cleft intervenes, this fusion cannot occur, so for the sake of convenience we call the isolated bone which is separated from the maxilla a 'premaxilla.' "

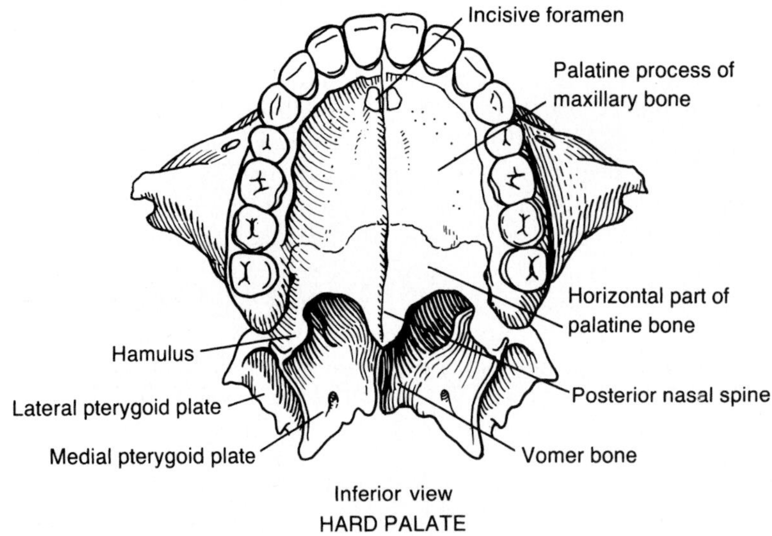

Figure 3-1 Inferior view of hard palate. Note that structures anterior to the incisive foramen make up the primary palate, whereas those posterior form the secondary palate. *(From Dickson DR, and Maue W:* Human vocal anatomy. *Springfield IL: CC Thomas, 1970.)*

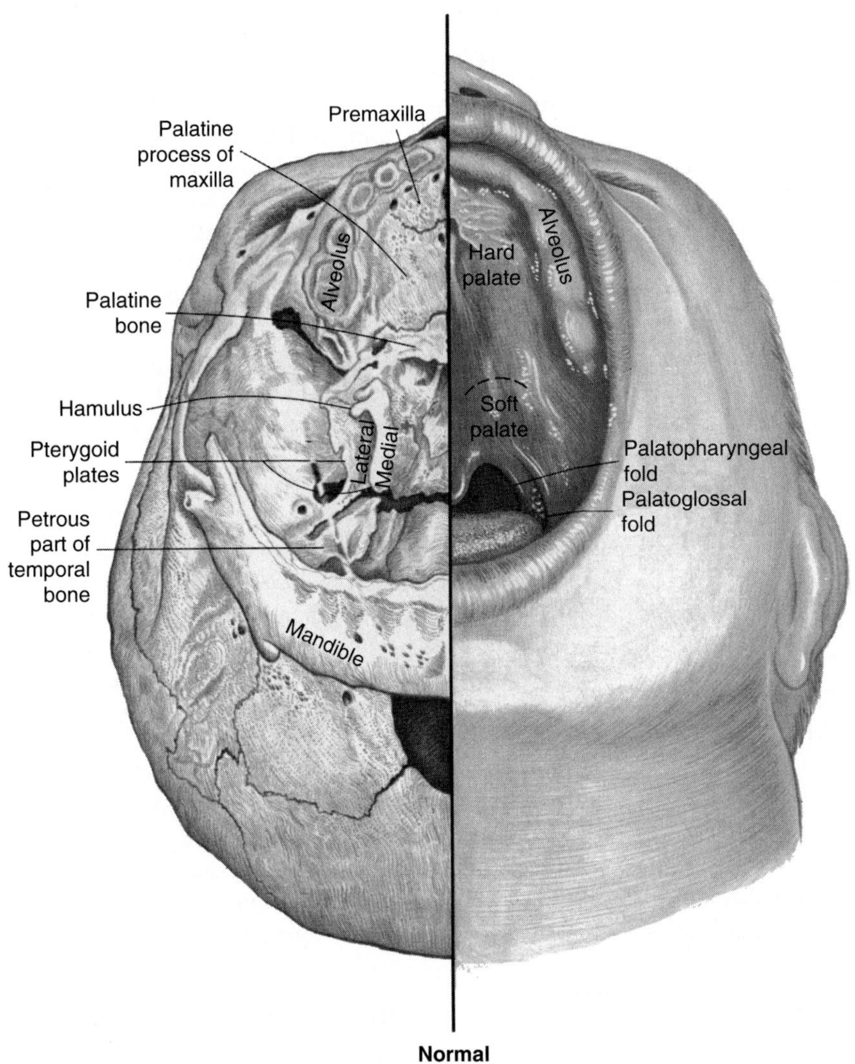

Figure 3-2 Inferior view-newborn palate and related structures. *(From Millard DR:* Cleft craft: the evolution of its surgery, III: alveolar and palatal deformities. *Boston: Little, Brown, 1980.)*

constrictor, the palatopharyngeus, and the palatoglossus. The function of some of these is well accepted, whereas others are less well understood. They are all paired muscles.

Tensor veli palatini. The ribbon-shaped tensor veli palatini (Figs. 3-3 and 3-4) originates from the base of the medial pteryoid plate of the sphenoid bone and the lateral sides of the membranous and cartilaginous portions of the auditory (eustachian) tube. The muscle becomes narrow and tendinous as it travels downward around the hamulus of the sphenoid bone where it takes on a fan-like appearance and becomes the palatine aponeurosis, a fibrous connective tissue that extends from the hard palate to the free border of the soft palate. The anteriormost fibers insert into the posterior border of the hard palate, whereas the more posterior fibers insert into the palatine aponeurosis of the opposite side (Fig. 3-4). The aponeurosis serves as a firm structure to which other muscles attach and against which they pull.

Kuehn and Kahane (1990) described a prominent tendon from the tensor veli palatini muscle that emerges from the hamulus and extends to the midline near the nasal surface of the soft palate in the area just posterior to the hard palate. They suggested that a possible function of this tendon may be to relieve stress that occurs at the "hinge" between the hard and soft palates as the velum elevates and lowers.

During contraction, the tensor opens the auditory tube, permitting equalization of middle ear air pressure with atmospheric pressure. Abnormal function of the tensor contributes to inadequate auditory tube opening, which may lead to accumulation of middle ear fluid and possibly infection. The tensor does not appear to contribute to velopharyngeal closure for speech (Fritzell, 1969; Kuehn and Kahane, 1990).

The tensor receives motor innervation from a branch of the mandibular division of the trigeminal nerve (fifth cranial nerve). Blood supply is provided by the ascending palatine branch of the facial artery and the descending palatine branch of the maxillary artery.

Levator veli palatini. The levator veli palatini (Figs. 3-3 and 3-4) originates from the lower surface of the petrous portion of the temporal bone and from the medial cartilaginous surface of the auditory tube. It descends in a frontomedial direction to insert into the upper surface of the palatal aponeurosis and to blend together with levator fibers from the opposite side. In children with palatal clefts the course and insertion of levator fibers is abnormal (Figs. 3-5 and 3-6).

The levator receives motor innervation from the pharyngeal plexus, which includes contributions from the glossopharyngeus, the pharyngeal branch of the vagus, and the cranial portion of the accessory nerves. Like the tensor, blood supply is provided by the ascending palatine branch of the facial artery and the descending palatine branch of the maxillary artery.

The paired levator muscles form a muscular sling that

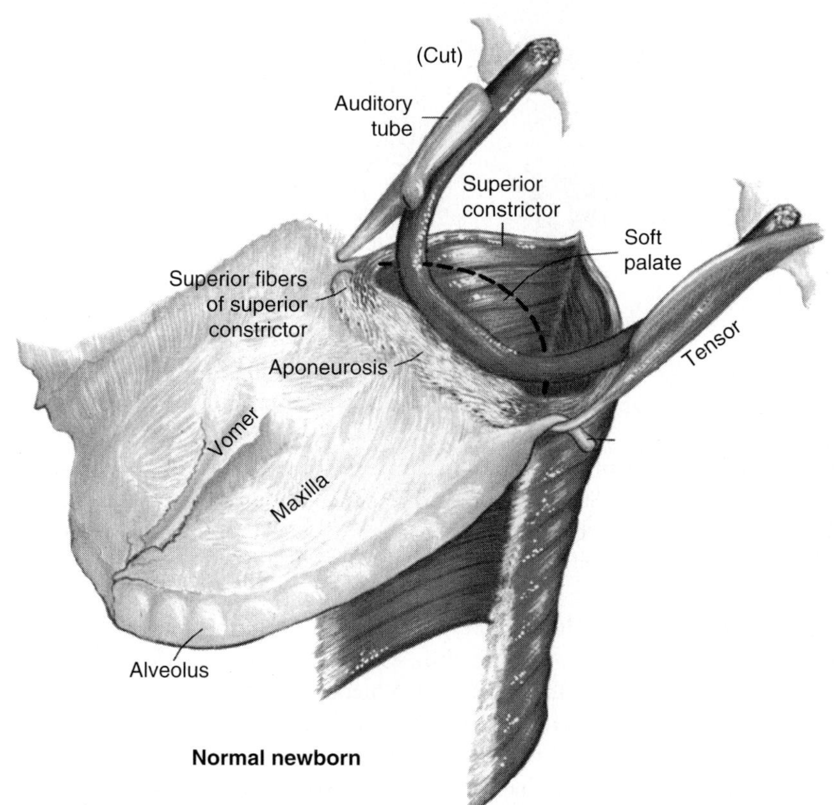

Figure 3-3 Superolateral view of the palate and pharynx, showing position of auditory tube and the tensor veli palatini, levator veli palatini, and superior constrictor muscles in a normal newborn. *(From Millard DR:* Cleft craft: the evolution of its surgery, III: alveolar and palatal deformities. *Boston: Little, Brown, 1980.)*

A

Hamulus

Tensor m. of velum palatinum

Palatal aponeurosis

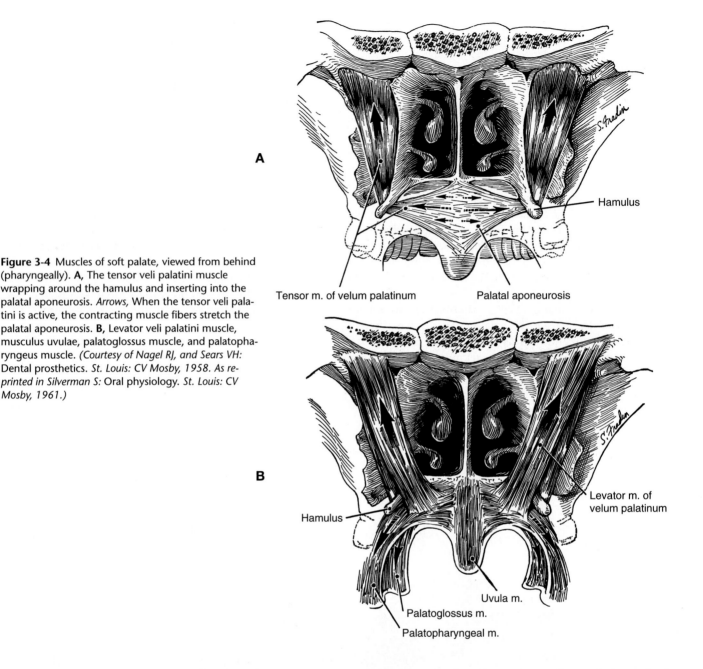

Figure 3-4 Muscles of soft palate, viewed from behind (pharyngeally). **A,** The tensor veli palatini muscle wrapping around the hamulus and inserting into the palatal aponeurosis. *Arrows,* When the tensor veli palatini is active, the contracting muscle fibers stretch the palatal aponeurosis. **B,** Levator veli palatini muscle, musculus uvulae, palatoglossus muscle, and palatopharyngeus muscle. *(Courtesy of Nagel RJ, and Sears VH:* Dental prosthetics. *St. Louis: CV Mosby, 1958. As reprinted in Silverman S:* Oral physiology. *St. Louis: CV Mosby, 1961.)*

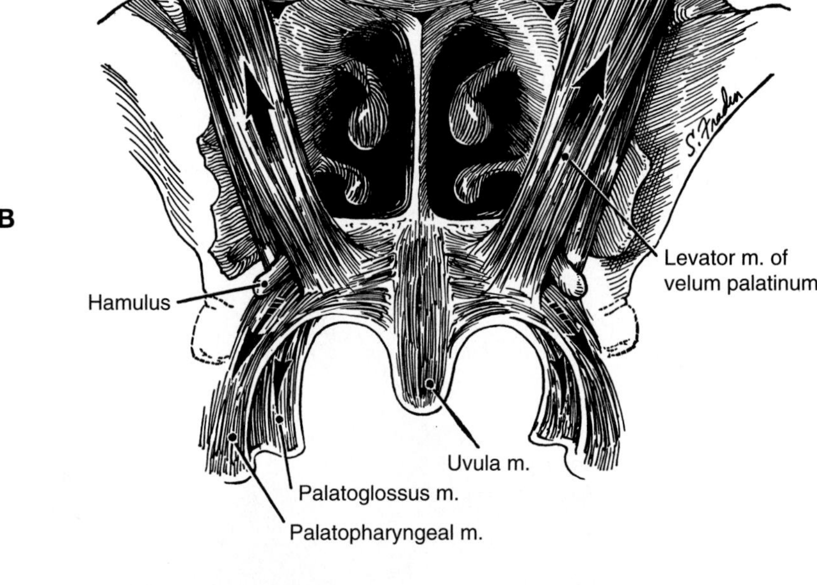

serves to raise the velum upward and backward to contact the posterior wall of the pharynx during speech and nonspeech activities such as swallowing, blowing, coughing, and sneezing. Although the levator is clearly the primary muscle responsible for velar elevation (Bell-Berti, 1976; Fritzell, 1969), several reports suggest that velar position during speech is controlled through interactions among the levator, palatoglossus, and palatopharyngeus muscles (Fig. 3-7) (Moon et al., 1994; Seaver and Kuehn, 1980). Inadequate function of the levator will likely result in velopharyngeal inadequacy.

Musculus uvulae. The musculus uvulae (Fig. 3-8) lies along the midline of the dorsal surface of the velum and has been described as a paired muscle (Azzam and Kuehn, 1977), although some anatomy texts describe it as unpaired. It originates just lateral to the midline of the palatal aponeurosis posterior to the hard palate and anterior to the insertion of the levator. It extends posteriorly over the levator bundles to converge with fibers of the musculus uvulae of the opposite side and insert into the mucous membrane of the uvula. This muscle is thought to contribute to the shape of the dorsal surface of the velum during function. There is general agreement that the musculus uvulae gives needed midline bulk to the velum (Azzam and Kuehn, 1977; Croft et al., 1978; Dickson, 1975; Langdon and Klueber, 1978; Maue-Dickson and Dickson, 1980). Kuehn, Folkins, and Linville (1988) reported supporting data also, including electromyographic findings that indicate the role of the muscle in healthy subjects is to provide velar extension during speech. Azzam

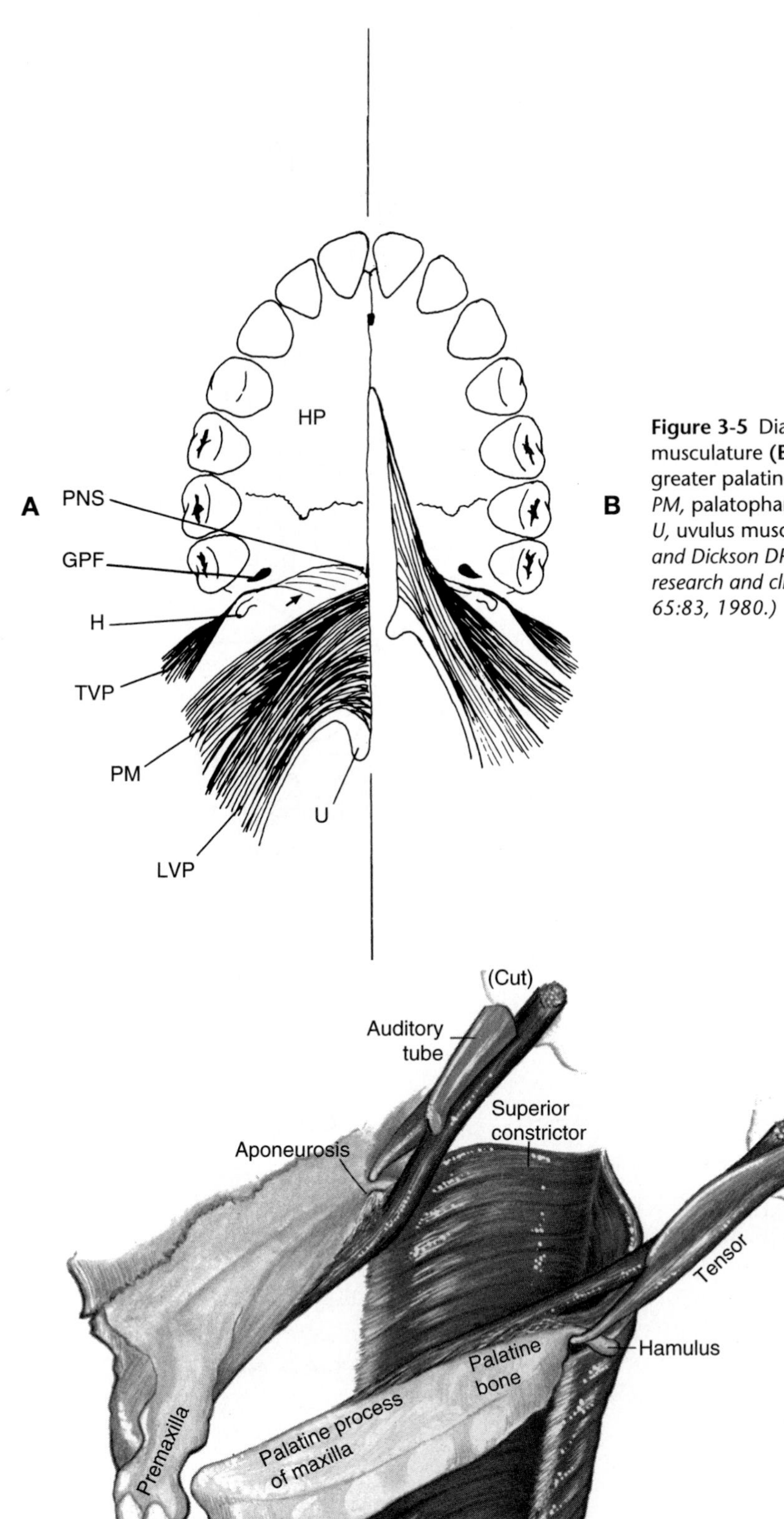

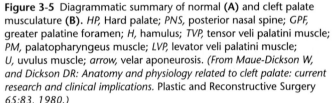

Figure 3-5 Diagrammatic summary of normal **(A)** and cleft palate musculature **(B)**. *HP,* Hard palate; *PNS,* posterior nasal spine; *GPF,* greater palatine foramen; *H,* hamulus; *TVP,* tensor veli palatini muscle; *PM,* palatopharyngeus muscle; *LVP,* levator veli palatini muscle; *U,* uvulus muscle; *arrow,* velar aponeurosis. *(From Maue-Dickson W, and Dickson DR: Anatomy and physiology related to cleft palate: current research and clinical implications.* Plastic and Reconstructive Surgery *65:83, 1980.)*

Figure 3-6 Superolateral view of the palate and pharynx, showing position of auditory tube and the tensor veli palatini, levator veli palatini, and superior constrictor muscles in a newborn with a cleft. *(From Millard DR:* Cleft craft: the evolution of its surgery, III: alveolar and palatal deformities. *Boston: Little, Brown, 1980.)*

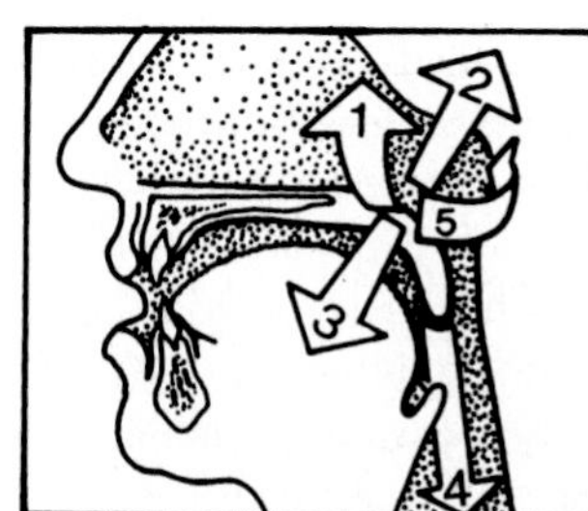

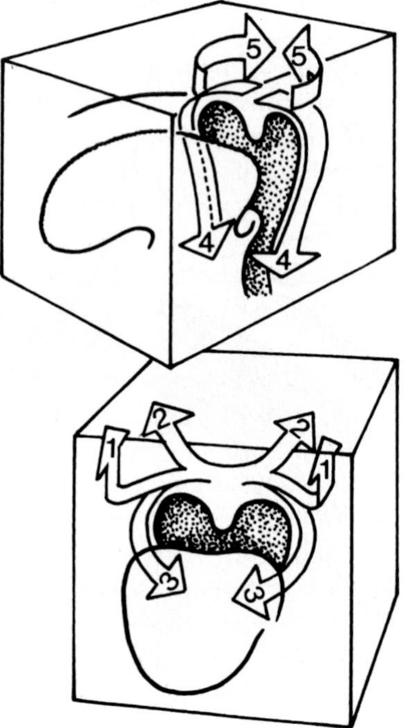

Figure 3-7 Schematic representation of the function of the muscles of the soft palate. *Arrows,* The approximate direction of their action and influence on the soft palate. *(From Fritzell B: The velopharyngeal muscles in speech.* Acta Otolaryngology Supplement *250, 1969.)*

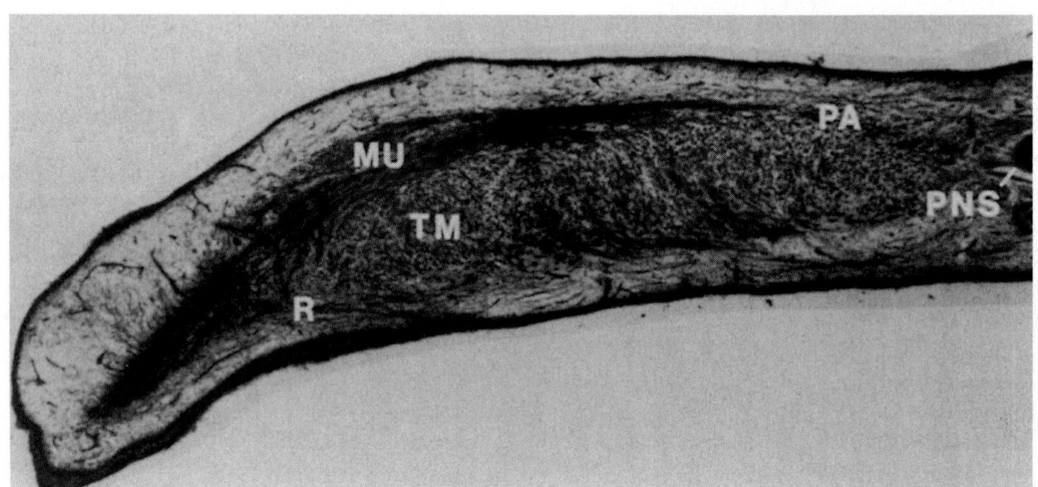

Figure 3-8 Sagittal section through velum illustrating the course and relationships of musculus uvulae. *(From Langdon HL, and Klueber K: The longitudinal fibromuscular component of the soft palate in the fifteen-week human fetus: musculus uvulae and palatine raphe.* Cleft Palate Journal *15:337, 1978.)*

and Kuehn (1977) concluded from a study of adult cadavers that two separate bundles of musculus uvulae are joined together by a midline septum.

Palatopharyngeus. The two palatopharyngeus muscles (Figs. 3-4 and 3-7) form the posterior pillars of the fauces. Each arises from the pharyngeal wall and the side of the soft palate and reach the midline of the soft palate between the levator and tensor muscles. It is difficult at dissection to differentiate between the fibers of the palatopharyngeus and other muscles, including the superior constrictor.

Palatopharyngeus functions include adduction of the posterior pillars, constriction of the pharyngeal isthmus, narrowing of the velopharyngeal orifice, raising of the larynx, and lowering of the pharynx. They are believed to be antagonists of the levator and, as such, active participants in fine control of the position of the soft palate during speech (Moon et al., 1994; Seaver and Kuehn, 1980). Some data suggest that the palatopharyngeus is more active in swallowing than in speech (Trigos et al., 1988).

Palatoglossus. The palatoglossus (Figs. 3-4 and 3-7) extends from the oral surface of the soft palate to the side of the tongue. The two palatoglossus muscles form the anterior pillars of the fauces. They serve to pull the tongue upward and backward and to constrict the faucial pillars. Like the palatopharyngeus, there are some data supporting an antagonistic relationship between the palatoglossus and the levator (Moon et al., 1994; Seaver and Kuehn, 1980). However, another study (Kuehn and Azzam, 1978) suggested that elastic fibers found in the anterior faucial pillar that intermingle with palatoglossus fascicles could provide a passive restorative force in lowering the palate, helping to keep the nasopharyngeal airway open for nasal respiration.

Superior constrictor. The superior constrictor muscle (Figs. 3-6, 3-7, and 3-9) arises from the velum, medial pterygoid plate and hamulus, pterygomandibular raphe, mylohyoid line and adjacent alveolar processes of the mandible, and the sides of the tongue. It inserts into the median pharyngeal raphe. Dickson and Maue-Dickson (1980) indicated that the superior fibers of the superior constrictor enter the velum with fibers of the levator veli palatini. Many of the origins of the superior constrictor are variable, and the anatomy of the muscle is variable from person to person (Bosma, 1953).

The superior constrictor may contribute to medial movement of the lateral walls and anterior movement of the posterior pharyngeal wall. Controversy regarding its contribution to medial movement of the lateral walls is discussed later. The superior constrictor may also contribute to movement of the velum, tongue, hyoid bone, and larynx and to the formation of Passavant's ridge. The superior constrictor, along with middle and inferior constrictors, is part of the pharyngeal tube.

Middle constrictor. The fan-shaped middle constrictor muscle (Figs. 3-9 and 3-10) extends from the median pharyngeal raphe to insert into the hyoid bone and stylohyoid ligament. This muscle overlaps the lower portion of the superior constrictor muscle and, in turn, is overlapped by the inferior constrictor muscle. It is thought to constrict the pharynx during deglutition and to move the hyoid bone posteriorly.

Inferior constrictor. The inferior constrictor muscle (Figs. 3-9 and 3-10) consists of thyropharyngeal and cricopharyngeal portions. It extends from the median pharyngeal raphe to the thyroid and cricoid cartilages of the larynx. The inferior constrictor contributes to constriction of the pharynx in deglutition and to movement of the larynx upward and backward. Its most inferior fibers form the cricopharyngeus, which exists in a state of constant contraction to maintain closure of the upper esophageal sphincter. During the swallow response the cricopharyngeus relaxes to permit opening of the upper esophageal sphincter to accept the bolus (Kahrilas et al., 1988). The cricopharyngeus is also thought to be important in esophageal and tracheoesophageal speech (Pruszewicz et al., 1992).

Stylopharyngeus. The stylopharyngeus muscle (Figs. 3-9 and 3-10) extends from the styloid process downward between the superior and middle constrictor muscles into the lateral pharyngeal wall. It attaches to the thyroid cartilage of the larynx and is thought to raise and widen the pharynx.

Salpingopharyngeus. The highly variable salpingopharyngeus muscle is not always identified at dissection and may not even be present in some people (Fritzell, 1969; Trigos et al., 1988). It arises from the torus tubarius at the opening of the eustachian tube and descends to join the palatopharyngeal fibers in the lateral pharyngeal wall. It may contribute to motion of the lateral pharyngeal wall in a manner similar to that in which the musculus uvulus may contribute to velar extension. Its location is compatible with influence on the eustachian tube.

Muscles That Form the Velar Eminence

As we have seen, elevation of the velum is attributed to the levator veli palatini muscles. The knuckled appearance of the nasal surface of the velum in sagittal radiographs has been called the levator eminence because it was thought to reflect the activity of the levator fibers, which insert into the region of the velum that is part of the eminence. For example, Shprintzen et al. (1975) wrote that the levator is positioned to contribute to the formation of the velar eminence. Other evidence suggests that the musculus uvulae contributes to the velar eminence (Azzam and Kuehn, 1977; Simpson and Austin, 1972).

Simpson and Austin (1972) noted that contraction of the uvular muscle may account for an observed increase in

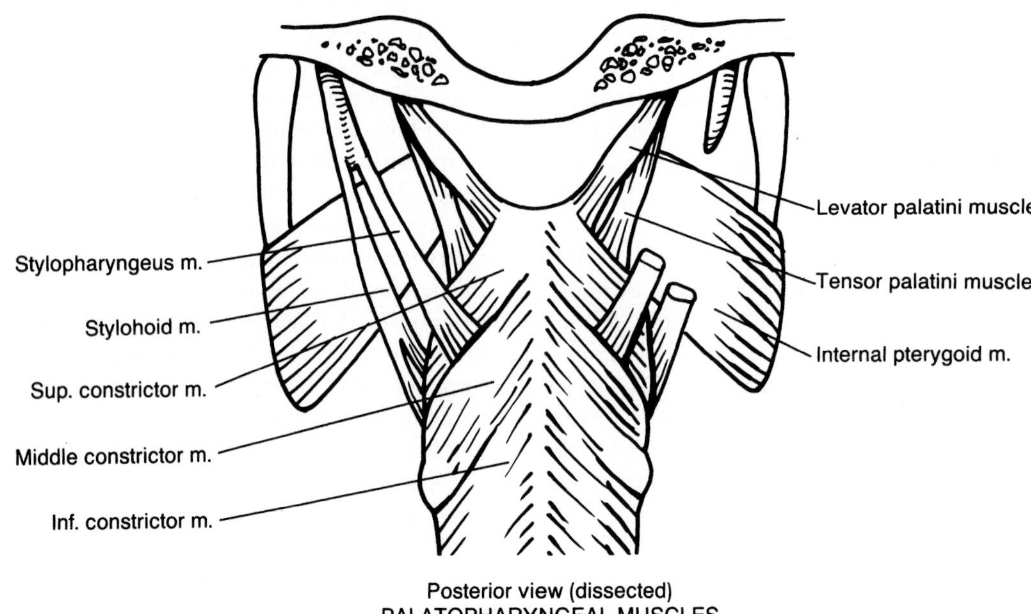

Figure 3-9 Palatopharyngeal muscles, posterior view (dissected). *(From Dickson DR, and Maue W:* Human vocal anatomy. *Springfield IL: CC Thomas, 1970.)*

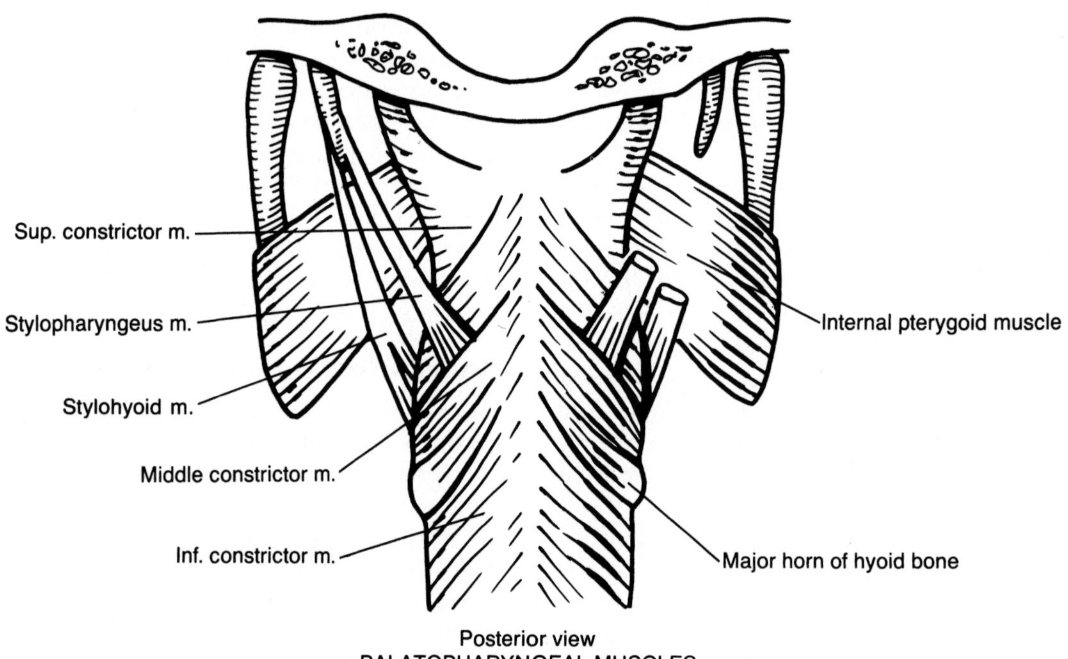

Figure 3-10 Palatopharyngeal muscles, posterior view. *(From Dickson DR, and Maue W:* Human vocal anatomy. *Springfield IL: CC Thomas, 1970.)*

the thickness of the soft palate during sustained /s/. Dissection and histological studies led Azzam and Kuehn (1977) to conclude that contraction of the musculus uvulae may contribute bulk to the dorsal surface of the velum. Langdon and Klueber (1978) concluded from their anatomical studies in 15-week fetuses that the "combined vectors of the musculi levator veli palatini and palatopharyngeus" are such that they may serve as antagonists to the musculus uvulae. Interaction among these muscles may be responsible for the knuckled eminence of the elevated velum, and the eminence should probably be called the velar eminence.

In addition, the levator fibers enter the velum at the most inferior level of that muscle, that is, at the bottom of the sling, which, when contracted, pulls the velum upward and backward. Because the mechanism of the eminence is not clear, we subscribe to the view that "levator eminence" should probably be called the "velar eminence."

Kuehn, Folkins, and Linville (1988) reported electromyographic findings that related the function of the musculus uvulae and the levator during speech. They found similar patterns of electromyographic activity for the musculus uvulae and the levator veli palatini in three healthy subjects. When differences in electromyographic activity between the two muscles were found, the tasks did not involve speech. These authors further suggested that the musculus uvulae may be important in filling the space between the elevated velum and the posterior pharyngeal wall. This explanation has clinical implications because the musculus uvulae is almost always lacking in patients with palatal clefts.

VELOPHARYNGEAL MOTOR INNERVATION

Fritzell (1969) wrote that all palatal and upper pharyngeal muscles except the tensor and uvular muscles are innervated by the pharyngeal plexus, which is composed of branches from the *glossopharyngeus, vagus,* and *accessory* cranial nerves (Fig. 3-11). The tensor is innervated by the mandibular branch of the trigeminal cranial nerve and, according to Fritzell (1969), is probably not involved in speech. Zemlin (1997) also wrote that fibers from the mandibular branch of the *trigeminal* nerve and cranial branch of the accessory nerve supply the palate and uvula along with fibers from the pharyngeal plexus, which arises from the sphenopalatine ganglion, and provide motor input to the pharynx and soft palate.

There has been some debate about a possible role for the facial nerve in palatal motor innervation of the palate. Nishio et al. (1976b) studied motor innervation of the velopharyngeal mechanism in rhesus monkeys by means of electrical stimulation of facial, glossopharyngeal, accessory, and vagus nerves and electromyographic recording of responses from levator, uvula, and superior constrictor muscles. They reported that stimulation of the vagus nerve resulted in the greatest electromyographic amplitude, followed by the glossopharyngeal and facial nerves. No electromyographic response was observed when the accessory nerve was stimulated. The authors concluded that "the levator veli palatini, uvula, and superior constrictor pharyngeus muscles are double innervated by the facial nerve and branches of the pharyngeal plexus derived from the glossopharyngeal and vagus nerves and that the facial nerve plays an important role as one of the motor nerves in movements responsible for velopharyngeal closure" (p. 30).

In a follow-up study, Nishio et al. (1976a) examined velopharyngeal movements, observed by means of a nasal fiberscope, in response to electrical stimulation of facial, glossopharyngeal, and vagus nerves. Movements were greatest when the vagus was stimulated, followed by the glossopharyngeal and the facial nerves, respectively. They further reported that stimulation of the glossopharyngeal and the vagus nerves resulted in upward movements of the velopharyngeal structures while facial nerve stimulation resulted in upper nasopharyngeal contraction in a more horizontal plane. The authors conclude, "Considering the degree and pattern of movements seen, it is assumed that the facial nerve controls finer movements of the velopharyngeal muscles than do the glossopharyngeal or the vagus nerve" (p. 212).

Dickson and Maue-Dickson (1980) interpreted the findings of Nishio et al. as evidence that the uvular, levator, and superior constrictor muscles are innervated by both the facial nerve and the pharyngeal plexus. They suggested that facial nerve stimulation resulted in closure patterns similar to those associated with speech, whereas stimulation of the vagus or glossopharyngeus resulted in swallow-like patterns. This echoed an interpretation offered earlier by Sedlackova, Lastovia, and Sram (1973) and others. Bosma (1986) rejected this hypothesis: "I would challenge the interpretation of Sedlackova and others that the levator is activated via the facial innervation during speech and via the vagal innervation during swallow." He went on to argue ". . . the motor innervation and the peripheral motor effector apparatus of the oral and pharyngeal area are pluripotential, apropos of performances" (pp. 390-391), suggesting that these peripheral motor nerves are capable of supporting more than one type of task, as are the muscles they innervate.

VELOPHARYNGEAL SENSORY INNERVATION

Bass and Morrell (1992) reported that the sensory innervation of the tonsils, pharynx, and soft palate is provided by the pharyngeal branch of the *vagus* nerve. Zemlin (1997) wrote that sensory fibers from the pharyngeal plexus supply the mucous membrane of the pharynx, the faucial pillars, the pharyngeal orifice of the auditory tube, and the soft palate. Fibers from the internal pharyngeal branches of the *vagus* and *glossopharyngeal* nerves are also involved.

Additional data are needed to define the exact nature of

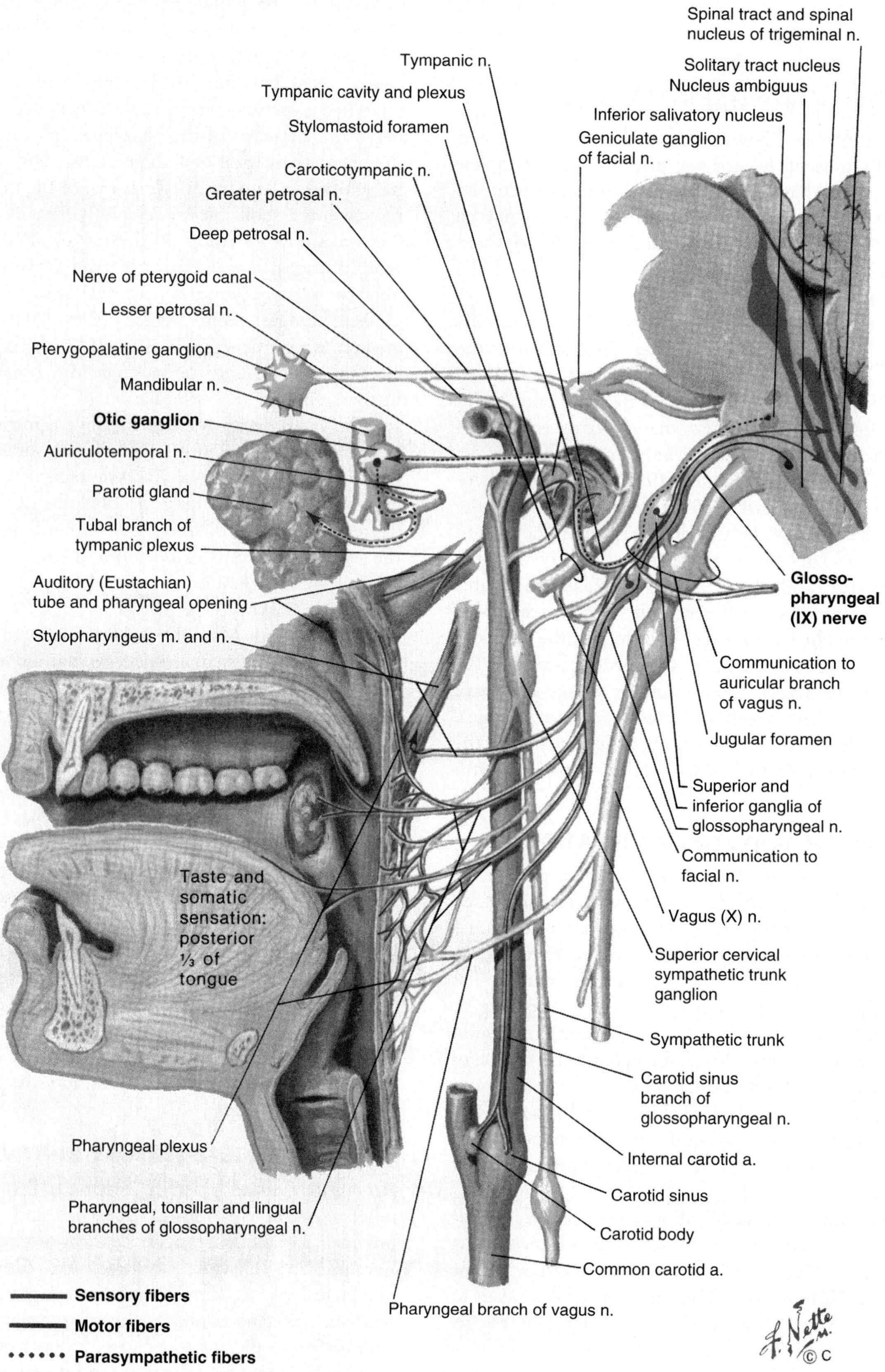

Figure 3-11 Glossopharyngeal (IX) nerve and otic ganglion. *(From Netter FH: The Ciba collection of medical illustrations. Volume 1:* Nervous system—I: anatomy and physiology. *West Caldwell, NJ: CIBA Pharmaceuticals Company, 1983.)*

motor and sensory innervation of the velopharyngeal musculature in humans. Considerable information is available about velopharyngeal physiologic features.

VELOPHARYNGEAL PHYSIOLOGY

Knowledge about the structure and function of the normal velopharyngeal valving mechanism is required if the speech pathologist is to evaluate and understand abnormal mechanisms and plan effective treatment approaches. We are interested here in function of the velopharyngeal mechanism, the relative contributions of the normal velum and pharyngeal walls, and the velopharyngeal closure requirements for normal speech.

Velar Movement for Speech

There is clear consensus that the levator veli palatini is the primary muscle responsible for velar elevation for speech and swallowing. Tensor veli palatini and salpingopharyngeus appear to have little, if any, effect on velar position for speech. The palatopharyngeus and palatoglossus may work in opposition to the levator to achieve a high degree of control over velar position although there is considerable interindividual variability (Moon et al., 1994). Moon and Canady (1995) found less levator activity associated with velar elevation when speakers were in a supine position than when they were upright. This suggests a small gravitational effect on velar muscle activation.

Radiographic studies indicate that, in healthy individuals, displacement of the velum upward and backward contributes to closure of the velopharyngeal port. Bzoch, Graber, and Aoba (1959) studied 44 healthy young adults during production of /p/, /b/, /f/, /w/, and /m/ and reported that the velum is highest at its middle segment and that its third quadrant meets the posterior wall of the pharynx in sealing the velopharyngeal port. They reported that, usually, the midpoint of contact between the velum and the posterior pharyngeal wall was 3 to 4 mm below the palatal plane. The highest point of contact was approximately at the palatal plane, and the highest point of the velar eminence was 4 to 5 mm above the palatal plane. Mazaheri, Millard, and Erickson (1964) found velopharyngeal contact to be below the palatal plane in eight of ten normal subjects.

Velopharyngeal closure, as observed in the sagittal view from lateral radiographs, is completed before onset of phonation and is maintained until the person produces either a nasal consonant or a vowel adjacent to a nasal consonant or stops talking (Fig. 3-12). Although velopharyngeal closure is maintained throughout the oral portions of an utterance, the velum does not remain immobile but rather moves upward and downward with variations in phonetic character of the oral sounds produced (Moll, 1960; Karnell, Folkins, and Morris, 1985; Karnell, Linville, and Edwards, 1988) (Fig. 3-13). Moon et al. (1994) and Moon, Kuehn, and Huisman (1995) reported similar variations in force of velopharyngeal closure.

Variation in velar displacement in different speech contexts has been of special interest to speech pathologists. Harrington (1944) was among the first to publish measurements showing differences in the extent of velar movement related to vowel type. Warren and Hofmann (1961) found from cineradiographic research that the velum did not maintain firm contact with the posterior wall during the production of isolated sounds, a finding that suggests limited clinical value of observing velar movement during sustained oral vowel sounds.

Moll (1962) studied velar height, the extent of contact between velum and posterior pharyngeal wall, and the gap between velum and posterior pharyngeal wall for four vowels produced by 10 healthy adults. Data were obtained from cinefluorographic films exposed at 24 frames per second. The vowels /i/, /æ/, /u/, and /æ/, were studied in isolation and in [CVC] syllables produced in the carrier phrase, "Say CVC again." Each syllable was initiated or

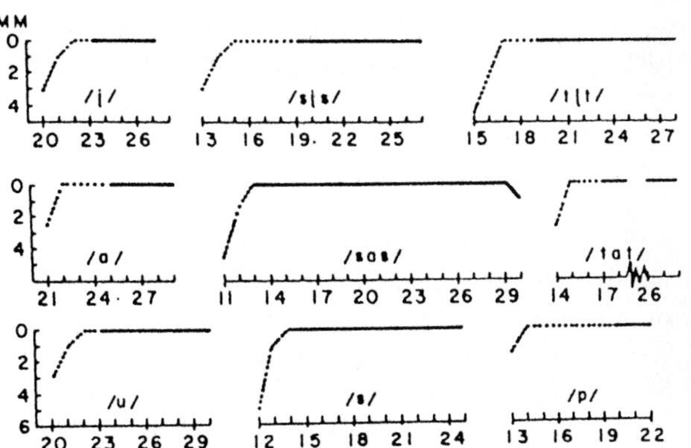

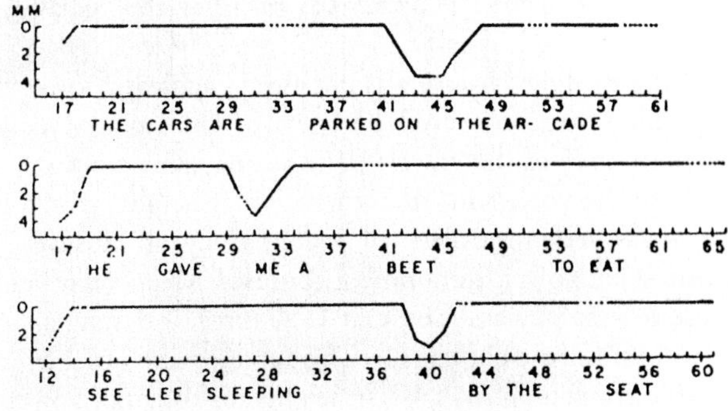

Figure 3-12 Curves illustrate palatopharyngeal gap in millimeters for each cine frame. Nonphonation frames are indicated by dotted lines. Frame numbers are indicated along the abscissa. Palatopharyngeal closure is complete except during utterance of nasal consonants. The subject is a normal speaker. *(Redrawn from Shelton RL, Brooks AR, and Youngstrom KA: Articulation and patterns of palatopharyngeal closure.* Journal of Speech and Hearing Disorders *29:395, 1964. © American Speech-Language-Hearing Association. Adapted with permission.)*

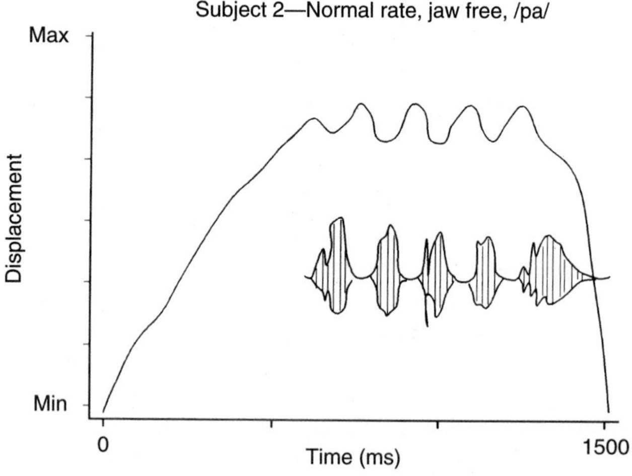

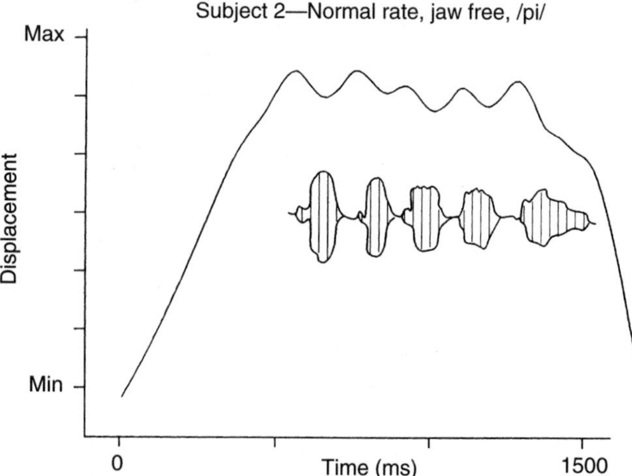

Figure 3-13 Plots of /pa/ and /pi/ repetition during the jaw free condition. *(From Karnell MP, Linville RN, and Edwards BA: Variations in velar position over time: a nasal videoendoscopic study.* Journal of Speech and Hearing Research *31:417-424, 1988. © American Speech-Language-Hearing Association. Reprinted with permission.)*

arrested with /p/. Fricatives, plosives, affricates, the liquid /l/, and the nasal /n/ appeared in either the releasing or arresting of each syllable.

Interestingly, closure was not always achieved for vowels. Openings were observed on 30% of the isolated vowels, 13% to 15% of the vowels in oral consonant contexts, and 89% of the vowels in /n/ context. Velar height, which may be measured regardless of velopharyngeal closure, was greatest for vowels in nonnasal contexts. Mean velar heights were lowest in nasal contexts (8.4 mm) and ranged from 11.6 mm for the contexts free from consonants to 12.3 mm for the consonant /ʤ/. Velar heights for the high vowels /i/ and /u/ averaged 12.4 mm each compared with 10.5 for /æ/, and 10.6 mm for /ɑ/. Differences between high and low vowels were statistically significant, whereas differences among the high vowels were not. Data for extent of velopharyngeal contact were similar in pattern to those for velar height. Only the isolated vowel data were analyzed because the consonant context data were skewed.

Distance between the velum and the posterior wall was studied only for vowels in nasal contexts because most of the measures in other contexts were 0; that is, the velopharyngeal port was closed. Mean gaps were 2.45 mm for /i/, 2.03 mm for /u/, 4.6 for /æ/, and 4.0 for /ɑ/. High vowels were not significantly different from one another; neither were the low vowels. However, the high vowels differed from the low vowels.

These data indicate that the function of the velum varies systematically with phonetic context. Moll (1962) noted that covariability in velar height with the tongue height (which determines vowel position) may reflect the influence of the palatoglossus muscle. The palatoglossus inserts into both the velum and tongue and may influence the muscles that elevate the velum. Different vowels may require different degrees of velar elevation to produce the desired acoustic and perceptual result.

Pharyngeal Wall Movement

There is controversy relative to the contribution of the levator veli palatini and the superior constrictor muscles to lateral velopharyngeal wall movement. Selected literature pertinent to this issue is considered here.

An explanation of lateral pharyngeal wall movements which emphasized the levator muscles was presented by Dickson (1972, 1975) and by Dickson and Maue-Dickson (1972). As summarized by Dickson and Maue-Dickson (1980), "the inferior tip of the torus tubarius" is near the level of the hard palate and the levator "crosses lateral to it." Thus the levator is positioned to influence the lateral walls of the pharynx by its action on the torus tubarius, whereas the superior constrictor is too low to contribute to velopharyngeal closure. They note that this is the most parsimonious explanation of lateral wall contribution to velopharyngeal closure. Movements of the torus tubarius have been described by Bosma (1953) and Lavorato and Lindholm (1976).

Other authors attribute anterior movement of the posterior pharyngeal wall and medial movement of the lateral walls at the level of velopharyngeal closure to the superior constrictor. Shprintzen et al. (1975) interpreted videofluoroscopic images to indicate that shelves form on the lateral walls during speech, that those shelves reflect the greatest range of motion of the lateral walls, and that they occur below the level of the most inferior fibers of the levator veli palatini muscles. These authors interpreted the literature to indicate that the most superior fibers of the superior constrictor are located where they could contribute to the shelf-like projections of the lateral walls. Iglesias, Kuehn, and Morris (1980) described simultaneous assessment of pharyngeal wall and velar displacement in normal subjects by lateral radiography and frontal tomography. They anticipated that if the levator was solely responsible for lateral wall and velar movements, those movements should be highly correlated. To the contrary, they reported low correlations between velar and pharyngeal displacement. They concluded that the superior constrictor muscle is an important contributor to velopharyngeal activity in normal speakers and that their findings did not support the hypothesis that the levator veli palatini muscle is solely involved in movements of the lateral pharyngeal walls. They concluded that levator may *assist* lateral wall movement in some, but not all, individuals.

Bell-Berti (1980) disagreed with that interpretation. Like Dickson and Maue-Dickson (1980), she disputed the contribution of superior constrictor to lateral pharyngeal wall movement because the superior constrictor is positioned below the level where velopharyngeal closure usually occurs. Her 1976 electromyographic data indicated that the superior constrictor contributed little to velopharyngeal closure. Contrary to the data reported by Iglesias et al. (1980), Niimi, Bell-Berti, and Harris (1982) reported very high correlations (r = 0.86 to r = 0.99, depending on phonemic context) between velar movement and lateral wall movement, leading them to the conclusion that levator was the muscle responsible for lateral wall movement at the level of velopharyngeal closure.

The controversy surrounding muscular activity responsible for lateral wall movement may be a result of the three-dimensional character of the velopharyngeal mechanism, intersubject variability in velopharyngeal physiology, and the methods used to examine these issues. Karnell, Folkins, and Morris (1985) found that views of the velopharyngeal port from oral endoscopy tended to better represent posterior wall movement, whereas views from nasal endoscopy tended to better represent lateral wall movement. Such differences are likely the result of anatomic and physiologic differences within individuals along the vertical dimension of the velopharyngeal port. Niimi, Bell-Berti, and Harris (1982) concluded their report with the following statement:

> Finally, we must also expect some individual differences, even among normal speakers, and thus it may be that some speakers use the superior constrictor in addition to levator palatini when they constrict the velopharyngeal port. (p 255)

Astley (1958) described what was probably the first use of frontal view cinefluorography to evaluate movement of the lateral walls. Symmetrical mesial movement of the lateral walls was described during speech and blowing tasks, with evidence of more extensive mesial movement for blowing than for speech. Similar descriptions were provided by Griffith et al. (1968), Isshiki, Honjow, and Morimoto (1969), and others. Minifie et al. (1970) reported lateral wall movement was greater for high vowels than for low vowels.

Intersubject differences in the relative contributions of the velum, lateral pharyngeal walls, and posterior pharyngeal wall have been long recognized. Zwitman, Sonderman, and Ward (1974) described four patterns of velopharyngeal closure on the basis of oral endoscopic observations of normal subjects.

1. Lateral walls move medially and make contact with one another as the velum touches the approximated section of the lateral walls.
2. Lateral walls almost approximate, with the velum contacting the lateral walls and partly occluding the space between them. A small medial opening is observed in some cases.
3. Lateral walls move medially, filling the lateral pharyngeal gutters and fusing with the raised velum as it contacts the posterior walls.
4. Lateral walls move slightly or not at all. Velum touches posterior wall at midline, and lateral openings are observed during phonation.

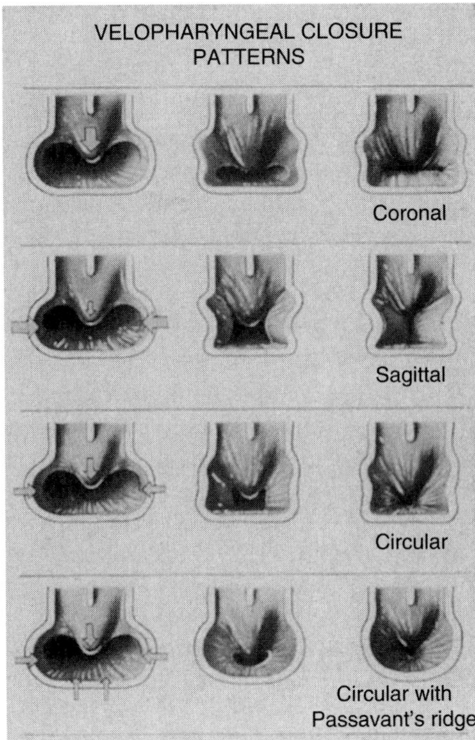

Figure 3-14 Patterns of velopharyngeal valving. *(From Siegel-Sadewitz VL, and Shprintzen RJ.* Cleft Palate Journal *19:196, 1982.)*

Skolnick et al. (1975) described three patterns of velopharyngeal closure on the basis of videofluoroscopic evaluations of normal subjects.

1. Simultaneous displacement of velum and lateral pharyngeal walls with roughly equal contributions from each or perhaps with a "somewhat greater velar than pharyngeal motion."
2. Circular motion (with or without Passavant's ridge), characterized by relatively great medial motion of the lateral walls and a "shortened velum or reduced velar movement."
3. Sagittal pattern where the lateral walls move markedly toward midline and the palate touches those lateral walls rather than the posterior wall.

Croft, Shprintzen, and Rakoff (1981) described these patterns of closure with the terms "coronal," "circular," "circular with Passavant's ridge," and "sagittal" as category names (Fig. 3-14). They found that the coronal pattern was the most common pattern in both normal individuals and individuals with velopharyngeal insufficiency.

In summary, there is little debate that the extent of lateral pharyngeal wall movement varies among individuals. With few exceptions, however, the extent of right and left lateral wall movement is symmetrical within individuals. Maximum lateral wall movement occurs at the level of contact between the velum and the posterior pharyngeal wall, and, similar to velar movement, the extent of lateral wall movement varies somewhat depending on phonetic context.

Posterior Pharyngeal Wall Movement and Passavant's Ridge

There has long been debate about the muscular activity associated with the anterior movement of the posterior pharyngeal wall during speech first described by Passavant (1863, 1869). Passavant's ridge is also variably named a "pad" or a "bar" in the literature. Calnan (1957) provided a thorough historical review of the controversy among nineteenth and twentieth century physicians who studied this phenomenon. The issue involved whether the superior pharyngeal constrictor and palatopharyngeus muscles were responsible for formation of the structure or perhaps whether the structure was formed by passive folding of mucosal tissue. The bulk of the research reviewed by Calnan credited superior constrictor with formation of Passavant's ridge. Calnan also described the controversy over the function of Passavant's ridge. The majority of the reports reviewed agreed with Calnan's position that Passavant's ridge was not essential for speech because the ridge occurred too low to be of use for velopharyngeal closure. As strong as Calnan's argument appeared to be, it does not enjoy widespread acceptance today.

Glaser et al. (1979) defined Passavant's ridge as:

> a localized anterior projection of the posterior pharyngeal wall as opposed to the generalized posterior pharyngeal wall motion seen within a broad inferior-superior range with little, if any, localized movement [Fig. 3-15]. The ridge is not a permanent projection, but instead is a "functional structure" which appears during certain velopharyngeal valving activities such as speech.

Glaser et al. (1980) reported that in 81.8% of their subjects the ridge was usually perpendicular to the velum (parallel to the palatal plane). In the remaining subjects the ridge was directed upward or downward. The authors reported that, among their subjects who exhibited a Passavant's ridge, a common pattern was for the ridge to take a crescent shape continuing along the lateral pharyngeal walls. In patients with this pattern, as viewed through baseview videofluorography, the velopharyngeal closure configuration was circular.

Croft, Shprintzen, and Rakoff (1981) noted that Passavant's ridge was a common component of velopharyngeal closure in both normal subjects and in individuals with velopharyngeal inadequacy (Table 3-1). These data supported current thinking that, although the muscular mechanism and appearance of Passavant's ridge is variable among individuals, it does play a role in velopharyngeal closure for some speakers.

Table 3-1 Relative Distribution of Velopharyngeal Closure Patterns Among Normal Individuals (n = 80) and Individuals with Velopharyngeal Inadequacy (n = 500)

Normals (80)	*Pattern*	*Pathologics (500)*
55% (44)	Coronal	45% (225)
16% (13)	Sagittal	11% (55)
10% (8)	Circular	20% (100)
19% (15)	Circular with Passavant's ridge	24% (120)

From Croft CB, Shprintzen RJ, and Rakoff SJ: Patterns of velopharyngeal valving in normal and cleft palate subjects: a multi-view videofluoroscopic and nasoendoscopic study. *Laryngoscope* 91:265-271, 1981.

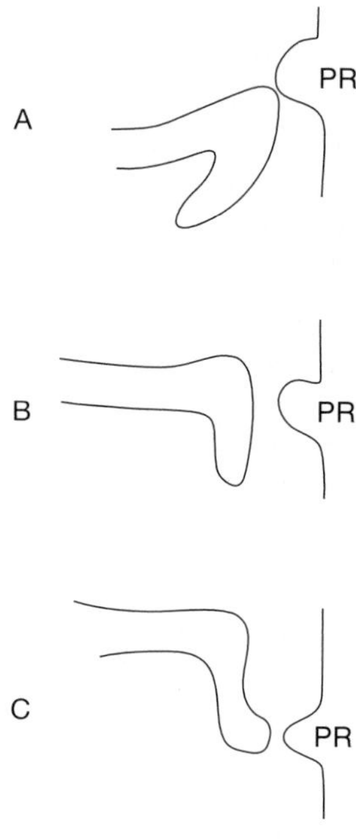

Figure 3-15 Passavant's ridge as a primary source of velopharyngeal narrowing or closure. *Pattern A,* Velar eminence to Passavant's ridge; *pattern B,* vertical portion of velum to Passavant's ridge; *pattern C,* uvula to Passavant's ridge. *(From Glaser ER, Skolnick ML, McWilliams BJ, and Shprintzen RJ: The dynamics of Passavant's ridge in subjects with and without velopharyngeal insufficiency—a multiview videofluoroscopic study.* Cleft Palate Journal *16:24, 1979.)*

Theories of Velopharyngeal Function

Speech scientists consider velopharyngeal function in terms of how the central and peripheral nervous systems control muscle function to move the velopharyngeal structures in coordination with other speech activities. For example,

Moll and Shriner (1967) hypothesized that the velum may function in only two modes, on and off. When the velum is "on," it elevates to achieve velopharyngeal closure. When it is "off," it lowers for nasal respiration or nasal sound production. Although velar postures between the elevated and rest positions were acknowledged, Moll and Shriner explained these intermediate positions as being related to timing variables and constraints inherent in the biomechanics of the structures.

Moll and Shriner's "binary" hypothesis stimulated a considerable body of research and discussion. Later studies combining cinefluorography and electromyography failed to support the binary theory. Lubker's data (1968) supported Moll's (1962) earlier observation that systematic variation in velar motion and position occur with changes in vowel height. In addition, his data and those of Fritzell (1969) indicated that electrical activity in palatal muscles, as measured with electromyography, is continuous rather than intermittent. Such electromyographic data supported the notion that variations in velar height, including velar lowering, are controlled by neuromotor signals and are not simply the result of biomechanical influences.

Moll and Daniloff (1971) studied velar *coarticulation,* that is, the interaction of velar movements and phonetic requirements for speech in syllables made up of oral consonants, vowels, and nasal consonants. Examining frame-by-frame tracings of high-speed (150 frames/sec) lateral cinefluorographic recordings in four adult subjects, they reported "extensive" evidence of anticipatory coarticulation. For example, they reported regarding VN and VVN sequences:

> in sequences in which a nasal consonant is preceded by one or two vowels sounds, the velar-opening gesture for the nasal is initiated near the beginning of primary articulatory movement toward the first vowel in the sequence. (p 683)

These authors further emphasized that this effect was not influenced by the presence of word boundaries within the sequence. They argued that these findings were consistent with a model of speech production where the phoneme is the basic unit of speech production (Henke, 1966). They further held that velar movements could be modeled according to the binary model of Moll and Shriner (1967) where the velum is (1) elevated for nonnasal sounds, (2) lowered for nasal sounds, and (3) unspecified for vowels.

Kent, Carney, and Severeid (1974) supported many of the general findings of Moll and Daniloff (1971) but refuted the binary model of velar control. They cited examples where velar elevation was noted during nasal consonants when followed by oral consonants (e.g., the [nt] sequence in the word "contract"). They suggested that velar control and articulatory movements in general are programed as "coordinated structures."

Lubker (1975) presented electromyographic data in support of a theory of velopharyngeal function that stressed the importance of the coordinated function of several velopharyngeal muscles with other, nonvelar, speech movements. Consistent with his earlier study and with the findings of Moll and Daniloff (1971), he asserted that the velopharyngeal mechanism must be centrally coordinated with other speech articulators. We agree with these authors. The velopharyngeal mechanism does not simply close for oral speech and then fall open when turned off for nasal consonants or silence. Rather, it closes to different degrees, depending on such variables as vowel height, voicing, and proximity to nasal consonants.

Kuehn (1976) examined variability of velar movements in two normal speakers. He found that the trajectory of normal palatal movement was relatively constant, even when the magnitude and speed of movement varied. Curvilinearity of velar trajectories varied across speakers. He reported less variability in velar movement patterns across consonant sequences that differed in *place* of consonant production than across consonant sequences that differed in *manner* of production. Not surprisingly, velar movement was found to be slower than tongue movement. Kuehn noted a powerful influence of vowel identity on velar movement:

> It appears that the entire locus of normal palatal movement between lowered and elevated positions rather than just the highest point of elevation is shifted depending on the particular vowel or vowel category within the phonetic environment. (p 99)

Subsequent findings would cast further doubt on the binary model of velar control. Seaver and Kuehn (1980) used electromyography to measure action potentials simultaneously in the levator, palatoglossus, and palatopharyngeus muscles at the same time that velopharyngeal movement was also filmed with sagittal cinefluorography. This study of normal velopharyngeal function was designed to examine variations in velar height when the velopharyngeal port is closed during production of nonnasal utterances. The authors wrote:

> The data from this investigation suggest that changes in velar positioning during the production of non-nasal speech are a result of the interaction of a number of variables operating simultaneously. Any attempt to relate only one of these variables to the activity of the velum may represent an oversimplification of this complex mechanical system (pp. 225-226).

Among their findings was the previously noted observation that velar height is greater for high vowels than for low vowels, even when nasal consonants were not present. As with Lubker's earlier findings (1975), Seaver and Kuehn's results are not compatible with the parsimonious on-off or binary hypothesis. They described variability in movement patterns both within and between subjects and suggested that other variables such as tissue mass and elasticity should be considered.

Kunzel (1979) used the velograph to study velar height in normal German speakers. He found velar heights to be greater for oral consonants than for vowels. He also reported greater height for plosives than for liquids. He found velar height to be greater in voiceless than in voiced plosives and in orally than in nasally released plosives. For example, in /lapn/ the release is oral, whereas in /lapm/ it is nasal. In the latter word, the position for /p/ is assumed but is not released. Rather, the syllable is released with the /m/. He described anticipatory and carryover coarticulation of velar movement, and he postulated that two types of coarticulation occur—passive and active. The difference in velar height for nasally and orally released stops was thought to reflect active neuromotor programming, whereas the modification of velar height during a vowel in anticipation of a consonant was seen by Kunzel as passive.

Others have attempted to understand the importance of the speech movement variability, such as that reported by Kuehn (1976) and by Seaver and Kuehn (1980). Attention has been given to the viewpoint that different individuals may achieve a common speech motor goal in different ways. For example, Folkins (1985) discussed the concepts of *flexibility* and *plasticity* relative to achievement of perceptually acceptable speech. Flexibility permits the talker to take alternate routes to perceptually acceptable speech. That is, there may be a range of movements within which an individual can achieve the same perceptible result, provided that those movements are *constrained* within the limits imposed by the motor control system. The coordinated movements of the velum, tongue, lips, jaw, and respiratory system are not perfectly stereotyped even when a speaker repeats the same words. However, when the movements fail to produce an acceptable speech outcome, plasticity may come into play. In such cases, working within the constraints of the motor control system is not adequate. Instead, the speaker must alter the motor control system to achieve a desired result. Flexibility allows for some variability in performance without resulting in failure; plasticity allows for correction of errors when failure occurs. These motor control concepts are consistent with the theory that speech motor control is accomplished, at least in part, by the learned ability to control muscle subgroups that have been described as coordinative structures (Fowler et al., 1980).

To test the theory of coordinative structures in speech motor control, it is necessary to first understand how the speech motor control system might *constrain* velopharyngeal movements during speech. Does the central nervous system monitor and control the actual biomechanical movements of the velum or is there an indirect control variable that has an impact on how we manage speech production? Do passive aeromechanical events have any effect on velopharyngeal movements? All of these questions have been the focus of various research efforts.

Warren (1986) suggested that velopharyngeal function for speech may be programmed according to a speech regulating system that adjusts its performance depending on *aerodynamic* demands (Fig. 3-16). This argument was based, in part, on the observation that speakers with cleft palate who have severely impaired velopharyngeal closure frequently attempt to articulate pressure consonants at the larynx or pharynx instead of within the oral cavity. This phenomenon, referred to as *compensatory articulation,* will be described in greater detail later in this volume.

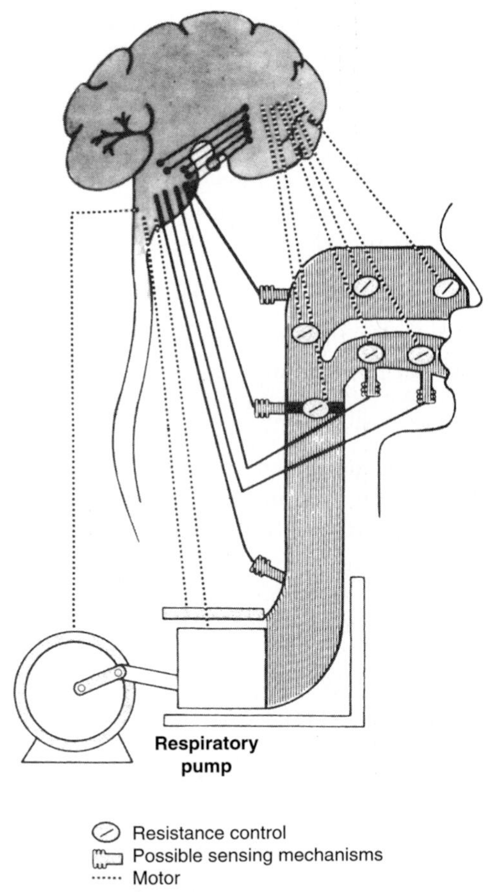

Figure 3-16 Theoretical representation of a possible feedback system to regulate speech pressures. Possible sensors send error messages to resistance controllers via the brain. *(From Warren DW: Compensatory speech behaviors in cleft palate: a regulation/control phenomenon.* Cleft Palate Journal *23:258, 1986.)*

Warren's aerodynamic theory implies that speech motor control is constrained, in part, by aerodynamic demands for speech. This theory accounts nicely for velopharyngeal opening for nasal consonants as well as for velopharyngeal closing for oral pressure consonants because management of nasal air flow and oral air pressure is necessary for appropriate production of these speech sounds. The theory fails, however, to explain velar position during vowel and semivowel (w, r, l) production when management of aerodynamic demands is less critical and management of acoustic resonance and perceived speech quality seems of paramount importance. Given the previously described findings of Moll (1962) and Lubker (1968, 1975) and the fact that vowel durations are longer than consonant durations in speech, failure to account for velar position during vowels is a major limitation of the aerodynamic theory.

Moon and Jones (1991) and Moon, Kuehn, and Huisman (1995) found support for Folkins' theory of velar motor control (1985). They noted that, given adequate performance feedback, individuals could learn to control velar position in novel ways during vowel production and that articulatory goals are specified for vowels. These data seem inconsistent with the pressure-regulation theory suggested by Warren (1986) because the primary source of pressure resistance during vowels is the larynx.

Can increases in aeromechanical forces during consonant production serve to lift the palate? Does jaw lowering influence velar lowering? To examine these mechanical influences on velar elevation, Karnell et al. (1988) measured the relative timing of intraoral pressure peaks, jaw movement, and velar movement during speech production with and without a bite block in place. They found that the temporal relationships between air pressure and velar movement did not support the possibility that momentary peaks in velar elevation were a passive mechanical result of increases in subvelar intraoral air pressure. The data also did not support the possibility that velar lowering was caused by jaw lowering resulting from a downward mechanical force placed on the velum by palatoglossus and palatopharyngeus muscular linkage with the jaw. A more plausible explanation is that velar displacement peaks were the result of momentary increases in levator muscular contraction coordinated by the central nervous system to produce increases in the force of velopharyngeal closure to prevent air leakage during pressure consonant production (Lubker, 1975; Seaver and Kuehn, 1980).

Additional data supporting this point of view were reported by Bell-Berti and Krakow (1991) who described velar lowering after oral consonant production as follows:

> the relatively shallow early part of the lowering movement observed in the CV_nN sequences matches that observed in minimally contrastive CVC sequences that end with an oral, rather than a nasal, consonant. (p. 121)

Bell-Berti and Krakow used these findings to refute the findings of previous studies (Kent, Carney, and Severeid, 1974; Moll and Daniloff, 1971; Ohala, 1971) that had suggested that anticipatory nasal coarticulation caused the onset of velar lowering for nasal consonants to occur throughout vowel productions before the onset of the nasal. Data consistent with those of Bell-Berti and Krakow were reported by LaVelle (1994), who observed variations in velopharyngeal closure pressures consistent with the velar movement observations reported by Karnell et al. (1988) and by Bell-Berti and Krakow (1991). Kuehn and Moon (1998) similarly reported variations in closure pressure within the velopharyngeal port during normal speech.

All of this detailed analysis appears to ultimately yield conclusions consistent with those described in the previously referenced report by Lubker (1975), who so eloquently wrote:

> velopharyngeal closure appears to be a complex and highly coordinated act. The muscles responsible function more or less forcefully to achieve more or less tight velopharyngeal closure. The tightness of the closure achieved is not a random variable, but is dictated by the speaker's needs, i.e., the production of a phoneme that is perceptually acceptable, and by certain physical constraints such as timing. Likewise, the variability of muscle effort is not random, but is also dependent partly upon the speaker's needs and partly upon what the velopharyngeal system has been required to do for the preceding phonemes. The clear implication is that of precise programming required in the central nervous system (p. 254).

It is difficult to improve on Lubker's interpretation of normal velopharyngeal physiology for speech. There remains a need for additional research to improve our understanding of the effects of anatomical variability as well as the nature of the central nervous system "programming" to fully grasp the manner in which the central nervous system learns how to successfully execute motor commands to the velopharyngeal mechanism in coordination with the many other speech movements that occur during normal speech production.

REFERENCES

Astley R: The movement of the lateral walls of the nasopharynx: a cine-radiographic study. *Journal of Laryngology* 72:325-328, 1958.

Azzam NA, and Kuehn DP: The morphology of musculus uvulae. *Cleft Palate Journal* 14:78-87, 1977.

Bass NH, and Morrell RM: The neurology of swallowing. In Groher ME (ed.): *Dysphagia: diagnosis and management.* Boston: Butterworth-Heinemann, 1992.

Bell-Berti F: An electromyographic study of velopharyngeal function in speech. *Journal of Speech and Hearing Research* 19:225-240, 1976.

Bell-Berti F: A spatial-temporal model of velopharyngeal function. In Lass NJ (ed.): *Speech and language: advances in basic research and practice.* Volume 4. New York: Academic Press, 1980, pp. 291-316.

Bell-Berti F, and Krakow RA: Anticipatory velar lowering: a coproduction account. *Journal of the Acoustical Society of America* 90:112-123, 1991.

Bosma JF: Correlated study of anatomy and motor activity of upper pharynx by cadaver dissection and by cinematic study of patients after maxillo-facial surgery. *Annals of Otology, Rhinology and Laryngology* 62:51-72, 1953.

Bosma JF: *Anatomy of the infant head.* Baltimore: Johns Hopkins University Press, 1986.

Bzoch KR, Graber TM, and Aoba T: A study of normal velopharyngeal valving for speech. *Cleft Palate Bulletin* 9:3, 1959.

Calnan JS: Modern views of Passavant's ridge. *British Journal of Plastic Surgery* 10:89-113.

Croft CB, Shprintzen RJ, and Rakoff SJ: Patterns of velopharyngeal valving in normal and cleft palate subjects: a multi-view videofluoroscopic and nasendoscopic study. *Laryngoscope* 91:265-271, 1981.

Croft CB, Shprintzen RJ, Daniller A, and Lewin ML: The occult submucous cleft palate and the musculus uvulae. *Cleft Palate Journal* 15:150-154, 1978.

Dickson DR: Normal and cleft palate anatomy. *Cleft Palate Journal* 9:280-293.

Dickson DR: Anatomy of the normal velopharyngeal mechanism. *Clinics in Plastic Surgery* 2:235-248, 1975.

Dickson DR, and Maue-Dickson W: Velopharyngeal anatomy. *Journal of Speech and Hearing Research* 15:372-381, 1972.

Dickson DR, and Maue-Dickson W: Velopharyngeal structure and function: a model for biomechanical analysis. In Lass NJ (ed.): *Speech and language: advances in basic research and practice.* Volume 3. New York: Academic Press, 1980, pp. 168-222.

Ettema SL, and Kuehn DP: A quantitative histologic study of the normal human adult soft palate. *Journal of Speech and Hearing Research* 37:303-313, 1994.

Folkins JW: Issues in the motor control of speech and their relation to speakers with a repaired palatal cleft. *Cleft Palate Journal* 22:106-122, 1983.

Fowler CA, Rubin P, Remez RE, and Turvey MT: Implications for speech production of a general theory of action in language production. In Butterworth B (ed.): *Speech and talk.* Volume 1. New York: Academic Press, 1980, pp. 372-420.

Fritzell B: The velopharyngeal muscles in speech. *Acta Otolaryngology* 250(Supplement):1-81, 1969.

Glaser ER, Skolnick ML, McWilliams BJ, and Shprintzen RJ: The dynamics of Passavant's ridge in subjects with and without velopharyngeal insufficiency—a multiview videofluoroscopic study. *Cleft Palate Journal* 16:24-33, 1979.

Griffith BH, Monroe CW, Hill BJ, Waldrop WF, and White H: Motion of the lateral pharyngeal wall during velopharyngeal closure. *Journal of Plastic and Reconstructive Surgery* 41:338-342, 1968.

Harrington R: A study of the mechanism of velopharyngeal closure. *Journal of Speech Diseases* 9:325-345, 1944.

Henke W: Dynamic articulatory model of speech production using computer simulation [dissertation]. Cambridge, MA: Massachusetts Institute of Technology, 1966.

Iglesias A, Kuehn DP, and Morris HL: Simultaneous assessment of pharyngeal wall and velar displacement for selected speech sounds. *Journal of Speech and Hearing Research* 23:429-446, 1980.

Isshiki N, Honjow I, and Morimoto M: Cineradiographic analysis of movement of the lateral pharyngeal wall. *Journal of Plastic and Reconstructive Surgery* 44:357-363, 1969.

Kahrilas PJ, Dodds WJ, Dent J, and Logemann JA: Upper esophageal sphincter function during deglutition. *Gastroenterology* 95:52-62, 1988.

Karnell MP, Folkins JW, and Morris HL: Relationship between perceived and kinematic aspects of speech production in cleft palate speakers. *Journal of Speech and Hearing Research* 28:63-72, 1985.

Karnell MP, Linville RN, and Edwards BA: Variations in velar position over time: a nasal videoendoscopic study. *Journal of Speech and Hearing Research* 31:417-424, 1988.

Kent RD, Carney PJ, and Severeid LR: Velar movement and timing: evaluation of a model of binary control. *Journal of Speech and Hearing Research* 17:470-488, 1974.

Kuehn DP: A cineradiographic investigation of velar movement variables of two normals. *Cleft Palate Journal* 13:88-103, 1976.

Kuehn DP, and Azzam NA: Anatomical characteristics of palatoglossus and the anterior faucial pillar. *Cleft Palate Journal* 15:349-359, 1978.

Kuehn DP, and Kahane JC: Histologic study of the normal human adult soft palate. *Cleft Palate Journal* 27:26-34, 1990.

Kuehn DP, and Moon JB: Velopharyngeal closure force and levator veli palatini activation levels in varying phonetic contexts. *Journal of Speech and Language Hearing Research* 41:451-462, 1998.

Kuehn DP, Folkins JW, and Linville RN: An electromyographic study of the musculus uvulae. *Cleft Palate Journal* 25:348, 1988.

Langdon HL, and Klueber K: The longitudinal fibromuscular component of the soft palate in the fifteen-week human fetus: musculus uvulae and palatine raphe. *Cleft Palate Journal* 15:337-348, 1978.

LaVelle CA: Coarticulatory effects on velar contact force [thesis]. Iowa City: University of Iowa, 1994.

Lavorato AS, and Lindholm CE: Fiberoptic visualization of the motion of the eustachian tube cartilage. Proceedings of the annual meeting of the American Academy of Ophthalmology and Otology, Las Vegas, 1976.

Lubker JF: An electromyographic-cinefluorographic investigation of velar function during normal speech production. *Cleft Palate Journal* 5:1-17, 1968.

Lubker JF: Normal velopharyngeal function in speech. *Clinics in Plastic Surgery* 2:249-259, 1975.

Maue-Dickson W, and Dickson DR: Anatomy and physiology related to cleft palate: current research and clinical implications. *Plastic and Reconstructive Surgery* 65:83-90, 1980.

Mazaheri M, Millard RT, and Erickson DM: Cineradiographic comparison of normal to noncleft subjects with velopharyngeal inadequacy. *Cleft Palate Journal* 1:199-210, 1964.

Minifie FD, Hixon TJ, Kelsey CA, and Woodhouse RJ: Lateral pharyngeal wall movement during speech production. *Journal of Hearing and Speech Research* 13:584-594, 1970.

Moll KL: Cinefluorographic techniques in speech research. *Journal of Hearing and Speech Research* 3:227-241, 1960.

Moll KL: Velopharyngeal closure on vowels. *Journal of Speech and Hearing Research* 5:30-37, 1962.

Moll KL, and Daniloff RG: Investigation of the timing of velar movements during speech. *Journal of the Acoustical Society of America* 50:678-684, 1971.

Moll KL, and Shriner TH: Preliminary investigation of a new concept of velar activity during speech. *Cleft Palate Journal* 4:58-69, 1967.

Moon JB, Canady JW: Effects of gravity on velopharyngeal muscle activity during speech. *Cleft Palate-Craniofacial Journal* 32(5):371-375, 1995.

Moon JB, and Jones DL: Motor control of velopharyngeal structures during vowel production. *Cleft Palate Journal* 28:267-273, 1991.

Moon J, Kuehn D, and Huisman J: Measurement of velopharyngeal closure force during vowel production [response to Piggot]. *Cleft Palate Journal* 32:263, 1995.

Moon JB, Smith AE, Folkins JW, Lemke JH, and Gartlan M: Coordination of velopharyngeal muscle activity during positioning of the soft palate. *Cleft Palate Journal* 31:45-55, 1994.

Niimi S, Bell-Berti F, and Harris KS: Dynamic aspects of velopharyngeal closure. *Folia Phoniatrica* 34:246-257, 1982.

Nishio J, Matsuya T, Ibuki K, and Miyazaki T: Roles of the facial, glossopharyngeal and vagus nerves in velopharyngeal movement. *Cleft Palate Journal* 13:201-214, 1976a.

Nishio J, Matsuya T, Machida J, and Miyazaki T: The motor nerve supply of the velopharyngeal muscles. *Cleft Palate Journal* 13:20-30, 1976b.

Ohala JJ: Monitoring soft palate movements in speech. Project on Linguistic Analysis Reports, Phonology Laboratory, Department on Linguistics, University of California, Berkeley, J01-J015, 1971.

Passavant G: On the closure of the pharynx in speech. *Archiv Heilk* 3:305, 1863.

Passavant G: On the closure of the pharynx in speech. *Virchows Archiv* 46:1, 1869.

Pruszewicz A, Woznica B, Kruk-Zagajewska A, and Obrebowski A: Electromyography of cricopharyngeal muscles in patients with oesophageal speech. *Acta Otolaryngology* (Stockholm) 112:366-369, 1992.

Seaver EJ, and Kuehn DP: A cineradiographic and electromyographic investigation of velar positioning in non-nasal speech. *Cleft Palate Journal* 17:216-226, 1980.

Sedlackova E, Lastovia M, and Sram F: Contribution to knowledge of soft palate innervation. *Folia Phoniatrica* 25:434-441, 1973.

Shprintzen RJ, McCall GN, Skolnick ML, and Lencione RM: Selective movement of the lateral aspects of the pharyngeal walls during velopharyngeal closure for speech, blowing, and whistling in normals. *Cleft Palate Journal* 12:51-58, 1975.

Simpson RK, and Austin AA: A cephalometric investigation of velar stretch. *Cleft Palate Journal* 9:341-351, 1972.

Skolnick ML, Shprintzen RJ, McCall GN, and Rakoff S: Patterns of velopharyngeal closure in subjects with repaired cleft palate and normal speech: A multi-view videofluoroscopic analysis. *Cleft Palate Journal* 12:369-376, 1975.

Trigos I, Ysunza A, Vargas D, and Vazquez MC: The San Venero Roselli pharyngoplasty: an electromyographic study of the palatopharyngeus muscle. *Cleft Palate Journal* 25:385-388, 1988.

Warren DW: Compensatory speech behaviors in cleft palate: a regulation/control phenomenon. *Cleft Palate Journal* 23:251-260, 1986.

Warren DW, and Hofmann FA: A cineradiographic study of velopharyngeal closure. *Plastic and Reconstructive Surgery* 28:656-669, 1961.

Zemlin WR: *Speech and hearing science: anatomy and physiology.* 4th ed. Englewood Cliffs (NJ): Prentice-Hall, 1997.

Zwitman DH, Sonderman JC, Ward PH: Variations in velopharyngeal closure assessed by endoscopy. *Journal of Speech and Hearing Disorders,* 39:366-372, 1974.

Chapter 4

Surgical Management of Cleft Lip and Palate

The child with cleft lip and palate will most likely undergo a minimum of four or five surgical procedures designed to create a lip and nose that are esthetically pleasing and functional, an intact palate, and an intact alveolar ridge that provides good bony support for the lip and nasal base. In general, these procedures include the initial closure of the lip, initial closure of the palate, a lip and nose revision in the preschool or early schoolage years, alveolar bone grafting somewhat later, and, if necessary, additional procedures on the palate to close an oronasal fistula or to lengthen the velum to provide better velopharyngeal closure. Lip and nose revisions may be repeated as the child matures. Finally, in many patients surgical advancement of the maxilla is performed in the early teenage years to improve the alignment of the upper and lower jaws.

The terminology applied to surgical procedures is often confusing. For example, in Chapter 1 you learned that the median portion of the upper lip and alveolus are formed from a structure often called the "primary palate." Yet a "primary palatoplasty" refers to the first (and perhaps only) surgical closure of the palate, not a surgical closure of the primary palate alone. In addition, within each category or generic label for a surgical procedure there are usually "brand names" specifying a particular technique and often named after the person(s) who developed the technique. You are not expected to memorize the brand names, but the following glossary of terms should help you in navigating your way through the medical histories and treatment recommendations for your patients. These definitions are drawn from treatment regimens or team practices common to the United States; specific terms may carry very different meanings in different parts of the world even if English is the shared language for scientific communication. When you encounter a term not included in the following glossary, consult your on-line resources for an update on new procedures or revisions of older techniques.

GLOSSARY OF TERMS

Alveolar bone grafting use of bone harvested from other parts of the body (usually from the cranium or the iliac crest) to fill in the alveolar clefts.

Primary alveolar bone grafting grafting of the alveolar cleft(s) in the infant or young toddler, sometimes done at the same time as the repair of the lip or rest of the palate.

Secondary alveolar bone grafting bone grafting of the alveolar cleft(s) in the older child or young teenager, when grafting of the alveolus has not been carried out as part of the initial palatal procedures in infancy.

Cheiloplasty or cheilorrhaphy surgery on the lip (Fig. 4-1).

LeFort I osteotomy advancement of the maxilla only, with a transverse cut just above the tooth roots of the teeth, as illustrated in Fig. 4-2.

LeFort II osteotomy a type of midface advancement with incisions and movement of segments, as illustrated in Fig. 4-3.

LeFort III osteotomy a type of midface advancement with incisions and movement of segments, as illustrated in Fig. 4-4.

Orthognathic surgery a generic term for any surgery to improve the relationship between the upper and lower jaws ("ortho" meaning straight, "gnathic" meaning jaws). Surgical advancement of the maxilla fits this category, as do many other procedures performed on patients with or without clefts. For a full list and explanations of the various types of jaw surgery, refer to current texts on oral and maxillofacial surgery.

Palatoplasty or palatorrhaphy surgery on the palate. ("Uranoplasty" is an antiquated term that was used for surgery on the hard palate.)

Primary palatoplasty the first surgery performed to close the palate; often the only procedure required to accomplish this goal (Fig. 4-5).

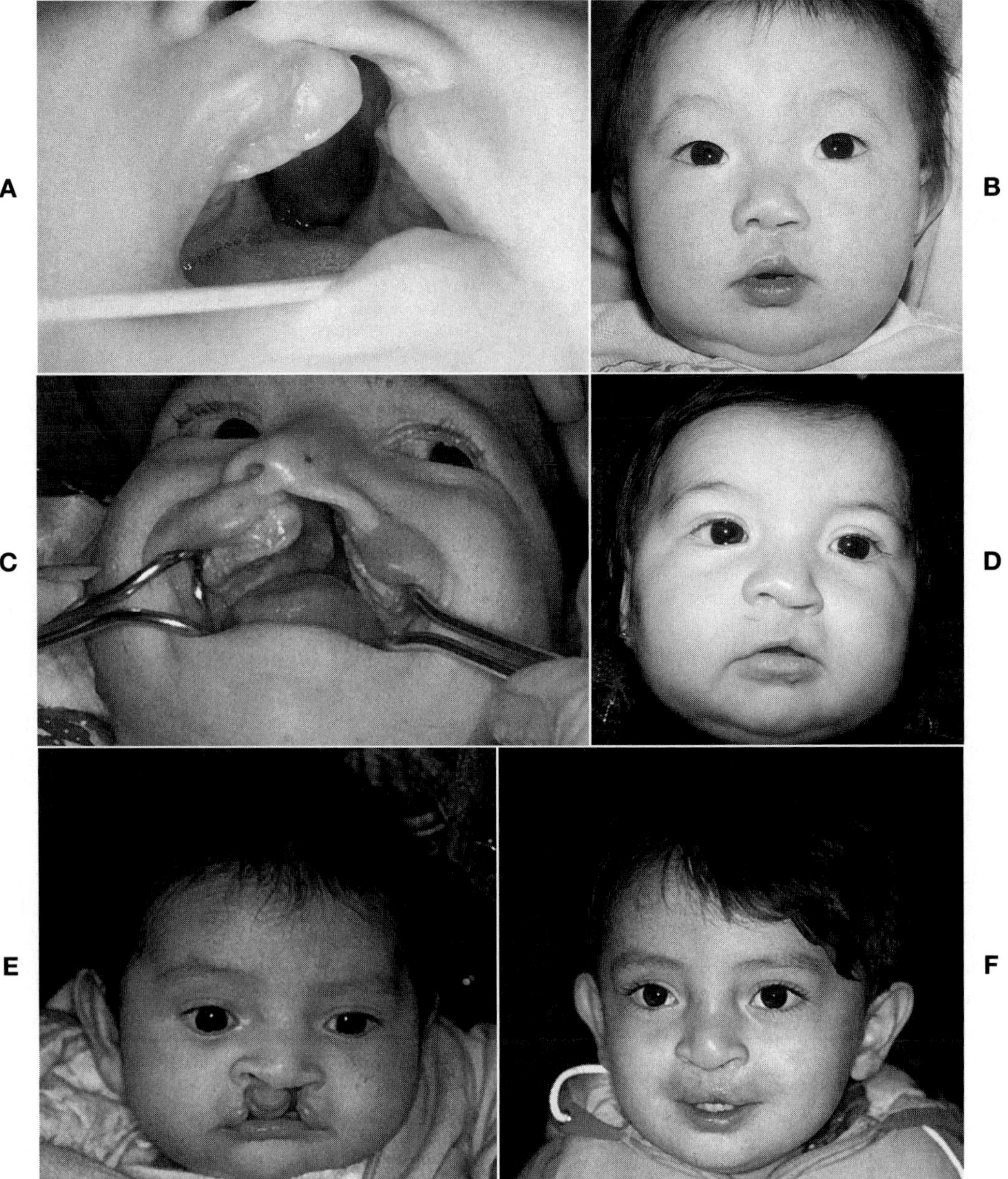

Figure 4-1 **A** to **F**, Preoperative and postoperative photos of two babies with unilateral clefts of the lip and one baby with a bilateral cleft.

Pharyngeal flap a designation for several different procedures that are themselves forms of "pharyngoplasty," usually involving some type of tissue bridge between the velum and the posterior pharyngeal wall (discussed in Chapter 13).

Pharyngoplasty a generic term applied to many different procedures for improving velopharyngeal closure by altering the physical structures of the pharynx and sometimes the velum (discussed in Chapter 13).

Primary veloplasty surgery in which the goal is to close only the soft palate cleft, leaving the cleft of the hard palate to be closed at a later time.

A PERSPECTIVE ON LIP AND PALATE SURGERY

For the beginning clinician, it can be very difficult to conceptualize what physical management procedures (surgery, orthodontics, prosthodontics) are likely to take place at what time in the child's life and in what combinations. Surgeons will generally try to limit the number of times a child is subjected to general anesthesia and will thus combine procedures when possible or desirable. However, philosophies about what surgical procedures are necessary, and at what age or time in the child's growth, vary widely. Furthermore, the philosophies or perspectives vary *over time* as surgeons and clinical teams revise their thinking in

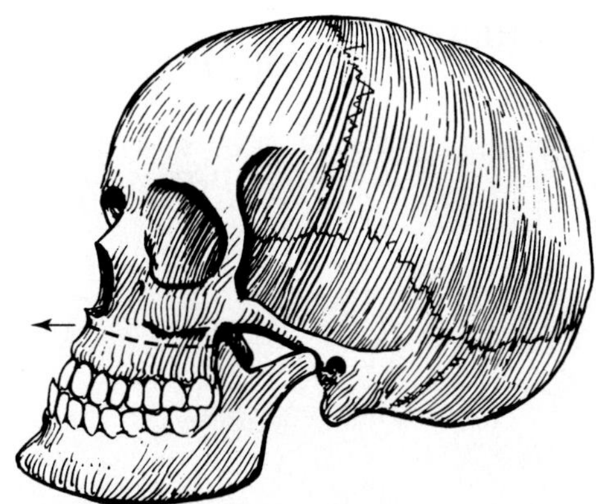

Figure 4-2 Schematic representation of a Le Fort I osteotomy, which moves the maxilla forward to improve occlusion and esthetic appearance of the face. In addition to the forward movement of this segment of the facial skeleton, the surgery may be modified to rotate the maxilla from side to side or back to front, accomplishing a better fit to the mandible. *(From Whitaker LA: Principles and methods of management. In Bluestone CD, Stool SE [eds.]:* Pediatric otolaryngology. *Philadelphia: WB Saunders, 1983.)*

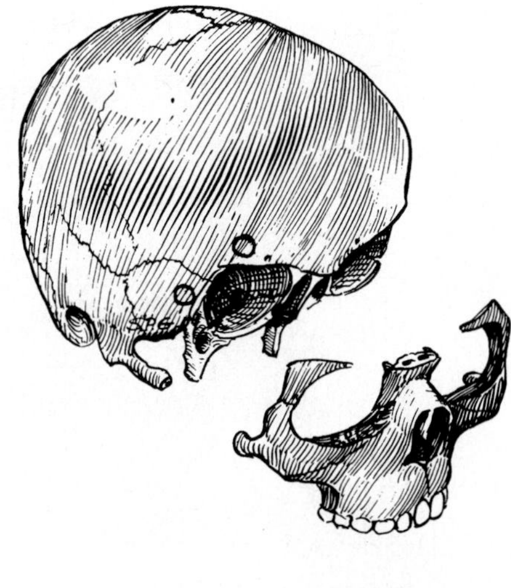

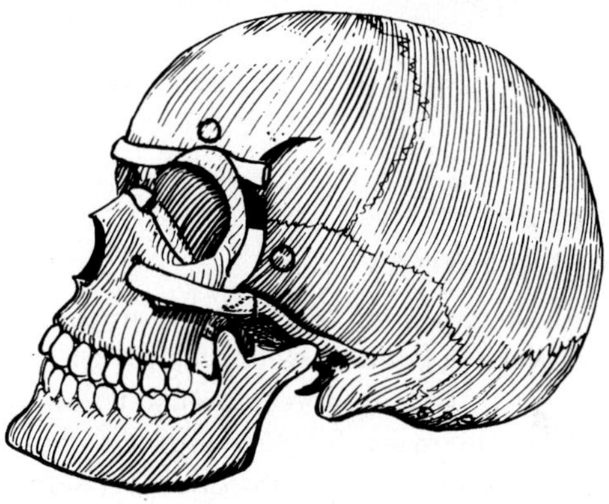

Figure 4-4 The Le Fort III osteotomy, advancing the facial bones from the superior orbital rims down through the maxilla. *(From Whitaker LA: Principles and methods of management. In Bluestone CD, Stool SE [eds.]:* Pediatric otolaryngology. *Philadelphia: WB Saunders, 1983.)*

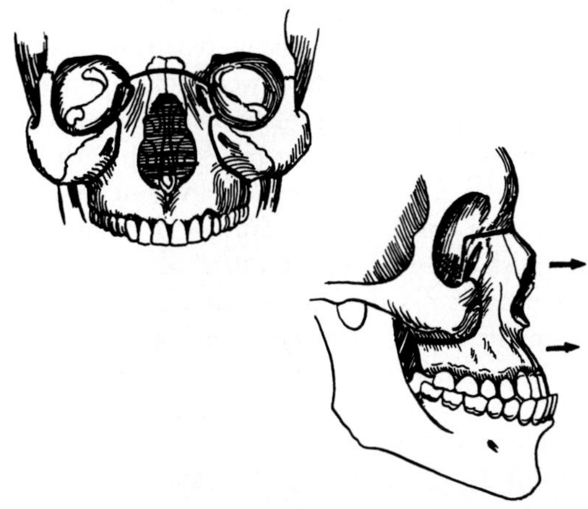

Figure 4-3 Schematic representation of a Le Fort II osteotomy, moving the midface (nasal bones and maxilla) forward. *(From Converse JM, et al: Deformities of the jaws. In Converse JM [ed.]:* Reconstructive plastic surgery: principles and procedures in correction, reconstruction and transplantation. *2nd ed. Volume 4. Philadelphia: WB Saunders, 1977, p. 2480.)*

accordance with their own increasing experience and with what they learn from a growing, shared body of clinical knowledge.

As a platform for approaching the theories or preferences affecting surgical planning for children with cleft lip and palate, it should help to keep the following in mind:

1. In most treatment programs, surgical closure of the lip precedes that of the palate. One notable exception occasionally takes place when surgical teams visit third-world countries and intentionally close the palate first (whatever the age of the infant or child) with the thought that, if they close the lip first, the family may never return for closure of the palate. Other exceptions occur when closure of the lip is combined with surgical closure of the soft palate only (primary veloplasty) and in programs advocating very early closure of the palate so that the lip and palate are actually done simultaneously.
2. For several generations, a controversy has raged that still affects current treatment philosophies, namely, a theory that early surgery (particularly on the palate) leads to impairment of midfacial growth. Of all the disagreements over the surgical treatment of clefts, none has commanded more attention in terms of printed pages (in articles and books) or presentations at professional meetings. There is still very little in the way of a worldwide consensus, and many specialists are still embroiled in what they see as a "speech versus appearance" issue. As a result of these issues and others that will be discussed, you will find that the surgical planning for children with clefts does not follow a straight line.

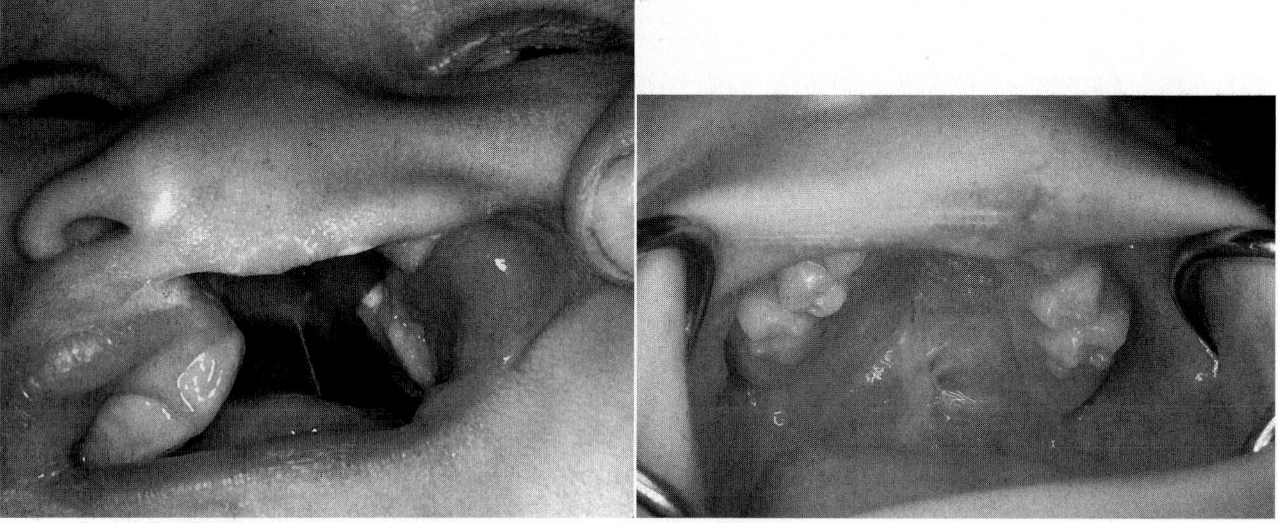

Figure 4-5 A baby with a wide unilateral cleft lip and palate before and after lip and palate surgery.

LIP SURGERY

Goals of Lip Surgery

Surgery on the lip aims to create an upper lip that is esthetically pleasing not only by uniting the two portions of the lip but also by creating good muscular continuity across the cleft. There are many different surgical techniques used both in initial lip surgery and subsequent revisions. We will not go into detail on all the different techniques here but will briefly describe some of the more popular approaches so that you can seek further information in the literature or on-line data systems. In addition, clinicians should be aware that, for individuals with van der Woude syndrome (described in Chapter 2), there will usually be one or more operations to improve the appearance of the lower lip and remove the sinuses or tracts that may drain onto the vermilion surface.

Age at Lip Surgery

In most treatment centers in the United States and Canada, surgical closure of the lip is performed within the first few months of life, usually around 2.5 or 3 months of age. For the child's safety, particularly because surgery requires a general anesthetic, many surgeons still follow the "rule of 10s" (Wilhelmsen and Musgrave, 1966) in setting a time for surgery when the child is 10 pounds in weight and 10 weeks of age and has 10 g of hemoglobin. When the cleft is bilateral, depending on the degree of severity of each side and the surgeon's preferences in management, one side may be closed first and the second side a few weeks later. A few surgeons both in the United States and Europe currently practice very early closure of the lip *and* palate, within the first few weeks of life, but this has not become a widely accepted approach (Denk and Magee, 1996; Nunn et al., 1995).

Some surgeons and teams prefer to try to bring the two sides of the lip and alveolar cleft into better alignment *before* surgical closure. The goal is to create a smaller space from side to side so that there is less tension across the line of the cleft at the time of the definitive lip repair. In bilateral clefts and in some unilateral clefts as well, these approaches may also bring the protrusive prolabium and premaxilla back into a better anterior-posterior relationship with respect to the rest of the maxilla. There are two main *nonsurgical* techniques and one surgical technique that have been used to accomplish this goal. The nonsurgical approaches are (1) simple taping across the line of the cleft or (2) a slightly more complex orthopedic device such as a bonnet with a band of stretchable material across the lip or prolabium (Figs. 4-6 and 4-7). A completely intraoral appliance for retraction of the premaxilla may also be used (Figueroa et al., 1996). In any of these approaches care must be taken so as not to apply too much pressure, or pressure in the wrong direction, to the cleft segment. In the case of the protrusive premaxilla in a bilateral cleft, the pressure can result in the premaxilla being bent back on itself or bent to one side, torquing the vomer bone. A similar result may occur if too much pressure is applied to the cleft segment in a unilateral cleft. Clinicians have claimed to measure the amount of pressure applied by orthopedic "bonnets" or similar devices, but the measures have too often proved to be erroneous because of the multiple vectors of motion that need to be taken into account. That is, the force applied by the device is not necessarily active in only one direction. Thus, use of taping or bonnets does not really constitute a clinical science, and when one of these approaches is used the baby must be monitored very closely (biweekly or more often) so that too much movement in a disadvantageous direction does not take place.

The surgical approach to the same goal of modifying the position of the two segments of the lip is called a "lip adhesion" (Cohen et al., 1995; Meijer and Cohen, 1990; Randall, 1965, 1990a, 1996; Randall and Graham, 1971;

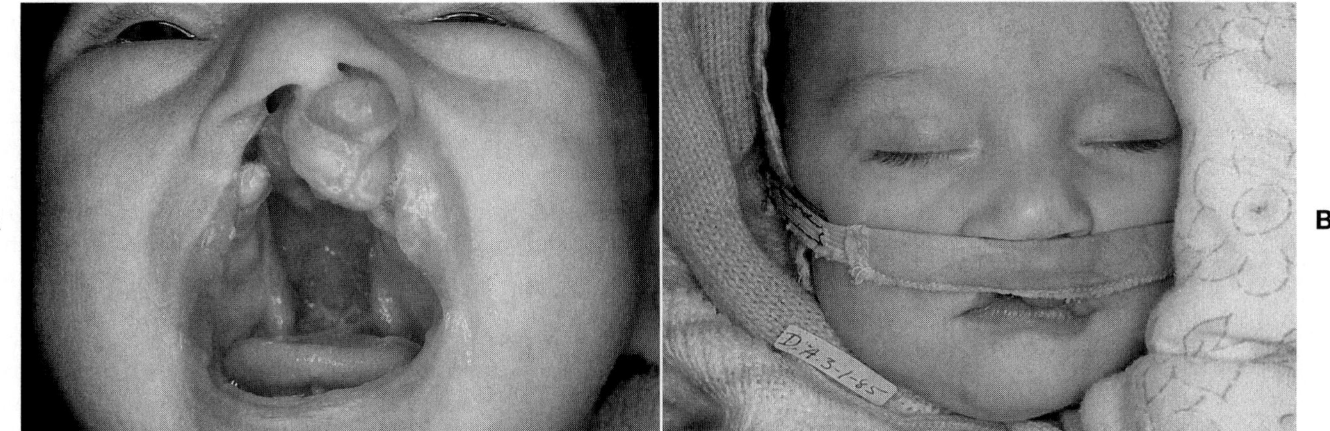

Figure 4-6 **A** and **B,** A baby with an incomplete bilateral cleft lip and palate (complete cleft of the lip on the baby's right and incomplete cleft on the baby's left). In the second picture, a taping device has been placed in the effort to bring the premaxilla into a more favorable position for surgical closure of the lip. (Note: The taping seen here is more aggressive [stronger] than that currently used.)

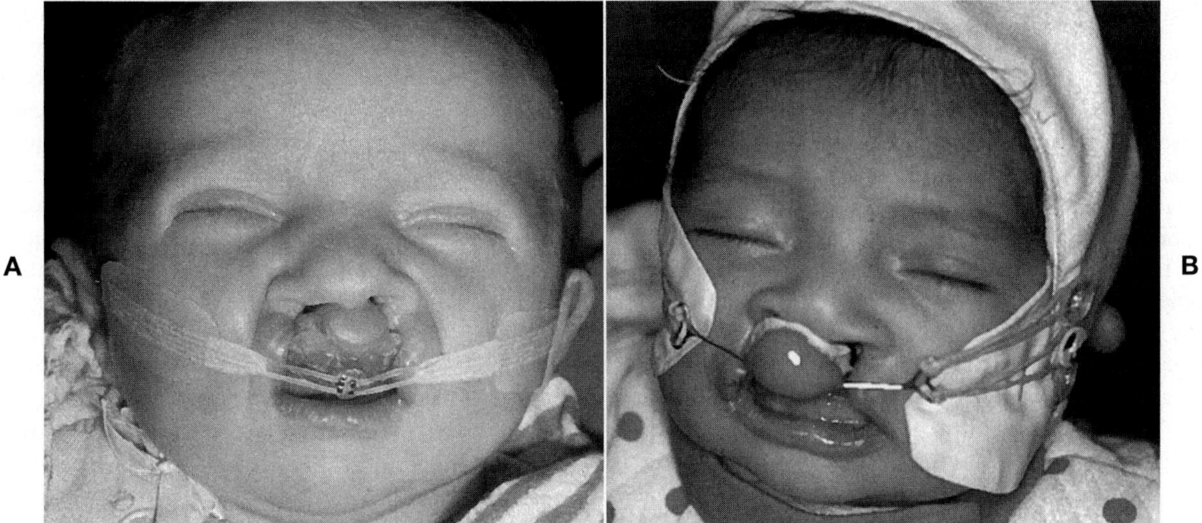

Figure 4-7 **A** and **B,** Two babies for whom extraoral acrylic devices have been molded to fit over the premaxilla and attached to taping **(A)** or a bonnet with strapping. The device seen in **B** is chronologically older (this patient is now out of high school) than the more modest taping procedures used today.

Rintala and Haataja, 1979). This is a simple repair almost equivalent to gluing the two sides together by surgically freshening the edges, creating two raw surfaces that then adhere to each other (Fig. 4-8). This becomes, in effect, a surgical "Band-aid," done with the hope of bringing the two segments of the lip (or three in bilateral clefts) into better alignment and making the definitive lip closure easier as well as bring the segments of the primary palate closer together. Undergoing this procedure means an extra general anesthetic and surgical experience for the child, and it has gained only limited acceptance. However, in some centers the lip adhesion is combined with another surgical procedure such as primary veloplasty or placement of ventilating tubes in the ears (Lohmander-Agerskov et al., 1990).

The age at which the definitive lip repair is performed is unlikely to be delayed when taping or a bonnet is used, but it may be delayed in some centers where the lip adhesion surgery or more complicated orthopedic repositioning of the cleft segments (the latter usually termed "presurgical orthopedics") are performed. The topic of presurgical orthopedics is discussed in Chapter 5.

Primary Repairs of the Lip and Nose

There are three main "name-brand" or widely recognized surgical techniques used in definitive surgical closure of the

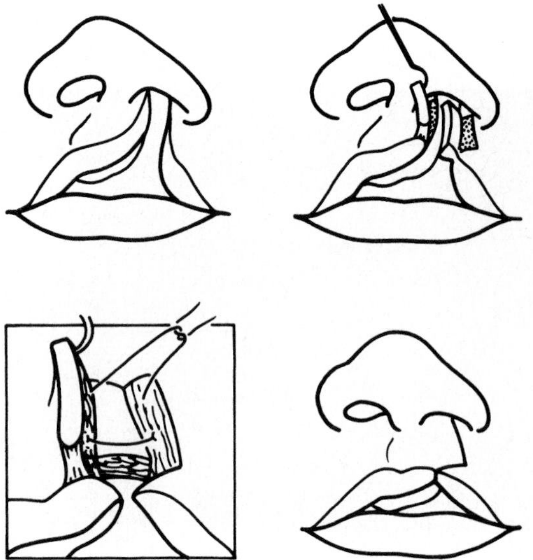

Figure 4-8 A schematic of the lip adhesion operation, as devised by Randall (1965). This technique creates two raw surfaces that are then allowed to adhere, without reorienting the muscles of the lip (left for later definitive lip repair). *(Adapted from Musgrave RH, and Garrett WS: The unilateral cleft lip. In Converse JM [ed.]:* Reconstructive plastic surgery: principles and procedures in correction, reconstruction, and transplantation. *Philadelphia: WB Saunders, 1977, p. 2033.)*

lip. These are the triangular-flap procedure introduced by Tennison in 1952 and later modified by Randall (Bardach, 1994; Bardach and Salyer, 1987; Randall, 1959, 1971, 1990b; Skoog, 1958, 1971) (Fig. 4-9), the quadrilateral flap of LeMesurier (1962), and the Millard rotation-advancement technique (Fig. 4-10) (Bardach, 1994; Millard, 1958, 1966b, 1971a, 1971b, 1976, 1977). The triangular flap and the rotation-advancement are the most popular, and both have been designed or modified for use in both unilateral and bilateral clefts (Millard 1971a, 1971b, 1976, 1977; Noordhoff, 1994; Skoog, 1971). New innovations or modifications are introduced frequently, and the likelihood of any of these becoming another standard approach in the surgeon's repertoire is influenced by how well the procedure seems to hold up or perform over time, that is, to produce the desired results in larger numbers of patients. Currently, the Millard rotation-advancement is being challenged by a modified straight-line repair in the hope of reducing hypertrophic scarring and asymmetry of the vermilion border (Salomonson, 1998). Salyer (1986, 1994) demonstrated the esthetic benefits of careful reconstruction of the nose as part of the initial lip repair in unilateral cases. Similarly, a series of studies in England and Germany demonstrated the importance of re-establishing the continuity of *all* the muscles involved in the cleft lip deformity, including the perinasal and perioral muscles, not just the horizontal portions of the orbicularis oris (Adcock and Markus, 1997; Delaire, 1971, 1975; Joos, 1987, 1989, 1995; Markus and Delaire, 1993). This was a concept first advanced by Veau (1938). The European studies carried out 40 to 50 years after the time of Veau showed how proper reconstruction of the muscles around the lip and nose could help to facilitate more normal forward growth of the maxilla in children with clefts.

The results of lip repair are generally assessed in terms of esthetic appearance, and to some extent the mobility of the lip, the latter particularly with respect to the direction of muscular pull or function (Mortier et al., 1997; Schendel, Pearl, and DeArmond, 1991). The surgeon attempts to "orient" the muscles around the lip and nose so that the vectors of muscular motion in speech, smiling, etc., are similar to what they would have been if there was no cleft. In addition, with specific regard to the nose, surgeons try to minimize the asymmetric slope or "collapse" of the alar wing on the cleft side (Fig. 4-1, *D*), or bilateral droop of the alae and nasal dome in bilateral clefts (McComb, 1975a, 1975b, 1985; Salyer, 1986, 1994). Some surgeons use nasal stents or "conformers" to provide a more pleasing shape to the nose (Salomonson, 1996).

Secondary Lip and Nose Surgery

Most children with cleft lips undergo some secondary surgery in early childhood to reduce scar tissue on the lip, improve the symmetry of the vermilion border, and improve the appearance and symmetry of the nose. Many undergo secondary surgery on the lip before beginning school, but secondary surgery on the nose typically does not take place until age 6 years or so because there are major midfacial growth sites in the nose and surgery can potentially interfere with that growth if it is performed too early. Cronin (1977) and Cronin and Upton (1978) devised a procedure for lengthening the columella, which tends to be very short with little to no cartilage, in bilateral clefts. This procedure provides better support for the dome of the nose, and it improves the size of the nares. Secondary surgery to improve the nasal airway often involves straightening the nasal septum for patients with unilateral clefts because the septum tends to buckle toward the non-cleft side, but such surgery is not usually done until the teenage years because the septum is a major growth site. The septum in bilateral clefts is usually straight (Fig. 4-11) unless there was partial attachment of one of the cleft segments to the vomer bone.

In the individual with a bilateral cleft, the repaired lip may be intact but quite short and immobile as a result of deficiency of tissue and the fact that the lip is often poorly differentiated from the premaxilla in the infant (Fig. 4-12). Surgery to create an adequate labial sulcus may be performed in early childhood or later, and a procedure to lengthen the central portion of the lip may be performed in the later childhood or teenage years. The latter procedure is called an "Abbe flap" or "cross-lip flap" (Fig. 4-13) and involves a staged transposition of tissue from the lower lip—which tends to be protrusive and "patulous" (drooping and poutlike in appearance)—to the upper lip (Kapetansky, 1971; Kawamoto, 1979; Lewis, 1994; Millard, 1977). A flap of tissue is lifted off the lower lip, leaving it attached to the lip to maintain adequate blood supply,

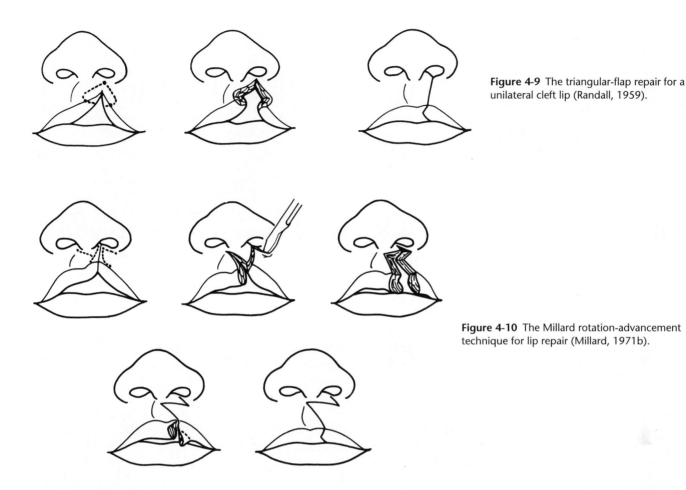

Figure 4-9 The triangular-flap repair for a unilateral cleft lip (Randall, 1959).

Figure 4-10 The Millard rotation-advancement technique for lip repair (Millard, 1971b).

and attached like a bridge to the upper lip. The two lips are left semiattached in this fashion until a second blood supply is established from the upper lip, usually about 2 weeks, and then the lower attachment is severed. The transposed tissue adds bulk and length to the upper lip.

Effect of the Repaired Lip on Speech

The literature contains little systematic information on the effect of the repaired lip on speech, most likely indicating that few clinicians have observed significant effects on lip function. Occasionally, a repaired lip, particularly in a bilateral cleft, may be too short for bilabial closure to be obtained easily in speech, so intended bilabial consonants become labiodentals in terms of placement. Surgeons term shortness of the lip in the central portion a "whistle deformity." In very wide bilateral cleft lips with a very small prolabium, there may be a whistle deformity of the repaired lip in early childhood (Fig. 4-14). This may improve as the lip grows, or it may require later revision. Severe shortness of the lip that persists despite growth and surgical revision is occasionally seen in older patients (Fig. 4-15). The perceptual effect on speech is usually minimal: the bilabial nasal and stop consonants may be produced as labiodentals. However, the speaker's conversational partner may be confused by the visual signal if he or she is actually looking at the speaker. Another factor related to the lips is the possibility of poor lip competency as a result of retroposition of the maxilla with respect to the mandible (maxillary retrusion or maxillary hypoplasia), placing the upper lip so far posteriorly that normal labiodental fricatives are in essence "inverted," produced with the lower incisors against the upper lip. This is seen in some cases of cleft lip and palate and also in those craniofacial syndromes in which midface hypoplasia is present.[1]

PALATAL SURGERY

Despite the relatively long history of palatal surgery, little consensus has been reached regarding the best surgical techniques, and even less regarding optimal timing. What to do, and when to do it, remains a constant concern of teams and surgeons.

Goals of Palatal Surgery

The goal of surgical closure of the palate is to establish an intact division between the oral and nasal cavities, including a fully functioning velopharyngeal system. In the baby, the hope is that an intact system will facilitate feeding; reduce the occurrence of upper respiratory infections; improve otologic health[2] ; and provide adequate physical structures

[1]These observations are based on our own clinical experience and are not documented by research studies or by interexaminer reliability data.

[2]However, studies on just how beneficial palatal surgery is for otologic health have not consistently shown an effect, as discussed in Chapter 6.

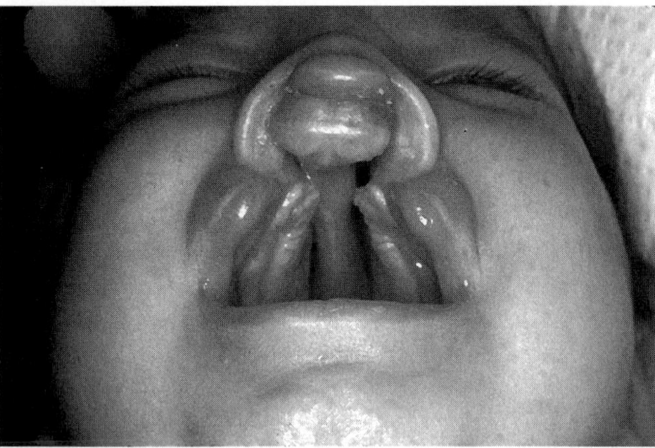

Figure 4-11 The straight vomer bone (and very protuberant premaxilla, with the palatal shelves collapsed medially being it) in an infant with a complete bilateral cleft.

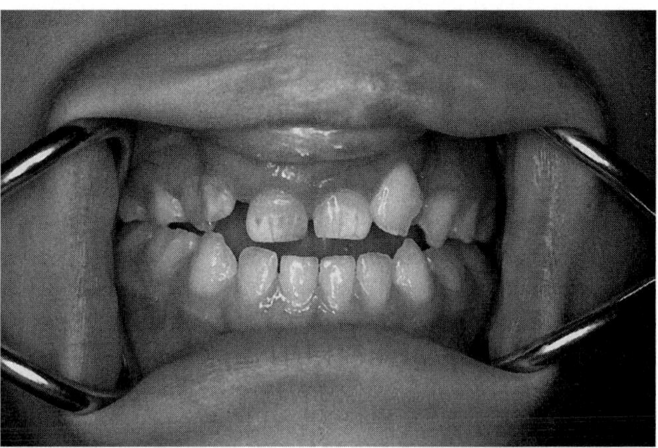

Figure 4-12 In this child with a bilateral cleft, the lip remains poorly differentiated from the premaxilla. Surgery to create a better lip sulcus can be undertaken at a later time.

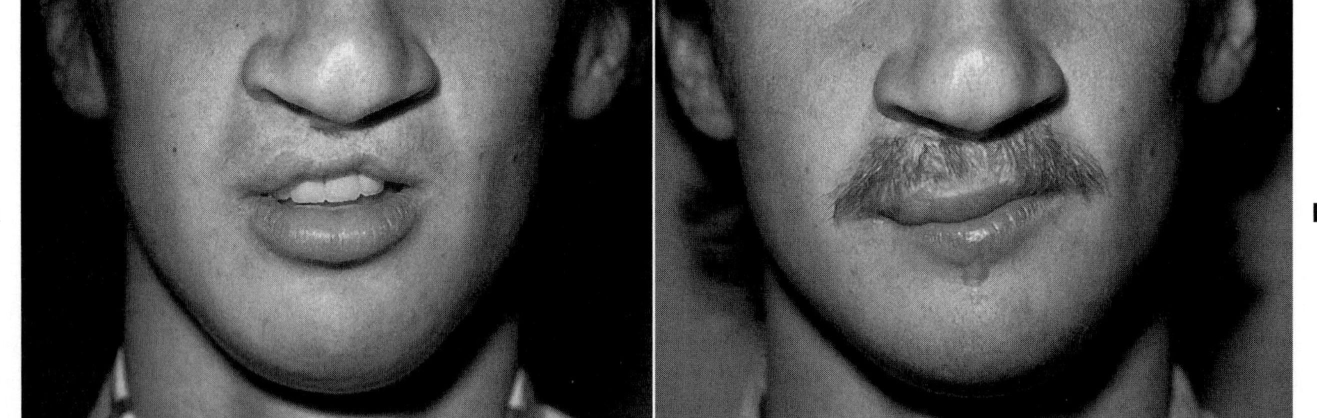

Figure 4-13 **A** and **B,** Young man with a bilateral cleft lip before and after an Abbe flap procedure to lengthen the lip. The lip is still asymmetrical in this patient. The little nubbin below the vermilion of the lower lip is the site from which the tissue was taken to add length to the upper lip.

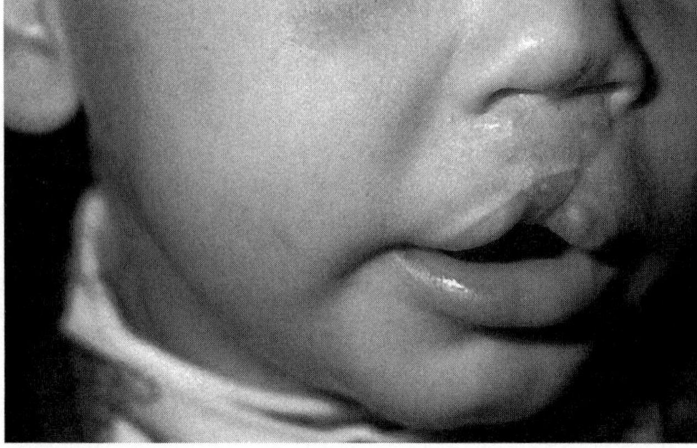

Figure 4-14 Child with a "whistle deformity" after bilateral lip repair in infancy. This deficiency in length may or may not improve as the child grows.

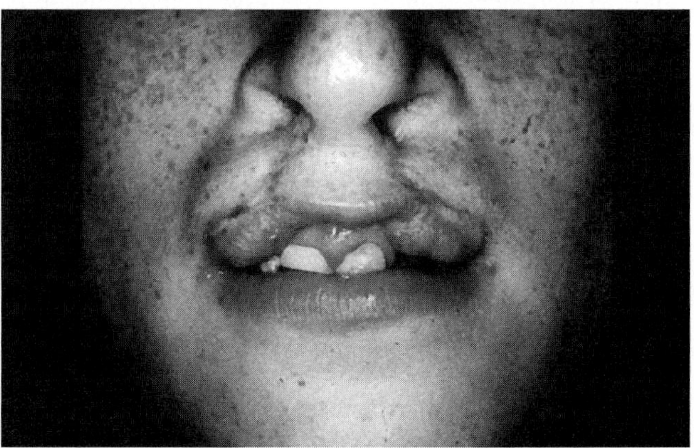

Figure 4-15 This teenager has a poor result from lip repair, with deep grooves along the lines of repair, depressions in the bases of the nostrils, and severe shortening (whistle deformity) in the central portion of the lip.

for the establishment of oral articulatory placements, oral direction of the vocal airstream, and normal resonance balance.

Age at Palatal Surgery

If speech development were the only focus of concern, speech-language pathologists would advocate palatal closure before the onset of babbling, when the infant is learning to use oral placements (articulatory targets) and needs to be able to direct the air stream orally to produce such early pressure consonants as /b/ and /d/. Kemp-Fincham, Kuehn, and Trost-Cardamone (1990) reviewed the literature on the development of speech motor control and phonetic development in infants and concluded that there is a particularly sensitive period or state of readiness between the ages of 4 and 6 months. They conjectured that it may thus be important to close the palate before or during the 4- to 6-month time frame to avoid development of maladaptive compensatory articulations. Interestingly, in that same year Copeland (1990) reported speech results in 100 children who underwent palatal surgery between the ages of 9 and 25 weeks (mean 16.4 weeks), an age bracket comparable to the sensitive period suggested by Kemp-Fincham, Kuehn, and Trost-Cardamone (1990). The Copeland report was essentially a follow-up of an earlier report by Desai (1983), the operating surgeon.[3] The speech of these children was evaluated only once, purportedly "at the time of the 5 year clinical review," but the age range was 3.8 to 6.3 years. The results as presented by Copeland (1990) were difficult to interpret: although 87 children were said to have acceptable speech, 16 of 100 had clinical signs of velopharyngeal inadequacy. The author reported differential effects of age at palatal surgery compared across 3 months, 4 months, 5 months, and 6 months. None of the children operated on at 3 months were exhibiting compensatory articulations, but an increasing number of children did exhibit these behaviors as age at palatal surgery increased. Although these findings would seem to fit well with the theoretical framework of Kemp-Fincham, Duehn, and Trost-Cardamone (1990), there were very uneven numbers of children in the four groups. In addition, the short time separating the ages at surgery and the nebulous nature of the speech data warrant caution in considering the results and conclusions.

It is helpful to gain an historical perspective on how the thinking regarding optimal age at palatal closure has evolved over the last few decades because (1) there are many surgeons who have not changed their surgical regimen regardless of new data, (2) the concerns about a potential trade-off between speech and facial growth have been given different levels of importance across studies, and (3) it is likely that clinicians currently entering the field will themselves encounter this issue any time they deal with infants with clefts. The amount of detail in this discussion may seem burdensome, but is included to help you reach your own conclusions.

Up through the mid to late 1970s, textbooks in pediatrics and surgery in the United States commonly cited an age range of 18 to 24 months as the appropriate time for palatal surgery. Little information on normal speech and language development was cited in support of this recommended age. The majority of the articles, although not all, were focused on surgical techniques, with relatively few data on speech outcome other than the surgeon's own observations. The focus was on postoperative healing (e.g., absence of fistulae) and, oddly, adequacy of velopharyngeal closure as judged on the oral examination. Many articles lacked any objective data on speech (Battle, 1967; Evans and Renfrew, 1974; Holdsworth, 1954; Jolleys, 1954; Koberg and Koblin, 1973; Lindsay, LeMesurier, and Farmer, 1962; Peet, 1961).

The role of speech-language pathologists in evaluating surgical results became increasingly prominent in the 1960s, and this was gradually reflected in the literature (Evans and Renfrew, 1974; McWilliams, 1960), although articles written solely by surgeons continued to predominate. Some publications addressed the issue of timing of palatoplasty, but there was troubling variation in what was considered to be an "early" age for surgery. Also, some articles compared speech outcomes across very large age ranges, from children who underwent surgery within the first year or two of life to patients for whom surgery was delayed until the teenage years. Finally, in the majority of articles the assessment of surgical results was highly confounded by the variables of type of surgery (often not consistent within a single study), age at surgery, age at evaluation, and methods of assessment.

Bearing in mind all of the limitations just listed, a cautious summary of the information and opinions found in the literature through the end of the 1970s follows[4]:

1. There was a general trend of better speech results (higher percentage of children reported to have normal or acceptable speech) with earlier ages at surgery (Evans and Renfrew, 1974; Holdsworth, 1954; Jolleys, 1954; Koberg and Koblin, 1973; Lindsay, LeMesurier, and Farmer, 1962; McWilliams, 1960; Peet, 1961), but what was considered early in some reports was comparable to the middle or later ages in other reports. Very few reports included children operated on before 1 year of age.
2. The highest reported percentage of good speech results was that of Jolleys (1954), who claimed that approximately 90% of children operated on before 2

[3]Desai (1983) reported "no velopharyngeal incompetency" in 100 children operated on by 16 weeks of age, but he offered no objective data and there was no speech-language pathologist involved in making this judgment.

[4]The attitudes and opinions are listed by relevant decades here because, even in many relatively recent texts and articles in journals, summaries of information on this topic are based on old information.

years of age had good or excellent speech, but the author offered no objective speech data.

3. Several authors, usually surgeons, concluded their reports by recommending specific age ranges for surgery: 6 to 9 months (Holdsworth, 1954), before the age of 8 months (Evans and Renfrew, 1974), in the "1-year range" (Lindsay, LeMesurier, and Farmer, 1962), and between the ages of 2 and 3 years (Koberg and Koblin, 1973).

The following decade began with an extensive review of the literature by Kaplan (1981), who tried to synthesize the articles on age-at-palatoplasty from the stand point of speech, midfacial growth, and types of surgical procedures. But many of the studies he included had been marred or completely invalidated by methodological flaws. To his credit, Kaplan attempted to bring the attention of fellow surgeons to the fact that children exhibit significant development of prespeech vocalizations and subsequent emergence of meaningful speech far earlier than had been assumed by previous authors. He advocated palatoplasty between the ages of 3 and 6 months so that there would be adequate time for wound healing and reduction of swelling and so that the palate could be functionally normal by the age of 9 months. However, he had no supporting data.[5]

Dorf and Curtin (1982) reported startlingly different speech results between a group of 21 children operated on before 12 months of age and another group of 59 children operated on at more than 12 months 15 days. Speech was assessed solely for the presence or absence of compensatory articulations. Only 10% of the children in the first group had these maladaptive patterns, compared with 86% of those operated on after the age of 12.5 months. In a later follow-up study of an expanded series of patients divided by the same criterion, the same authors (1990) reported an even greater discrepancy in speech outcome between the two surgical groups. In both articles Dorf and Curtin stressed the importance of the child's stage of *phonemic development*, or what they called "articulation age," as opposed to chronological age, in deciding on the appropriate age for surgery. They felt that a child more than 1 year old showing a lag in speech-language development might not be as vulnerable to the effects of delayed palatal surgery because he or she is not making the same demands on the oral and velopharyngeal system as a child targeting the phonemes that normally develop at this time. Ironically, although the work of Dorf and Curtin (1982, 1990) is still widely cited in the literature on palatoplasty, their caveat about a discrepancy between chronological age and "articulation age" is often ignored.

Throughout the remainder of the 1980s, articles on this topic continued to emerge, but the titles were sometimes misleading because some surgeons still seemed to have little idea how early surgery would have to take place to have a positive effect on early speech and language development. For example, Blijdorp and Muller (1984) set out to see whether there was a differential effect on speech development between children who underwent closure between the ages of 2 years 6 months and 3 years 6 months in comparison to children who underwent closure between 5 years 6 months and 6 years 6 months.[6] It is little wonder that they found no significant difference. Other surgeons attempted to move the time of surgery into the first few months of life (Ainoda, Yamashita, and Tsukada, 1985; Barimo et al., 1987; Desai, 1983; Randall et al., 1983) but often gave little information on how speech was assessed. Barimo et al. (1987) published one of the few interdisciplinary articles on speech results as related to age of surgery. They reported impressive results in 22 children randomly selected from a larger group of more than 190 whose palates were repaired between the ages of 3 and 8 months. These subjects were followed up from the toddler age to nearly 9 years of age; they reportedly exhibited no glottal stops or pharyngeal fricatives and no nasal emission. The authors concluded that early surgery (mean age 6 months), *together with parental involvement and speech stimulation,* produced virtually normal speech development in all 22 children.[7]

By the late 1980s there was a parallel development in the study of early acquisition of phonology and phonetic skills that helped to boost the interest in the relationship between age at palatoplasty and subsequent speech development. Before this time there existed only a modicum of information about the prelinguistic vocalizations produced by infants with clefts before their palatal surgery. Reports by Grunwell and Russell (1987, 1988) and O'Gara and Logemann (1988, 1990) provided a framework for understanding how the physical constraints that the cleft imposed on early vocal output could influence postclosure vocal output, a line of study that continued to progress in the 1990s.

At the end of the 1980s there was a fairly solid movement toward performing palatal surgery before the end of the first year of life if the child was nonsyndromic and exhibiting otherwise normal development, but confusion continued in terms of what qualified as "early" surgery. Unfortunately, studies that followed the reports of Dorf and Curtin (1982, 1990) failed to yield results validating 12 months of age as a "watershed" (Dalston, 1992; Peterson-

[5]The same was true of a slightly later literature review by Egyedi (1985), who opted for 12 to 18 months for surgery to suit what he thought was a necessary compromise between issues relating to speech and those relating to growth. However, his review of the literature was flawed by misinterpretation of many of the original articles and he thus reached illogical conclusions.

[6]The speech assessment in the Blijdorp and Muller article (1984) consisted of watching the amount of fogging on a mirror held beneath the child's nose during speech.

[7]Unfortunately, even when "parental involvement" and "speech stimulation" are stipulated in such reports, it is impossible to meaningfully assess the possible effects on outcome because of the variability in type, intensity, and quality of stimulation.

Table 4-1 **Comparison of the Overall Prevalence of Compensatory Articulations**

Cleft Type	*Dalston (1992)*	*Peterson-Falzone (1990)*	*Totals (Dorf and Curtin [1990])*
UCLP	13/53 = 24.5%	20/132 = 15.1%	33/185 = 17.8% (vs. 25/44 = 56.8%)*
BCLP	12/29 = 41.4%	24/63 = 38.1%	36/92 = 39.1% (vs. 23/26 = 88.4%)*
CPO	20/77 = 26.0%	8/45 = 17.8%	28/122 = 23.0% (vs. 25/61 = 40.9%)*
Totals	45/159 = 28.3%	52/240 = 21.7%	97/399 = 24.3% (vs. 73/131 = 55.7%)*

*Inferred from the bar graphs in the Dorf and Curtin article (1990) because only percentages are given in the text and shown in the graphs, with no actual numbers given in either the graphs or text. (UCLP, unilateral cleft lip and palate; BCLP, bilateral cleft lip and palate; CPO, cleft palate only.)

Falzone, 1990). But of equal importance was the fact that a large multicenter study by Ross (1987) on the effects of palatal surgery on midfacial growth provided data that argued *against* the age-old fear that early palatal surgery would interfere more with midfacial growth than delayed surgery would. Specifically, Ross (1987) studied large numbers of cephalometric measurements and reported slightly better facial growth for children with unilateral cleft lip and palate who underwent surgery in the first year of life compared with children operated on in any of several later age groups of repair. (The topic of midfacial growth and the possible relationship to palatal surgery is discussed on pp. 107-108.)

In the early 1990s knowledge regarding prespeech vocalizations and early speech development in babies with clefts continued to expand. Some of these studies indirectly addressed the question of timing of surgery. O'Gara and Logemann (1988, 1990) monitored 23 babies from the ages of 3 to 36 months. These babies were divided, posthoc, into an "earlier closure–greater tissue" group (mean age at surgery 9.3 months) and a later closure–lesser tissue group (mean age at surgery 16.1 months). The infants in the earlier repair group showed an earlier decrease in the use of abnormal speech sounds after palatal closure, but it must be borne in mind that these babies had their surgery earlier precisely *because* their clefts were less severe than those in the later closure group. The findings of O'Gara and Logemann (1988, 1990) essentially paralleled those of the slightly earlier reports by Grunwell and Russell (1987, 1988) in terms of the changes found in vocal output before and after palatal surgery in babies with cleft palate.

Studies by Peterson-Falzone (1990) and Dalston (1992), reporting on an aggregate of 399 children between them, failed to confirm the findings of Dorf and Curtin (1982, 1990) regarding 12 months as a critical age for palatal surgery. The overall prevalence of compensatory articulations in these studies was 24.3%, compared with 87.8% in the report of Dorf and Curtin (1990) (Table 4-1).[8] Although the age at surgery was known for only 90 of the children in the retrospective Peterson-Falzone report, the results in comparison to the Dorf and Curtin reports were disparate: there was only a small difference in the prevalence of compensatory articulations between those children operated on at less than 12.5 months of age and those operated on at an older age (Table 4-2). The mean age at surgery for those who had these maladaptive patterns was 24.2 months, whereas the mean for those who did not develop these patterns was 21.2 months, far beyond the expected 12-month boundary. In the Dalston study (1992), only 13 of the 159 children had undergone repair before the age of 12.5 months, and of these 5 (38.5%) were exhibiting compensatory articulations. In the latter study 146 children underwent closure over the age of 12.5 months, and 40 (27.4%) were using compensatory articulations. It should be pointed out that all four of these studies had one or more of the following methodological problems.

1. Not all the children were examined by the authors at the time of the first clinical examination after surgery, so it was not known whether the velopharyngeal system at that time was in fact competent and thus whether the compensatory articulations were simply residuals of earlier velopharyngeal inadequacy.
2. The age at the time of postoperative examination was not given in the first Dorf and Curtin (1982) report.
3. The criteria for determining that compensatory articulations were present in a given child were not

[8]Simple presence or absence of compensatory articulations in a patient's speech is only one possible indication of velopharyngeal inadequacy for speech, the others being nasal air loss on pressure consonants with consequent weakening of those consonants, and hypernasal resonance. Furthermore, compensatory articulations can persist after VPI is successfully treated, and so are not a reliable indication of *ongoing* inadequacy.

Table 4-2 **Comparison of the Results in Children Operated on at Less Than or More Than 12.5 Months Old in the Dalston (1992), Peterson-Falzone (1990), and Dorf and Curtin (1990) Reports**

	Dalston (1992)		*Peterson-Falzone (1990)*		*Dorf and Curtin (1990)**	
Cleft Type	*<12 m*	*>12 m*	*<12 m*	*>12 m*	*<12 m*	*>12 m*
UCLP			10	36	15	29
CAs +			4	7	1	24
% age			40.0	19.4	6.6	82.7
BCLP			5	21	2	24
CAs +			2	15	0	23
% age			40.0	71.4	0	95.8
CPO			2	16	32	29
CAs +			1	3	1	24
% age			50.0	18.8	3.1	82.7
Totals	13	146	17	7	49	82
CAs +	5	40	7	25	2	72
% age	38.4	27.4	41.2	34.2	4.1	87.8
					73/131 with CAs (55.7%)	

*It is difficult to derive actual numbers from the Dorf and Curtin report. For example, they state that 5% of the 15 children with UCLP who were operated on before 12.5 months had compensatory articulations, but the lowest possible number would be 1 child of the 15, which equals 6.66%, not "less than 5%" as stated in the text of the article. (UCLP, unilateral cleft lip and palate; CAs +, compensatory articulations present: BCLP, bilateral cleft lip and palate; CPO, cleft palate only.)

specified in either of the Dorf and Curtin reports (1982, 1990) and were not consistent between the Peterson-Falzone (1990) and Dalston (1992) reports. In the Peterson-Falzone report specific compensatory articulations were counted as "present" if they recurred in an identifiable pattern in the child's speech, whereas in the Dalston (1992) report any compensatory articulation was counted as "present" in the child's speech even if it occurred only once in the recorded speech sample.

4. All four reports lacked interexaminer reliability data because all four were based on the perceptual speech evaluations performed by a single experienced examiner.

Finally, the percentage of subjects with each type of cleft was not similar among the studies. Nevertheless, the similarity between the Peterson-Falzone and Dalston reports, and the dissimilarity of those two data sets to those of the Dorf and Curtin reports, stimulated the comment by Dalston (1992) that "the patient population studied by Dorf and Curtin may have been atypical."

A study by Haapanen and Rantala in 1992 did little to clarify the age-at-surgery question because of small, uneven numbers of subjects. They reported better speech results in children operated on between the ages of 16 and 20 months in comparison to children operated on earlier (12 to 15 months) or later (21 to 24 months). The percentage of children in the latter two groups who had normal or "practically normal" speech was essentially the same (73% and 72%), but none of the children operated on between 16 and 20 months had compensatory articulations. Unfortunately, the number of children in this group was less than half the number in the other two groups, making the results tenuous at best. The authors concluded ". . . the age of about 18 months seemed optimal for the repair, but the numbers were too small to come to any firm conclusions." Their suggestion of 18 months being a possible optimal age for surgery was reminiscent of common clinical practices 30 years before the article was published.

Although Haapanen and Rantala (1992) had no data on children operated on before the end of the first year of life, a 1994 study from Mexico did (Ysunza et al., 1994). The latter authors reported that a significantly greater percentage of children undergoing surgery between the ages of 24 and 36 months had compensatory articulations than did children operated on at the ages of 6, 12, or even 18 months. However, the total number of children who had these maladaptive patterns was very high in this study (23 of 38, 60.5%), far greater than is acceptable in current practice.

Studies by Chapman and Hardin in 1992 and by O'Gara, Logemann, and Rademaker in 1994 on early speech development in youngsters with clefts noted the important role of time as a determinant of what we hear in their speech and alerted clinicians to the dangers of relying on studies for which results are based only on one-time assessments. Chapman and Hardin (1992) found that children with repaired clefts who had shown significant delays in speech development before the age of 2 years eventually showed "catch-up," although at a later age than typically seen in children without clefts. In a follow-up of the children first studied by O'Gara and Logemann (1988, 1990), O'Gara, Logemann, and Rademaker (1994) also emphasized the factor of time, stating ". . . time is an even stronger variable than age of palatoplasty for development of palatal, alveolar and velar place features, oral stops, and oral fricatives." Changes over time in the 23 babies they studied seemed to gradually erase the earlier discrepancy in speech sound development between those in the early closure group and those in the later closure group. However, it is important to note that all the children in this study had been consistently monitored and treated by an interdisciplinary craniofacial team, and the treatment included active intervention in the form of parent counseling to increase stimulation in the home.[9]

In summary, the knowledge gained in recent years regarding the effects of early structural constraints on later phonetic and phonological development in children with clefts supports efforts toward earlier palatal surgery when those children are otherwise developmentally normal. To date, we do not have sufficient data to support a need for palatoplasty in the first few weeks of life, a time when surgery might be possible but inherently more dangerous to the child (anesthetic risk) and the closure technically more difficult (smaller baby with a smaller area in which the surgeon must work, less available tissue). More treatment centers are continuing to collect longitudinal outcome data on babies operated on within the first 4, 6, 9, or 12 months of life. If their results show a consistent advantage in speech outcome and if these babies can be shown to have a degree of midface deformity that is no worse than in babies operated on at later ages, there is little doubt that earlier surgery will become a widely accepted norm.

Primary Veloplasty: A Very Different Variation on a Theme

Although the trend toward earlier definitive palatoplasty continues to grow in many centers, there is nearly an equally strong and persistent advocacy for primary veloplasty and later closure of the hard palate in other centers. This approach first came to prominence in Germany in the 1950s (Schweckendiek, 1966; Schweckendiek and Kruse, 1990) and gained devotees among surgeons in other countries as well, chiefly in Europe (Fara and Brousilova, 1969; Herfert, 1963; Hotz et al., 1984; Perko, 1974, 1979; Poupard et al., 1983; Robertson and Jolleys, 1974). The theory behind primary veloplasty is that putting off surgery on the hard palate will help reduce interference with forward growth of the maxilla as the child grows. The effort to conduct research on this approach has been hampered by several problematic sources of variation among studies, among them (1) the ages at which the primary veloplasty and later definitive palatal closure were carried out, (2) whether the children wore obturating plates until the entire palate was closed, (3) speech therapy, (4) surgical technique, (5) methods of speech assessment, and (6) types of measurements used to assess facial growth and the period of time over which the measurements were made. The timing for the primary veloplasty has variously been recommended at the ages of 3 months, 6 to 8 months, before 12 months, 12 to 18 months, and even as high as 2 years 6 months (DeLuke et al., 1997; Dingman and Argenta, 1985; Fara and Brousilova, 1969; Friede, Lilja, and Johanson, 1980; Friede et al., 1991; Greminger, 1981; Harding, 1979; Harding and Campbell, 1989[10]; Herfert, 1963; Lohmander-Agerskov, 1998; Lohmander-Agerskov and Soderpalm, 1993; Lohmander-Agerskov et al., 1993, 1995, 1996, 1997; Meijer and Cohen, 1990; Noordhoff et al., 1987; Poupard et al., 1983; Schweckendiek and Kruse, 1990; Tanino et al., 1997; Vedung, 1995; Wu, Chen, and Noordhoff, 1986). The majority of practitioners have advocated hard palate closure in the preschool years or early school years, but the patients of Meijer and Cohen (1990) underwent closure between 12 and 22 months, with a mean age of 20 months. At the other extreme, Schweckendiek waited until ages 11 to 13 years (1966, 1978). His reports contained little mention of use of obturating plates over the residual cleft in the years between the primary veloplasty and the palatoplasty. Later clinical studies either omitted mention of plates or stated that such plates were used in some patients and did not document consistency of use nor differentiate the speech results in obturated patients from nonobturated patients.

Two studies did attempt to look at obturator use. Noordhoff et al. (1987) examined articulation development in 71 children *before* repair of the hard palate. These children had undergone primary veloplasty at an average age of 18 months and were 2 to 6 years old at the time of the study. Of these, 51 patients had worn palatal plates in the past, and 10 were wearing one at the time of the study. The authors stated they could not find an advantage in articulation for those who had had plates. All the children showed significantly poorer articulation skills than did children without clefts at each age studied, and the authors concluded ". . . to date, this study and all but one of the other reports assessing the effects of delayed hard palate

[9]See footnote 7.

[10]The Harding and Campbell study (1989) was badly flawed by several factors, among them the fact that the "early complete" palatal closures were not done until age 15 months. This group had a 30% prevalence of abnormal speech patterns that were described as "incorrect airstream and errors of tongue placement," the same types of errors found in the late repair group.

closure on speech lead any conscientious clinician to seriously question the advantages of delayed closure over early complete palate closure."[11] Van Demark et al. (1989) conducted a retrospective study on children with unilateral clefts who had had primary veloplasty at an average age of 18.9 months and hard palate repair at little more than 5 years 6 months (range 47 to 163 months, mean 67.2 months). At the time of the speech evaluation from which the study data were drawn, one patient had already had a Teflon injection pharyngoplasty for velopharyngeal inadequacy. The authors reported that no subject had either a severe articulation problem or a severe nasality problem, and that 94.5% had marginal to adequate velopharyngeal closure. The prevalence of compensatory articulations was low, and no child exhibited nasal grimacing in speech. None of the children had worn palatal obturators before hard palate closure, but all (with one exception) had had intensive speech therapy. The authors felt that the relatively favorable speech results, in comparison to those of other studies on primary veloplasty, were due in part to the particular type of soft palate closure that had been used and also to the intensive speech therapy. In contrast, in the study of Bardach, Morris and Olin (1984) on the "Marburg" project, 44% of children who had had delayed closure of the hard palate demonstrated nasal grimacing and also a high prevalence of glottal and pharyngeal placements in speech.

Lohmander-Agerskov et al. (1996) reported speech findings on 12 patients between the ages of 6.5 and 8 years who still had an unoperated cleft of the hard palate. This study was part of the database on primary veloplasty developed in Scandinavia over a period of two decades. At the time of the study, four (44%) of the children were using "retracted articulation" (articulation accomplished with abnormally posterior placement) and one additional child was using "glottal compensations." These children used these patterns regardless of whether the anterior palatal defect was covered with an "oral bandage." The patterns seemed to reflect the articulatory patterns the children had learned as a result of years of speaking with inadequately closed palates, patterns that did not change automatically once the anterior defect was obturated.

Many different techniques have been used for the hard palate closure in children first having primary veloplasty. For example, Schweckendiek and Kruse (1990) dissected the soft palate into its three layers (oral mucosa, muscle, nasal mucosa) and placed a rubber band from one side of the cleft to the other (through a needle) to help pull the two sides together before suturing each of the layers together with the same layers on the opposite side of cleft. They felt that the elastic action was needed to help approximate (in this case, literally "pull together") the sides of the cleft. Kriens (1969) advocated reconstruction of the levator sling in closing the soft palate, a principle that has been popular both in primary veloplasties and one-stage definitive palatoplasties. Similarly, techniques for later closure of the hard palate have varied, even within a single report. Meijer and Cohen (1990, page 323), for example, used a "von Langenbeck technique with or without the use of a vomer flap for two-layer closure, or occasionally a modified Widmaier technique (one-layer vomer flap closure) . . . when the palatal shelves [had] progressed medially until only a very narrow space [remained]." It is not known to what extent variations in technique may have produced different results across studies, although there have been many studies on differences in speech results associated with specific techniques used in one-stage palatal closures (discussed in the next section) and perhaps some inferences to two-stage closure are appropriate. However, as in all studies of results of surgery, caution is necessary in making cause-and-effect conclusions. First, in such studies we are not always told that the palatoplasty in fact produced an intact, functioning palate (e.g., what was the fistula rate or dehiscence rate?). Second, the length of time and rigor of follow-up are not always specified. Third, a "name-brand" technique recommended by one surgeon may be performed somewhat differently by another surgeon. Fourth, as stated previously, speech therapy or stimulation is often not documented or quantifiable. Finally, many factors are in place even preoperatively (amount of tissue, the skill and experience of the surgeon) that influence outcome.

Those who advocated primary veloplasty in older reports as well as those offering more current data (Lohmander-Agerskov, 1998; Lohmander-Agerskov et al., 1990, 1993, 1995, 1996, 1997) generally reported what they considered to be "acceptable" or "intelligible" speech with acknowledged nasal air loss of varying degrees. Other clinicians have reached different conclusions. A cautionary report about the effect of primary veloplasty on speech was published by Cosman and Falk in 1980. Jackson, McLennan, and Scheker (1983) compared the speech and facial growth results in children who had had primary veloplasty with results from primary palatoplasty; they reported that speech was inferior in the first group and that there was no difference between the two groups in the incidence of midface retrusion. They concluded, "This procedure does not offer enough to warrant its routine application." Witzel, Salyer, and Ross (1984) reviewed all the published studies on primary veloplasty and concluded that delaying hard palate repair past the age of 12 years produced good skeletal relationships but results on repairs done between

[11]The "one other" report they were referring to was the 1978 study by Hotz et al., which compared speech results in 40 children who had had soft palate closure at 18 months and hard palate closure at 6 to 8 years to speech in 30 who had had complete closure of the palate between 2 years 6 months and 3 years. These authors reported no advantage for the "early" complete closure of the cleft in terms of speech outcome, but the study was fraught with serious methodological errors, beginning with the fact that the age of 2 to 3 years for palatal closure places the child at a disadvantage for acquisition of phonology and phonetic skills. In addition, this study contained no description of how speech was assessed, and no data on inter- or intra-judge reliability.

the ages of 4 and 8 years were contradictory. These authors also concluded that severe speech problems were prevalent in the patients included in the studies they reviewed. Bardach, Morris, and Olin (1984) studied 45 patients operated on by Schweckendiek, and also reported generally acceptable facial growth but a high prevalence (52%) of velopharyngeal inadequacy.

In the study of Lohmander-Agerskov et al. of 1996, the children wore intraoral appliances only during the first 12 to 18 months of life to facilitate feeding, "stabilise [sic] the alveolar processes, and enhance the development of anterior sounds." At the time of the study, the children were 7 years old and it was reported that 6 of 20 had "functionally closed" hard palates (meaning no observable residual opening) and 14 had open palates. The speech results as given by the authors were difficult to interpret. They stated that there was only mild hypernasality present in both groups of children and thus they both had "acceptable velopharyngeal function." Not surprisingly, the children with open clefts had more nasal escape and a higher prevalence of compensatory articulations. In the children with the "functionally closed" clefts, the closure seemed to have taken place at about 18 to 36 months of age. The only other report of spontaneous "functional" closure of a cleft was that of Cosman and Falk (1980).

Rohrich et al. (1996) compared speech results in two groups of children, one with complete palate repair at a mean age of 10.8 months and the other with a primary veloplasty at 11 months and hard palate repair at a mean age of 48.6 months. They reported persistent palatal fistulae in 35% of the late-closure group versus 5% of the early-closure group. There were statistically significant greater speech deficiencies in the late-closure group with regard to articulation, nasal resonance, intelligibility, and substitution patterns. These authors also reported that there were no significant differences between the two groups in maxillofacial growth.

By the end of the 1990s some surgeons and even teams were still advocating the use of primary veloplasty (Hotz et al., 1984; Lohmander-Agerskov, 1998; Lohmander-Agerskov and Soderpalm, 1993; Lohmander-Agerskov et al., 1990, 1993, 1995, 1996, 1997), but reports of poor speech results in comparison to results from complete palatoplasties signaled a need for continued skepticism (Bardach, Morris, and Olin, 1984; Cosman and Falk, 1980; Jackson, McLennan, and Scheker, 1983; Noordhoff et al., 1987; Rohrich, 1996; Witzel, Salyer, and Ross, 1984). Some reports from Europe (Lohmander-Agerskov et al., 1990, 1993, 1996, 1997; Van Demark et al., 1989) underscored the necessity for rigorous speech therapy from early in life until the rest of the palate is closed; provision of such continuing intervention is not always possible. Effects on facial growth have not conclusively shown a better result in terms of facial growth compared with earlier, complete palatoplasty (Jackson, McLennan, and Scheker, 1983; Rohrich et al., 1996; Ross, 1987).

As pointed out by Van Demark (1995), advocates of this approach have ignored the financial and psychosocial costs of increased number of surgical procedures, clinic visits for the fitting and maintenance of palatal plates, speech therapy, etc. Nevertheless, it is likely that some speech-language pathologists will be dealing with children well past the year 2000 who have had primary veloplasty and delayed hard palate closure.[12] This forecast seems especially pertinent given a recent report by Lohmander-Agerskov (1998), who may have pointed the way toward eventual resolution of this seemingly "us versus them" issue. She reviewed the regimen of treatment for children with clefts at the center in Goteborg, where primary veloplasty and late hard palate closure has been the approach for many years. In that center velar repair is achieved at 6 to 8 months and the hard palate is closed at 8 to 10 years of age. The children in this report had been routinely fitted with intraoral plates to cover the hard palate cleft up through the ages of 12 to 18 months, but it is unclear from the article just how consistently the plates were worn. Speech was evaluated at five ages from 3 to 16 years (not all children were seen at all five ages). After hard palate closure, about 7% of the children required a pharyngeal flap because of residual hypernasality. Only three of the 59 children in the study exhibited "glottal articulation" even when their hard palates were still open (but presumably closed by the intraoral plates). After surgical palate closure, the one speech problem that did seem to persist was retracted (backed) articulation of "alveo-dental pressure plosives. . . ." This last finding caused the team to alter their surgical approach in terms of technique but not timing: they changed their method of closure of the velum "slightly" by moving forward the point of insertion of the vomer flap they used as part of the closure of the posterior cleft, hoping to encourage narrowing of the cleft in the hard palate. The photographs of a few dental casts included in the article showed narrowing of the hard palate cleft, perhaps to the extent that the residual effect on speech would have been minimal, but no actual measurements (case by case or averages) were given. A few profile photos were included to demonstrate good forward growth of the midface, an important achievement for the surgeon and orthodontist planning the physical management of cases. At the time of the report (1998), the team was satisfied with the facial growth outcome of their approach and dissatisfied only with the persistence of retracted "alveo-dental" pressure plosives. Speech results in terms of low incidence of glottal articulations and hypernasality seemed to be substantially improved over earlier studies and approaches.

[12]Some surgeons use a different type of two-staged palatal surgery, closing the hard palate first and the soft palate at a later date. The ages for these two stages vary: Enemark, Bolund and Jorgenson (1990) closed the hard palate at 10 weeks of age and the soft palate at an average of 22 months of age, a disturbingly late age from the stand point of speech development. To date, there have been no systematic investigations of speech results from centers using this "hard palate first" approach.

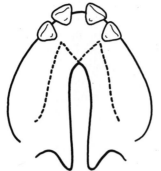

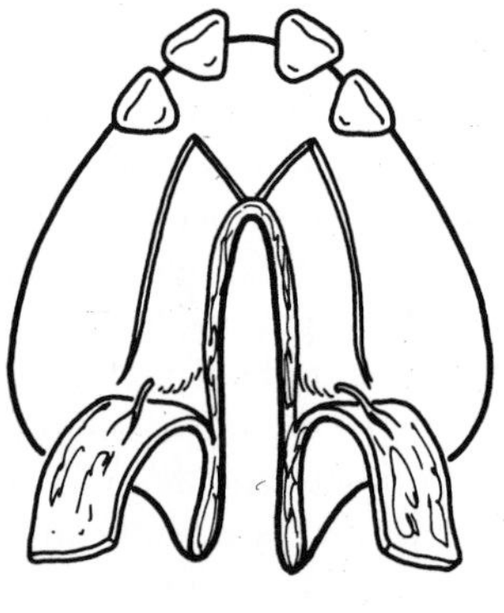

Figure 4-16 The V-Y retroposition procedure for the repair of palatal clefts. *(Adapted from Stark RB: Cleft palate. In Converse JM [ed.]:* Reconstructive plastic surgery: principles and procedures in correction, reconstruction, and transplantation. *2nd ed. Volume 4. Philadelphia: WB Saunders, 1977, p. 2096.)*

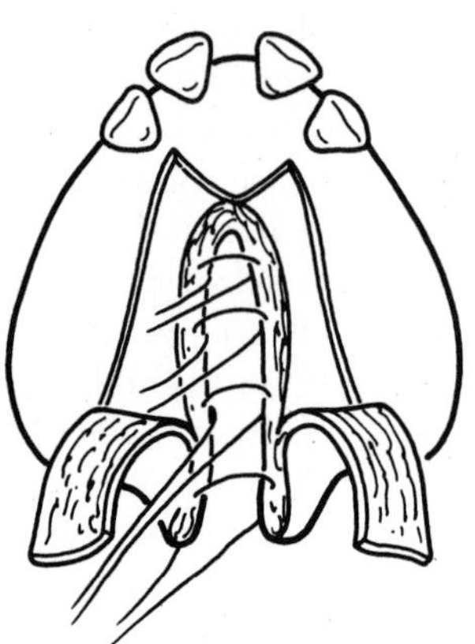

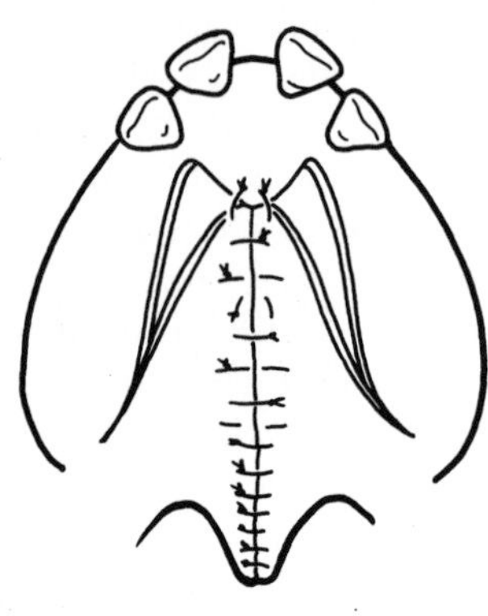

It is our opinion that primary veloplasty (1) *may* protect or enhance midfacial growth, although the data are not universally accepted, let alone conclusive, (2) in most treatment centers still poses an unnecessary hazard on communication development (because anterior or lateral crossbites are easily fixed by routine orthodontics in most cases), but (3) probably deserves the continued attention, development, and close surveillance suggested in the recent report by Lohmander-Agerskov (1998), especially when the veloplasty enhances narrowing of the residual hard palate cleft. It would be ideal if obturating plates could be shown to routinely facilitate the development of normal articulatory placement in these children with residual palatal openings, but that has not been demonstrated and seems unlikely to be, given the fact that even the strongest proponents of primary veloplasty have now ceased routine use of the plates.

Procedures for Initial Palatoplasty

A few techniques for closure of palatal clefts[13] have been popular for several decades and continue to be the "old standards" used by many surgeons and often modified by others into "new" (redesigned) techniques. Probably the oldest known technique for palatal repair is the von Langenbeck (1861) technique, also sometimes called a "straight-line repair" to contrast it to some other procedures that result in more of a zigzag line of closure. Lindsay (1971) described the modifications of the von Langenbeck technique that had been devised up through the late 1960s; other modifications have emerged since that time, usually in an attempt to reduce the amount of exposed or "denuded" bone. The French surgeon Victor Veau (1931) strongly criticized this straight-line suturing of the palatal halves in the midline. Dorrance (1925, 1932, 1933; Dorrance and Bransfield, 1946) designed a pushback procedure that freed the palatal mucosa and mucoperiosteum anteriorly (virtually all of the mucosa and mucoperiosteum of the secondary palate) and moved it backward in the attempt to obtain better palatal length than had been achieved with the straight-line repair. Later, Kilner (1937) and Wardill (1937) devised what came to be known as a "V-Y" pushback closure, now variously known as the Oxford technique, the Wardill-Kilner, the Veau-Wardill-Kilner, or the Veau-Wardill-Kilner-Peet method (Bardach, 1990; Calnan, 1976; Grabb, 1971). This approach has generated variations based on the number of unipedicled mucoperiosteal[14] flaps raised in the palate and moved into positions to provide closure of the cleft (Fig. 4-16). Both the modified von Langenbeck (Fig. 4-17) and the V-Y

[13]Not including the cleft of the alveolus, discussed in a following section.

[14]"Unipedicled" means "single footed," denoting a flap left attached at one end. "Mucoperiosteal" refers to the layer of tissue between the mucosal surface and the bone itself. In palatal surgery it is the mucoperiosteum that is moved, not bone.

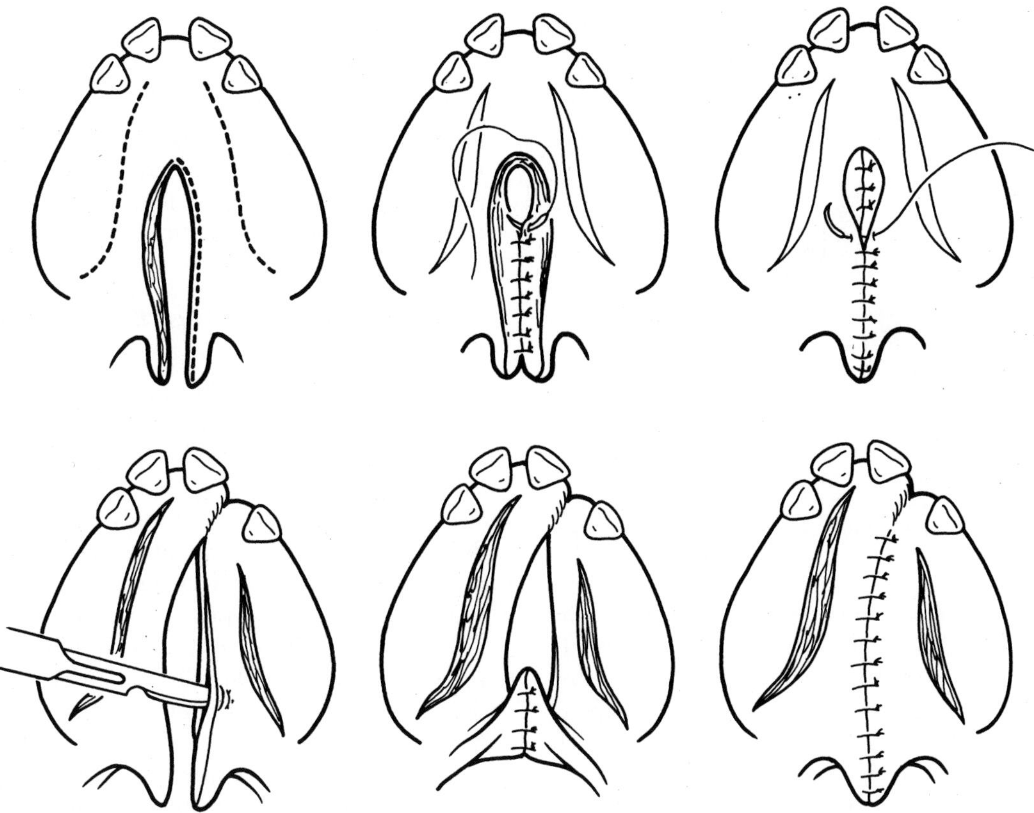

Figure 4-17 The von Langenbeck method of closing palatal clefts, shown for incomplete clefts (top three schematics) and complete clefts (bottom three schematics). This procedure is often referred to as a "straight-line" repair.

pushback closures are still in wide use. The Veau-Wardill-Kilner-Peet V-Y method mobilizes a total of four flaps, which are then moved posteriorly, leaving a relatively large area of bare bone on each side (nasal and oral) of the hard palate. The same is true of the traditional von Langenbeck approach, which depended on rather large lateral incisions next to the alveolar bone to free up tissue for movement to the midline.[15]

In the original "vomer flap" technique for palatal surgery (Wynn, 1974, 1976), a portion of the base of the vomer bone was mobilized to close the cleft. This technique gradually diminished in use because the suture line[16] of the vomer bone is an important growth center or site in the growing child's face (Delaire and Precious 1985, 1986), and reports of apparent interference with midfacial growth in children subjected to vomer flaps led to decreasing use of this approach.[17] However, many contemporary surgeons do use a portion of the vomer bone mucoperiosteum in closing the bony portion of the cleft (Butow and Steinhauser, 1989; Enemark, Bolund, and Jorgensen, 1990; Kobus, 1984; LaRossa et al., 1990; Tanino et al., 1997).

To close unilateral or bilateral clefts of the lip and palate or complete clefts of the secondary palate, surgeons often combine procedures, using one particular technique for closing the hard palate and another for closure of the soft palate. For example, the hard palate might be closed by a von Langenbeck procedure or a modified vomer flap and the soft palate by a Furlow double reversing Z-plasty (Furlow, 1986; Millard, 1980) or perhaps an intravelar veloplasty, also known as levator retropositioning (Braithwaite and Maurice, 1968; Brown, Cohen, and Randall, 1983; Edgerton and Dellon, 1971; Kriens, 1970; Trier and Dreyer, 1984). Furlow's Z-plasty repair of the palate (Figs.

[15]Bardach (1990) summarized the research that had shown the growth of the maxilla (including, of course, the palate) after surgery to be negatively influenced by the amount of bone left exposed or denuded in palatal surgery. He designed a two-flap technique of palatal closure in the 1960s (Bardach, 1990; Bardach and Salyer, 1987) that is currently popular.

[16]"Suture" lines do not necessarily refer to surgery. In anatomy, the line along which two bones or two parts of a bone meet is also called a suture line.

[17]Although Marks and Wynn (1985) stated that "risk of postpuberty maxillary retrusion is reduced" [in Wynn's vomer flap], they did not specify the comparison (e.g., in comparison to patients operated on by other techniques). Several studies did report unfavorable growth results with this technique (Aduss and Pruzansky, 1971; Bergland and Sidhu, 1974; Blocksma, Leuz, and Mellerstig, 1975; Friede and Johanson, 1977).

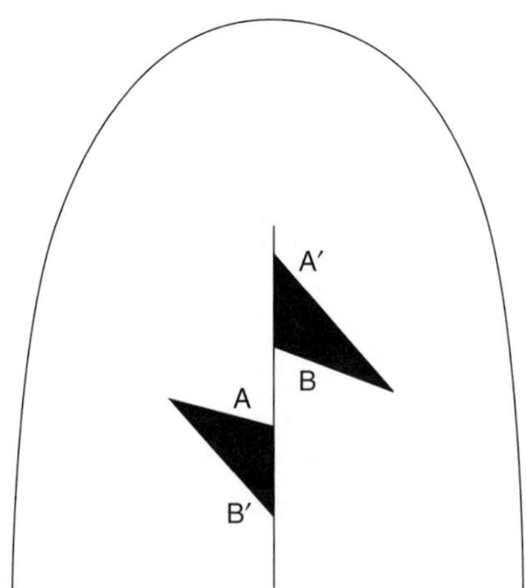

Figure 4-18 Where the flaps go in a Z-plasty. After the cuts are made and the flaps are raised, "A" is fitted into the upper gap labeled as "A′ " and "B" is fitted into the lower gap labeled "B′."

4-18 and 4-19) produces greater palatal length but at the expense of width; Furlow originally proposed using it only in clefts of minimal or moderate width. Mann and Fisher (1997) proposed the use of bilateral buccal flaps (flaps of tissue taken from the insides of the cheeks) into the cleft area combined with a Z-plasty for closure of wider clefts. They used this procedure in 76 patients with wide palatal clefts and reported that there had been only a 4% occurrence of postoperative dehiscence, but they had no speech data.

Several decades ago there were some advocates of incorporating a centrally placed pharyngeal flap into the initial palatoplasty in the hopes of lowering the chances of postpalatoplasty velopharyngeal inadequacy (Bingham et al., 1972; Buchholz et al., 1967; Dalston and Stuteville, 1975; Fara et al., 1970; Stark and DeHaan, 1960; Stark et al., 1969; Stellmach, 1985; Trigos and Ysunza, 1988). This procedure was termed a "primary" pharyngeal flap. It never reached the status of being a standard approach in palatal surgery and fell into disrepute, particularly when it was realized that, if this approach were to be applied to every patient, a large number would be receiving pharyngeal flaps who never would have needed them. For example, Morris (1973) reviewed the speech results of initial palatoplasties—regardless of specific type—as published up through 1971 and found that the majority of studies were yielding success rates between 66% and 75%. If these numbers were valid, then performing a primary pharyngeal flap in every cleft palate closure would mean that 25% to 33% of patients would be getting a procedure they would never have needed.

Currently, both levator retropositioning and the Furlow Z-plasty are popular in repair of clefts of the soft palate (whether occurring alone or in conjunction with anterior clefts), and craniofacial teams continue to develop databases to document their short-term and long-term effectiveness (Brothers et al., 1995; Butow and Jacobs, 1991; Coston et al., 1986; LaRossa, 1994; LaRossa et al., 1990; Marsh, Grames, and Holtman, 1989; Poole and Nunn, 1989; Randall et al., 1986). The "long-term" information is important not only because children grow and the velopharyngeal closure changes as they do so but also because any procedure may initially seem to provide good results but then, over time, fail to show sustained velopharyngeal adequacy.[18]

Ostensible Relationships Between Type of Palatoplasty and Speech Outcomes

This section is intentionally titled very cautiously because so many erroneous assumptions have been made in trying to relate specific types (brand names) of palatal surgery to subsequent speech results. From the preceding section on age at palatal surgery, you already have a sense of what a difficult and misleading question "What surgery produces the best speech results?" may be. Establishing a cause-effect relationship means taking into account a long list of difficult variables: severity and extent of the original defect, success in complete closure of the cleft without residual fistulae, postoperative healing (specifically, occurrence of fistulae and/or scarring), overall developmental level of the child, types of objective speech measurements taken, length of time between surgery and assessment, and short-term versus long-term follow-up.[19] Still another variable is the experiential base of the surgeon(s): the less experienced the

[18]This was the fate of the "island flap" or "island push-back" that was designed and reported simultaneously by Edgerton (1962) and Millard (1962), with later modification. The "island flap" was a flap of palatal mucoperiosteum taken from the oral surface of the velum and transposed to the nasal surface to compensate for the soft tissue deficit on this surface, in the attempt to make the palate longer. This procedure was initially exciting to surgeons (Batstone and Millard, 1971; Hoge, 1966; McNeill, 1967; Millard, 1966a, 1980; Millard et al., 1970; Noordhoff, 1970) but was gradually found to be no particular improvement over other procedures (Berkowitz, 1996; Georgiade et al., 1969; Greminger, 1981; Lewin, Heller, and Kojak, 1975; Luce, McClinton, and Hoopes, 1976). Edgerton (1965) later combined the island flap with a "suspensory pharyngeal flap" for patients with clefts of the soft palate only, in an attempt to obtain maximum length of the velum. However, he reported no preoperative or postoperative measurements of the palate, and he had no objective speech data.

[19]As children grow, at least three factors change the physical mechanism of velopharyngeal closure: the change in angulation of the palate in relationship to the pharynx and the cranial base (the soft palate in the infant is nearly parallel to—and hanging closer to—the posterior pharyngeal wall); the natural downward and forward growth of the face, which carries the hard and soft palate further away from the posterior pharyngeal wall and the cranial base; and the involution of the adenoids. The latter two factors, in particular, may lead to deterioration in velopharyngeal closure over time as the child grows, especially during the pubertal growth spurt. This deterioration is often reflected in longitudinal studies of speech results (Hardin-Jones et al., 1993; Karnell and Van Demark, 1986), something that will be missed in studies relying only on a one-time postoperative assessment.

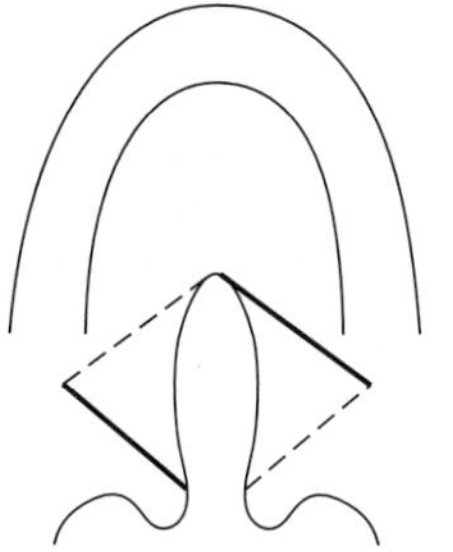
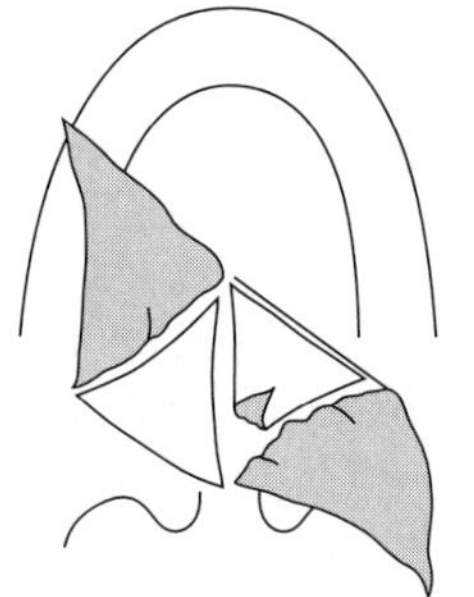
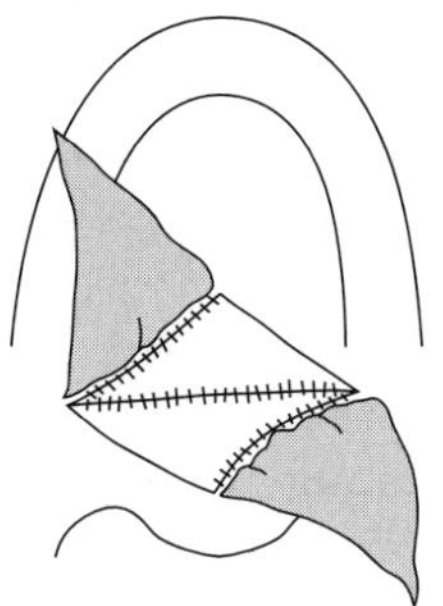
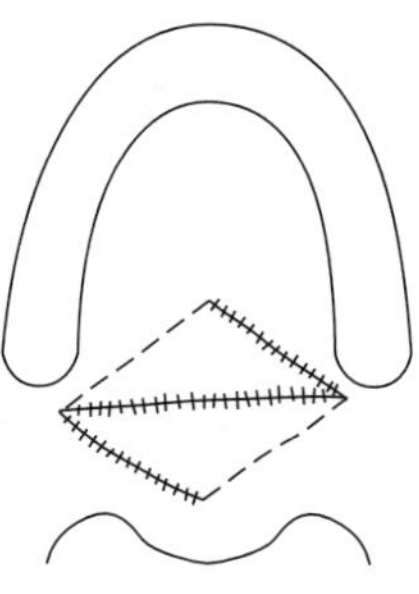

Figure 4-19 Adaptations of the schematics from Furlow (1986) showing how the transpositions of the flaps makes the palate longer in a Z-plasty. *(Redrawn from Furlow LT: Cleft palate repair by double opposing z-plasty.* Plastic and Reconstructive Surgery *78:724-736, 1986.)*

surgeon, the greater the likelihood of unsatisfactory results (Emory et al., 1997; Morris et al., 1993; Rintala and Haapanen, 1995; Ross, 1987). Following is a review of most of the pertinent studies published to date. However, as a clinician working with patients with cleft palate, it will always be important for you to access—and assess—new studies.

Because they are two of the most widely used techniques of palatoplasty, studies on the success of the Veau-Wardill-Kilner "V-Y" pushback and the von Langenbeck repair have been appearing since the 1960s. By the late 1970s, the studies that had been published on the results of the V-Y pushback had reported success rates ranging from 21% to 95%, with the majority reporting an average of more than 70% (Battle 1967; Blocksma, Leuz, and Mellerstig, 1975; Braithwaite, 1964; Calnan, 1971; Evans and Renfrew, 1974; Greene, 1960; Krause, Tharp, and Morris, 1976; Krause, Van Demark, and Tharp, 1975; McWilliams, 1960; Morris, 1973; Musgrave, McWilliams, and Matthews, 1975; Trauner and Trauner, 1967). A 1993 report on 27 years' experience with the V-Y technique stated that, in 230 patients, the dehiscence rate was 4% and the need for secondary surgery for speech problems was 11% (Elander et al., 1993). Success rates reported with the von Langenbeck up to the late 1970s fell in a somewhat narrower range (51% to 73%) (Blocksma, Leuz, and Mellerstig, 1975; Kaplan et al., 1978; Krause Van Demark, and Tharpe, 1975; McEvitt, 1971; Musgrave, McWilliams, and Matthews, 1975). Myklebust and Abyholm (1989) reported speech results on 203 patients who had had a von Langenbeck repair at a mean age of just over 2 years (24.4 years)—very late by current standards. Articulation was judged "good" in 86.2%, and nasality was similarly judged "good" in 80.5.

Several studies directly compared the V-Y and the von Langenbeck procedures. The majority of these demonstrated no significant differences in speech outcomes between these two procedures (Hardin-Jones et al., 1993; Marrinan, LaBrie, and Mulliken, 1998; Witzel et al., 1979).[20,21] An earlier study by Palmer et al. (1969) purportedly indicated an advantage for the von Langenbeck over the V-Y pushback, but the speech results were condensed into only "acceptable" and "unacceptable," and there was a high fistula rate in both. Three studies in the mid-1970s showed a better success rate for the V-Y pushback than for the von Langenbeck (Krause, Van Demark, and Tharp, 1975; Krause, Tharp, and Morris, 1976; Musgrave, McWilliams, and Matthews, 1975). Dreyer and Trier (1984) compared results among patients whose palatoplasties had been performed according to three different regimens: von Langenbeck with no palatal lengthening, palatal lengthening consisting of either a V-Y pushback or an island flap, and von Langenbeck with the addition of levator reconstruction. They found no differences between the first two groups: approximately 30% of the patients in each group had excellent speech, 35% acceptable speech, and about 38% poor speech. However, in the von Langenbeck plus levator reconstruction patients, excellent speech was achieved in 50% and acceptable speech in 41%. In comparison to more current reports, these success rates are not particularly impressive.[22] In a companion study on the same patient population, Moore et al. (1988) reported that fewer secondary operations for

[20]O'Riain and Hammond (1972) found no significant differences in speech outcomes between the von Langenbeck and the four-flap version of a pushback. However, the speech data they reported were uninterpretable.

[21]Holtmann, Wray, and Weeks (1984) also set out to compare the V-Y procedure with the von Langenbeck procedure, but they always combined the latter with a primary pharyngeal flap, and the anterior palatal defect was not closed in either procedure, leaving an open hard palate cleft. Thus the speech results were meaningless.

[22]There were several possible sources of contamination in this study. The second group of patients was a mix of two different types of palatal lengthening, one of which (the island flap) has been reported to show unstable results over time. Also, no information was given on how the judgments of excellent speech, acceptable speech, or poor speech were made.

velopharyngeal inadequacy (pharyngeal flaps) were required for patients receiving the levator reconstruction than the other procedures and that postoperative fistulae were slightly more frequent in the Wardill-Kilner patients than in the other groups.

Three studies from the University of Iowa indicated that the von Langenbeck yielded poorer speech results than the Wardill pushback and its various modifications (Hardin-Jones et al., 1993; Krause, Tharp, and Morris, 1976; Van Demark and Hardin, 1985). These studies led to a change toward the Bardach two-flap operation at that particular institution.

The much later study of Marrinan, LaBrie, and Mulliken (1998) also compared speech outcomes between the von Langenbeck and V-Y procedures. They used the McWilliams-Philips perceptual scale (1979) to rate speech in 228 patients, looking at how many children were judged to need a pharyngeal flap by the age of 4 years. It is important to note that the presence or absence of compensatory articulations was not a part of the judgment regarding need for a flap because the authors wisely realized that such aberrant articulations can persist even when velopharyngeal competency is present and also that the presence of compensatory articulations should be perceptually delineated from the presence of other speech stigmata such as hypernasal resonance and nasal emission. The authors found no difference between the two groups in the need for secondary velopharyngeal management (14% versus 15%). However, they did report that *age* at closure, as opposed to technique, was a factor in later speech results: flaps were judged to be necessary in 11% of the children who underwent closure at 8 to 10 months of age, 14% at 11 to 13 months, 19% at 14 to 16 months, and in 32% of those beyond the age of 16 months.

Three studies attempted to compare speech results among a larger variety of techniques of palatal repair, but each was flawed by methodological errors. Seyfer and Simon (1989) compared results across the von Langenbeck, the V-Y pushback, a pushback combined with an island flap, and a pushback combined with a pharyngeal flap (primary pharyngeal flap). Their 109 patients were distributed among four types of clefts (unilateral cleft lip and palate [UCLP], bilateral cleft lip and palate [BCLP], cleft palate only [CPO], and submucous clefts), and 10 different surgeons. No speech pathologist was involved in making the judgment of "good," "improved," or "unimproved" speech. Eighty-eight percent of the patients receiving a primary pharyngeal flap were rated as having "good" speech compared with 27% to 39% in the other groups, but in the total of 109 patients only 45% of the patients had good results. In his commentary on the article, Peterson (1989) pointed out the unfortunate number of variables, the lack of a speech pathologist in making the speech ratings, and the fact that the speech evaluation had been reduced to the "terrible terms" of good, improved, and unimproved. He felt that the defects in the report produced "a fairly meaningless set of numbers." A study limited to clefts of the soft palate only (Grobbelaar et al., 1995) used five different types of surgery distributed over 184 patients. The surgical procedures were the Dorrance pushback, the Wardill pushback, the Perko repair, the von Langenbeck, and the Furlow Z-plasty. However, the operations had been done over a span of 24 years, and both the Dorrance and the Wardill procedures had already been discarded (because of unfavorable effects on growth) by the time the study was conducted. Seventy-seven patients were operated on at less than 6 months old and 107 over this age. The authors reported better results with the children operated on at less than 6 months old and also better results with the Perko and Furlow procedures than with the older approaches. None of the children (24 operated on at less than 6 months old, 15 over this age) operated on by either of these two procedures demonstrated problems in velopharyngeal closure. However, it must be considered that, if the same surgeons were performing all the operations over the 24 years of this study, their own expertise had undoubtedly grown and it is only to be expected that their results would be better with the procedures they adopted as they matured in their skills.

A few studies have examined speech results in the use of intravelar veloplasty or levator repositioning for closure of the soft palate.[23] Dreyer and Trier (1984) reported that 89% of their patients who had levator reconstruction exhibited velopharyngeal competency for speech. Coston et al. (1986) reported speech outcomes on 60 patients who had had levator reconstruction, 11 of them as a primary procedure in palate closure and 49 as a secondary procedure when the original palatal surgery had not provided adequate velopharyngeal closure. Although they reported a 60% success level, they did not indicate the comparative success in primary versus secondary surgery. Also, the speech judgments were based only on presence or absence of hypernasality and nasal escape. If either hypernasality or nasal escape was present, multiview videofluoroscopy or flexible fiberoptic nasopharyngoscopy was done, and only if the authors saw a gap on these imaging studies was the subject considered to be a failed case. The authors did not state whether compensatory articulations were present or absent, an important consideration because a speaker who uses such articulations may simply bypass a potentially competent velopharyngeal system and even the most sophisticated imaging studies may therefore be invalid. In addition, the age range of patients at the time of surgery was fairly broad (5 months to 7 years), and the article does not specify how many of the noninfant cases were either primary or secondary palatal procedures. Marsh, Grames, and Holtman (1989) were unimpressed with their own

[23]Butow and Jacobs (1991) designed seven different modifications of this procedure to "fit the anatomical defect" and to prevent fistulae formation, but they had no speech data.

results when they compared one group of children who had this procedure with another group who had palatal closure without levator reconstruction: They could not demonstrate better speech results in the latter group, and pointed out that the procedure required a significantly longer operating time. Brown, Cohen, and Randall (1983) reported finding better speech results only in "Veau class II" clefts (cleft of the hard and soft palate without cleft lip), but their study was flawed by methodological problems, among them the fact that they used four surgical variations distributed over 85 patients with four different types of clefts, analyzed speech only by screening for hypernasality and nasal escape, and classified the speech results only as "abnormal" or "normal." Hartel, Gundlach, and Ruickholdt (1994) looked at the incidence of "need for velopharyngoplasty" as an index to the success of four different types of types of surgery across 109 patients and reported the best results (least percentage of need for secondary surgery) in the Kriens intravelar veloplasty. Again, their exact criteria for establishing the need for secondary surgery were not specified.[24]

Attempting to draw meaningful conclusions about the probable benefits of one type of palatoplasty over another will always be fraught with methodological pitfalls, and the judgments that are made at any given time will (and should) be re-examined as more clinical data are accrued on newer techniques. There are conflicting data sets regarding the possible advantage of a modified von Langenbeck over a V-Y pushback, or vice versa, but both are still in frequent use and it seems obvious that either can produce good results in the right surgical hands. The Bardach two-flap procedure is widely used, and new procedures or modifications continue to be developed (e.g., Onizuka et al., 1996). The Furlow Z-plasty is currently growing in usage, and is particularly popular for use in clefts of the soft palate only (Grobbelaar et al., 1995). However, Brothers et al. (1995) compared the results from 21 patients operated on by the Furlow technique with those of 10 operated on with a modified Wardill-Kilner pushback and reported quite similar results for each.[25] They also made the point that the Furlow procedure is not appropriate when the palatal cleft is more than 1 cm in width because the increase in velar length in this procedure is obtained at the expense of width. A recent study by Gunther et al. (1998) compared speech results between children who had had intravelar veloplasties versus a group with velar repair with the Furlow double-reversing Z-plasty. All types of clefts were represented in both groups: UCLP, BCLP, and CPO. The children in both groups had had the hard palate portions of their clefts repaired either by modified von Langenbeck or Wardill procedures. Mean age at palatoplasty was similar in both groups (11.3 and 12.1 months). The speech evaluations from which the outcome data were drawn took place at 3 years of age. Twenty-nine percent of the 52 children in the intravelar veloplasty group were judged to be in need of a secondary pharyngoplasty compared with 8% of the 24 Furlow patients. Postoperative fistulae were present in about 12% of the intravelar veloplasty group and 19% of the Furlow group. The authors felt that the Furlow procedure provided better outcome for speech. The information they presented did not include width of the cleft and whether this factor might have played a role in occurrence of postoperative fistulae or inadequate velopharyngeal function.

Ostensible Relationships Between Timing and Type of Palatoplasty and Facial Growth

Finding appropriate data and reaching valid conclusions about this topic is nearly as difficult as reaching conclusions about the best palatal surgery for producing good speech results. The topic of facial growth after palatal surgery has historically spawned massive numbers of studies—far more than can be covered here.[26] Before the development of more advanced imaging studies (e.g., three-dimensional computerized tomography scans), most studies used dental casts and cephalometric films to document facial growth and occlusion after palatal surgery. The concern is not only about the forward growth of the maxilla but maxillary arch width as well. Reliance on cephalometric data for assessing facial growth has recently engendered criticism (Posnick, 1997), but as of this writing the bulk of the information available on postoperative facial growth is that derived from older techniques.

Although cleft lip and palate are known to be not just divisions and distortions of structures but deficiencies in tissue as well, surgeons, orthodontists, and researchers such as anthropometricians have long struggled to determine how much of the growth deficiency in the midface in individuals with clefts was due to the cleft condition itself versus how much was due to surgery. Some researchers compared facial growth in older children and adults with operated clefts with that in individuals with unoperated clefts and usually concluded that surgery does indeed have a deleterious effect on growth (e.g., Bishara, 1973; Bishara

[24]Hartel, Gundlach, and Ruickholdt (1994) also had 36 children in their study who had had primary pharyngeal flaps and concluded that "primary velopharyngoplasty should be the exception," echoing the earlier conclusion of Morris (1973).

[25]The success rates in the study of Brothers et al. (1995) were actually not very impressive: nasal emission was eliminated in only 52% of Furlow patients and 40% of Wardill patients and hypernasality in 62% and 70%, respectively. Also, note that the number of subjects is small.

[26]There is some evidence that even surgical closure of the lip has a negative effect on maxillary growth. In one recent study (Kapucu et al., 1996), maxillary retrusion was essentially equal in adult patients who had had only lip repair and another group of adults who had had lip and palate repair. However, this study did not include patients who had had no lip or palate repair and may have simply reflected the inherent deficiencies in tissue and growth potential in patients with cleft lip and palate, rather than effects of lip repair.

et al., 1976b). Many clinicians attributed unfavorable maxillary growth to early palatal closure, leading them to champion primary veloplasty and delayed closure of the hard palate (Gnoinski, 1982; Hotz and Gnoinski, 1979; Hotz et al., 1984; Jorgenson, Shapiro, and Odinet, 1984; Schweckendiek, 1966). Several decades ago surgeons were convinced that they could help to protect against midface retrusion in their patients by preserving the integrity of the posterior neurovascular bundle. However, a multidisciplinary investigation of children who had been operated on by a technique that involved severance of the neurovascular bundle did *not* find severe midface deformities (Demjen and Krause, 1978; Morris, 1978a, 1978b).

The large multicenter study by Ross (1987) failed to substantiate a relationship either between palatoplasty performed within the first year of life and aggravation of the growth deficit of the midface in males with unilateral cleft lip and palate or between the type of palate repair and subsequent growth measurements. Ross also reported that approximately 25% of the patients went on to have maxillary advancements in the teenage years. This indicates that, at least in the minds of the professionals in those centers, midfacial growth was not satisfactory. Although neither type nor timing of palatoplasty differentiated between those who would later need maxillary advancement and those who would not, Ross (1987) did find that repair of the alveolus in infancy appeared to adversely affect maxillary growth. Alveolar repair is discussed on p. 108.

Two studies, both involving primary veloplasty, indicated increased problems with facial growth and occlusion when the method of hard palate repair was a V-Y pushback as opposed to the von Langenbeck method (Friede et al., 1991) or a modified vomer flap (Tanino et al., 1997). In contrast, Nystrom and Ranta (1994) reported better maxillary arch width in patients who had V-Y closure in comparison to patients in whom the "Cronin" procedure was performed (a pushback with nasal flaps used to line the upper surface) (Cronin 1957, 1971; Cronin et al., 1964). They also reported better results in patients operated on at 1.8 years as opposed to 1.1 years. Secondary pharyngoplasties were required for more patients in the V-Y group than in the Cronin group; however all their subjects were in the 3- to 6-year age range at the time of the study, possibly too young for definitive judgments about the ultimate need for secondary palatal surgery, especially since no detailed speech analysis was performed. An earlier study on the comparative effects of the Wardill-Kilner and von Langenbeck operations (carried out for complete closure of clefts in the initial palatoplasty) did not show a significant difference between the two in terms of the effects on facial growth (Bishara, Enemark, and Tharp, 1976).

Research continues in the attempt to determine which type of palatal procedure (and performed at what age) is least likely to interfere with the forward and lateral growth of the maxilla. As surgeons and other team members study this problem, they continue to devise surgical modifications to lessen the amount of denuded bone and postoperative scarring. Knowing that there will almost inevitably be some degree of midface deficiency or lateral crossbite no matter how ideal the surgery, treatment teams aim for reaching a postoperative result that will require a minimum amount of orthodontic correction to provide good occlusion and pleasing facial proportions. Additional information on this topic will be found in the section on orthognathic surgery (pp. 112-114).

Repair of the Alveolar Cleft in Infancy: Periosteoplasty, Primary Bone Grafting

Surgeons have struggled for several decades to decide how best to handle the alveolar portion of a cleft of the lip and palate, knowing that there is the potential for interfering with the normal forward growth of the maxilla and thus contributing to a possible "dished-in face" appearance of their patients. This is a multistep clinical decision. In the infant the surgeon and team may decide (1) to leave the alveolar cleft unoperated, (2) to close it by a primary periosteoplasty, or (3) to close it by primary bone grafting.[27] In any of these three choices, they may decide to use early (presurgical) orthopedics to reposition the premaxilla and cleft segments before lip or palate surgery. If the alveolar cleft is not operated on in infancy, "secondary" bone grafting will typically be done in the later childhood or early teenage years. Those who advocate either periosteoplasty or primary bone grafting in infancy argue that these procedures provide an intact anterior palate and lead to better tooth position without serious adverse effects on midfacial growth (Brauer and Cronin, 1964; Dado, 1993; Pickrell, Quinn, and Massengill, 1968; Rosenstein et al., 1982; Skoog, 1965). Early surgical repair of the alveolus (with or without presurgical orthopedics) has historically been more popular in Europe and Scandinavia than in the United States (Larson and Nilsson, 1983; Larson, Ideberg, and Nordin, 1983; Nordin et al., 1983; Smahel and Mullerova, 1988).[28] Those who oppose early alveolar surgery argue that creating a solid bony bridge early in childhood keeps the palatal arch from expanding in a

[27]Periosteoplasty means raising periosteal flaps and moving them into position to close the alveolar cleft (Hellquist and Ponten, 1979; Hellquist, 1982). In bone grafting autogenous bone (bone from the patient, not from a another person) is taken from another site in the body (e.g., a rib). The donor site varies with the age of the child. Rib grafts are more common in infants, whereas bone from the iliac crest is often used in older children and teenagers. In some articles the term "bone grafting" is used for the movement of periosteal flaps (e.g., Brattstrom et al., 1991), which makes interpreting this literature additionally confusing.

[28]Smahel and Mullerova (1988) compared three groups of boys with UCLP, one with primary periosteoplasty, one with primary bone grafting, and one who had had neither in infancy. However, the palate in each case had been repaired with a pushback procedure and a primary pharyngeal flap. Although the authors reported that facial retrusion was milder in the cases of primary periosteoplasty and least satisfactory in the children who had had primary bone grafting, they in essence sabotaged their own study because the palatal repairs included primary pharyngeal flaps.

normal fashion both laterally and in the anterior-to-posterior dimension, contributing to maxillary retrusion and constriction of maxillary width (Berkowitz, 1996; Pruzansky, 1964). They are also concerned about the limitations imposed on the later possibilities for orthodontic expansion of the maxilla.

More than a quarter of a century ago, Koberg (1973) reviewed 160 papers on primary bone grafting, and concluded that there was unanimous agreement that this procedure led to severe impairment of maxillary growth. Hellquist (1982) looked at infant (up to the age of 2 years) versus delayed periosteoplasty (between 4 and 7 years of age), and reported more satisfactory results in the latter with regard to bone formation and incidence of crossbite. Robertson and Jolleys (1983) were early enthusiasts of primary bone grafting but were disappointed with the long-term results and warned against using it. Other groups reported similar experiences. For example, Nordin et al. (1983) studied children with UCLP in the 7 to 13 year age group who had had presurgical orthopedics and primary bone grafting and another who had had the bone grafting but without the presurgical orthopedics. They reported, "The development of the skeletal profile, especially in our [presurgical orthopedics] group, was well within the limits of non-grafted US cases. . . ." In a companion study that also included a group of children with bilateral clefts (Larson, Ideberg, and Nordin, 1983), the authors similarly reported that the early bone grafting (after presurgical orthopedics) produced dental occlusion comparable to that in ungrafted children. However, when Brattstrom et al. (1992) looked at facial growth results in patients who had been treated according to four regimens, including that used by Nordin et al. (1983), they concluded that regimens that included primary bone grafting (at or before 6 months of age) resulted in inhibited maxillary growth. McCarthy, Cutting, and Hogan (1990) voiced the same opinion: "Primary bone grafts do not grow as originally postulated but instead hinder growth with a significant limitation of maxillary development and a dramatic increase in crossbite, malocclusion, and pseudoprognathism. . . . As the story unfolded, it tended to confirm the prescience of Pruzansky who in 1964 condemned the unscientific and unsubstantiated use of primary bone grafting. . . ."

One team in the United States that remains unconvinced on this point is that at Northwestern University (Dado, 1993; Rosenstein et al., 1982, 1991a, 1991b). Rosenstein et al. (1991b) concluded that early bone grafting of the maxilla did not adversely affect facial growth in their patients, stating that 22.2% ultimately needed orthognathic surgery to correct jaw relationships, whereas Ross's multicenter study (1987) had shown that about 25% of all patients with unilateral clefts needed such surgery. Posnick (1991), in his commentary on the Rosenstein et al. (1991b) study, said the need for orthognathic surgery can vary between 25% and 75%, depending on the criteria applied.

Posnick's point (1991) was an important one: teams and clinicians vary in what they view as an acceptable facial profile and occlusal result in their patients, and some may decide that orthognathic surgery is necessary in individuals whose results would be judged as "acceptable" by other teams. Of course, the same is true in speech. As of this writing there is a countrywide (United States) effort, under the auspices of the American Cleft Palate–Craniofacial Association, to pool outcome data with the hope of eventually agreeing on criteria for results in *all* areas of cleft and craniofacial care. However, such "standards" do not currently exist. At the end of the 1990s, the argument about whether to surgically repair the alveolar cleft(s) in infancy, and how best to do so, continues with fervor.

Secondary Alveolar Bone Grafting

Secondary bone grafting, typically done in later childhood or early adolescence, is much less controversial than primary bone grafting and is a routine part of cleft care in most US and Canadian treatment centers, as well as in many parts of Europe (Abyholm, 1996; Abyholm, Bergland, and Semb, 1981; Bergland, Semb, and Abyholm, 1986; Boyne and Sands, 1976; Cohen, Polley, and Figueroa, 1993; Enemark, Krantz-Simonsen, and Schramm, 1985; Jansma et al., 1999; Posnick, 1997; Turvey et al., 1984). The usual plan is to graft the alveolar cleft before eruption of the canine teeth, which may take place any time between the ages of 9 and 11 years. The sequence of treatment consists of orthodontic alignment of the palatal segments (when necessary), followed by alveolar bone grafting, although some aspects of orthodontic treatment may not be completed until after bone grafting (Abyholm, 1996; Abyholm et al., 1981; Boyne and Sands, 1976; Enemark, Krantz-Simonson, and Schramm, 1985; Posnick, 1997).

You will remember from your anatomy classes that teeth will erupt only into bone. The reason for doing alveolar bone graft before eruption of the canine is that this tooth (on the cleft side) will not erupt at all or will erupt into an abnormal position if there is insufficient bone. When teeth are congenitally absent, as discussed in Chapter 5, the bone graft serves as "housing" for placement of endosseous implants, on which prosthetic teeth will later be anchored. This approach to the prosthetic replacement of congenitally missing or poorly formed teeth in children with clefts has gradually replaced older treatment approaches such as the use of partial dental bridges (Kearns et al., 1997).

In the older child or adolescent with a cleft, secondary alveolar bone grafting may be the last, or nearly the last, requirement on that child's life for surgical reconstruction of the cleft. Although the importance to the speech-language pathologist may be minimal, a teenager rarely perceives any surgical procedure as minimal either in terms of potential impact on appearance or potential interference with school and daily life. For the patient and for the parents, the most important role of the speech-language pathologist may be counseling them regarding what to expect in terms of temporary effects of the physical management (braces, surgery) on the oral environment and thus on speech.

Oronasal Fistulae

The topics of secondary alveolar bone grafting and oronasal fistulae are sometimes the *same* topic because bone grafting may close an open path from the oral cavity into the nose (Abyholm, Borchgrevnik, and Eskeland, 1979; Cohen, Polley, and Figueroa, 1993; Jackson, 1972; Jackson, Jackson, and Christie, 1976; Rintala, 1980). However, this is not always the case. There are two reasons: (1) Some fistulae are not in the alveolus but in other locations in the palate. (2) Some residual alveolar clefts are not actually "patent" (open) into the nasal cavity, although there is no solid bony bridge across the cleft until the grafting is done. Rather, what would be an open pathway is essentially plugged by soft tissue (mucosa). At the other extreme, some anterior fistulae are so large that they consist of an opening through the alveolus from the labial sulcus into the oral cavity and then upward into the nasal cavity (Fig. 4-20).

Folk, D'Antonio, and Hardesty (1997) provided an excellent tutorial on (1) the variability in the size and position of fistulae, (2) the ways in which the configuration of a fistula may change from the oral surface to the nasal cavity, and (3) the ways in which fistulae may or may not be significant factors in speech. They iterated the fact that a fistula after palatoplasty may represent a failure in healing or a portion of the original cleft that was unintentionally left unrepaired. They used the terms "primary" for any fistula present after repair of the palatal cleft and "recurrent" for fistulae associated with multiple previous palatal incisions, in other words, failures of multiple surgical attempts to completely close a cleft. Folk, D'Antonio, and Hardesty (1997) also stressed the "three-dimensional structure" of a fistula versus the conceptualization of a palatal defect as simply an open hole of a given diameter or location. They pointed out that it may be difficult to discern between a fistula and a blind pouch on the intraoral view alone and suggested either "gentle probing" or transillumination by placing a nasopharyngoscope in the nose (however, any small bright light source will do so long as it cannot overheat). Simply estimating the size of a fistula from the intraoral view alone is fraught with clinical pitfalls. Often, the course of a fistula is irregular, and the narrowest part of the opening may not be observable from the oral surface. While the study of Folk, D'Antonio, and Hardesty (1997) was not a data-based investigation of the effects of palatal fistulae on speech, it alerted surgical, dental, and speech clinicians to the wide variability in fistulae and to the need for multifaceted evaluations of the effects on speech.

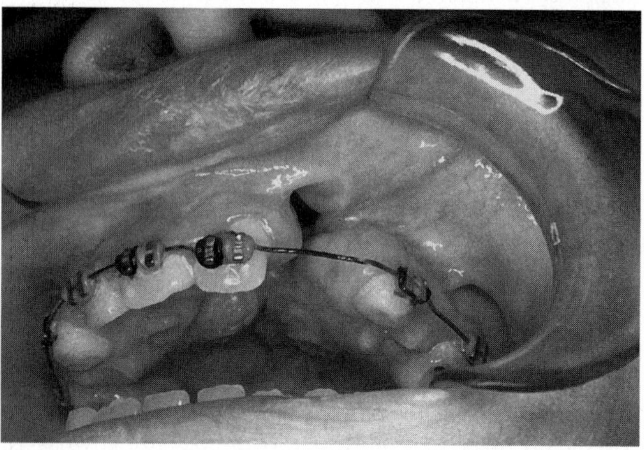

Figure 4-20 Labionasal defect extending upward through the alveolus and into the nasal cavity.

Fistulae can occur in the following locations and scenarios: (1) unoperated, open pathways into the nasal cavity through the labial sulcus and alveolus, (2) intentionally unrepaired or postsurgical fistulae in the anterior portion of the hard palate, primarily in the region of the incisive foramen (left open because the original cleft was so large that the surgeon did not attempt complete closure, or fistulae that opened spontaneously after surgery), (3) fistulae opening spontaneously after surgery at the juncture of the hard and soft palate, and (4) fistulae in the soft palate itself. In addition, any combination of these defects is possible. The effects on speech will be dependent at least in part on the size the opening, the location, and the developmental time in the child's acquisition of communication skills in which the fistula is or was present.[29] Many authors writing on this topic have emphasized that the functional significance of any fistula must be evaluated for each patient individually (Folk, D'Antonio, and Hardesty, 1997; Oneal, 1971; Shelton and Blank, 1984; Witt and D'Antonio, 1993).

Cohen et al. (1991) attempted to examine the rate of fistula occurrence as related to (1) severity of the original cleft, (2) type of palatoplasty, (3) age at surgery, and (4) the specific surgeon doing the palatoplasty. They found 30 fistulae (detected only by visualization of the oral cavity) in 129 consecutive cases of palatal clefts. They did not include patients in whom there was either a nasal-alveolar fistula or an anterior palatal fistula that had been intentionally left unrepaired. Unfortunately, their article did not specify the actual number of patients in each category of severity of cleft (given according to the Veau classification) or in each category of surgical procedure. There were a total of 17 variables (four categories of severity, four surgeons, four types of palatoplasties, three types of soft palate surgical closures) yielding $4 \times 4 \times 4 \times 3 = 192$ possible combinations distributed across the 129 patients, making the study subject to statistical flaws and the results thus difficult to interpret. The factor of age at surgery was examined only in the sense that the authors reported no statistically significant difference in the mean age at surgery for those children who had fistulae (15.1 months $\pm$ 5.7 months) versus those who did not (16.6 months $\pm$ 12.5 months).

[29]As a precautionary step in your oral examination, have the patient sniff forcefully to clear mucus out of the oral cavity. Either mucus or food particles can obscure the oral opening of a fistula.

The other three major variables were reported to show significant effects. Fistulae were more apt to occur in patients with more severe clefts and in the hands of less experienced surgeons.[30] With respect to type of palatoplasty, the authors reported a 43% fistula rate with the Veau-Wardill-Kilner pushback procedure, 10% with the Furlow double opposing Z-plasty, 22% with the van Langenbeck procedure, and 0 with the Dorrance pushback. However, it is clear that there were not equal numbers of patients with an even distribution of types of clefts receiving these procedures, and it is also quite probable that Furlow Z-plasty was used in smaller as opposed to larger clefts. Although the authors stated that they had "sought to clarify some of the existing confusion" with regard to the prevalence and etiology of clefts, the methodological flaws in their study rendered it highly questionable.

If there is a question as to whether it is necessary to try to close a fistula for the purpose of improving speech, try temporary obturation as suggested by Reisberg, Gold, and Dorf (1985), who used a skin barrier adhesive patch, specifically HolliHesive (Hollister Inc., Libertyville, Ill.). Other types or brands of skin barrier materials are available, and most will adhere to the oral mucosa when the protective covering is removed and the patch is briefly held in place until the adhesive takes effect. Have your patient produce speech samples containing both anterior and posterior oral pressure consonants. In theory, if the fistula is the sole route of nasal air loss, that loss will occur only on consonants anterior to the location of the fistula. If all pressure consonants continue to be produced with nasal air loss, it is possible that the cause is inadequate velopharyngeal function and not the fistula alone. But beware of two behaviors that may invalidate this comparison. First, if the patient is substituting glottal stops for some or all pressure consonants, the velopharyngeal system may well be "bypassed," even if closure is physically possible (Henningsson and Isberg, 1987; Isberg and Henningsson, 1987). Second, on posterior pressure consonants such as /k/ and /g/, the patient may unknowingly use a lingual assist to lift the velum or "plug" the velopharyngeal port. Once you have completed your exploration of what the patient can do with the adhesive in place, it can be easily dislodged and discarded. However, for a variety of reasons, it is best to carry out such temporary obturation in a medical or dental setting.[31,32]

The surgical closure of a fistula can be quite difficult because of scar tissue in the operative site (all surgery except prenatal surgery [still experimental as of this writing] causes the formation of scar tissue) and a lack of what Witt and D'Antonio (1993) termed "virgin local tissue." Several techniques have been described for the movement of soft tissue to close oronasal fistulae, the choice being to some extent dependent on the location and medical history of the defect (e.g., initial versus recurrent). The approaches have included local "turnover" flaps, various versions of "island" mucoperiosteal flaps of palatal tissue, buccal flaps (from the inside of the cheek), and "tongue flaps" (a portion of the mucosal surface of the tongue) (Argamaso, 1990; Emory et al., 1997; Leonard, 1979; Oneal, 1971; Pigott, Rieger, and Moodie, 1984). When the fistula is located more posteriorly in the palate, a very long pharyngeal flap may serve both purposes of closing the fistula and decreasing the size of the velopharyngeal port (Emory et al., 1997). Recurrence rates of operated fistulae are relatively high (Cohen et al., 1991; Oneal, 1971), again related to the difficulties of reoperation on scarred tissue.

SURGERY FOR SUBMUCOUS CLEFT PALATE AND NONCLEFT VPI[33]

Much of what you have just read about surgical treatment of overt clefts also pertains to surgery for submucous clefts and noncleft velopharyngeal inadequacy. You will read in Chapter 8 that treatment for submucous clefts (obvious or occult) is warranted only when there is evidence of true velopharyngeal inadequacy (VPI) in speech, not just on the basis of physical signs alone (bifid uvula, dehiscence of the musculature of the soft palate, anterior insertion of the levator palatini, submucous bony defect of the hard palate). The surgical approaches that have been used to repair submucous clefts include the von Langenbeck procedure, either alone or together with a centrally based pharyngeal flap (Abyholm, 1976; Crikelair, Striker, and Cosman, 1970), pharyngeal flaps (Crockett, Bumsted, and Van Demark, 1988; Garcia-Velasco et al., 1985; Hoopes et al., 1970), pushback procedures (Abyholm, 1976; Calnan, 1954; Gylling and Soivio, 1965; Massengill, Pickrell, and Robinson, 1973; Porterfield and Trabue, 1965), the Millard island flap (Lewin, Heller, and Kojak, 1975), reconstruction of the levator sling (intravelar veloplasty) (Coston et al., 1986; Kriens, 1969, 1970; Pensler and Bauer, 1988), and combinations of procedures such as a pushback and a pharyngeal flap (Porterfield, Mohler, and Sandel, 1976) or levator sling reconstruction + palatal pushback + a pharyngeal flap (Fisher and Edgerton, 1975; Kaplan, 1975; Minami et al., 1975). More recently, the Furlow double-reversing Z-plasty has gained popularity

[30]The distribution of patients across the four surgeons was very uneven: two of the surgeons performed 74% of the procedures, one performed 15%, and the remaining one 11%.

[31]A patch that is too small may become accidentally wedged into the opening or move upward through it. A medical or dental professional should be present who can extract it without endangering the youngster.

[32]Several studies on patients with oronasal fistulae have demonstrated changes in the behavior of the velopharyngeal system between the "open" (unobturated) condition and a closed condition (Isberg and Henningsson, 1987; Karling, Larson, and Henningsson, 1993; Lohmander-Agerskov et al., 1996; Tachimura et al., 1997).

[33]There is some necessary overlap between this section and Chapter 13, which presents information on physical management of "secondary" VPI, that is, when initial palatoplasty has failed to provide adequate velopharyngeal closure for speech.

in treatment of submucous clefts (Chen et al., 1996; D'Antonio, 1997; Lindsey and Davis, 1996). In addition, virtually all the forms of pharyngoplasty discussed in Chapter 13 have been used—sphincter pharyngoplasties, augmentation pharyngoplasties, and superiorly based and inferiorly based central pharyngeal flaps. In fact, historically, the first surgery of choice in submucous clefts or noncleft velopharyngeal inadequacy was often a pharyngeal flap. As surgeons gained more expertise in recreating the levator sling and lengthening the velum, flaps became less of a panacea in these cases. This evolution in surgical approaches was typified by the remarks of Velasco et al. (1988, p. 173), "In the past, we treated velopharyngeal insufficiency associated with submucous cleft palate by performing a primary pharyngeal flap with simultaneous palatal muscle correction. Our previous speech results with a simple push-back procedure were discouraging. . . . At the present time we are using a Z-plasty as described by Furlow . . . in submucous cleft palate patients." Their more recently published results (Ysunza et al., 1994) indicated an advantage for the Z-plasty over the prior technique.

The choice of the type of surgical procedure, or combination of procedures, should be made on the basis of adequate visualization of the velopharyngeal system in function, typically by nasopharyngoscopy and/or videofluoroscopy, to ascertain the amount of motion present in the velum and the pharyngeal walls and to determine the vertical level of attempted closure (Peat et al., 1994; Pigott, 1974, 1979; Shprintzen et al., 1979; Witzel and Stringer, 1990).[34] If the velopharyngeal deficit is deemed too large to be successfully treated by palatal or pharyngeal augmentation, some type of pharyngeal flap may be selected. A central pharyngeal flap depends on inward motion of the lateral pharyngeal walls for closure, and if no motion of those walls is seen preoperatively a sphincter flap may be chosen. The most difficult patients to treat are those in whom there is little or no motion of the velopharyngeal system, which is often the case in neurologically based VPI. Witt et al. (1995) termed this "the hypodynamic velopharynx" or "the black hole." Before 1989 their team treated such cases with a "lateral port control" pharyngeal flap (Hogan, 1973); subsequently, sphincter pharyngoplasties were added to their repertoire. Witt et al. (1995) recommended superiorly based pharyngeal flaps for patients with narrow to moderate gaps (in the lateral dimensions) and a circular pattern of closure.[35] Sphincter pharyngoplasties were recommended for patients with large gaps and coronal, circular, or "bow-tie" patterns of velopharyngeal movement and in cases of velopharyngeal paresis. Surgical outcomes were reported for 18 patients; success was defined as "acceptable resonance." This result was achieved in 63.6% of the patients receiving sphincter pharyngoplasties and 41.9% of those receiving superiorly based lateral port control flaps. Although these numbers may seem unimpressive, it must be emphasized that the authors were reporting on some of the most difficult to manage cases. Other reports on the problems in trying to surgically alter the speech of patients with neurologically based VPI include those of Cadieux et al. (1984); Calnan (1976); Crikelair et al. (1964); Davison, Razzell, and Watson (1990); Heller et al. (1974); Jackson, McGlynn, and Huskie (1980); Jafek et al. (1979); Johns (1985); Salomonson, Kawamoto, and Wilson (1988); and Younger and Dickson (1985).

MAXILLOFACIAL SURGERY FOR PATIENTS WITH CLEFTS

Midface Advancement

Many patients with repaired clefts require surgical advancement of the midface to establish and maintain an appropriate maxilla-to-mandible relationship (Epker and Wolford, 1975, 1976; Eskenazi and Schendel, 1992; Houston and James, 1989; Posnick, 1997). Individuals without clefts may also require this surgical realignment of the jaws as a result of underdevelopment of the maxilla for a variety of reasons. There have been many studies of the effects of maxillary advancement on articulation and other aspects of speech production in both noncleft and cleft palate speakers (Bralley and Schoeny, 1977; Dalston and Vig, 1984; Garber, Speidel, and Marsh, 1981; Kummer et al., 1989; Maegawa, Sells, and David, 1998a, 1998b; Mason and Turvey, 1980; McCarthy, Coccaro, and Schwartz, 1979; Okazaki et al., 1993; Poole, Robinson, and Nunn, 1986; Ruscello, et al., 1986; Schendel et al., 1979; Schwartz et al., 1979; Schwarz and Gruner, 1976; Turvey, Warren, and Dalston, 1990; Vallino, 1990; Watzke et al., 1990; Witzel and Munro, 1977; Witzel, Ross, and Munro, 1980). For patients with clefts, the concern is that advancement of the maxilla may cause (or reinstigate) inadequate velopharyngeal closure.[36]

[34]Before the late 1960s or early 1970s, most of the surgeons reporting on their preferences for treatment of patients with submucous clefts, as well as other types of VPI, had little if any visual information on the performance of the mechanism either before or after surgery. There were some early studies with lateral cinefluorography, but these did not provide the same quality or quantity of information as multiview videofluoroscopy. Nasopharyngoscopy or endoscopy for viewing the velopharyngeal mechanism was developed in 1969 (Pigott, Bensen, and White, 1969) and gradually grew in use during the next two decades.

[35]See Chapter 10 for a discussion of the patterns of velopharyngeal closure as seen on endoscopic and multiview videofluoroscopic studies.

[36]Some of the literature on the need for jaw surgery in patients with clefts is misleading. For example, DeLuke et al. (1997) discussed only the need for "orthognathic surgery" without specifying the surgical procedure, much less the measurements or other data that led them to decide that orthognathic surgery was necessary. Posnick and Thompson (1995) presented clinical information on 166 adolescents who had had Le Fort I: 116 with UCLP, 33 with BCLP, 17 with CPO. Thirty-two of these also had simultaneous sagittal split osteotomies of the mandible. However, they did not address the issue of how many patients with clefts require such surgery, and the article contained no information on speech.

In general, studies on the danger of onset of VPI subsequent to midface advancement in *noncleft* patients indicate that the possibility is negligible, although not unknown, whereas the risk of either onset or exacerbation of VPI is higher in patients with clefts (Dalston, 1996; Kummer et al., 1989; Maegawa, Sells, and David, 1998a, 1998b; Mason, Turvey, and Warren, 1980; McCarthy, Coccaro, and Schwartz, 1979; Okazaki et al., 1993; Poole, Robinson, and Nunn, 1986; Schwartz, et al., 1979; Schwarz and Gruner, 1976; Witzel, 1989; Witzel and Munro, 1977).[37] The early report of Schwarz and Gruner on this topic was highly detailed (1976) but misleading in stating that velopharyngeal function had deteriorated in both cleft and noncleft patients after maxillary advancement: In some of their noncleft patients, nasal resonance had actually improved from hyponasality to normal resonance balance. Witzel and Munro (1977) reported deterioration in velopharyngeal function in one child with a repaired cleft. The studies by McCarthy, Coccaro, and Schwartz (1979) and Schwartz et al. (1979) were actually two reports on the same study and included a poorly delineated mix of nonsyndromic and syndromic patients (Apert and Crouzon) in both of the patient groups (cleft palate and "maxillary hypoplasia alone"), all of which made the results difficult to interpret. The authors reported that none of the patients had VPI, but did not specify either the exact amount of maxillary advancement or the length of postoperative follow-up.[38] They did state that hyponasality was eliminated in several patients with Crouzon disease. The report of Mason, Turvey, and Warren (1980) was limited to two patients with clefts, one of whom adapted well to a maxillary advancement of 7 mm and another who had had borderline closure before the advancement and, not surprisingly, deteriorated in velopharyngeal closure after advancement.

Poole, Robinson, and Nunn (1986) reported results of Le Fort I maxillary advancements in seven patients with cleft palate and used a variety of techniques to assess the results "at least 4 months postoperatively" (perceptual assessment, nasendoscopy, Doppler flow studies, and radiographic assessment of skeletal relapse). Only one patient had postoperative deterioration in speech; this patient had an oronasal fistula as a result of the procedure.

Kummer et al. (1989) studied changes in articulation, resonance, and velopharyngeal function in 16 patients with clefts who underwent Le Fort I maxillary advancements. Eleven had preoperative articulation errors, and seven of these improved in articulation skills. The results with regard to velopharyngeal function in both the noncleft and cleft patients were questionable, at least as reported in the publication. Two noncleft subjects reportedly showed "slight change in nasal resonance" 3 to 6 months postoperatively, and two (one with cleft lip and palate and one with reported cleft lip only) had mild nasal emission. Kummer et al. (1989) concluded that there was no significant effect on velopharyngeal function in the cleft patients, but the way in which they chose to analyze the results in their patients was highly questionable, as pointed out by Witzel (1989) in her comments on the article. She pointed out that the study clearly demonstrated a deterioration in velopharyngeal closure in 9 patients, and even if that deterioration was not severe enough to cause symptomatic hypernasality the patient sample was very small and the lack of a significant perceptual effect on speech could have been related to the extent of the surgery (amount of advancement) and/or the preoperative velopharyngeal competence in each patient. In addition, Witzel (1989) provided new data on a sample of 41 patients without clefts and 50 with repaired clefts. The patients without clefts had a very low risk for deterioration of velopharyngeal function, as did patients with clefts who demonstrated good closure before maxillary advancement. Of the 15 patients in Witzel's group who showed "borderline" closure before maxillary advancement, 11 demonstrated postoperative VPI. Watzke et al. (1990), Okazaki et al. (1993), and Maegawa, Sells, and David (1998a, 1998b) similarly showed that patients with clefts were at risk for postoperative VPI after maxillary advancement. Maegawa, Sells, and David (1998b) also reported that articulation improved in about one fourth of their patients and that, of those who were hyponasal because of pharyngoplasties performed before advancement, hyponasality was reduced in about one third. However, there were serious design flaws in these companion studies. (1) Although the average amount of maxillary advancement was about 3 mm greater in those patients who demonstrated "deteriorated intelligibility" after surgery compared with the amount of advancement who showed "improved" or "unchanged intelligibility," the authors did not deal with the fact that age range at surgery was very large (13 to 41 years), meaning that some patients were obviously smaller than others and thus that an advancement of "x" mm in an adult patient might be the equivalent of a "$x + 3$" amount of advancement in a young teenager. (2) The amount of time between the procedure and the postoperative assessment ranged from 1 month to 5 years (remember that advancements do not necessarily stay stable over time). (3) Of the 20 patients whose articulation improved after advancement, seven had had a combined procedure of maxillary advancement and mandibular setback.[39]

[37]Schendel et al. (1979) reported only some angular and distance changes in the velopharynx at rest and in function. The "need ratio" they reported (velar length to pharyngeal depth) was similar to that reported by Subtelny more than 40 years earlier (1957).

[38]Maxillary advancements can "relapse" over time, so the ultimate amount of advancement is not what the surgeon intended.

[39]Maegawa, Sells, and David (1998b, p. 181) conjectured that the mandibular setback may "reduce tension on the muscles (superior constrictor and palatopharyngeus) of velopharyngeal closure" but had no actual data relating to this hypothesis.

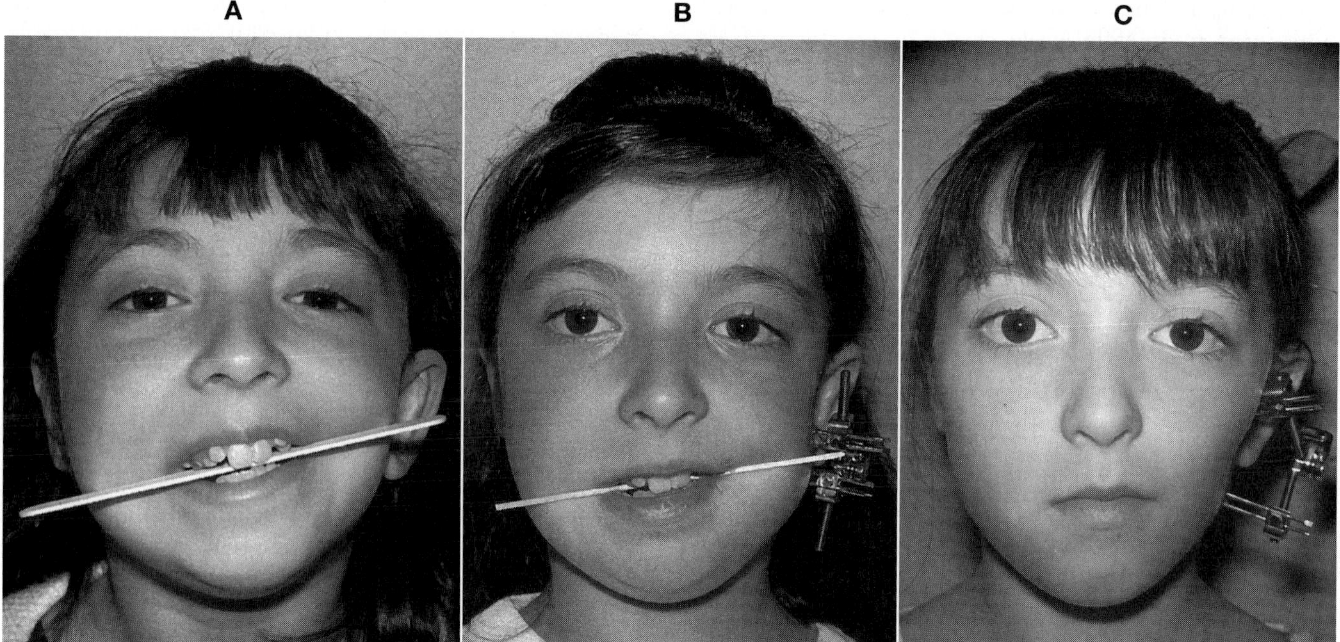

Figure 4-21 Girl with hemifacial microsomia proceeding through mandibular distraction osteogenesis. **A,** Occlusal cant before treatment. **B,** Midway through treatment. **C,** Near the end of treatment. Note the improvement in the symmetry of the mouth (position of the oral commissures) in the last picture.

In summary, it seems that a substantial number of patients with clefts will continue to require midface advancements and that the potential effects on speech may include improvement in articulation but a risk of postadvancement VPI. In patients who have had prior pharyngoplasties, there may be some reduction in hyponasality. There are many variables, not just the obvious one of the expected or planned number of millimeters of advancement. Fox (1996) summarized most of the published studies on the effects of orthognathic surgery on speech and concluded her comments with a warning that speech should be evaluated on a case-by-case basis as each patient progresses through treatment. One additional concern *may* be patients who have already had a pharyngeal flap because in theory the flap could be a tethering force to the posterior pharyngeal wall and surgical advancement of the maxilla could be inhibited by the flap. However, surgeons have developed methods for lengthening or revising pre-existing pharyngeal flaps to allow for the necessary advancement of the midface (Braun and Sotereanos, 1983; Maegawa, Sells, and David, 1998a; Ruberg, Randall, and Whitaker, 1976).[40,41] At the very least, future reports must be rigorous about segregating postoperative speech results on patients with prior pharyngeal flaps from the results in the remainder of the study population.

Distraction Osteogenesis

A relatively recent development in reconstruction of the craniofacial complex in patients with clefts, as well as in patients with more complex disorders, is called "distraction osteogenesis," an umbrella term for several different techniques for moving facial bones into more normal positions. The surgeon first makes certain strategic cuts in the bony structure that is to be repositioned and then places either an external or internal metal device that is used to "crank" the divided segments of bone further apart. The gap that is created by the surgery is gradually increased by turning a screw in the distraction device to lengthen the bone (Fig. 4-21). Then the gap is filled in by the natural formation of new bone, creating a maxilla or mandible that is longer in the horizontal plane, vertical plane, or a combination of both. There have been several published reports (and many more oral reports at professional meetings) on distraction osteogenesis of the maxilla or mandible in patients with cleft lip and palate, patients with midface hypoplasia and retrusion of unknown etiology, and patients with some of the complex disorders discussed in Chapter 2 (Robin sequence, hemifacial microsomia, mandibulofacial dysostosis, Nager syndrome, Apert syndrome, Crouzon syndrome, and Pfeiffer syndrome) (Britto et al., 1998; Chin and Toth, 1996, 1997; Cohen, Rutrick, and Burstein, 1995; Cohen et al., 1997; Dogliotti, Nadal, and Ulfe, 1998; Guyette et al., 1996; Guyette et al., 1998; McCarthy et al., 1992; Molina and Ortiz-Monasterio,

[40]Millard (1980) pointed out that it was actually Paul Tessier who first devised a method of lengthening a pre-existing pharyngeal flap in patients needing midface advancement and that the report by Ruberg, Randall, and Whitaker (1976) engendered no small amount of animus on the part of the originator of the procedure.

[41]Barker (1987) reported changes in auditory tube function and audiometric results in both cleft and noncleft patients subsequent to orthognathic surgery. Gotzfried and Thumfart (1988) reported that Le Fort I osteotomies could have a beneficial effect on the ventilation function of the middle ear.

1996; Polley and Figueroa, 1997; Rodriguez and Dogliotti, 1998; Toth et al., 1998).

There have been a few reports of deterioration in velopharyngeal adequacy pursuant to distraction osteogenesis and one report of some of improvement in articulation, particularly apical consonants and palatal fricatives with secondary improvement in labiodental fricatives (Guyette et al., 1996). In a report on 19 children with clefts, Guyette et al. (1998) reported that maxillary distraction led to a deterioration in velopharyngeal closure in three, the worst case being a child whose maxilla was gradually brought forward by more than 15 mm.

The collective database on the effects on speech of distraction osteogenesis on the maxilla or mandible is in its infancy, as is the procedure itself. It is tempting to think that, because the procedure is gradual, the velopharyngeal system might have more time to adapt to changing (increasing) requirements than may be the case in surgical advancements. To some extent, clinicians may be able to predict outcomes on the basis of the projected amount of advancement and the time over which it will occur. Reassurance to patients and families will depend on the amount of carefully documented clinical outcomes.

REFERENCES

Abyholm FE: Submucous cleft palate. *Scandinavian Journal of Plastic and Reconstructive Surgery* 10:209-212, 1976.

Abyholm FE: Secondary bone grafting of alveolar clefts. In Berkowitz S (ed.): *Cleft lip and palate: perspectives in management.* Volume 2: *An introduction to other craniofacial anomalies.* San Diego: Singular, 1996, pp. 111-117.

Abyholm FE, Bergland O, and Semb G: Secondary bone grafting of alveolar clefts. *Scandinavian Journal of Plastic and Reconstructive Surgery* 15:127-140, 1981.

Abyholm FE, Borchgrevnik HH, and Eskeland G: Palatal fistulae following cleft palate surgery. *Scandinavian Journal of Plastic and Reconstructive Surgery* 13:295-300, l979.

Adcock S, and Markus AF: Mid-facial growth following functional cleft surgery. *British Journal of Oral and Maxillofacial Surgery* 35:1-5, 1997.

Aduss H, and Pruzansky S: Craniofacial growth in complete unilateral cleft lip and palate. *Angle Orthodontist* 41:202-213, 1971.

Ainoda N, Yamashita D, and Tsukada S: Articulation at age 4 in children with early repair of cleft palate. *Annals of Plastic Surgery* 15:415-422, 1985.

Argamaso RV: The tongue flap: placement and fixation for closure of postpalatoplasty fistulae. *Cleft Palate Journal* 27:402-410, 1990.

Bardach J: Cleft palate repair: two flap palatoplasty, research philosophy, technique and results. In Bardach J, and Morris HL (eds.): *Multidisciplinary management of cleft lip and palate.* Philadelphia: WB Saunders, 1990, pp. 352-365.

Bardach J: Unilateral cleft lip. In Cohen M (ed.): *Mastery of plastic and reconstructive surgery.* Volume 1. Boston: Little, Brown, 1994, pp. 548-565.

Bardach J, and Salyer K: *Surgical techniques in cleft lip and palate.* Chicago: Year Book, 1987.

Bardach J, Morris HL, and Olin WH: Late results of primary veloplasty: the Marburg project. *Plastic and Reconstructive Surgery* 73:207-215, 1984.

Barimo JP, Habal MB, Scheuerle J, and Ritterman SI: Postnatal palatoplasty, implications for normal speech articulation—a preliminary report. *Scandinavian Journal of Plastic and Reconstructive Surgery* 21:139-143, 1987.

Barker GR: Auditory tube function and audiogram changes following corrective orthognathic maxillary and mandibular surgery in cleft and non-cleft patients. *Scandinavian Journal of Plastic and Reconstructive Surgery* 23:133-138, 1987.

Batstone J, and Millard DR: Pushback palatorraphy with island flap to the nasal surface. In Grabb W, Rosenstein S, and Bzoch KR (eds.): *Cleft lip and palate: surgical, dental and speech aspects.* Boston: Little, Brown, 1971, pp. 441-447.

Battle RJV: Speech results of palate repair when performed before two years of age. *Transactions of the Fourth International Congress on Plastic and Reconstructive Surgery.* 1967, pp. 425-238.

Bergland O, and Sidhu SS: Occlusal changes from the deciduous to the early mixed dentition in unilateral complete clefts. *Cleft Palate Journal* 11:317-326, 1974.

Bergland O, Semb G, and Abyholm FE: Elimination of residual alveolar cleft by secondary bone grafting and subsequent orthodontic treatment. *Cleft Palate Journal* 23:175-205, 1986.

Berkowitz S: *Cleft lip and palate: perspectives in management.* Volume I. San Diego: Singular, 1996.

Bingham HG, Suthunyarat P, Richards S, and Graham M: Should the pharyngeal flap be used primarily with palatoplasty? *Cleft Palate Journal* 9:319-325, 1972.

Bishara S: The influence of palatoplasty and cleft length on facial development. *Cleft Palate Journal* 10:390-398, 1973.

Bishara S, Enemark H, and Tharp R: Cephalometric comparisons of the results of the Wardill-Kilner and von Langenbeck palatoplasties. *Cleft Palate Journal* 13:319-329, 1976.

Bishara S, Krause CJ, Olin WH, Weston D, Van Hess J, and Felling C: Facial and dental relationships of individuals with unoperated clefts of the lip and/or palate. *Cleft Palate Journal* 13:238-252, 1976b.

Blijdorp P, and Muller H: The influence of the age at which the palate is closed on speech in the adult cleft palate patient. *Journal of Maxillofacial Surgery* 12:239-246, 1984.

Blocksma R, Leuz C, and Mellerstig K: A conservative program for managing cleft palates without the use of mucoperiosteal flaps. *Plastic and Reconstructive Surgery* 55:160-169, 1975.

Boyne PJ, and Sands NR: Combined orthodontic-surgical management of residual palato-alveolar cleft defects. *American Journal of Orthodontics* 70:20-37, 1976.

Braithwaite E: Cleft palate repair. In Gibson T (ed.): *Modern trends in plastic surgery.* London: Butterworth, 1964, pp. 30-49.

Braithwaite E, and Maurice D: The importance of the levator palati muscle in cleft palate closure. *British Journal of Plastic Surgery* 21:60-62, 1968.

Bralley RC, and Schoeny ZG: Effects of maxillary advancement on the speech of a submucosal cleft palate patient. *Cleft Palate Journal* 14:98-101, 1977.

Brattstrom V, McWilliam J, Larson O, and Semb G: Craniofacial development in children with unilateral clefts of the lip, alveolus and palate treated according to four different regimes. II: Mandibular and vertical development. *Scandinavian Journal of Plastic and Reconstructive Surgery* 25:55-63, 1992.

Brauer RO, and Cronin TD: Maxillary orthopedics an anterior palate repair with bone grafting. *Cleft Palate Journal* 1:31-42, 1964.

Braun T, and Sotereanos G: Pharyngeal flap extension as an adjunct to maxillary advancement in patients with cleft palate. *Journal of Oral and Maxillofacial Surgery* 41:411, 1983.

Britto JA, Evans RD, Hayward RD, and Jones BM: Maxillary distraction osteogenesis in Pfeiffer's syndrome: urgent ocular protection by gradual midfacial skeletal advancement. *British Journal of Plastic Surgery* 51:343-349, 1998.

Brothers DB, Dalston RW, Peterson HD, and Lawrence WT: Comparison of the Furlow double-reversing z-palatoplasty with the Wardill-Kilner procedure for isolated clefts of the soft palate. *Plastic and Reconstructive Surgery* 95:969-977, 1995.

Brown AS, Cohen MA, and Randall P: Levator muscle reconstruction: does it make a difference? *Plastic and Reconstructive Surgery* 72:1-6, 1983.

Buchholz R, Chase R, Jobe R, and Smith H: The use of the combined palatal pushback and pharyngeal flap operation: a progress report. *Plastic and Reconstructive Surgery* 39:554-561, 1967.

Butow K-W, and Jacobs FJ: Intravelar veloplasty: surgical modification according to anatomical defect. *International Journal of Oral and Maxillofacial Surgery* 20:296-300, 1991.

Butow K-W, and Steinhauser EW: Follow-up investigation of palatal closure by means of a one-layer cranially-based vomer-flap. *International Journal of Oral Surgery* 13:396-400, 1984.

Cadieux RJ, Kales A, McGlynn TJ, Jackson D, Manders EK, and Simmonds MA: Sleep apnea precipitated by pharyngeal surgery in a patient with myotonic dystrophy. *Archives of Otolaryngology* 110:611-613, 1984.

Calnan JS: Submucous cleft palate. *British Journal of Plastic Surgery* 7:264-282, 1954.

Calnan JS: V-Y pushback palatorraphy. In Grabb W, Rosenstein S, and Bzoch KR (eds.): *Cleft lip and palate: surgical, dental and speech aspects.* Boston: Little, Brown, 1971, pp. 422-431.

Calnan JS: Surgery for speech. In Calnan JS (ed.): *Recent advances in plastic surgery, I.* Edinburgh: Churchill Livingstone, 1976, pp. 39-57.

Chapman KL, and Hardin MA: Phonetic and phonologic skills of two-year-olds with cleft palate. *Cleft Palate–Craniofacial Journal* 29:535-443, 1992.

Chen PK-T, Wu J, Hung K-F, Chen Y-R, and Noordhoff MS: Surgical correction of submucous cleft palate with Furlow palatoplasty. *Plastic and Reconstructive Surgery* 97:1136-1146, 1996.

Chin M, and Toth BA: Distraction osteogenesis in maxillofacial surgery using internal devices: report of five cases. *Journal of Oral and Maxillofacial Surgery* 54:45-53, 1996.

Chin M, and Toth BA: Le Fort III advancement with gradual distraction using internal devices. *Plastic and Reconstructive Surgery* 100:819-830, 1997.

Cohen M, Polley JW, and Figueroa AA: Secondary (intermediate) alveolar bone grafting. *Clinics in Plastic Surgery* 20:691-705, 1993.

Cohen SR, Rutrick RE, and Burstein FD: Distraction osteogenesis of the human craniofacial skeleton: initial experience with new distraction system. *Journal of Craniofacial Surgery* 6:368-374, 1995.

Cohen SR, Burstein FD, Stewart MG, and Rathburn MA: Maxillary-midface distraction in children with cleft lip and palate: a preliminary report. *Plastic and Reconstructive Surgery* 99:1421-1428, 1997.

Cohen SR, Corrigan M, Wilmot J, and Trotman CA: Cumulative operative procedures in patients aged 14 years and older with unilateral or bilateral cleft lip and palate. *Plastic and Reconstructive Surgery* 96:267-271, 1995.

Cohen SR, Kalinowski J, LaRossa D, and Randall P: Cleft palate fistulas: a multivariate statistical analysis of prevalence, etiology, and surgical management. *Plastic and Reconstructive Surgery* 87:1041-1047, 1991.

Copeland M: The effects of very early palatal repair on speech. *British Journal of Plastic Surgery* 43:676-682, 1990.

Cosman B, and Falk AS: Delayed hard palate repair and speech deficiencies: a cautionary report. *Cleft Palate Journal* 17:27-33, 1980.

Coston GN, Hagerty RF, Jannarone RJ, McDonald V, and Hagerty RC: Levator muscle reconstruction: resulting velopharyngeal competency—a preliminary report. *Plastic and Reconstructive Surgery* 77:911-918, 1986.

Crikelair GF, Kastein S, Fowler EP, and Cosman B: Velar dysfunction in the absence of cleft palate. *New York State Journal of Medicine* 15:263-269, 1964.

Crikelair G, Striker P, and Cosman B: The surgical treatment of submucous cleft palate. *Plastic and Reconstructive Surgery* 45:58-65, 1970.

Crockett DM, Bumsted RM, and Van Demark DR: Experience with surgical management of velopharyngeal incompetence. *Otolaryngology–Head and Neck Surgery* 99:1-9, 1988.

Cronin TD: Method of preventing raw area on the nasal surface of the soft palate in push-back surgery. *Plastic Reconstructive Surgery* 20:474-484, 1957.

Cronin TD: Pushback palatorraphy with nasal mucosal flaps. In Grabb W, Rosenstein S, and Bzoch KR (eds.): *Cleft lip and palate: surgical, dental and speech aspects.* Boston: Little, Brown, 1971, pp. 432-440.

Cronin TD: The bilateral cleft lip with bilateral cleft of the primary palate. In Converse JM (ed.): *Reconstructive plastic surgery.* volume 4: *Cleft lip and palate, craniofacial deformities.* Philadelphia: WB Saunders, 1977, pp. 2048-2089.

Cronin TD, and Upton J: Lengthening the short columella associated with bilateral cleft lip. *Annals of Plastic Surgery* 1:75-95, 1978.

Cronin TD, Brauer RO, Alexander J, and Taylor W: Pushback repair using nasal mucosal flaps: results. *Cleft Palate Journal* 1:269-274, 1964.

Dado DV: Primary (early) alveolar bone grafting. *Clinics in Plastic Surgery* 20:683-689, 1993.

Dalston RM: Timing of cleft palate repair: a speech pathologist's viewpoint. *Problems in Plastic and Reconstructive Surgery: Cleft Palate Surgery* 2:30-38, 1992.

Dalston RM: Velopharyngeal impairment in the orthodontic population. *Seminars in Orthodontics: Cleft Lip and Palate* 2:220-227, 1996.

Dalston RM, and Stuteville O: A clinical investigation of the efficacy of primary nasopalatal pharyngoplasty. *Cleft Palate Journal* 12:177-192, 1975.

Dalston RM, and Vig PS: Effects of orthognathic surgery on speech: a prospective study. *American Journal of Orthodontics* 86:291-298, 1984.

D'Antonio LL: Correction of velopharyngeal insufficiency using the Furlow double-opposing Z-plasty. *Western Journal of Medicine* 157:101-102, 1997.

Davison PM, Razzell RE, and Watson ACH: The role of pharyngoplasty in congenital neurogenic speech disorders. *British Journal of Plastic Surgery* 43:187-196, 1990.

Delaire J: Considerations sur la croissance faciale en particulier du maxillaire superieur. *Revue de Stomatologie et de Chirurgie Maxillo-Faciale* 72:57-76, 1971.

Delaire J: La cheilorhinoplastie primaire pour fente labiomaxillaire congenitale unilaterale. *Revue de Stomatologie et de Chirurgie Maxillo-Faciale* 76:193, 1975.

Delaire J, and Precious DS: Avoidance of the use of vomerine mucosa in primary surgical management of velpalatine cleft. *Oral Surgery, Oral Medicine, Oral Pathology* 60:589-597, 1985.

Delaire J, and Precious DS: Influence of the nasal septum on maxillonasal growth in patients with congenital labiomaxillary clefts. *Cleft Palate Journal* 23:270-277, 1986.

DeLuke DM, Marchand A, Robles EC, and Fox P: Facial growth and the need for orthognathic surgery after cleft palate repair: literature review and report of 28 cases. *Journal of Oral and Maxillofacial Surgery* 55:694-697, 1997.

Demjen SE, and Krause CJ: The W/V-Y palatoplasty procedure: a step-by-step description. In Morris HL (ed.): *The Bratislava project: some results of cleft palate surgery.* Iowa City: University of Iowa Press, 1978, pp. 27-49.

Denk MJ, and Magee WP: Cleft palate closure in the neonate: preliminary report. *Cleft Palate–Craniofacial Journal* 33:57-61, 1996.

Desai S: Early cleft palate repair completed before the age of 16 weeks: observations on a personal series of 100 children. *British Journal of Plastic Surgery* 36:300-304, 1983.

Dingman R, and Argenta L: The correction of cleft palate with primary veloplasty and delayed repair of the hard palate. *Clinics in Plastic Surgery* 12:677-684, 1985.

Dogliotti P, Nadal E, and Ulfe I: Oral-acral syndrome and its correction using maxillary bone distraction osteogenesis. *Journal of Craniofacial Surgery* 9:123-126, 1998.

Dorf DS, and Curtin J: Early cleft palate repair and speech outcome. *Plastic and Reconstructive Surgery* 68:153-157, 1982.

Dorf DS, and Curtin J: Early cleft palate repair and speech outcome: a ten-year experience. In Bardach J, and Morriss HL (eds.): *Multidisciplinary management of cleft lip and palate.* Philadelphia: WB Saunders, 1990, pp. 341-348.

Dorrance GM: Lengthening of the soft palate operations. *Annals of Surgery* 82:208-211, 1925.

Dorrance GM: The repair of cleft palate. *Annals of Surgery* 95:641-658, 1932.

Dorrance GM: *The operative story of cleft palate.* Philadelphia: WB Saunders, 1933.

Dorrance GM, and Bransfield JW: The push-back operation for repair of cleft palate. *Plastic and Reconstructive Surgery* 1:145-169, 1946.

Dreyer TM, and Trier WC: A comparison of palatoplasty techniques. *Cleft Palate Journal* 21:251-253, 1984.

Edgerton MT: Surgical lengthening of the cleft palate by dissection of the neurovascular bundle. *Plastic and Reconstructive Surgery* 29:551-560, 1962.

Edgerton MT: The island flap pushback and the suspensory pharyngeal flap in surgical treatment of the cleft palate patient. *Plastic and Reconstructive Surgery* 36:591-602, 1965.

Edgerton MT, and Dellon AL: Surgical retrodisplacement of the levator palatini muscle: preliminary report. *Plastic and Reconstructive Surgery* 47:154-167, 1971.

Egyedi P: Timing of palatal closure. *Journal of Maxillofacial Surgery* 13:177-182, 1985.

Elander A, Lilja J, Friede H, Persson E-C, Lohmander-Agerskov A, and Soderpalm E: Surgical treatment of cleft palate: 27 years' experience of the Wardill-Kilner technique. *Scandinavian Journal of Plastic and Reconstructive Surgery* 27:291-295, 1993.

Emory RE, Clay RP, Bite U, and Jackson IT: Fistula formation and repair after palatal closure: an institutional perspective. *Plastic and Reconstructive Surgery* 99:1535-1538, 1997.

Enemark H, Bolund S, and Jorgensen I: Evaluation of unilateral cleft lip and palate treatment: long term results. *Cleft Palate–Craniofacial Journal* 27:354-361, 1990.

Enemark H, Krantz-Simonsen E, and Schramm JE: Secondary bonegrafting in unilateral cleft lip palate patients: indications and treatment procedure. *International Journal of Oral Surgery* 14:2-10, 1985.

Epker BN, and Wolford LM: Middle-third facial osteotomies: their use in the correction of acquired and developmental dentofacial and craniofacial deformities. *Journal of Oral Surgery* 33:491-514, 1975.

Epker BN, and Wolford LM: Middle-third facial osteotomies: their use in the correction of congenital dentofacial and craniofacial deformities. *Journal of Oral Surgery* 34:324-342, 1976.

Eskenazi LB, and Schendel SA: An analysis of LeFort I maxillary advancement in cleft lip and palate patients. *Plastic and Reconstructive Surgery* 90:779-786, 1992.

Evans D, and Renfrew C: The timing of primary cleft palate repair. *Scandinavian Journal of Plastic and Reconstructive Surgery* 8:153-155, 1974.

Fara M, and Brousilova M: Experiences with early closure of velum and later closure of hard palate. *Plastic and Reconstructive Surgery* 44:134-141, 1969.

Fara M, Sedlackova E, Klaskova O, Hrivnakova J, Chmelova A, and Supacek I: Primary pharyngofixation in cleft palate repair. *Plastic and Reconstructive Surgery* 45:449-458, 1970.

Figueroa AA, Reisberg DB, Polley JW, and Cohen M: Intraoral-appliance modification to retract the premaxilla in patients with bilateral cleft lip. *Cleft Palate–Craniofacial Journal* 33:497-500, 1996.

Fisher J, and Edgerton MT: Combined use of levator retrodisplacement and pharyngeal flap for congenital palate insufficiency. *Cleft Palate Journal* 12:270-273, 1975.

Folk SN, D'Antonio LL, and Hardesty RA: Secondary cleft deformities. *Clinics in Plastic Surgery: Secondary Management of Craniofacial Disorders* 24:599-611, 1997.

Fox DR: Speech considerations for orthognathic surgeons. In Berkowitz S (ed.): *Cleft lip and palate: perspectives in management.* Volume II: *An introduction to other craniofacial anomalies.* San Diego: Singular, 1996, pp. 171-176.

Friede H, and Johanson B: A follow-up study of cleft children treated with vomer flap as part of a three-stage soft tissue surgical procedure. *Scandinavian Journal of Plastic and Reconstructive Surgery* 11:45-57, 1977.

Friede H, Lilja J, and Johanson B: Cleft lip and palate treatment with delayed closure of the hard palate. *Scandinavian Journal of Plastic and Reconstructive Surgery* 14:49-53, 1980.

Friede H, Enemark H, Semb G, Paulin G, Abyholm F, Bolund S, Lilja J, and Ostrup L: Craniofacial and occlusal characteristics in unilateral cleft lip and palate patients from four Scandinavian centres. *Scandanavian Journal of Plastic and Reconstructive and Hand Surgery* 25:269-276, 1991.

Furlow LT: Cleft palate repair by double opposing Z-plasty. *Plastic and Reconstructive Surgery* 78:724-736, 1986.

Garber S, Speidel T, and Marse G: The effects on speech of surgical premaxillary osteotomy. *American Journal of Orthodontics* 79:54-62, 1981.

Garcia-Velasco M, Galvez-Perez F, Ysunza-Rivera A, and Ortiz-Monasterio F: Conceptos actuales sobre el paladar hendido submucoso. *Boletin Medicina Hospital de Infant de Mexico* 42:657-661, 1985.

Georgiade NG, Mladick R, Thorne R, and Massengill R: Preliminary evaluation of the island flap in cleft palate repair. *Cleft Palate Journal* 6:488-494, 1969.

Gnoinski WM: Early maxillary orthopedics as a supplement to conventional primary surgery in complete cleft lip and palate patients. *Journal of Maxillofacial Surgery* 10:165-172, 1982.

Gotzfried HF, and Thumfart WF: Pre- and postoperative middle ear function and muscle activity of the soft palate after total maxillary osteotomy in cleft patients. *Journal of Cranio-Maxillo-Facial Surgery* 16:64-68, 1988.

Grabb WC: General aspects of cleft palate surgery. In Grabb W, Rosenstein S, and Bzoch KR (eds.): *Cleft lip and palate: surgical, dental and speech aspects.* Boston: Little, Brown, 1971, pp. 373-392.

Greene M: Speech analysis of 263 cleft palate cases. *Journal of Speech and Hearing Disorders* 25:43-48, 1960.

Greminger R: Island soft palatoplasty for early reconstruction of the posterior muscular ring. *Plastic and Reconstructive Surgery* 68:871-877, 1981.

Grobbelaar AO, Hudson DA, Fernandes DB, and Lentin F: Speech results after repair of the cleft soft palate. *Plastic and Reconstructive Surgery* 95:1150-1154, 1995.

Grunwell P, and Russell J: Vocalisations before and after cleft palate surgery: a pilot study. *British Journal of Disorders of Communication* 22:1-17, 1987.

Grunwell P, and Russell J: Phonological development in children with cleft lip and palate. *Clinical Linguistics and Phonetics* 2:75-95, 1988.

Gunther E, Wisser JR, Cohen MA, and Brown AS: Palatoplasty: Furlow's double reversing z-plasty versus intravelar veloplasty. *Cleft Palate–Craniofacial Journal* 35:546-549, 1998.

Guyette TW, Polley JW, Figueroa AA, and Cohen MN: Mandibular distraction osteogenesis: effects on articulation and velopharyngeal function. *Journal of Craniofacial Surgery* 7:186-191, 1996.

Guyette TW, Polley JW, Figueroa AA, and Smith B: Changes in the speech of cleft palate patients following maxillary distraction. Presented before the 55th annual meeting of the American Cleft Palate-Craniofacial Association, Baltimore, April 25, 1998.

Gylling U, and Soivio AI: Submucous cleft palate. *Acta Chirugica Scandinavia* 129:282-287, 1965.

Haapanen M-L, and Rantala S-L: Correlation between the age at repair and speech outcome in patients with isolated cleft palate. *Scandinavian Journal of Plastic, Reconstructive and Hand Surgery* 26:71-78, 1992.

Hardin-Jones MA, Brown CK, Van Demark DR, and Morris HL: Long-term speech results of cleft palate patients with primary palatoplasty. *Cleft Palate–Craniofacial Journal* 30:55-63, 1993.

Harding R: Surgery. In Cooper H, Harding R, Drogman W, Mazaheri M, and Millard DR (eds.): *Cleft palate and cleft lip: a team approach to clinical management and rehabilitation of the patient.* Philadelphia: WB Saunders, 1979, pp. 163-262.

Harding A, and Campbell RC: A comparison of the speech results after early and delayed hard palate closure: a preliminary report. *British Journal of Plastic Surgery* 42:187-192, 1989.

Hartel H, Gundlach KKH, and Ruickoldt K: Incidence of velopharyngoplasty following various techniques of palatoplasty. *Journal of Cranio-Maxillo-Facial Surgery* 22:272-275, 1994.

Heller JC, Gens GW, Moe DG, and Lewin ML: Velopharyngeal insufficiency in patients with neurologic, emotional and mental disorders. *Journal of Speech and Hearing Disorders* 39:350-359, 1974.

Hellquist R: Experiences with infant and delayed periosteoplasty. *Swedish Dental Journal Supplement* 15:79-87, 1982.

Hellquist R, and Ponten B: The influence of infant periosteoplasty on facial growth and dental occlusion from five to eight years of age in cases of complete unilateral cleft lip and palate. *Scandinavian Journal of Plastic and Reconstructive Surgery* 13:305-312, 1979.

Henningsson G, and Isberg A: Influence of palatal fistulae on speech and resonance. *Folia Phoniatrica* 39:183-191, 1987.

Herfert O: Two-stage operation for cleft palate. *British Journal of Plastic Surgery* 16:37-45, 1963.

Hogan VM: A clarification of the surgical goals in cleft palate speech and the introduction of the lateral port control (L.P.C.) pharyngeal flap. *Cleft Palate Journal* 10:331-345, 1973.

Hoge J: Millard's island flap in secondary lengthening of cleft soft palates. *British Journal of Plastic Surgery* 19:317-321, 1966.

Holdsworth WG: Early treatment of cleft-lip and cleft-palate. *British Medical Journal* 1:304-308, 1954.

Holtmann B, Wray R, and Weeks P: A comparison of three techniques of palatorraphy: early speech results. *Annals of Plastic Surgery* 12:514-519, 1984.

Hoopes JE, Dellon AL, Fabrikant JI, and Soliman AH: Cineradiographic assessment of combined island flap pushback and pharyngeal flap in the surgical management of submucous cleft palate. *British Journal of Plastic Surgery* 23:39-44, 1970.

Hotz M, and Gnoinski W: Effects of early maxillary orthopaedics in coordination with delayed surgery for cleft lip and palate. *Journal of Maxillofacial Surgery* 7:201-210, 1979.

Hotz MM, Gnoinski WM, Nussbaumer H, and Kistler E: Early maxillary orthopedics in CLP cases: guidelines for surgery. *Cleft Palate Journal* 15:405-411, 1978.

Hotz MM, Gnoinski WM, Perko M, Nussbaumer H, Hof E, and Haubensak R (eds.): *Early treatment of cleft lip and palate.* Bern: Hans Huber, 1984.

Houston JB, and James DR: Le Fort I maxillary osteotomies in cleft palate cases: surgical changes and stability. *Journal of Cranio-Maxillo-Facial Surgery* 17:9-15, 1989.

Isberg A, and Henningsson G: Influence of palatal fistulae on velopharyngeal movements: a cineradiographic study. *Plastic and Reconstructive Surgery* 79:525-530, 1987.

Jackson IT: Closure of secondary palatal fistulae with intra-oral tissue and bone-grafting. *British Journal of Plastic Surgery* 25:93-105, 1972.

Jackson IT, McGlynn MJ, and Huskie CF: Velopharyngeal incompetence in the absence of cleft palate: results of treatment in 20 cases. *Plastic and Reconstructive Surgery* 66:211-213, 1980.

Jackson IT, McLennan G, and Scheker L: Primary veloplasty or primary palatal plasty: some preliminary findings. *Plastic and Reconstructive Surgery* 72:153-157, 1983.

Jackson MS, Jackson IT, and Christie FB: Improvement in speech following closure of anterior palatal fistulas with bone grafts. *British Journal of Plastic Surgery* 29:293-296, 1976.

Jafek B, Balkany T, Wong M, and Bryant K: Surgical management of the hypodynamic palate. *Archives of Otolaryngology* 105:347-350, 1979.

Jansma J, Raghoebar GM, Batenburg RHK, Stellingham C, and van Oort RP: Bone grafting of cleft lip and palate patients for placement of endosseous implants. *Cleft Palate–Craniofacial Journal* 36:67-72, 1999.

Johns DF: Surgical and prosthetic management of neurogenic velopharyngeal incompetency in dysarthria. In Johns DF (ed.): *Clinical management of neurogenic communicative disorders.* 2nd ed. Boston: Little, Brown, 1985, pp. 153-177.

Jolleys A: A review of the results of operations on cleft palates with reference to maxillary growth and speech function. *British Journal of Plastic Surgery* 7:229-241, 1954.

Joos U: The importance of muscular reconstruction in the treatment of cleft lip and palate. *Scandinavian Journal of Plastic and Reconstructive Surgery* 21:109-113, 1987.

Joos U: Evaluation of the result of surgery on cleft lip and palate and skeletal growth determinants of the cranial base. *Journal of Cranio-Maxillo-Facial Surgery* 17:23-25, 1989.

Joos U: Skeletal growth after muscular reconstruction for cleft lip, alveolus, and palate. *British Journal of Oral and Maxillofacial Surgery* 33:139-144, 1995.

Jorgenson RJ, Shapiro SD, and Odinet KL: Studies on facial growth and arch size in cleft lip and palate. *Journal of Craniofacial Genetics and Developmental Biology* 4:33-38, 1984.

Kapetansky DI: Double pendulum flaps for whistling deformities in bilateral cleft lips. *Plastic and Reconstructive Surgery* 47:321-323, 1971.

Kaplan E: The occult submucous cleft palate. *Cleft Palate Journal* 12:356-368, 1975.

Kaplan E: Cleft palate repair at three months? *Annals of Plastic Surgery* 7:179-190, 1981.

Kaplan I, Labandter H, Ben-Bassat M, Dresner J, and Nachmani A: Long-term follow-up of clefts of the secondary palate repaired by von Langenbeck's method. *British Journal of Plastic Surgery* 31:353-354, 1978.

Kapucu MR, Gursu KG, Enacar A, and Aras S: The effect of cleft lip repair on maxillary morphology in patients with unilateral complete cleft lip and palate. *Plastic and Reconstructive Surgery* 97:1371-1375, 1996.

Karling J, Larson O, and Henningsson G: Oronasal fistulas in cleft palate patients and their influence on speech. *Scandinavian Journal of Plastic and Reconstructive Surgery* 19:193-201, 1993.

Karnell MP, and Van Demark DR: Longitudinal speech performance in patients with cleft palate: comparisons based on secondary management. *Cleft Palate Journal* 23:278-288, 1986.

Kawamoto JH Jr: Correction of major defects of vermilion with a cross-lip vermilion flap. *Plastic and Reconstructive Surgery* 64:315-318, 1979.

Kearns G, Perott DH, Sharma A, Kaban LB, and Vargervik K: Placement of endosseus implants in grafted alveolar clefts. *Cleft Palate–Craniofacial Journal* 34:520-525, 1997.

Kemp-Fincham SI, Kuehn DP, and Trost-Cardamone JE: Speech development and the timing of primary palatoplasty. In Bardach J, and Morris HL (eds.): *Multidisciplinary management of cleft lip and palate.* Philadelphia: WB Saunders, 1990, pp. 736-745.

Kilner TP: Cleft lip and palate repair technique. *St. Thomas Hospital Report* 2:127, 1937.

Koberg WR: Present view of bone grafting in cleft palate (review of the literature). *Journal of Maxillofacial Surgery* 1:185-198, 1973.

Koberg WR, and Koblin I: Speech development and maxillary growth in relation to technique and timing of palatoplasty. *Journal of Maxillofacial Surgery* 1:44-50, 1973.

Kobus K: Extended vomer flaps in cleft palate repair: a preliminary report. *Plastic and Reconstructive Surgery* 73:895-901, 1984.

Krause CJ, Tharp RF, and Morris HL: A comparative study of results of the von Langenbeck and the V-Y pushback palatoplasties. *Cleft Palate Journal* 13:11-19, 1976.

Krause CJ, Van Demark DR, and Tharp RF: Palatoplasty: a comparative study. *Transactions of the American Academy of Ophthalmology and Otolaryngology* 80:551-559, 1975.

Kriens OB: An anatomical approach to veloplasty. *Plastic and Reconstructive Surgery* 43:29-41, 1969.

Kriens OB: Fundamental anatomic findings for an intravelar veloplasty. *Cleft Palate Journal* 7:27-36, 1970.

Kummer AW, Strife JL, Grau WH, Creaghead NA, and Lee L: The effects of LeFort I osteotomy with maxillary movement on articulation, resonance, and velopharyngeal function. *Cleft Palate Journal* 26:193-199, 1989.

LaRossa D: Cleft palate. In Cohen M (ed.): *Mastery of plastic and reconstructive surgery.* Volume 1. Boston: Little, Brown, 1994, pp. 595-604.

LaRossa D, Randall P, Cohen M, and Cohen S: The Furlow double reversing z-plasty for cleft palate repair: the first ten years of experience. In Bardach J, and Morris HL (eds.): *Multidisciplinary management of cleft lip and palate.* Philadelphia: WB Saunders, 1990, pp. 337-340.

Larson O, and Nilsson B: Early bone grafting in complete cleft lip and palate cases following maxillofacial orthopedics. *Scandinavian Journal of Plastic and Reconstructive Surgery* 17:209-223, 1983.

Larson O, Ideberg M, and Nordin K-E: Early bone grafting in complete cleft lip and palate cases following maxillofacial orthopedics. III: A study of the dental occlusion. *Scandinavian Journal of Plastic and Reconstructive Surgery* 17:81-92, 1983.

LeMesurier AB: *Harelips and their treatment.* Baltimore: Williams & Wilkins, 1962.

Leonard MS: Repair of oronasal fistula with mucoperiosteal flap: report of a case. *Journal of Oral Surgery* 37:511-512, 1979.

Lewin ML, Heller J, and Kojak D: Speech results after Millard island flap repair in cleft palate and other velopharyngeal insufficiencies. *Cleft Palate Journal* 12:263-269, 1975.

Lewis M: Secondary soft tissue procedures for cleft lip and palate. In Cohen M (ed.): *Mastery of plastic and reconstructive surgery.* Volume 1. Boston: Little, Brown, 1994, pp. 605-618.

Lindsay WK: von Langenbeck palatorraphy. In Grabb W, Rosenstein S, and Bzoch KR (eds.): *Cleft lip and palate: surgical, dental and speech aspects.* Boston: Little, Brown, 1971, pp. 393-403.

Lindsay WK, LeMesurier AB, and Farmer AW: A study of the speech results of a large series of cleft palate patients. *Annals of Otology, Rhinology, and Laryngology* 29:273-288, 1962.

Lindsey WH, and Davis PT: Correction of velopharyngeal insufficiency with Furlow palatoplasty. *Archives of Otolaryngology–Head and Neck Surgery* 122:881-884, 1996.

Lohmander-Agerskov A: Speech outcome after cleft palate surgery with the Goteborg regimen including delayed hard palate closure. *Scandinavian Journal of Plastic and Reconstructive and Hand Surgery* 32:63-80, 1998.

Lohmander-Agerskov A, and Soderpalm E: Evaluation of speech after completed late closure of the hard palate. *Folia Phoniatrica* 45:25-30, 1993.

Lohmander-Agerskov A, Dotevall H, Lith A, and Soderpalm E: Speech and velopharyngeal function in children with an open residual cleft in the hard palate, and the influence of temporary covering. *Cleft Palate–Craniofacial Journal* 33:324-332, 1996.

Lohmander-Agerskov A, Friede H, Lilja J, and Soderpalm E: Delayed closure of the hard palate: a comparison of speech in children with open and functionally closed residual clefts. *Scandinavian Journal of Plastic and Reconstructive and Hand Surgery* 30:121-127, 1996.

Lohmander-Agerskov A, Friede H, Soderpalm E, and Lilja J: Residual clefts in the hard palate: correlation between cleft size and speech. *Cleft Palate–Craniofacial Journal* 34:122-128, 1997.

Lohmander-Agerskov A, Havstam C, Soderpalm E, Elander A, Lilja J, Friede H, and Persson E-C: Assessment of speech in children after repair of isolated cleft palate. *Scandinavian Journal of Plastic and Reconstructive Surgery* 27:307-310, 1993.

Lohmander-Agerskov A, Soderpalm E, Friede H, and Lilja J: Cleft lip and palate patients prior to delayed closure of the hard palate: evaluation of maxillary morphology and the effect of early stimulation on pre-school speech. *Scandinavian Journal of Plastic and Reconstructive and Hand Surgery* 24:141-148, 1990.

Lohmander-Agerskov A, Soderpalm E, Friede H, and Lilja J: A longitudinal study of speech in 15 children with cleft lip and palate treated by late repair of the hard palate. *Scandinavian Journal of Plastic and Reconstructive and Hand Surgery* 29:21-31, 1995.

Luce E, McClinton M, and Hoopes J: Long-term results of the island flap palatal pushback. *Plastic and Reconstructive Surgery* 58:332-339, 1976.

Maegawa J, Sells RK, and David DJ: Pharyngoplasty in patients with cleft lip and palate after maxillary advancement. *Journal of Craniofacial Surgery* 9:330-335, 1998a.

Maegawa J, Sells RK, and David DJ: Speech changes after maxillary advancement in 40 cleft lip and palate patients. *Journal of Craniofacial Surgery* 9:177-182, 1998b.

Mann RJ, and Fisher DM: Bilateral buccal flaps with double opposing Z-plasty for wider palatal clefts. *Plastic and Reconstructive Surgery* 100:1139-1143, 1997.

Marks S, and Wynn S: Speech results after bilateral osteotomy surgery for cleft palate: a review of 413 patients. *Plastic and Reconstructive Surgery* 86:230-238, 1985.

Markus AF, and Delaire J: Functional primary closure of cleft lip. *British Journal of Oral and Maxillofacial Surgery* 31:281-291, 1993.

Marrinan EM, LaBrie RA, and Mulliken JB: Velopharyngeal function in nonsyndromic cleft palate: relevance of surgical technique, age at repair, and cleft type. *Cleft Palate–Craniofacial Journal* 35:95-100, 1998.

Marsh JL, Grames ML, and Holtman B: Intravelar veloplasty: a prospective study. *Cleft Palate Journal* 26:46-50, 1989.

Mason RM, Turvey TA, and Warren DW: Speech considerations with maxillary advancement procedures. *Journal of Oral Surgery* 38:752-758, 1980.

Massengill R, Pickrell K, and Robinson J: Results of pushback operations in treatment of submucous cleft palate. *Plastic and Reconstructive Surgery* 51:432-435, 1973.

McCarthy JG, Coccaro JP, and Schwartz MD: Velopharyngeal function following maxillary advancement. *Plastic and Reconstructive Surgery* 64:180-189, 1979.

McCarthy JG, Cutting CB, and Hogan VM: Introduction to facial clefts. In McCarthy JG (ed.): *Plastic surgery.* Volume 4: *Cleft lip & palate and craniofacial anomalies.* Philadelphia: WB Saunders, 1990, pp. 2437-2450.

McCarthy JG, Schreiber J, Karp N, Thorne CH, and Grayson BH: Lengthening the human mandible by gradual distraction. *Plastic and Reconstructive Surgery* 89:1-8, 1992.

McComb H: Primary repair of the bilateral cleft lip nose. *British Journal of Plastic Surgery* 28:262-267, 1975a.

McComb H: Treatment of the unilateral cleft lip nose. *Plastic and Reconstructive Surgery* 55:596-601, 1975b.

McComb H: Primary correction of unilateral cleft lip nasal deformity: a 10-year review. *Plastic and Reconstructive Surgery* 75:791-797, 1985.

McEvitt WG: The incidence of persistent rhinolalia following cleft palate repair. *Plastic and Reconstructive Surgery* 47:258-262, 1971.

McNeill KA: Experiences with island flap in palate surgery. *Archives of Otolaryngology* 85:75-77, 1967.

McWilliams BJ: Cleft palate management in England. *Speech Pathology and Therapy* 3:3-7, 1960.

McWilliams BJ, and Philips BJ: *Audio seminars in speech pathology: velopharyngeal incompetence.* Philadelphia: WB Saunders, 1979.

Meijer R, and Cohen S: Two-stage palatoplasty and evaluation of speech results. In Bardach J, and Morris HL (eds.): *Multidisciplinary management of cleft lip and palate.* Philadelphia: WB Saunders, 1990, pp. 321-327.

Millard DR: A radical rotation in single harelip. *American Journal of Surgery* 95:318-322, 1958.

Millard DR: The island flap in cleft palate surgery. *Surgery, Gynecology, and Obstetrics* 116:297-300, 1962.

Millard DR: A new use of the island flap in wide palatal clefts. *Plastic and Reconstructive Surgery* 30:330-355, 1966a.

Millard DR: Rotation-advancement method for cleft lip. *Journal of the American Medical Women's Association* 21:913-915, 1966b.

Millard DR: Rotation-advancement in the repair of bilateral cleft lip. In Grabb W, Rosenstein S, and Bzoch KR (eds.): *Cleft lip and palate: surgical, dental and speech aspects.* Boston: Little, Brown, 1971a, pp. 305-310.

Millard DR: Rotation-advancement in the repair of unilateral cleft lip. In Grabb W, Rosenstein S, and Bzoch KR (eds.): *Cleft lip and palate: surgical, dental and speech aspects.* Boston: Little, Brown, 1971b, pp. 195-203.

Millard DR: *Cleft craft: the evolution of its surgeries.* Volume I: *The unilateral deformity.* Boston: Little, Brown, 1976.

Millard DR: *Cleft craft: the evolution of its surgeries.* Volume II: *The bilateral deformity.* Boston: Little, Brown, 1977.

Millard DR: *Cleft craft: the evolution of its surgeries.* Volume III: *Alveolar and palatal deformities.* Boston: Little, Brown, 1980.

Millard DR, Batstone J, Heycock M, and Bensen J: Ten years with the palatal island flap. *Plastic and Reconstructive Surgery* 46:540-547, 1970.

Minami RT, Kaplan EN, Wu G, and Jobe RP: Velopharyngeal incompetence without overt cleft palate. *Plastic and Reconstructive Surgery* 55:573-587, 1975.

Molina F, and Ortiz-Monasterio F: Remodeling the craniofacial skeleton by distraction osteogenesis. In Berkowitz S (ed.): *Cleft lip and palate: perspectives in management.* Volume II: *An introduction to other craniofacial anomalies.* San Diego: Singular, 1996, pp. 287-297.

Moore MD, Lawrence WT, Ptak JJ, and Trier WC: Complications of primary palatoplasty: a twenty-one year review. *Cleft Palate Journal* 25:156-162, 1988.

Morris HL: Velopharyngeal competence and primary cleft palate surgery, 1960-1971: a critical review. *Cleft Palate Journal* 10:62-71, 1973.

Morris HL: Summary and discussion. In Morris HL (ed.): *The Bratislava project: some results of cleft palate surgery.* Iowa City: University of Iowa Press, 1978a, pp. 159-163.

Morris HL: Velopharyngeal competence and the Demjen W/V-Y technique. In Morris HL (ed.): *The Bratislava project: some cleft palate surgical results.* Iowa City: University of Iowa Press, 1978b, pp. 49-73.

Morris HL, Bardach J, Ardinger H, Jones D, Kelly KM, Olin WH, and Wheeler J: Multidisciplinary treatment results for patients with isolated cleft palate. *Plastic and Reconstructive Surgery* 92:842-851, 1993.

Mortier PB, Martinot VL, Anastossov Y, Kulik JF, Duhamel A, and Pellerin PN: Evaluation of the results of cleft lip and palate surgical treatment: preliminary report. *Cleft Palate–Craniofacial Journal* 34: 247-255, 1997.

Musgrave R, McWilliams BJ, and Matthews J: A review of the results of two different surgical procedures for the repair of clefts of the soft palate only. *Cleft Palate Journal* 12:281-290, 1975.

Myklebust O, and Abyholm FE: Speech results in CLP patients operated on with a von Langenbeck palatal closure. *Scandinavian Journal of Plastic and Reconstructive Surgery* 23:71-74, 1989.

Noordhoff MS: The island flap in secondary cleft palate surgery. *Plastic and Reconstructive Surgery* 46:463-467, 1970.

Noordhoff MS: Bilateral cleft lip. In Cohen M (ed.): *Mastery of plastic and reconstructive surgery.* Volume 1. Boston: Little, Brown, 1994, pp. 566-580.

Noordhoff MS, Kuo J, Wang F, Wuang H, and Witzel MA: Development of articulation before delayed hard-palate closure in children with cleft palate: a cross-sectional study. *Plastic and Reconstructive Surgery* 80:518-524, 1987.

Nordin E-E, Larson O, Nylen B, and Eklund G: Early bone grafting in complete cleft lip and palate cases following maxillofacial orthopedics. I: The method and skeletal development from seven to thirteen years of age. *Scandinavian Journal of Plastic and Reconstructive Surgery* 17:33-50, 1983.

Nunn DR, Derkay CS, Darrow DH, Magee W, and Strasnick B: The effect of very early cleft palate closure on the need for ventilation tubes in the first years of life. *Laryngoscope* 105:905-908, 1995.

Nystrom M, and Ranta R: Effect of timing and method of closure of isolated cleft palate on development of dental arches from 3 to 6 years of age. *European Journal of Orthodontics* 16:377-383, 1994.

O'Gara MM, and Logemann JA: Phonetic analyses of the speech development of babies with cleft palate. *Cleft Palate Journal* 25:122-134, 1988.

O'Gara MM, and Logemann JA: Phonological development in children with cleft lip and palate. In Bardach J, and Morris HL (eds.): *Multidisciplinary management of cleft lip and palate.* Philadelphia: WB Saunders, 1990, pp. 717-721.

O'Gara MM, Logemann JA, and Rademaker AW: Phonetic features by babies with unilateral cleft lip and palate. *Cleft Palate–Craniofacial Journal* 31:446-451, 1994.

Okazaki K, Satoh K, Kato M, Iwanami M, Ohokubo F, and Kobayashi K: Speech and velopharyngeal function following maxillary advancement in patients with cleft lip and palate. *Annals of Plastic Surgery* 30:304-311, 1993.

Oneal RM: Oronasal fistulas. In Grabb W, Rosenstein S, and Bzoch KR (eds.): *Cleft lip and palate: surgical, dental and speech aspects.* Boston: Little, Brown, 1971, pp. 490-498.

Onizuka T, Ohokubo F, Okazaki K, Hirakawa T, and Takahashi M: A new cleft palate repair. *Annals of Plastic Surgery* 37:457-464, 1996.

O'Riain S, and Hammond B: Speech results in cleft palate surgery: a survey of 249 patients. *British Journal of Plastic Surgery* 25:380-387, 1972.

Palmer C, Hamlen M, Ross RB, and Lindsay WK: Cleft palate repair: comparison of the results of two surgical techniques. *Canadian Journal of Surgery* 12:32-39, 1969.

Peat BG, Albery EH, Jones K, and Pigott RW: Tailoring velopharyngeal surgery: the influence of etiology and type of operation. *Plastic and Reconstructive Surgery* 93:948-953, 1994.

Peet E: The Oxford technique of cleft palate repair. *Plastic and Reconstructive Surgery* 28:282-294, 1961.

Pensler JM, and Bauer BS: Levator repositioning and palatal lengthening for submucous clefts. *Plastic and Reconstructive Surgery* 82:765-769, 1988.

Perko M: Primary closure of the cleft palate using a palatal mucosal flap: an attempt to prevent growth impairment. *Journal of Maxillofacial Surgery* 2:40, 1974.

Perko M: Two-stage closure of cleft palate. *Journal of Maxillofacial Surgery* 7:76-80, 1979.

Peterson HD: Commentary on Seyfer and Simon. *Plastic and Reconstructive Surgery* 83:791, 1989.

Peterson-Falzone SJ: A cross-sectional analysis of speech results following palatal closure. In Bardach J, and Morris HL (eds.): *Multidisciplinary management of cleft lip and palate.* Philadelphia: WB Saunders, 1990, pp. 750-757.

Pickrell K, Quinn G, and Massengill R: Primary bone grafting of the maxilla in clefts of the lip and palate: a four year study. *Plastic and Reconstructive Surgery* 41:438-442, 1968.

Pigott R: The results of nasopharyngoscopic assessment of pharyngoplasty. *Scandinavian Journal of Plastic and Reconstructive Surgery* 8:148-152, 1974.

Pigott RW: An assessment of some surgical techniques used in the management of palatal incompetence. In Ellis R, and Flack R (eds.): *Diagnosis and treatment of palato glossal malfunction.* London: College of Speech Therapists, 1979, pp. 67-60.

Pigott RW, Bensen JF, and White FD: Nasendoscopy in the diagnosis of velopharyngeal incompetence. *Plastic and Reconstructive Surgery* 43:141-147, 1969.

Pigott RW, Rieger FW, and Moodie AF: Tongue flap repair of cleft palate fistulae. *British Journal of Plastic Surgery* 37:285-293, 1984.

Polley JW, and Figueroa AA: Management of severe maxillary deficiency in childhood and adolescence through distraction osteogenesis with an external, adjustable, rigid distraction device. *Journal of Craniofacial Surgery* 8:181-185, 1997.

Poole MD, and Nunn M: Early experiences with Furlow's cleft palate technique. *British Journal of Plastic Surgery* 42:359, 1989.

Poole MD, Robinson S, and Nunn M: Maxillary advancements in cleft palate patients. *Journal of Maxillofacial Surgery* 14:123-127, 1986.

Porterfield HW, and Trabue JC: Submucous cleft palate. *Plastic and Reconstructive Surgery* 35:45-50, 1965.

Porterfield HW, Mohler LR, and Sandel A: Submucous cleft palate. *Plastic and Reconstructive Surgery* 58:60-65, 1976.

Posnick JC: Discussion of Rosenstein, Kernahan, Dado, Grasseschi, and Griffith, 1991. *Plastic and Reconstructive Surgery* 87:840-842, 1991.

Posnick JC: The treatment of secondary and residual dentofacial deformities in the cleft patient: surgical and orthodontic therapy. *Clinics in Plastic Surgery: Secondary Management of Craniofacial Disorders* 24:583-597, 1997.

Posnick JC, and Tompson B: Cleft-orthognathic surgery: complications and long-term results. *Plastic and Reconstructive Surgery* 96:255-266, 1995.

Poupard B, Coornaert H, Cebaere P, and Treanton A: Cleft lip and palate: can the hard palate be left open? A study of sixty-two cases with a follow-up of six years or more. *Annales de Chirurgie Plasticae Esthetique* 28:325-336, 1983.

Pruzansky S: Pre-surgical orthopedics and bone grafting for infants with cleft lip and palate: a dissent. *Cleft Palate Journal* 1:164-187, 1964.

Randall P: A triangular flap operation for the primary repair of unilateral clefts of the lip. *Plastic and Reconstructive Surgery* 23:331-347, 1959.

Randall P: A lip adhesion operation in cleft lip surgery. *Plastic and Reconstructive Surgery* 23:371-376, 1965.

Randall P: Triangular flap in the repair of unilateral cleft lip. In Grabb W, Rosenstein S, and Bzoch KR (eds.): *Cleft lip and palate: surgical, dental and speech aspects.* Boston: Little, Brown, 1971, pp. 204-214.

Randall P: Lip adhesion for wide unilateral and bilateral clefts of the lip. In Bardach J, and Morris HL (eds.): *Multidisciplinary management of cleft lip and palate.* Philadelphia: WB Saunders, 1990a, pp. 163-165.

Randall P: Long-term results with the triangular flap technique for unilateral cleft lip repair. In Bardach J, and Morris HL (eds.): *Multidisciplinary management of cleft lip and palate.* Philadelphia: WB Saunders, 1990b, pp. 173-183.

Randall P: A short history of cleft lip repair. In Berkowitz S (ed.): *Cleft lip and palate: perspectives in management.* Volume II: *An introduction to other craniofacial anomalies.* San Diego: Singular, 1996, pp. 25-32.

Randall P, and Graham W: Lip adhesion in the repair of bilateral cleft lip. In Grabb W, Rosenstein S, and Bzoch KR (eds.): *Cleft lip and palate: surgical, dental and speech aspects.* Boston: Little, Brown, 1971, pp. 282-287.

Randall P, LaRossa D, Fakhree SM, and Cohen MA: Cleft palate closure at 3 to 7 months of age: a preliminary report. *Plastic and Reconstructive Surgery* 71:624-627, 1983.

Randall P, LaRossa D, Solomon M, and Cohen MA: Experience with the Furlow double-reversing Z-plasty for cleft repair. *Plastic and Reconstructive Surgery* 77:569-576, 1986.

Reisberg DJ, Gold HO, and Dorf DS: A technique for obturating palatal fistulas. *Cleft Palate* 22:286-289, 1985.

Rintala AE: Surgical closure of palatal fistulae. *Scandinavian Journal of Plastic and Reconstructive Surgery* 14:235-238, 1980.

Rintala AE, and Haapanen ML: The correlation between training and skill of the surgeon and reoperation rate for persistent cleft palate speech. *British Journal of Oral and Maxillofacial Surgery* 33:295-298, 1995.

Rintala AE, and Haataja J: The effect of the lip adhesion procedure on the alveolar arch. *Scandinavian Journal of Plastic and Reconstructive Surgery* 13:301-304, 1979.

Robertson N, and Jolleys A: The timing of hard palate repair. *Scandinavian Journal of Plastic and Reconstructive Surgery* 8:49-51, 1974.

Robertson N, and Jolleys A: An 11-year follow-up on the effects of early bone grafting in infants born with complete clefts of the lip and palate. *British Journal of Plastic Surgery* 36:438-443, 1983.

Rodriguez JC, and Dogliotti P: Mandibular distraction in glossoptosis-micrognathic association: preliminary report. *Journal of Craniofacial Surgery* 9:127-129, 1998.

Rohrich RJ, Rowsell AR, Johns DF, Drury MA, Grieg G, Watson DJ, Godfrey AM, and Poole MD: Timing of hard palatal closure: a critical long-term analysis. *Plastic and Reconstructive Surgery* 98:236-246, 1996.

Rosenstein S, Dado D, Kernahan D, Griffith BH, and Grasseschi M: The case for early bone grafting in cleft lip and palate: a second report. *Plastic and Reconstructive Surgery* 87:644-654, 1991a.

Rosenstein S, Kernahan D, Dado D, Grasseschi M, and Griffith BH: Orthognathic surgery in cleft patients treated by early bone grafting. *Plastic and Reconstructive Surgery* 87:835-839, 1991b.

Rosenstein S, Monroe C, Kernahan D, Jacobson B, Griffith B, and Bauer B: The case for early bone grafting in cleft lip and cleft palate. *Plastic and Reconstructive Surgery* 70:297-305, 1982.

Ross RB: Treatment variables affecting facial growth in complete unilateral cleft lip and palate. *Cleft Palate Journal* 24:54-77, 1987.

Ruberg RL, Randall P, and Whitaker LA: Preservation of a posterior pharyngeal flap during maxillary advancement. *Plastic and Reconstructive Surgery* 57:336-337, 1976.

Ruscello CM, Tekieli ME, Jakomis T, Cook L, and Van Sickles JE: The effects of orthognathic surgery on speech production. *American Journal of Orthodontics* 89:237-241, 1986.

Salomonson J: Preserving aesthetic units in cleft lip repair. *Scandinavian Journal of Plastic and Reconstructive Surgery and Hand Surgery* 30:111-120, 1996.

Salomonson J: Minimizing external incisions in cleft lip and nasal reconstruction. Proceedings of the 55th annual meeting of the American Cleft Palate–Craniofacial Association, Baltimore, April 22, 1998.

Salomonson J, Kawamoto H, and Wilson L: Velopharyngeal incompetence as the presenting symptom of myotonic dystrophy. *Cleft Palate Journal* 25:296-300, 1988.

Salyer KE: Primary correction of the unilateral cleft nose: a 15-year experience. *Plastic and Reconstructive Surgery* 77:558-566, 1986.

Salyer KE: Primary correction of the nasal deformity associated with cleft lip. In Cohen M (ed.): *Mastery of plastic and reconstructive surgery.* Volume 1. Boston: Little, Brown, 1994, pp. 518-594.

Schendel SA, Pearl RM, and DeArmond SJ: Pathophysiology of cleft lip muscles following the initial surgical repair. *Plastic and Reconstructive Surgery* 88:197-200, 1991.

Schendel SA, Oeschlaeger M, Wolford LM, and Epker BN: Velopharyngeal anatomy and maxillary advancement. *Journal of Maxillofacial Surgery* 7:116-124, 1979.

Schwartz MF, McCarthy JG, Coccaro P, Wood-Smith D, and Converse JM: Velopharyngeal function following maxillary advancement. In Converse JM, McCarthy J, and Wood-Smith D (eds.): *Symposium on diagnosis and treatment of craniofacial anomalies.* St. Louis: Mosby, 1979, pp. 279-281.

Schwarz C, and Gruner E: Logopaedic findings following advancement of the maxilla. *Journal of Maxillofacial Surgery* 4:40-50, 1976.

Schweckendiek W: Primary veloplasty. In Schuchardt K (ed.): *Treatment of patients with cleft lip, alveolus, and palate.* Stuttgart: Thiem, 1966, pp. 85-87.

Schweckendiek W: Primary veloplasty: long-term results without maxillary deformity. *Cleft Palate Journal* 15:268-274, 1978.

Schweckendiek W, and Kruse E: Two-stage palatoplasty: Schweckendiek technique. In Bardach J, and Morris HL (eds.): *Multidisciplinary management of cleft lip and palate.* Philadelphia: WB Saunders, 1990, pp. 315-320.

Seyfer AE, and Simon CD: Long-term results following the repair of palatal clefts: a comparison of three different techniques. *Plastic and Reconstructive Surgery* 83:785-790, 1989.

Shelton RL Jr, and Blank J: Oronasal fistulas, intraoral air pressure, and nasal air flow during speech. *Cleft Palate Journal* 21:91-99, 1984.

Shprintzen RJ, Lewin ML, Croft C, Daniller A, Argamaso R, Ship A, and Strauch B: A comprehensive study of pharyngeal flap surgery: tailor made flaps. *Cleft Palate Journal* 16:46-55, 1979.

Skoog T: A design for the repair of unilateral cleft lips. *American Journal of Surgery* 95:223-226, 1958.

Skoog T: The management of the bilateral cleft of the primary palate (lip and alveolus). II: Bone grafting. *Plastic and Reconstructive Surgery* 35:140-147, 1965.

Skoog T: Skoog's methods of repair of unilateral and bilateral cleft lip. In Grabb W, Rosenstein S, and Bzoch KR (eds.): *Cleft lip and palate: surgical, dental and speech aspects.* Boston: Little, Brown, 1971, pp. 288-305.

Smahel Z, and Mullerova Z: Effects of primary periosteoplasty on facial growth in unilateral cleft lip and palate: 10-year follow-up. *Cleft Palate–Craniofacial Journal* 25:356-361, 1988.

Stark RB, and DeHaan CR: The addition of a pharyngeal flap to primary palatoplasty. *Plastic and Reconstructive Surgery* 26:378-387, 1960.

Stark RB, DeHaan CR, Frileck SP, and Burgess PD: Primary pharyngeal flap. *Cleft Palate Journal* 6:381-383, 1969.

Stellmach R: Prevention of velopharyngeal insufficiency following palatoplasty by velopharynx adhesion. *Fortschritte Kiefer Gesichts-chirurgie* 30:145-147, 1985.

Subtelny JD: A cephalometric study of the growth of the soft palate. *Plastic and Reconstructive Surgery* 19:49-62, 1957.

Tachimura T, Hara H, Koh H, and Wada T: Effect of temporary closure of oronasal fistulae on levator veli palatini muscle activity. *Cleft Palate–Craniofacial Journal* 34:505-511, 1997.

Tanino R, Akamatsu T, Nishimura M, Miyasaka M, and Osada M: The influence of different types of hard-palate closure in two-stage palatoplasty on maxillary growth: cephalometric analyses and long-term follow-up. *Annals of Plastic Surgery* 39:245-253, 1997.

Tennison CW: Repair of unilateral cleft lip by the stencil method. *Plastic and Reconstructive Surgery* 9:115-120, 1952.

Toth BA, Kim JW, Chin M, and Cedars M: Distraction osteogenesis and its application to the midface and bony orbit in craniosynostosis syndromes. *Journal of Craniofacial Surgery* 9:100-113, 1998.

Trauner R, and Trauner M: Result of cleft lip and palate operations. *Transactions of the Fourth International Congress on Plastic and Reconstructive Surgery,* 1967, pp. 429-434.

Trier WC, and Dreyer TM: Primary von Langenbeck palatoplasty with levator reconstruction: rationale and technique. *Cleft Palate Journal* 21:254-262, 1984.

Trigos I, and Ysunza A: A comparison of palatoplasty with and without primary pharyngoplasty. *Cleft Palate Journal* 25:163-166, 1988.

Turvey TA, Warren DW, and Dalston RM: Alterations in velopharyngeal function after maxillary advancement in cleft palate patients. *Journal of Oral and Maxillofacial Surgery* 48:685-689, 1990.

Turvey TA, Vig K, Moriarty J, and Hoke J: Delayed bone grafting in the cleft maxilla and palate: a retrospective multidisciplinary analysis. *American Journal of Orthodontics* 86:244-256, 1984.

Vallino LD: Speech, velopharyngeal function and hearing before and after orthognathic surgery. *Journal of Oral and Maxillofacial Surgery* 48:1274-1281, 1990.

Van Demark DR: Commentary on Vedung S: pharyngeal flaps after one- and two-stage repair of the cleft palate: a 25-year review of 520 patients. *Cleft Palate–Craniofacial Journal* 32:216, 1995.

Van Demark DR, and Hardin MA: Longitudinal evaluation of articulation and velopharyngeal competence of patients with pharyngeal flaps. *Cleft Palate Journal* 22:163-172, 1985.

Van Demark DR, Gnoinski W, Hotz MM, Perko M, and Naussbaumer H: Speech results of the Zurich approach in the treatment of unilateral cleft lip and palate. *Plastic and Reconstructive Surgery* 83:605-613, 1989.

Veau V: *Division palatine.* Paris: Masson et Cie., 1931.

Veau V: *Bec-de-lievre.* Paris: Masson et Cie, 1938.

Vedung S: Pharyngeal flaps after one- and two-stage repair of the cleft palate: a 25-year review of 520 patients. *Cleft Palate–Craniofacial Journal* 32:206-215, 1995.

Velasco MG, Ysunza A, Hernandez X, and Marquez C: Diagnosis and treatment of submucous cleft palate: a review of 108 cases. *Cleft Palate Journal* 25:171-173, 1988.

Von Langenbeck B: Operation der angeborenen totalen Spaltung des harten Gaumens nach either neuen Methode. *Deutsches Archiv fur Klinische Medizin* 13:231, 1861.

Wardill WEM: Technique of operation for cleft palate. *British Journal of Surgery* 25:117-130, 1937.

Watzke I, Turvey TA, Warren DW, and Dalston RM: Alterations in velopharyngeal function after maxillary advancement in cleft palate patients. *Journal of Oral and Maxillofacial Surgery* 48:685-689, 1990.

Widmaier W: A surgery procedure for the closure of palatal clefts. In Schuchardt K (ed.): *Treatment of patients with cleft lip, alveolus, and palate.* Stuttgart: Thiem, 1966, pp. 87-89.

Wilhelmsen HR, and Musgrave RH: Complications of cleft lip surgery. *Cleft Palate Journal* 3:223-231, 1966.

Witt PD, and D'Antonio LL: Velopharyngeal insufficiency and secondary palatal management: a new look at an old problem. *Clinics in Plastic Surgery* 20:707-721, 1993.

Witt PD, Marsh JL, Marty-Grames L, Muntz HR, and Gay HD: Management of the hypodynamic velopharynx. *Cleft Palate–Craniofacial Journal* 32:179-187, 1995.

Witzel MA: Commentary on Kummer AW, et al.: the effects of Le Fort I osteotomy with maxillary movement on articulation, resonance, and velopharyngeal function. *Cleft Palate Journal* 26:199-200, 1989.

Witzel MA, and Munro IR: Velopharyngeal insufficiency after maxillary advancement. *Cleft Palate Journal* 14:176-180, 1977.

Witzel MA, and Stringer DA: Methods of assessing velopharyngeal function. In Bardach J, and Morris HL (eds.): *Multidisciplinary management of cleft lip and palate.* Philadelphia: WB Saunders, 1990, pp. 763-776.

Witzel MA, Ross RB, and Munro IR: Articulation before and after facial osteotomy. *Journal of Maxillofacial Surgery* 8:195-202, 1980.

Witzel MA, Salyer KE, and Ross RB: Delayed hard palate closure: the philosophy revisited. *Cleft Palate Journal* 21:263-269, 1984.

Witzel MA, Clarke J, Lindsay WK, and Thomson H: Comparison of results of pushback or von Langenbeck repair of isolated cleft of the hard and soft palate. *Plastic and Reconstructive Surgery* 64:347-352, 1979.

Wu J, Chen YR, and Noordhoff MS: Articulation proficiency and error pattern of cleft palate children with delayed hard palate closure. *Annals of the Academy of Medicine of Singapore* 17:384-387, 1988.

Wynn S: Bone-flap technique in cleft palate surgery. In Georgiade N (eds.): *Symposium on cleft lip and palate and associated deformities.* St. Louis: Mosby, 1974.

Wynn S: Long-term results after cleft palate closure by bilateral osteotomy technique. *Plastic and Reconstructive Surgery* 58:71-79, 1976.

Younger R, and Dickson R: Adult pharyngoplasty for velopharyngeal insufficiency. *Journal of Otolaryngology* 14:158-162, 1985.

Ysunza A, Guerrero M, Pamplona M, Loreto F, and Garcia-Velasco M: Speech outcome of surgical repair of cleft palate: the effect of age at the time of surgery. Proceedings of the annual meeting of the Society for Ear, Nose, and Throat Advances in Children (SENTAC), Sacramento, December 2, 1994.

Chapter 5

Dental Management of Cleft Lip and Palate

Dental specialists participate in the physical habilitation of patients with clefts throughout the growing years of the child and adolescent and also in the adult years when not all the proper care was available in childhood. The "time-ordered agenda" of dental care may seem a little surprising to clinicians who are new to the care of children with clefts, in that it is actually the team *orthodontist* who meets with families of newborns as part of the first infant evaluations. This is because it is the orthodontist who is the specialist in the growth and development of the craniofacial complex, working with the surgeons in planning how various physical treatment strategies are likely to affect (and be affected by) that growth. As you would expect, the *family dentist* or *pediatric dentist* provides regular dental care for the child, which should start no later than the age of 2 years. The pediatric dentist may also be involved in the fabrication of early feeding plates, although the use of such plates is not universally accepted as a necessary part of the care of these infants. The orthodontist provides or makes the treatment plans for straightening the teeth and guiding the upper and lower jaws into the best possible occlusal relationship. This may involve active treatment at several ages in the child's life. The orthodontist also monitors the growth of the craniofacial complex. The involvement of the *prosthodontist* depends on the particular treatment plans for that child and may include early obturating plates used for a variety of purposes, a palatal lift or "speech bulb" obturator if surgical management has not provided adequate velopharyngeal function, and prosthetic replacement of missing teeth. Finally, an *oral surgeon* (often someone with double degrees, one in medicine and one in dentistry) participates in bone grafts, dental extractions, and the placement of endosseous dental implants. On some teams, oral surgeons repair the cleft itself, as discussed in Chapter 4. They may also be the surgeons who perform the midface advancements discussed in Chapter 4.

Because dental development and the dental anomalies that are frequent in children with clefts can affect speech production, it is important for you to have a basic understanding of normal development of the teeth and occlusion, discussed in the following section.

NORMAL DENTAL DEVELOPMENT

Normal Dentition

The *primary dentition* (also called "deciduous dentition" and sometimes "milk teeth" or "baby teeth") consists of 20 teeth (Fig. 5-1). The lower central incisors erupt first and then the remaining teeth according to the sequence indicated in Fig. 5-1. Most children have all of their primary dentition in place by the age of 2½ years. By the age of 6 or 7 years, they are beginning the "mixed dentition" phase, when the primary teeth are gradually being replaced by the permanent teeth.

There are 32 teeth in the *permanent dentition;* this number depends on whether the third molars or "wisdom teeth" (the most posterior teeth on each side of each dental arch) erupt (Fig. 5-2). Again, the lower central incisors erupt first, followed by the upper centrals, the lateral incisors, the canines (cuspids), and the first, second, and third molars in order. In general, the eruption of the lower or second teeth is slightly before the eruption of the maxillary teeth. Impacted wisdom teeth—teeth that do not erupt normally because they are malpositioned in the alveolar ridge or because there is not enough room in the arch for them to erupt—constitute one of the most common dental problems in adults, regardless of whether they have clefts.

Occlusion

The main reference points for describing occlusion are the maxillary and mandibular first molars. How these molars are positioned with respect to each other determines how the orthodontist categorizes the occlusion (Fig. 5-3). The

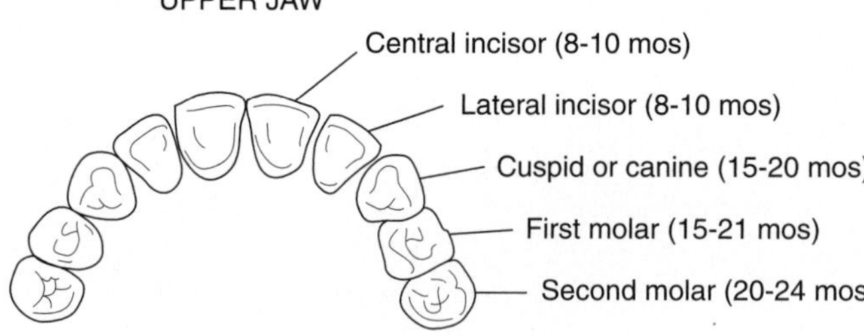

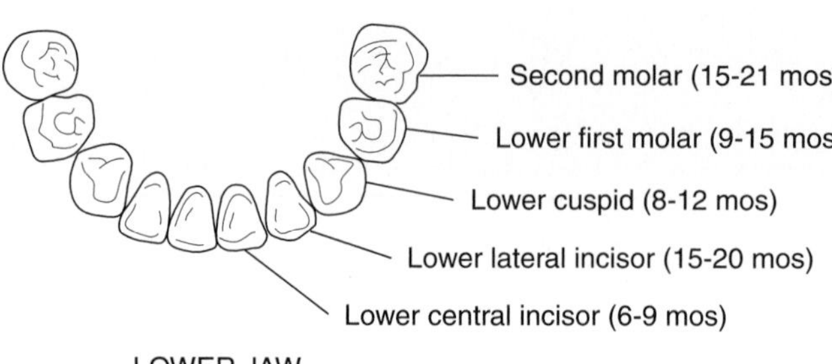

Figure 5-1 The primary dentition and the timing of normal tooth eruption.

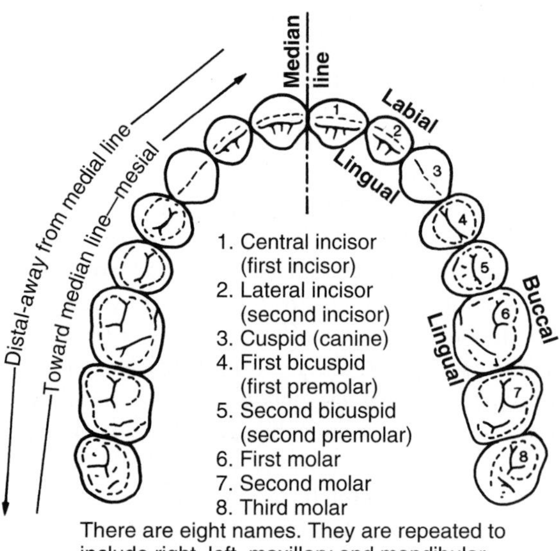

Figure 5-2 The permanent dentition in an adult dental arch and terms used for orientation (distal, medial, labial, buccal). *(Wheeler:* Textbook of dental anatomy and physiology. *Philadelphia: WB Saunders, 1940. p. 7.)*

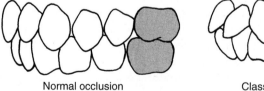

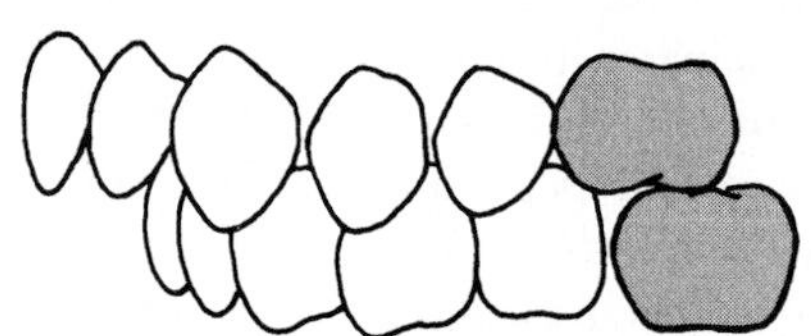

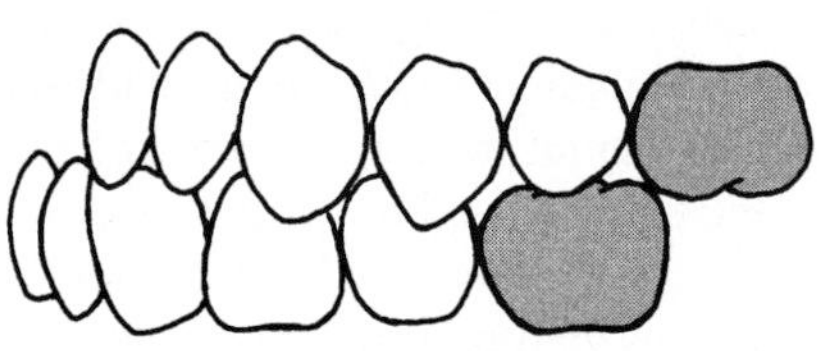

Class II malocclusion

Class III malocclusion

Figure 5-3 Normal occlusion and malocclusion classes as specified by Angle. *(From Proffit WR:* Contemporary orthodontics. *3rd ed. St. Louis: Mosby, 2000, p. 4.)*

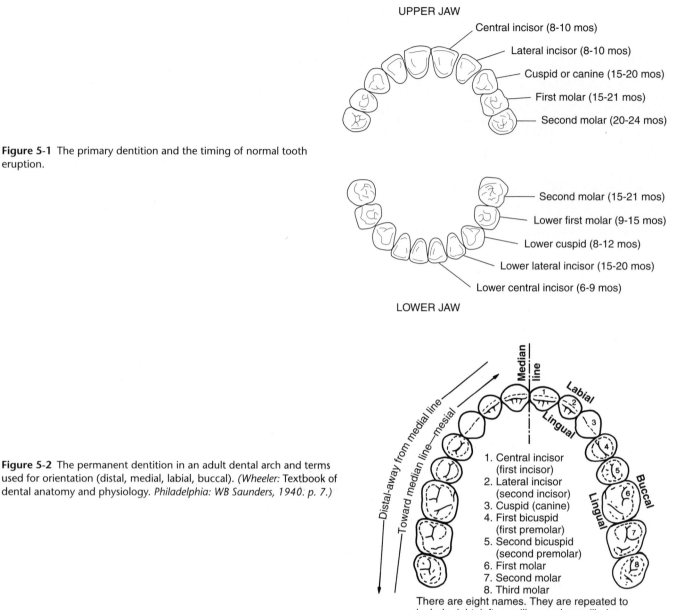

maxillary arch is normally slightly wider than the mandibular arch, so to some extent fits over it, as pictured in Fig. 5-3. That is, the teeth in the maxillary arch are expected to be about a half-tooth overlapping their counterparts in the mandibular arch, and the molar occlusion is such that the inner cusps (the cusps nearer the tongue) of the upper teeth fit into the central grooves between the cusps in the lower teeth. In normal occlusion, there is a *slight* "overjet" and also "overbite" of the anterior maxillary teeth in relationship to the anterior mandibular teeth, as illustrated in Fig. 5-4. Table 5-1 lists additional terms used in the description of normal and abnormal occlusion.

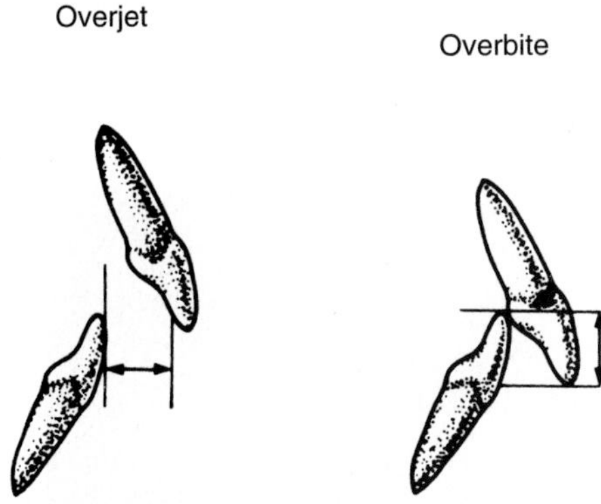

Figure 5-4 Relationship between the upper and lower incisors in overjet and overbite. *(From Hall DJ, and Warren DW:* Orthodontic problems in children. *In Bluestone CD, and Stool SE [eds.]:* Pediatric otolaryngology. *Volume 2. Philadelphia: WB Saunders, 1983, p. 966.)*

Additional Notes About Open Bites

An anterior open bite is more likely than a posterior open bite to be of concern to speech pathologists. Two of the most common causes of anterior open bites, unrelated to clefts, are (1) nasopharyngeal airway obstruction and (2) thumb sucking. When the nasopharyngeal airway is significantly crowded or obstructed, the child becomes an obligate oronasal breather or mouth breather.[1] Over time, the mouth-open posture can lead to overeruption of the posterior teeth, so that, even if the obstruction is resolved (by adenoidectomy, natural adenoid involution, nasoseptal reconstruction, or simply growth), the anterior teeth are still prevented from meeting. The mouth-open posture also leads to abnormal configuration of the palatal vault: With the mouth constantly open, there is not the normal apposition of the tongue against the vault, leading to inward or medial collapse of the lateral maxillary segments or to hypertrophy (overdevelopment) of alveolar tissue or to

[1]The commonly used term is "mouth breather." However, unless nasal airflow is documented by appropriate aerodynamic studies (see Chapter 10) to be nonexistent in a given individual, it cannot be assumed that *all* the airflow of breathing is going in and out the mouth simply because that individual breathes with the mouth open. Thus respiratory physiologists prefer the term "oronasal."

Table 5-1 **A Listing of Common Terms Used to Describe Dental and Occlusal Anomalies**

Term	*Description*
Crossbite	Maxillary teeth inside (or "lingual" to) mandibular teeth
Anterior crossbite (Fig. 5-5)	Maxillary incisors behind mandibular incisors, may describe only single teeth or all incisors
Canine crossbite	Crossbite of the canine teeth
Lateral crossbite (Fig. 5-6) (also called "buccal" or "lingual" crossbite)	Crossbite of the teeth in the lateral segment or segment nearest the cheek
Neutroclusion (Class I molar relationship) (Fig. 5-3)	The "sagittal" (front-to-back) relationship of the jaws is normal but there may be malalignment of individual teeth or a discrepancy in jaw position in the "transverse" or horizontal plane.
Class II molar relationship (Figs. 5-3 and 5-7)	Maxillary teeth more anterior to the mandibular teeth than normal, with a larger overjet. Often accompanied by excessive vertical overlap of the maxillary incisors over the mandibular incisors, also called "closed bite," "deep bite," or "overbite"
Class III molar relationship (Figs. 5-3 and 5-8)	Maxillary molars posterior to mandibular molars. Usually accompanied by anterior "crossbite" or "underbite," although sometimes the anterior mandibular teeth are tipped backward ("retroclined") so that they still fit behind the anterior maxillary teeth.*
Anterior open bite (Fig. 5-9)	Open space between the anterior maxillary and mandibular teeth. Often the result of finger habit or habitual open-mouth breathing
Posterior open bite (Fig. 5-10)	Open space between the maxillary and mandibular teeth (molars or molars plus bicuspids)

*As you may have suspected by now, nondentists often confuse the terms that should be used to describe only the molar relationship (Class I, Class II, Class III) with the terms used to describe the relationship between the anterior maxillary and mandibular teeth (overbite, overjet, underbite, crossbite).

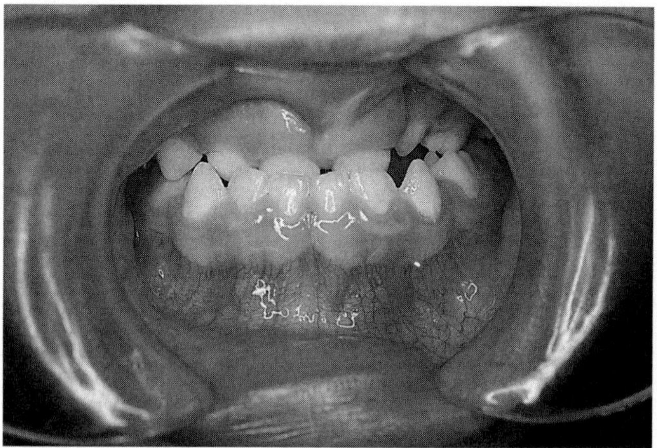

Figure 5-5 Patient with an anterior crossbite.

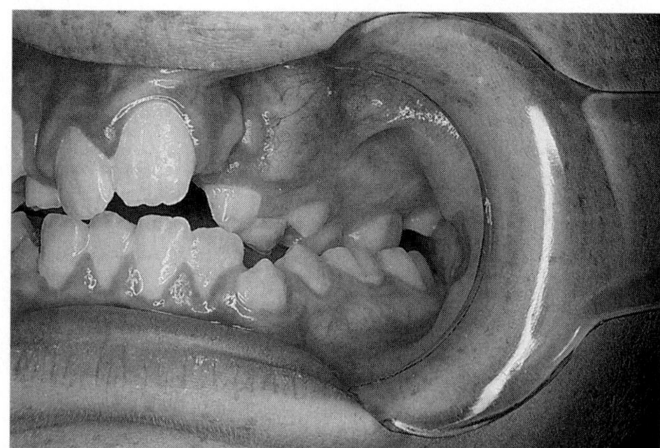

Figure 5-6 Patient with a canine and buccal crossbite.

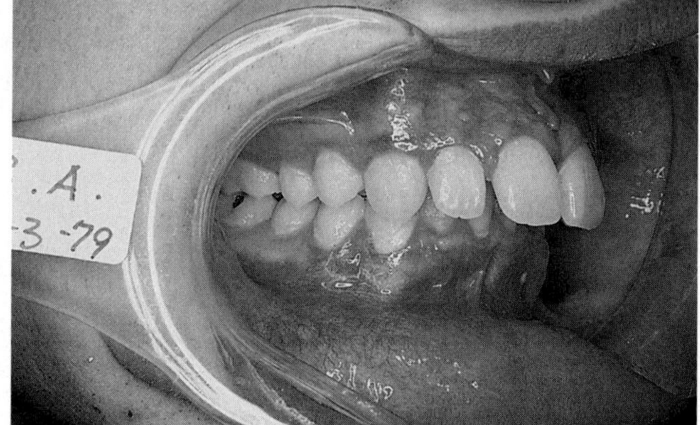

Figure 5-7 Patient with a Class II malocclusion.

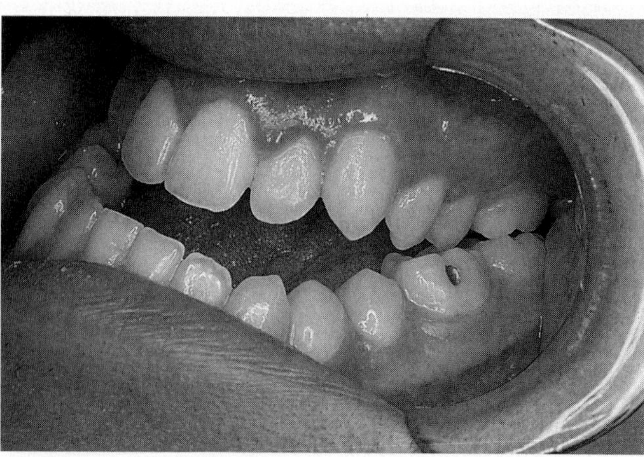

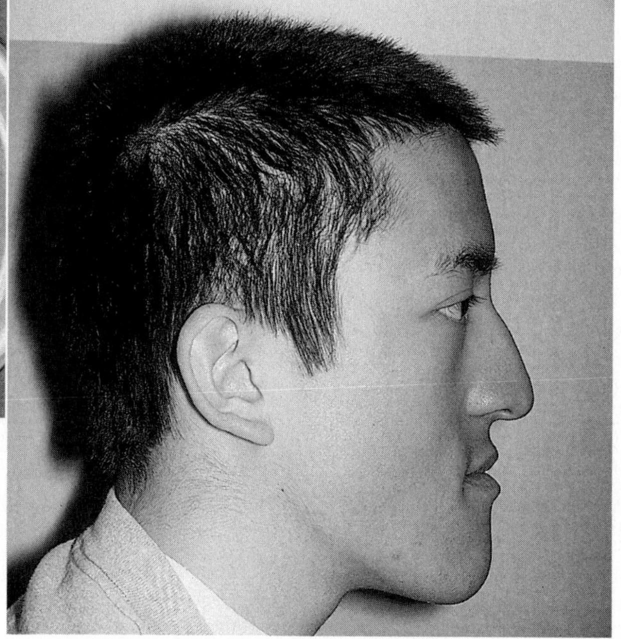

Figure 5-8 Intraoral and profile views of a patient with a Class III malocclusion.

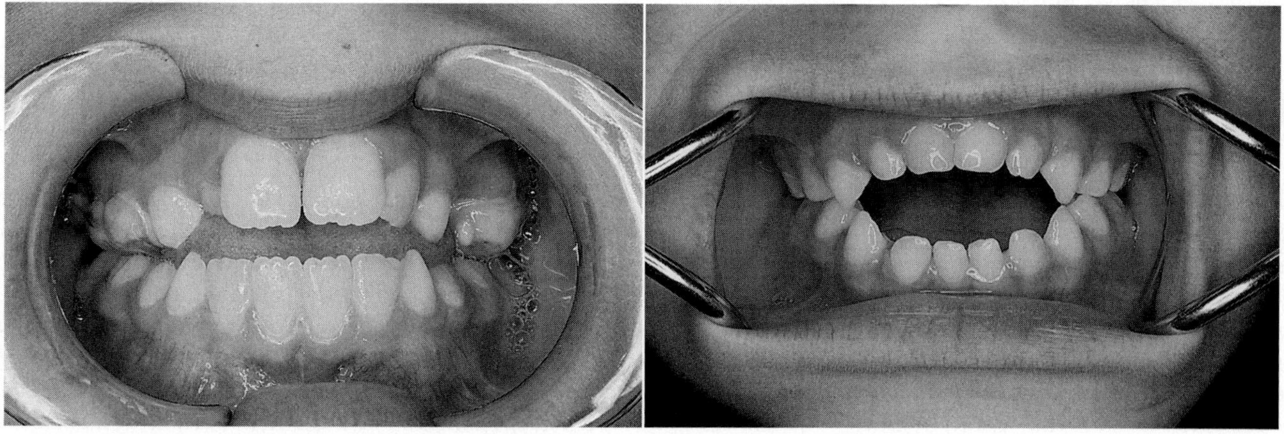

Figure 5-9 Two patients with anterior open bites, one far more severe than the other.

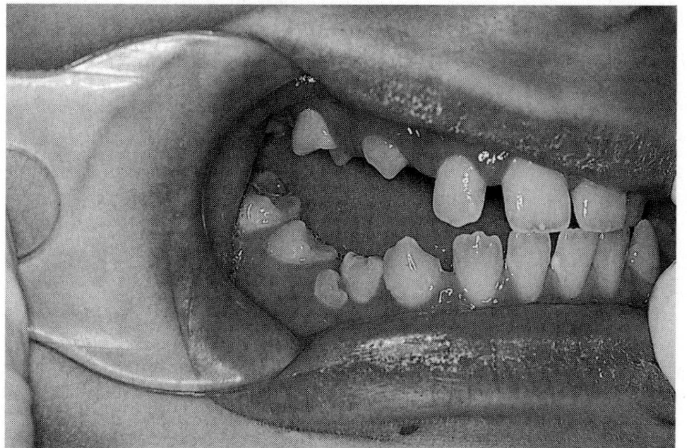

Figure 5-10 Patient with a posterior open bite.

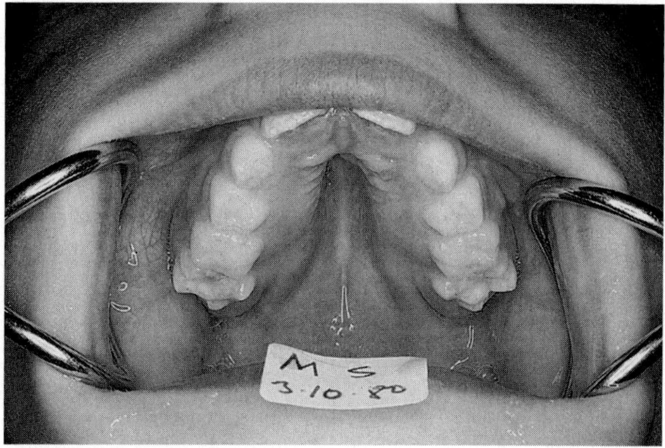

Figure 5-11 The intraoral view that often leads clinicians to use the term "high-arched palate."

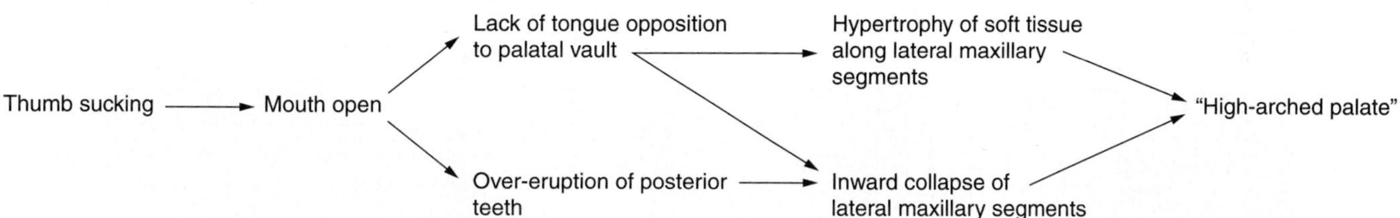

Figure 5-12 Sequence of events cascading from thumb sucking and leading to the subjective impression of a "high-arched palate," often mistakenly assumed to be a cause of speech problems.

both. On the intraoral examination the clinician gets the subjective impression of a "high-arched" palate even though the vertical level of the palatal plane is normal (Fig. 5-11).[2] A similar sequence of events can be initiated by thumb sucking, as diagramed in Fig. 5-12. Unfortunately, the inexperienced clinician may make an automatic assumption that a palatal vault such as that shown in Fig. 5-11 is responsible for speech problems. That is, the clinician may conclude (1) that a speech problem such as velopharyngeal inadequacy must be present even though he or she has not detected it perceptually, (2) that the abnormal vault is an adequate explanation for velopharyngeal inadequacy, or (3) that the abnormal vault is a cause of abnormal articulatory contacts in speech.

Posterior open bite occurs when there is an uneven plane

[2]"High-arched palate" is, at best, a descriptive term with limited meaning and should not be considered a diagnosis.

of the maxilla or mandible (side to side, or front to back), so that the teeth on one side of the mouth "meet first" as the jaws come together and the remaining teeth cannot meet. A unilateral posterior open bite is common in hemifacial microsomia, before all aspects of treatment are completed, because the transverse (horizontal) plane of the mandible is not even. Another cause of posterior open bite, unilateral or bilateral, is incomplete eruption of teeth, so that they do not meet the occlusal plane. Clinical insight tells us that the abnormal space between the maxillary and mandibular teeth such as that shown in Fig. 5-10 may result in lateral emission of the oral air stream in articulation and/or the tongue protruding into this space in speech, but there are no published data proving this to be true.

There may be asymmetrical jaw relationships (for example, normal occlusion on one side but a crossbite on the other). This is particularly common in clefts but occurs in individuals without clefts as well.

DENTITION AND OCCLUSION IN CLEFT LIP AND PALATE

Dental Anomalies

Dental eruption may be delayed in individuals with clefts, particularly boys with unilateral clefts, but no one has derived a unified theory for why dental eruption should be differentially affected by gender or by cleft-type subgroups (Jordon, Kraus, and Neptune, 1966; Loevy and Aduss, 1988; Prahl-Anderson, 1976; Ranta, 1971, 1972; Solis et al., 1998). Ross (1975) reported that children with cleft palate alone (with no cleft of the lip or alveolus) also have a high incidence of missing permanent lateral incisors. In data from older studies, there is always the "hindsight" doubt as to whether all the children in the study were actually free of any syndromes in which delayed dental development might have been part of the syndromic picture.[3] However, a recent comprehensive study of 109 patients with isolated cleft palate reported congenitally missing permanent teeth (third molars or "wisdom" teeth excluded) in 30% of patients and ectopic eruption of the first permanent molars in 37% (Larson, Hellquist, and Jakobsson, 1998).

Some of the dental problems in clefts affect the primary dentition, but more problems become apparent only when the permanent dentition erupts. There may be a fused central + lateral incisor in the primary dentition (Fig. 5-13), but this does not mean that the central and lateral incisors will be fused in the permanent teeth. A missing lateral incisor on the side of the cleft is quite common in the permanent dentition of children with clefts. It is something of a paradox that supernumerary teeth (Fig. 5-14) are also common (Vargervik, 1981); this is thought to be the result of the cleft dividing the developing tooth bud in two. Often the lateral incisor or canine erupts into the line of the alveolar cleft, sometimes "palatally," meaning that the tooth is behind the normal dental arch. It is important that palatally erupted teeth (or "lingually erupted," meaning toward the tongue) *not* be extracted simply because they are in the wrong place: they can be moved through orthodontic treatment, and all teeth should be preserved for the sake of jaw development.[4] Similarly, supernumerary teeth should not be extracted in growing children because they help to preserve the shape of the dental arch.

[3]Even in nonsyndromic children with clefts, there is a significantly greater probability of congenitally missing teeth, which can have worrisome effects on jaw development and facial proportions.

[4]When teeth are missing, the alveolar bone that would have been their "home" has no stimulus for development. Thus congenitally missing teeth produce a secondary deleterious effect on jaw growth and facial proportions.

A 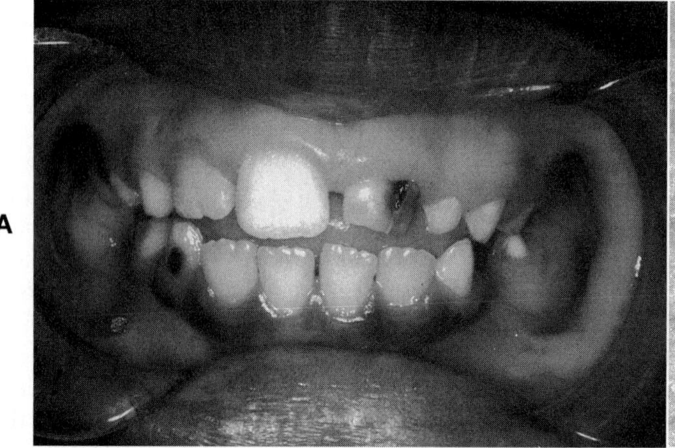

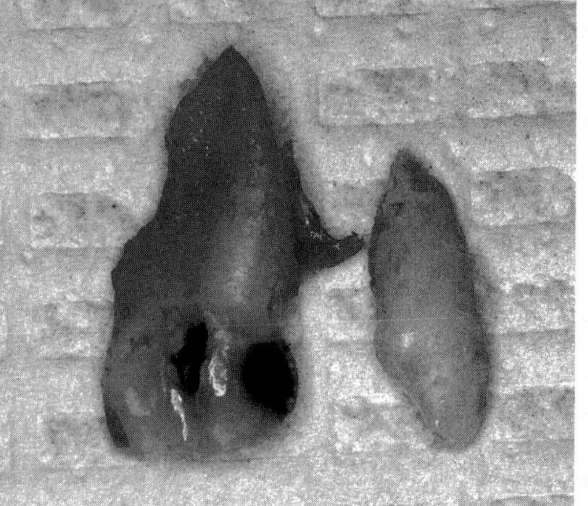 B

Figure 5-13 A fused central and lateral incisor (with a cavity) in the maxillary arch **(A)** and after extraction **(B)**, showing the two roots. A supernumerary tooth was also extracted.

In young children with clefts the spaces created by missing teeth or teeth that are late in erupting may contribute to oral distortion of complex consonants such as sibilants and affricates, but the effect is usually temporary. In our opinion, speech therapy to correct tongue placement on these consonants in the young child is not recommended because nature or the prosthodontist will fill the space.

Malocclusions[5]

Although there are individuals with clefts in whom the jaw relationships are normal, it is much more common for there to be a malocclusion, except in cases of cleft lip only. In unilateral cleft lip and palate there is often a lateral crossbite on the side of the cleft, that is, the lateral segment of the maxilla is positioned medially to its counterpart in the mandible. This is termed "arch collapse" (Fig. 5-15). In some children the malrelationship between the maxillary and mandibular teeth may be confined only to the teeth nearest the cleft, not affecting the rest of the dental arch, so that the molar relationship is in fact normal (Fig. 5-16), whereas in other children the entire lateral segment is medial to the teeth in the mandible, as shown in Fig. 5-15, *B.* Bilateral crossbite, meaning collapse of both arches in the maxilla, is often found in bilateral clefts but may also occur in unilateral clefts, particularly when there are congenitally missing teeth (Fig. 5-17). If the premaxilla is also positioned behind the anterior mandibular teeth, this is a full crossbite or a Class III malocclusion. In some cases the premaxilla may still be positioned anteriorly (in front of the mandibular teeth), with the lateral segments collapsed behind it (Fig. 5-18). Class II occlusions are relatively rare in clefts, except in those conditions in which the mandible is inherently small. Many children with Pierre Robin sequence show a Class II tendency in their early dentition because the mandible is small, but in the absence of a syndromic condition (see Chapter 2) the mandible in patients with Robin sequence usually grows forward. In contrast, in syndromes such as mandibulofacial dysostosis and Stickler syndrome maxillary-mandibular disproportion usually remains and may in fact become more marked with growth.

In Chapter 4, you learned about the controversy regarding the potential effects of timing and type of surgery on growth of the maxilla and thus on dental arch form and occlusion. Because clefts inherently involve not only a distortion in position of segments but a deficiency of tissue and growth potential, the controversy about effects of surgery is likely to continue well into the next century. For speech-language pathologists, it is helpful to keep in mind that dental and occlusal problems are likely to be present in nearly every schoolage or older child with a cleft until all orthodontic and surgical treatment has been completed. Although these problems may cause articulatory problems, they should be temporary. Consult with the treating team to learn what is likely to happen, and when, with respect to the patient's physical management.

Effects of Dental and Occlusal Problems on Speech

The dental and orthodontic literature contains some fairly consistent information regarding the effects of dental problems and malocclusions on speech. None of the information is particularly surprising. In general, this literature tells us that dental and occlusal problems are more likely to be causative factors in speech problems (1) when they occur in combination rather than singly, (2) when they are present during the speech-learning years as opposed to later years, and (3) when they influence the spatial relationship between the tip of the tongue and the incisors (Peterson-Falzone, 1994). The literature also indicates that speech problems are fairly common when there is a restriction in the size of the palatal vault and are more apt to be found in Class III occlusions compared with Class II (Peterson-Falzone, 1994). Children with clefts are obviously vulnerable to several of these problems: presence of dental or occlusal problems (possibly several at one time) during the speech-learning years, restriction in size of the palatal vault, and the possibility of Class III occlusions. The question is, Will the speech problems diminish as the dentition or occlusion improves? The literature indicates

[5]For nondentists, it is confusing that orthodontists assess two aspects of occlusion: the relationship between the jaws and the relationship of the teeth embedded in the jaws. The former is called the "skeletal" relationship and the latter the "dental" relationship. This distinction plays a role in assessing effects of treatment. For example, Peat (1982) found that presurgical orthopedics had a significant beneficial effect (in comparison to babies without such treatment) on the eventual incidence of dental crossbites but not on skeletal development. For speech-language pathologists, the difference may seem obscure and trivial. But the former (dental) problems are more easily treatable than the latter (skeletal) and thus are less likely to have long-term effects on speech.

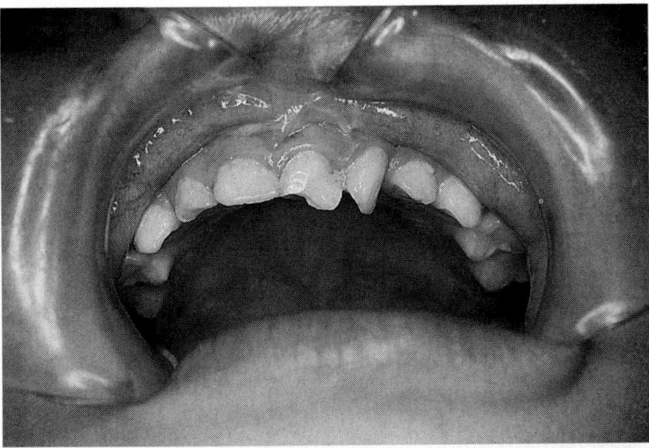

Figure 5-14 This individual has at least one supernumerary tooth (the fourth tooth from your right) and possibly two (note the anomalous central incisor, which appears to have an extra segment).

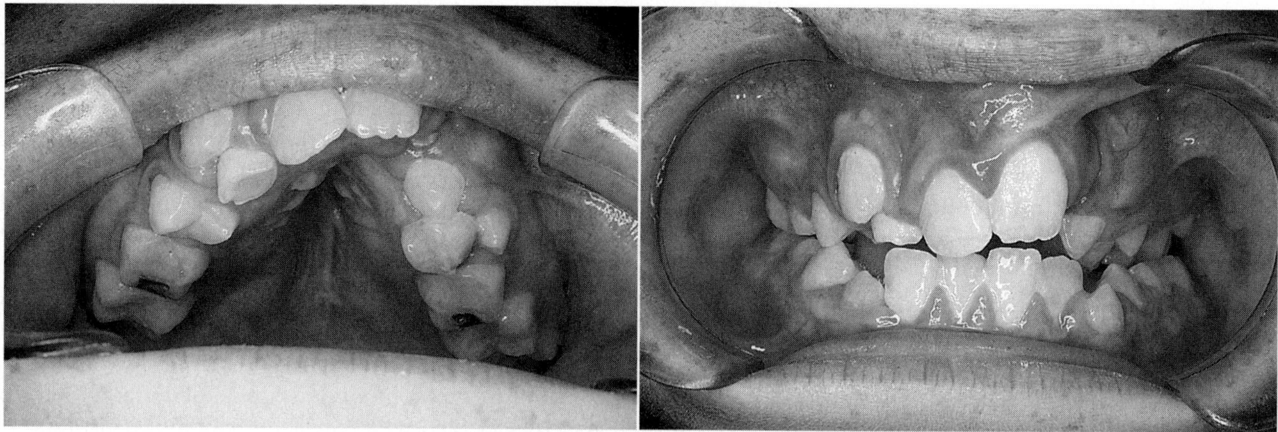

Figure 5-15 A patient with collapse of the left maxillary arch. This patient also has a labially erupted canine in the maxilla on his right side and a labially and distally erupted canine on his left.

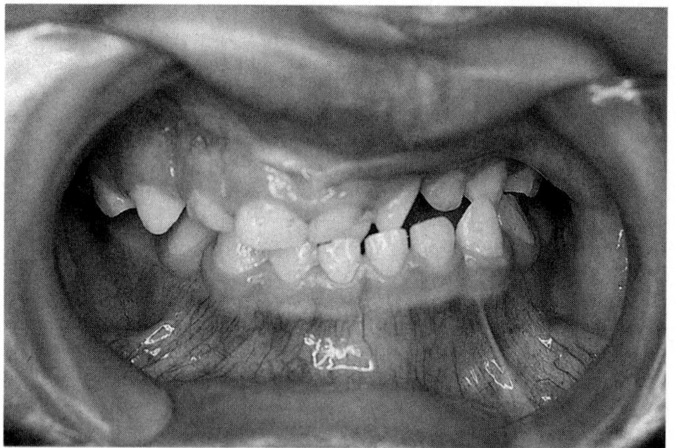

Figure 5-16 Patient with a crossbite only of the teeth nearest the cleft, with a normal molar relationship.

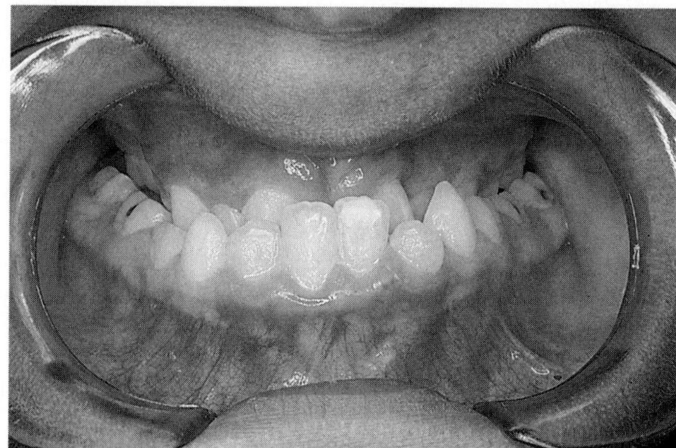

Figure 5-17 This patient had only a left unilateral cleft lip and palate but has a bilateral crossbite, a condition caused in part by multiple missing teeth in the maxillary arch.

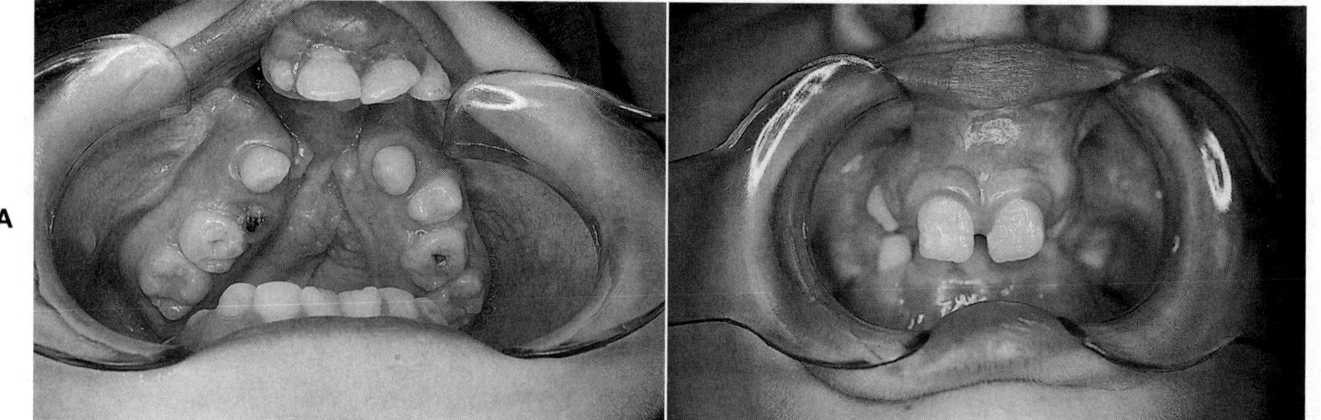

Figure 5-18 Both of these patients have a severely protrusive premaxilla, with the lateral segments collapsed behind it. In **A,** note also the alveolar defects and the pile-up of scar tissue (from the palatal repair) in the palatal vault. The alveolar clefts are also unrepaired in **B,** but the segments abut one another.

that in many children they will, but this remains a question that must be answered only through longitudinal follow-up with each child.

DENTAL PROBLEMS AND THEIR TREATMENT AS CHILDREN GROW

It is useful to consider dental or occlusal problems in children with clefts from a longitudinal perspective, that is, what problems or issues arise at what time in the child's development. Reviews of this type were offered by Cooper et al. (1979) and by Vargervik (1990, 1995), all of whom are orthodontists with extensive experience working in cleft palate–craniofacial treatment centers. This same developmental approach serves as the framework for the remainder of this chapter.

The First Few Months of Life

Feeding plates.[6] One of the most emotionally loaded issues in dealing with children with clefts is feeding and growth in the neonatal period. Parents need to feel that they can nourish and care for their babies, to bond with them, and to feel confident that their babies will thrive like noncleft babies. It has long been known that infants with clefts frequently exhibit problems in early weight gain and growth. These problems have most often been attributed to difficulties in establishing an adequate suckle-and-swallow sequence in the presence of an open cleft because of the inability to create negative intraoral pressure. Reviews of feeding issues were offered by Clarren, Anderson, and Wolf (1987), Jones (1988), Paradise and McWilliams (1974), and Seth and McWilliams (1988). Asher (1986) discussed the various approaches taken to feeding appliances or combination feeding/presurgical orthopedic appliances in European centers as of the mid-1980s. Ten years later Habel, Sell, and Mars (1996) found that use of "baby plates" had been standard in many British centers for 50 years and once again concluded that there had been no evidence to support or indeed refute any of the claims for the benefits of these plates with respect to speech and facial growth. As they put it, "The practice [using baby plates] remains empirical."[7]

Of some importance here is the concern for how feeding methods should or should not be altered as the baby goes through surgery. Historically, surgeons and other members of cleft palate/craniofacial teams felt that infants with clefts should not return to any form of nipple feeding immediately after cleft lip repair but should be exclusively spoon-fed for a set period of time. In 1992 a consortium of nurses from four cleft palate/craniofacial centers presented their results on post-cleft-lip-repair feeding, and concluded that there was no advantage for special feeding techniques during this period (Boekelheide et al., 1992). Babies who returned to their preoperative nipple feedings immediately after lip surgery did not exhibit any higher rates of postoperative lip dehiscences or decreases in oral fluid intake than did babies who were temporarily switched to other forms of feeding (e.g., spoon feeding). On a practical basis, surgeons and teams continue to recommend whatever technique for oral feeding they feel will be least likely to adversely affect the operative site, without causing anything more than a short-term interruption in the child's preoperative feeding routine.

Several studies have demonstrated growth deficiencies in children with clefts even beyond infancy (Cunningham and Jerome, 1997; Duncan et al., 1983; Jensen, Dahl and Kreiborg, 1983; Laron, Taube, and Kaplan, 1969; Ranalli and Mazaheri, 1975). It is important to note that an inborn growth hormone deficiency has been documented to occur in many children with clefts (Frances et al., 1966; Goumy, Dalens, and Malpuech, 1978; Raggazzini, La Cauza, and Marianelli, 1978; Rudman et al., 1978). The relationship is logical because the master gland for growth is the pituitary gland, the anterior portion of which (called the "hypophysis") (1) secretes growth hormone and (2) is embryologically the product of invagination of the end of the roof of the buccal cavity (called "Rathke's pouch"), which extends upward early during embryological migration. This development is closely related to that of the facial structures, so it is logical that congenital malformations of the facial bones could cause anatomical and functional disturbances of the anterior pituitary gland (Laron, Taube, and Kaplan, 1969; Raggazzini, La Causa, and Marinalli, 1978).[8] Earlier, Rintala and Gylling (1967) reported that birth weights for children with clefts were below average and seemed to be correlated with the severity of the anomaly, which caused the authors to speculate that birth weight was possibly also correlated with the "mechanism of production" of the anomaly. In total, there seems to be ample evidence that growth deficiencies in children with clefts are not necessarily the direct result of feeding problems.

Many kinds of feeding devices or schemes have been recommended for babies with clefts, including special nipples, special bottles, "feeding plates," and combinations

[6]The topic of feeding plates arises in this chapter because, when they are used, such plates are fitted by dental specialists (pediatric dentists, orthodontists, prosthodontists) and also because such plates are often multipurpose devices fabricated with the goal of guiding the early growth and development of the palatal segments and premaxilla.

[7]Kelly, Sorenson, and Turner (1978) designed an infant plate for obturation of the palate and a presumed aid in feeding for a baby with Pierre Robin sequence. Their plate also incorporated a posterior extension in the form of a wire loop fitted over the dorsum of the tongue that was supposed to position the dorsum further forward, creating a better airway for the child. However, no follow-up data were included and this report did not lead to a proliferation of reports of similar devices for Robin infants.

[8]Because clinicians see so many children with clefts who appear to be clinically normal apart from the cleft itself, it becomes difficult to remember that clefts are in essence midline defects (even those that are not truly "median" clefts [see Chapter 1]), which carry with them the potential for far-reaching functional disorders. This will be examined more closely in Chapter 14.

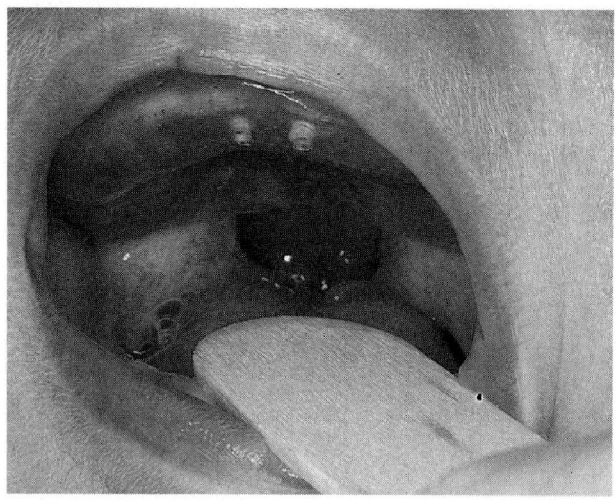

Figure 5-19 This baby has a small plate that resembles the "feeding plates" used in some cleft palate treatment programs.

of feeding plates and molding devices for control of the position of the lateral maxillary segments (Fig. 5-19) (Asher, 1986; Balluff and Udin, 1986; Choi et al., 1991; Fleming, Pielou, and Saunders, 1985; Graf-Pinthus and Bettex, 1974; Hotz, 1983; Hotz and Gnoinski, 1976; Huddart, 1967; Hummel, 1987; Jones, 1981; Jones and Kerkhof, 1984; Jones, Henderson, and Avery, 1982; Kelly, 1971; Komposch, 1986; Markowitz, Gerry, and Fleishner, 1979; Martin, 1983; Oliver, 1969; Paradise and McWilliams, 1974; Pashayan and McNab, 1979; Razek, 1980; Robertson and Hilton, 1971; Samant, 1989; Spira et al., 1969; Trankmann, 1986; Williams, Rothman, and Sedman, 1968). Some of these plates have been rather complicated in design. Claims of success in easing feeding and facilitating weight gain have varied from conservative to fervid, but many studies have been carried out only on small groups of dissimilar babies and often without control groups.

In general, depending on the location and severity of their clefts, infants with cleft lip and/or palate can do quite well in feeding once their caregivers are instructed in certain basic considerations such as placing the baby in a semi-upright position instead of a supine position (Delgado, Schaaf, and Emrich, 1992; Dunning, 1986; Paradise and McWilliams, 1974), use of soft-sided "squeezable bottles" and soft nipples perhaps with enlarged holes, and appropriate placement of that nipple on the tongue and into the noncleft side of the palate or, in bilateral clefts, against the larger palatine shelf.[9] Specialists in feeding problems of children with clefts caution caregivers to be certain that (1) the child is not expending so much energy in getting the milk or formula from the nipple that more calories are lost than gained during the feeding process and that (2) the flow of the formula is not so free that there is risk of choking, regurgitation, or aspiration. The one feeding method to be avoided in all but the most severely compromised babies is the use of a nasogastric tube, which bypasses the oral mechanism altogether and inhibits development of the necessary suckle-swallow feeding pattern, potentially leading to or contributing to oral aversion. Unfortunately, nasogastric tubes are still routinely resorted to in many neonatal nurseries where the personnel are not sufficiently knowledgable about feeding infants with clefts.

As of this writing, many speech-language pathologists are involved in the care of both pediatric and older patients without clefts who have a variety of feeding and swallowing disorders. In the context of a cleft palate or craniofacial team, it is more often the pediatrician or the nurse practitioner who assumes this responsibility (American Cleft Palate–Craniofacial Association, 1993). If you are dealing with an infant with a cleft whose feeding or weight gain is not satisfactory, you should (1) contact the child's pediatrician directly, (2) contact the cleft palate or craniofacial team caring for the child, and (3) if you cannot get appropriate help and support for the family locally, contact the Cleft Palate Foundation at 1-800-24-CLEFT. In any event, do not abandon the effort or assign the problem to someone else who may have little knowledge of the problem or of the resources.

Palatal plates before palatal surgery: a combined orthodontic-prosthodontic issue. In the chapter on surgical management of clefts, you were introduced to the controversy regarding whether better treatment results could be obtained in infants with clefts by using various means of manipulating the position of the cleft segments before surgical repair of the defects. This controversy is not likely to disappear. The literature is somewhat difficult to follow because many devices of different designs have been recommended for controlling or guiding the position of the lip, premaxilla, and palatal segments before surgery and because the "research" has been contaminated by the same variables that hamper efforts to document effects of treatment in virtually all areas of cleft lip and palate care: differences in clefts, differences in timing and length of intervention, differences in length of follow-up, etc. Although as a speech-language pathologist your involvement in this issue will be secondary, the topic is discussed here so that you will be familiar with the terms used in such treatment and the reasons why the controversy continues.

The goal of presurgical orthopedics in unilateral clefts of the lip and palate is to bring the cleft segment into alignment with the noncleft side to minimize the width of the defect. In bilateral clefts the goals are (1) to bring the unattached premaxilla into better alignment with both of the lateral alveolar segments and (2) to keep the lateral segments from moving inward behind the premaxilla both before and after lip surgery.

[9]Although infants with cleft palate may comprise a significant percentage of the infants that a feeding specialist might see, the inverse is *not* true, that is, the overall percentage of infants with clefts who have feeding problems is low once proper instruction has been provided to caregivers.

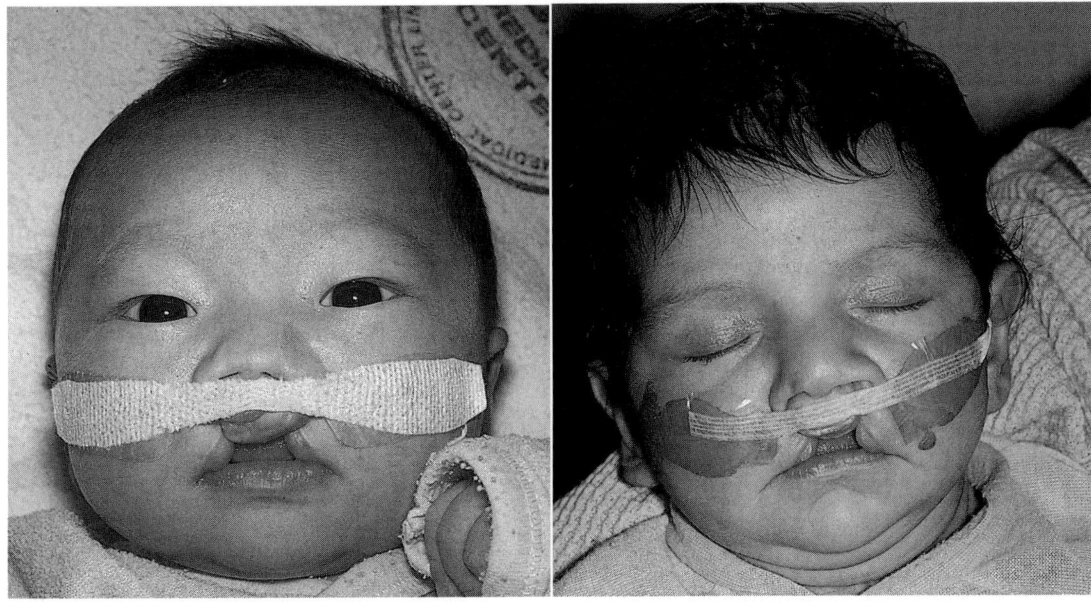

Figure 5-20 Taping to bring the premaxilla into a more advantageous position for lip repair in two babies with bilateral clefts.

The devices for accomplishing these goals vary from passive to active and from very simple to quite complex. For bringing the lip and premaxilla into better alignment, the taping procedure described in Chapter 4 probably qualifies as the simplest end of the continuum. It has been used in unilateral clefts when the cleft segment was severely rotated outward, with a wide soft tissue and alveolar defect as a result. In bilateral clefts (Fig. 5-20), taping can be quite effective in molding the premaxilla inward (Ross, 1989; Vargervik, 1995). Ross (1989) pointed out that tipping the premaxilla inward is "the exact movement required to reverse the forward rotation (tipping upward) of the premaxilla caused by the action of the tongue without the restraint of an intact lip." He also advocated taping because it flattens and widens the prolabium (the section of lip over the premaxilla), which can aid the surgeon in lip closure. But even this simple approach carries potential dangers of overcorrection if too much pressure is applied and the direction of movement is not adequately controlled.

The remaining approaches to optimizing the alignment of the soft tissue and maxillary segments in clefts fall generally into the following categories (progressing from simple to complex)[10]:

1. Passive intraoral plates for preventing medial movement (collapse) of the cleft segment(s) or guiding the growth of the palatal shelves and also partially obturating the cleft before palatal surgery (Figs. 5-21 and 5-22) (DiBiase and Hunter, 1983; Gnoinski, 1982; Graf-Pinthus and Bettex, 1974; Hayward, 1983; Hotz, 1973; Hotz and Gnoinski, 1976; Hotz and Perko, 1974; Hotz et al., 1978; Jacobson and Rosenstein, 1984; Jones and Kerkhof, 1984; Lennartsson, Friede, and Johanson, 1984; McNeil, 1954; Mishima, Sugahara, Mori, and Sakuda, 1996a, 1996b; Monroe and Rosenstein, 1971; Rosenstein, 1974a, 1974b).
2. Passive or active (that is, designed to accomplish expansion) intraoral plates plus extraoral taping, strapping, or an acrylic bridge over the premaxilla to

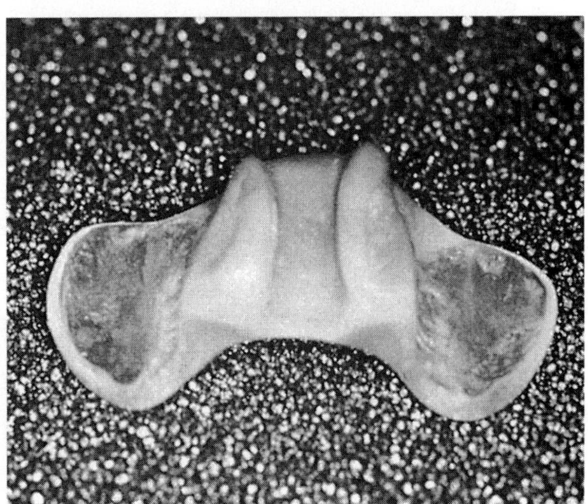

Figure 5-21 An intraoral plate for partially obturating a bilateral cleft in an infant and also for preventing inward collapse of the lateral segments. *(From Rutrick R, Black PW, and Jurkiewicz MJ: Bilateral cleft lip and palate: presurgical treatment.* Annals of Plastic Surgery *12:105-117, 1984.)*

[10]There are more details about presurgical orthopedics given in this section than you will need clinically. All the references and studies are cited so that, if you encounter a child being treated with a particular type of device, you will be able to look up original reports.

keep the unattached premaxilla in bilateral clefts from growing too far forward (Fig. 5-22)[11] (DiBiase and Hunter, 1983; Hayward, 1983; Jacobson and Rosenstein, 1965; McNeil, 1954; Monroe, 1974; Monroe and Rosenstein, 1971; Moore, 1976; Robertson, Shaw, and Volp, 1977; Rosenstein, 1969, 1974b; Troutman, 1974). In their survey of various aspects of cleft lip and palate management in England, Asher-McDade and Shaw (1990) noted that intraoral "moulding" appliances plus extraoral strapping were used in more than half of the centers surveyed and concluded "This method . . . remains popular in spite of doubts as to its long-term effects and even the possibility of some negative effects in growth with extra oral strapping techniques." Plint and Mars (1983) showed that the results produced by this approach, specifically as presented by DiBiase and Hunter (1983), could be produced without any type of presurgical orthopedics. In a recent small study of 10 babies with bilateral clefts, clinicians who used a "Hotz plate" plus an extraoral appliance consisting of a band and elastics reported bending of the vomer bone in two babies and twisting of the premaxilla in three (Mishima, Sugahara, Mori, Minami and Sakuda, 1998).

3. Passive intraoral plates plus extraoral mechanical traction. An intraoral plate plus an extraoral "T-traction" device is used to position the cleft segments in both unilateral and bilateral clefts in some Scandinavian centers (Fig. 5-23) (Friede and Lennartsson, 1981; Larson et al., 1993; Nordin et al., 1983).
4. Intraoral plates with jack-screws or spring devices to push the cleft segments laterally, particularly in bilateral clefts (Rutrick, Black, and Jurkiewicz, 1984).

[11]Some clinicians have used small intraoral plates simply to anchor a tape, bridge, or elastic material that is placed over the premaxilla in bilateral clefts (Figueroa et al., 1996; Reisberg, Figueroa, and Gold, 1988).

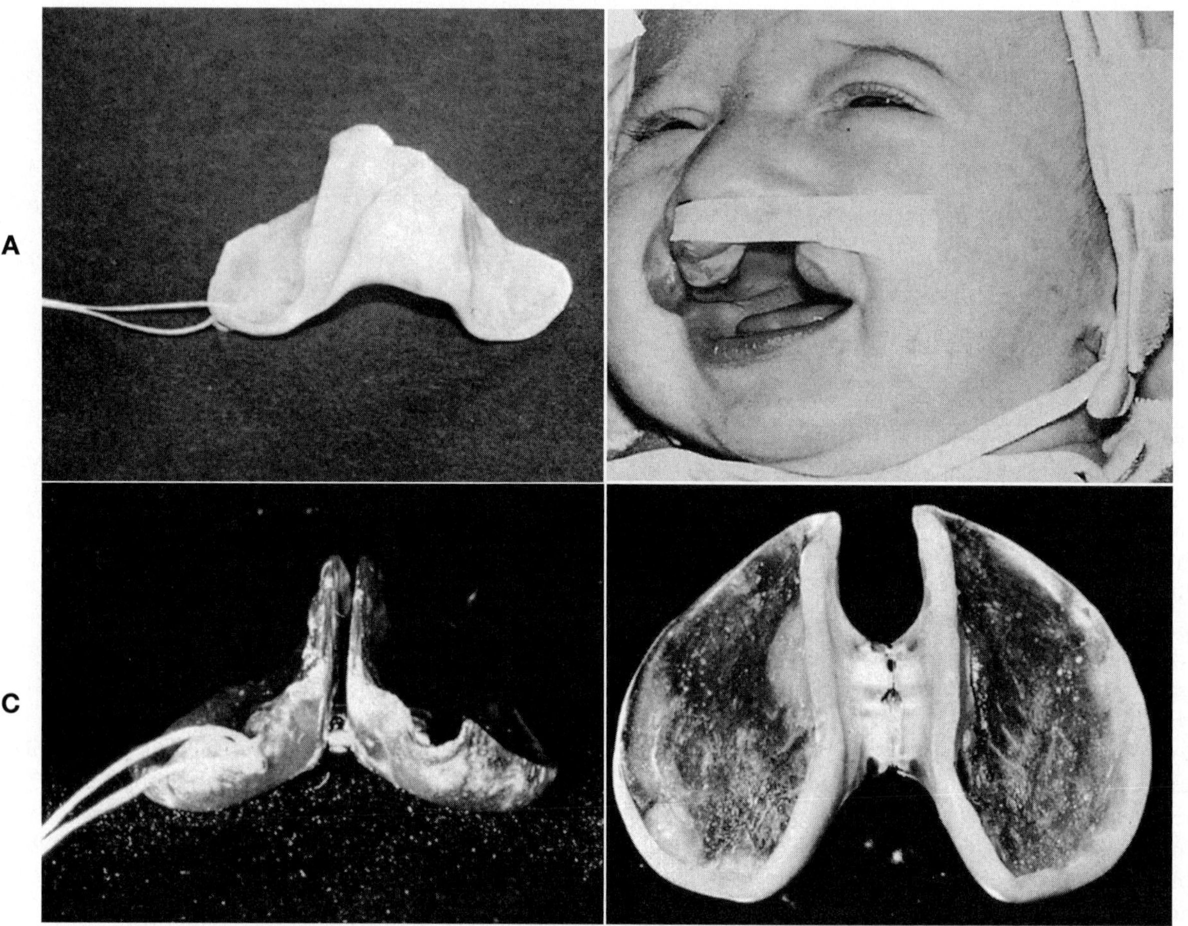

Figure 5-22 Extraoral taping. **(A)** A partial obturating plate **(B)** for an infant with an incomplete bilateral cleft. Here the tape is being used to try to narrow the cleft on the baby's left side. The device shown in **C** is an expansion device fabricated for another baby with a bilateral cleft in whom the palatal shelves had collapsed toward the midline. *(From Rutrick R, Black PW, and Jurkiewicz MJ: Bilateral cleft lip and palate: presurgical treatment.* Annals of Plastic Surgery *12:105-117, 1984.)*

5. Pin-retained appliances consisting of two acrylic pieces surgically pinned to the palatal segments with an external screw that is gradually cranked to move the segments laterally and retract the premaxilla (Georgiade, 1970; Georgiade and Latham, 1974, 1975; Georgiade et al., 1989; Latham, 1980; Latham, Kusy, and Georgiade, 1976; Sierra and Turner, 1995) (Figs. 5-24, 5-25, and 5-26). This approach is probably the most controversial type of presurgical orthopedics and has engendered many heated arguments. Ross (1989) cautioned that this appliance caused local damage to bone, teeth, and the premaxilla itself and tearing and slippage of the premaxillary-vomerine suture (a major growth site). Berkowitz (1996) offered longitudinal data showing the damage the device can cause and compared these results with the results of more conservative management. Nevertheless, a few orthodontists continue to use it.

Interestingly, a recent study conducted in a center where the use of presurgical orthopedic treatment is routine compared the short-term cost-effectiveness of such treatment in infants with complete unilateral clefts (Severens et al., 1998). The specific treatment was the "Hotz and Gnoinski plate," and the outcome measures were the overall cost of treatment and the time of surgical closure of the lip in babies who had had the presurgical plate compared with a control group with no plate. There was no difference in the operative time required for the surgical closure of the lip, and the overall cost of treatment was higher in the group treated with the presurgical plates.

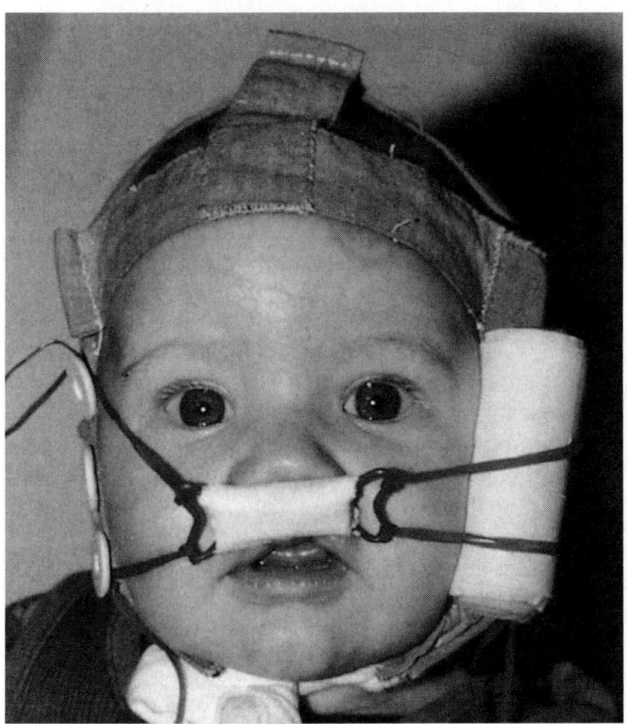

Figure 5-23 The "T-traction" device used in some centers in Scandinavia. *(From Larson M, Sallstrom K-O, Larson L, McWilliam J, and Ideberg M: Morphologic effect of preoperative maxillofacial orthopedics [T-traction] on the maxilla in unilateral cleft lip and palate patients.* Cleft Palate–Craniofacial Journal *30:29-34, 1993.)*

Despite the wide variation in types of appliances, much of the argument over presurgical orthopedics (sometimes also called premaxillary orthopedics) has taken on a simplistic "us-versus-them" flavor over the last 35 years. In 1964 Pruzansky wrote a vehement protest against both presurgical orthopedics and primary bone grafting for infants with clefts, arguing that the devices had no proven long-term benefit and could possibly impede growth of the premaxilla and palatal segments. His argument was systematic, sequentially taking on each of the claims that had been previously offered by proponents of both these treatments, but the argument was also flawed by unsubstantiated claims (e.g., that allowing the lateral palatine segments to collapse inward facilitated good velopharyngeal function). Pruzansky did make the point that the proponents of presurgical orthopedics, as of the mid-1960s, had no control subjects for proving that their methods provided superior results.[12] Subsequent publications by Pruzansky and others continued to fuel the controversy over presurgical orthopedics (Aduss, 1974; Aduss and Pruzansky, 1967, 1968; Aduss, Friede, and Pruzansky, 1974; Bergland, 1967; Berkowitz, 1978, 1996; Berkowitz and Pruzansky, 1968; Collito, 1974; Cooper et al., 1979; Fara, Mullerova, and Smahel, 1990; Gnoinski, 1982, 1990; Graf-Pinthus and Bettex, 1974; Gruber, 1990; Hotz and Perko, 1974; Huddart, 1990; Huebener and Marsh, 1990; Jolleys and Robertson, 1972; Larson and Nilsson, 1983; Moore, 1976, 1986; O'Donnell, Krischer, and Shiere, 1974; Oliver, 1969; Peat, 1982; Plint and Mars, 1983; Pruzansky and Aduss, 1964, 1967; Robertson, 1983; Robertson and Hilton, 1971; Robertson, Shaw, and Volp, 1977; Ross, 1989; Shaw, 1978). Berkowitz (1978, 1996) pointed out that several proponents of this treatment had reported instability of the results over time or had very little in the way of long-term results to discuss. Huddart and Bodenham (1972) and Huddart (1974) found that favorable short-term results in infants were no longer in evidence by age 5 years. Graf-Pinthus and Bettex (1974) and Moore (1986) also decried the lack of long-term results and similarly reported that presurgical orthopedics did not reduce the amount of time later required for orthodontic therapy. Ross (1975, 1987, 1989) similarly concluded that the long-term results of presurgical orthopedics appeared to offer no improvement in arch form beyond that which was

[12]Some proponents of presurgical orthopedics in the succeeding years have indeed had control groups, but most publishing their results, even into the 1990s, have not.

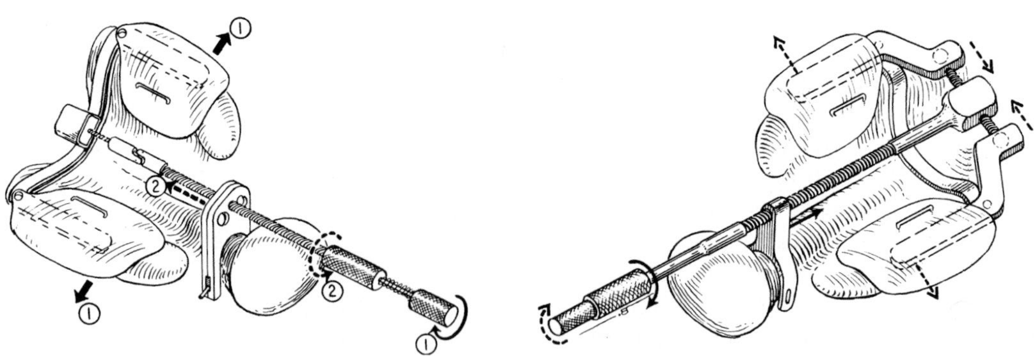

Figure 5-24 The pin-retained appliance of Georgiade and Latham. The two lateral acrylic plates are stapled to the palatal segments. Turning knob 1 clockwise expands the maxillary arches. Turning knob 2 counterclockwise retracts the premaxilla. *(From Georgiade NG, and Latham RA: Maxillary arch alignment in bilateral cleft lip and palate infant, using pinned coaxial screw appliance.* Plastic and Reconstructive Surgery *56:52-60, 1975.)*

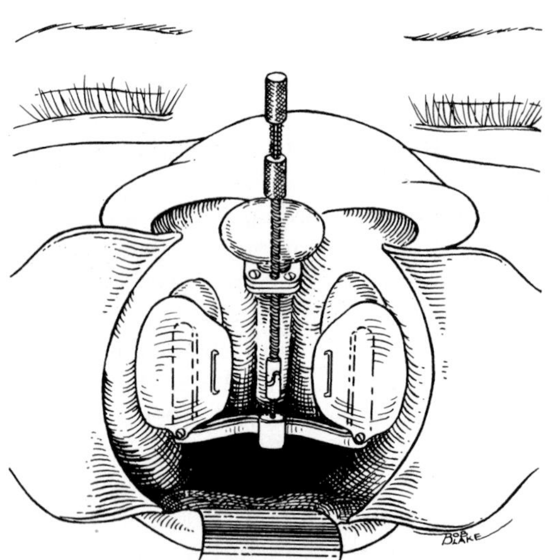

Figure 5-25 A schematic of the device shown in Fig. 5-24 after it has been inserted in the baby's mouth and stapled to the palatal shelves. *(From Georgiade NG, and Latham RA: Maxillary arch alignment in bilateral cleft lip and palate infant, using pinned coaxial screw appliance.* Plastic and Reconstructive Surgery *56:52-60, 1975.)*

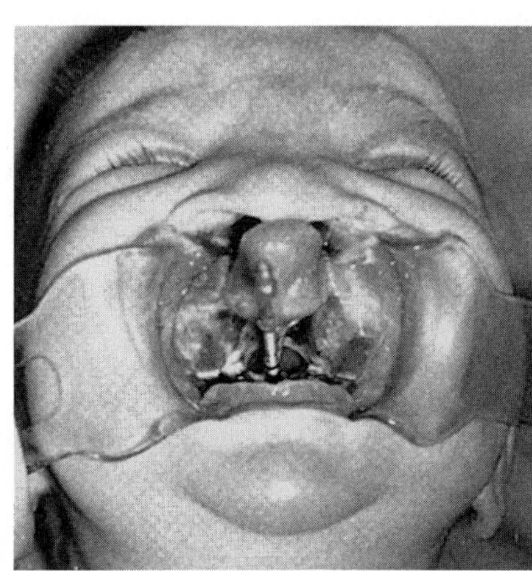

Figure 5-26 A baby with the device shown in Figs. 5-24 and 5-25 in place. *(From Georgiade NG, and Latham RA: Maxillary arch alignment in bilateral cleft lip and palate infant, using pinned coaxial screw appliance.* Plastic and Reconstructive Surgery *56:52-60, 1975.)*

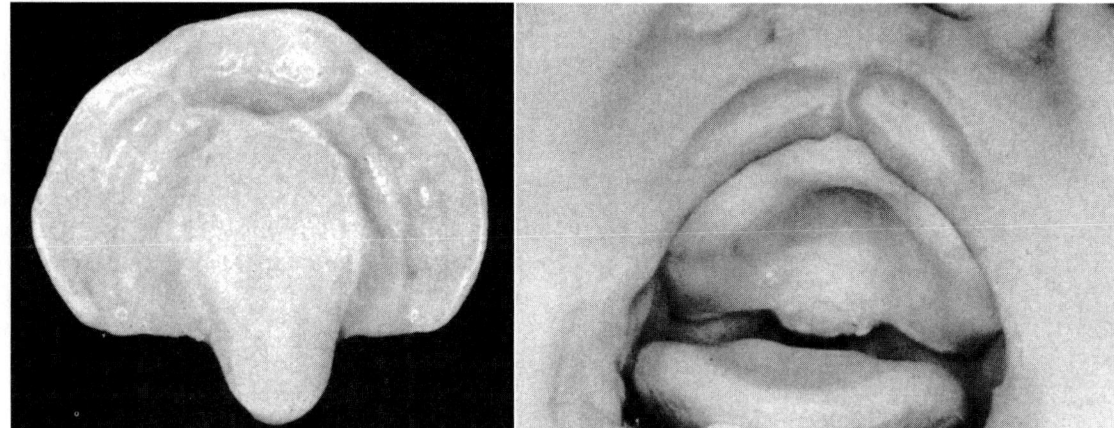

Figure 5-27 The "articulation development" prosthesis advocated by Dorf, Reisberg, and Gold (1985). Note that the prosthesis does not extend far enough posteriorly to completely obturate the clefts. *(From Dorf DS, Reisberg DJ, and Gold HO: Early prosthetic management of cleft plate. Articulation development prosthesis: a preliminary report.* Journal of Prosthetic Dentistry *3:222-226, 1985.)*

obtained by lip closure alone and did not decrease the amount of later orthodontic treatment.

Palatal plates used as "articulation development prostheses." As the speech-language pathologist involved in treatment decisions and provision of therapy for a child with a cleft, you will want to be sure that the child has the most normal oral-pharyngeal mechanism as soon as possible. Toward that end, you will be tempted to recommend surgical closure of the palate as soon as feasible (see Chapter 4), but you will often see the infant with a cleft go through the first year of life without an intact palate. The early infant plates discussed in the previous section of this chapter were often assumed, by their designers or advocates, to be beneficial for early speech development. Virtually none of the plates described in those articles fully obturated both the cleft in the oral cavity *and* the inevitable deficiency in the velopharyngeal system, but claims of benefits for speech nevertheless varied from cautious to fervid. In 1985 an attempt was made to document the effects of "articulation development prostheses" (Fig. 5-27) in infants whose definitive palatal surgeries, for various reasons, were being delayed beyond the ages at which speech-language pathologists would like to see the child have an optimum mechanism (Dorf, Reisberg, and Gold, 1985). As in the reports on early infant plates, the prostheses in this report were not designed to completely obturate the velopharyngeal port, primarily because of safety issues: a toddler is physically very active and subject to frequent falls. With a speech bulb fitting snugly against the posterior pharyngeal wall, falls and other jostling could result in injury to the tissues of the velopharyngeal port and possibly even to the cervical spine. Dorf, Reisberg, and Gold (1985) attempted this treatment in 11 toddlers, but only seven actually wore the prosthesis. Two of the seven did not return for all the necessary follow-up, and at the time the report was written three were still too young for conclusions about speech outcome. Of the two remaining children who actually wore the plate until the time of palatal surgery, one showed good articulatory placement but the other developed the use of compensatory articulations. Thus the study protocol was really carried out on only two children when the report was published, and the results were 50:50, no better than chance alone might have predicted. The disappointing results were probably more due to difficulties in fitting and maintaining such prostheses in toddlers than to any other factors.

Orthodontic Treatment: Early Childhood (Deciduous and Early Mixed Dentition)

Lip surgery in the infant has a molding effect on the position of the maxillary segments, usually bringing them into better alignment, and by the age or 4 or 5 years the maxillary segments are in contact with each other, although not physically attached, unless the treatment protocol included primary bone grafting. To some extent, the stability of the maxillary segments is dependent on the number and individual positions of the teeth nearest the cleft margin because an absent or badly positioned tooth may invite medial drift or collapse inward of the cleft segment, as seen in Figs. 5-15, *A,* and 5-18, *A.* In bilateral clefts the incisors in the premaxilla are usually in contact with the mandibular incisors by the age of 3 or 4 years, which means that the maxillary anterior teeth and the alveolar process will come forward as the mandible grows forward (Vargervik, 1983). That is, the growth of the lower jaw benefits the growth of the upper jaw during these early years so long as the lower incisors contact the upper incisors.

In the primary dentition, the most common deviation from a normal dental arch is a crossbite of one or more teeth on the cleft side, typically the canine or primary cuspid (Vargervik, 1981). In bilateral clefts, dental deviations of various types are likely to be present on both sides.

The primary focus of dental care during the deciduous dentition phase is on maintaining all the primary teeth (i.e., keeping the teeth healthy, preventing baby bottle caries, seeing to it that restorations are carried out when necessary, and intervening to prevent ill-advised dental extractions). Remember that, for the purposes of optimum jaw growth and good arch form, it is crucial that all the teeth be maintained. At times the orthodontist uses selective grinding of teeth to improve the bite relationship (Vargervik, 1995). The partial crossbite that is common in the deciduous dentition will usually be left untreated until the permanent maxillary incisors erupt. Vargervik (1990, 1995) suggested that orthodontic treatment may begin during this period, however, if there is a significant collapse of the maxillary segment on the side of the cleft and particularly if the mandible shifts into an occlusal relationship with the collapsed segment. If such a situation is left untreated, the functional shift of the mandible may lead to a permanent, unfavorable position of the lower jaw even after the permanent dentition erupts.

For the most part, however, orthodontic therapy is not undertaken in the deciduous dentition phase because the effects are unlikely to be sustained in the permanent dentition (Asher-McDade and Shaw, 1990; Bergland and Sidhu, 1974; Berkowitz, 1978, 1996; Ross, 1975; Ross and Johnston, 1967; Vargervik, 1981, 1983). As Cooper et al. (1979) stated, ". . . while primary dentition may appear close to normal, the cases most always require active orthodontic treatment at later stages, regardless of prior intervention." Moore (1986) pointed out that the need for long-term retention (long-term use of appliances to keep the teeth in the desired position) could, in the deciduous dentition, actually impede growth.

Orthodontic treatment is more likely to be considered when the child is in the early mixed dentition stage (roughly ages 6 to 9 years) (Berkowitz, 1978, 1996; Cooper et al., 1979; Ross, 1975; Vargervik, 1981, 1983, 1990, 1995). Bergland and Sidhu (1974) recommended delaying treatment until complete eruption of the permanent anterior teeth (notwithstanding the fact that one or more teeth may be congenitally absent). They reported that virtually 90% of their subjects with unilateral clefts had a malocclusion in the early mixed dentition stage that required treatment.

There may be several areas of concern for the orthodontist at this stage. Vargervik (1990, 1995) pointed out that, in addition to missing lateral incisors, the central incisors are often narrower than normal. Both lateral and anterior crossbites increase in frequency in comparison to the situation in the deciduous dentition, primarily because the mandible is growing normally while the maxilla is not. Vargervik (1990, 1995) recommended that treatment to correct the position of the maxillary segments and maxillary incisors start when the 6-year molars have erupted and the permanent incisors are in the process of eruption. She also pointed out that the position of the tongue is one of the factors that influences the growth patterns of the maxilla and mandible. If the tongue is positioned below the maxillary teeth, for example as the result of inward collapse of the lateral segment or an open-mouth posture due to nasal obstruction, there will be effects on the development of the maxillary alveolus: with a lack of normal apposition[13] of the tongue against the oral surface of the maxilla, the alveolus in effect "overgrows," leading to a progressive lowering of the mandible and a more retruded position of the chin.

The first goals of treatment in the early mixed dentition phase will include expansion of the maxilla and straightening of the incisors, something that will take a few months to achieve (Vargervik, 1995). The maxillary expansion is typically accomplished with a lingual appliance (meaning an appliance placed on the lingual side or inside of the maxillary teeth), sometimes with a spring that gives more of a push to the anterior part of the lateral maxillary segment than the posterior part. Subsequently, as the child progresses into the later mixed dentition stage, a lingual fixed appliance is used for retention of the maxillary segments in the positions into which they have been moved (Vargervik, 1995) (Fig. 5-28).

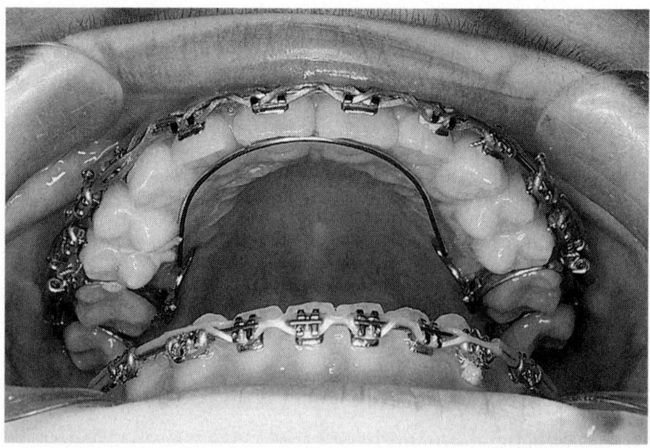

Figure 5-28 A lingual fixed appliance to maintain the maxillary segments in the proper position.

Orthodontic Treatment: Later Childhood (Late Mixed Dentition)

In the age range of 9 to 12 years, orthodontic treatment focuses on maintenance of improved positions of the teeth and maxillary segments obtained in earlier treatment. The orthodontist will be focusing on correction of maxillary width in preparation for alveolar bone grafting. If maxillary expansion and/or protraction was begun earlier, that treatment can continue while the remaining permanent teeth erupt. As pointed out by Vargervik (1995), expansion of the maxilla and proclination of the incisors may have to be undertaken more than once as the mandible continues to grow forward normally while the maxilla does not.[14] For some children a face mask may be used in the effort to bring the maxilla forward (Fig. 5-29); such a device is usually worn only at night or during the child's nonschool, less active hours of the day (Berkowitz, 1996; Rygh and Tindlund, 1982). Some of the fixed appliances used for maxillary expansion and correction of the position of individual teeth are illustrated in Figs. 5-30 and 5-31. Edentulous spaces during this period may be treated by an orthodontic appliance to maintain the space for later placement of an implant, because implants will generally not be placed until after eruption of all the permanent dentition. If edentulous spaces are a hazard to speech production or a source of embarrassment to the child, temporary plates carrying the missing tooth or teeth can be placed. Sometimes these spaces may be filled by allowing or encouraging forward drift of the teeth posterior to the space, so that, for example, the space left by a missing lateral incisor may be filled by letting the cuspid move forward.

In the late childhood or early teenage years, treatment teams are frequently drawn into virtually "salvage" situations for children whose early treatment did not provide the optimum result either in terms of the position of the orofacial structures or functional considerations such as speech. In such cases clinicians try to meet the challenges of orthodontic treatment and necessary prosthetic treatment at the same time. The treatment may thus become simultaneously "orthodontic" and "prosthetic." For example, LaVelle and Van Demark (1976) presented a combination orthodontic-prosthodontic appliance for treatment during the childhood years (age unspecified) that incorporated (1) initially, a split palatal plate to expand the maxilla with an attached posterior speech bulb to obturate

[13]"Apposition" means positioning of one structure against or next to another; it is not the equivalent of "opposition."

[14]Expansion devices usually involve wires that effectively lower or flatten the amount of "operating room" for the tongue in the oral cavity and thus often interfere with speech on a temporary basis.

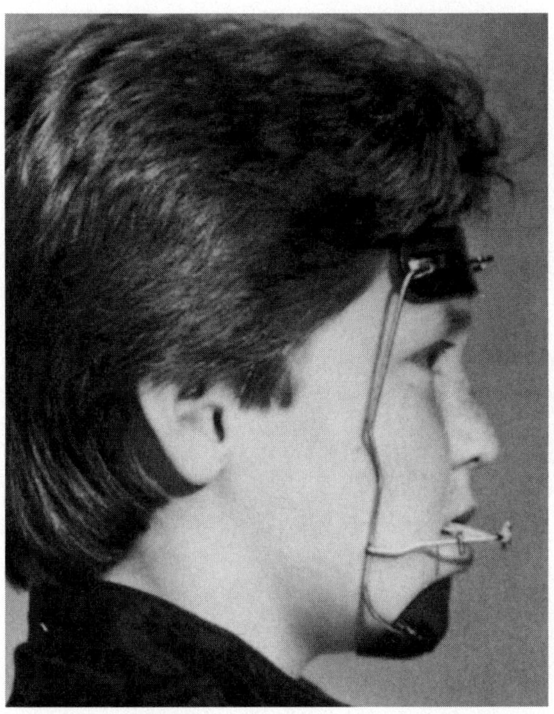

Figure 5-29 A face mask designed to help bring the maxilla forward. *(From Proffit WR:* Contemporary orthodontics. *3rd ed. St. Louis: Mosby, 2000, p. 271.)*

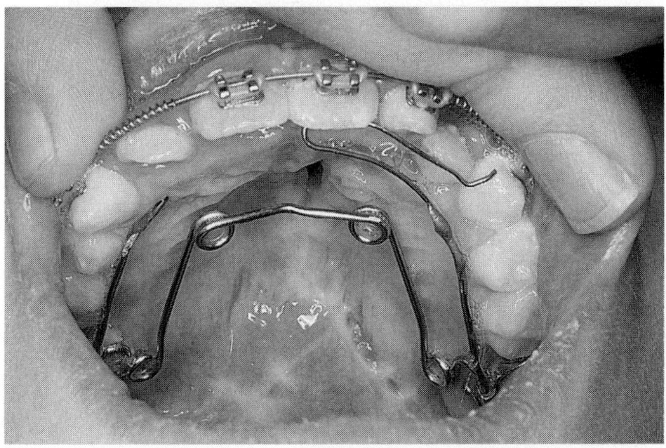

Figure 5-30 A quad-helix appliance.

an incompetent velopharyngeal port, which was later modified to become (2) a single anterior palatal plate plus speech bulb (Fig. 5-32). Fortunately, as surgery improves the need for such appliances diminishes.

Orthodontic Treatment: Teenage Years and Adulthood

Systematic orthodontic treatment in the later childhood and teenage years, without lapses or delays, produces young adults with better jaw relationships (Smahel, 1994), but there can still be troublesome problems in these years. Vargervik (1995) pointed out that, during the adolescent

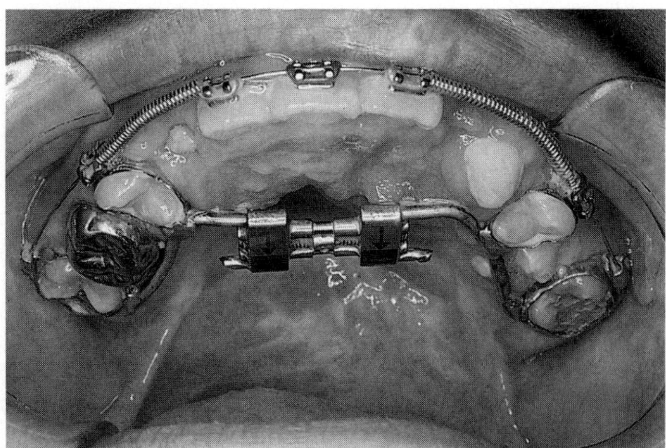

Figure 5-31 A Hyrax appliance.

growth spurt, the maxilla often falls behind in growth and development and may become significantly hypoplastic in all three dimensions of space. This disproportion can upset facial esthetics. Posnick (1997) offered details on orthodontic treatment for patients with clefts in the age range of 15 to 25 years; many of the patients he presented had apparently come late to treatment or had had poor results from earlier intervention, an experience shared by most craniofacial treatment centers. The last stages of orthodontic treatment may take 2 to 2½ years (Habel, Sells, and Mars, 1996). Once alveolar bone grafting and all remaining phases of orthodontic treatment have been completed, missing teeth are replaced in a more permanent fashion, either with a fixed bridge or through the use of osseointegrated implants. If the maxillary expansion or protraction performed at an earlier age did not provide the optimum jaw relationship, the patient becomes a candidate for the midface advancement surgery discussed in Chapter 4. In some cases the continued forward growth of the mandible in the teenage years leads to such a discrepancy in jaw position that "two-jaw surgery" is needed, combining advancement of the maxilla with a setback of the mandible (Fig. 5-33). All such surgery requires the evaluation and guidance of the orthodontist working with the surgeon(s) to plan the amount of advancement or setback needed to achieve an optimum jaw relationship.

In the patients you see, the timing and sequence of various aspects of orthodontic intervention may differ from the general framework given in this chapter, especially as clinical research continues to lead to new treatment techniques. Aduss (1990), in his comments on an article by Enemark, Bolund, and Jorgensen (1990) on long-term results of treatment in unilateral clefts, observed that successful treatment protocols are not rigid but in a constant state of evaluation and modification to improve patient care. His comment, although not original or unique, gave emphasis to the necessity of on-going evaluation of treatment results, a theme that continues pervade the clinical literature.

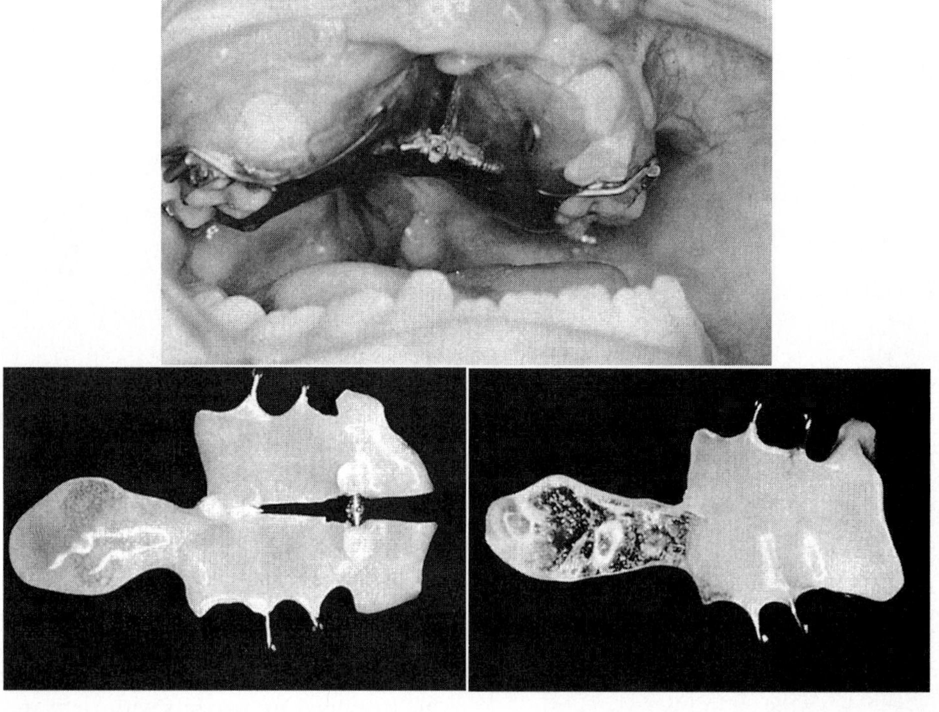

Figure 5-32 A combination appliance for maxillary expansion and obturation of a cleft. *(From LaVelle WE, and Van Demark DR: Construction of a maxillary orthopedic prosthesis for simultaneous maxillary expansion and obturation.* Journal of Prosthetic Dentistry *35:665-670, 1976.)*

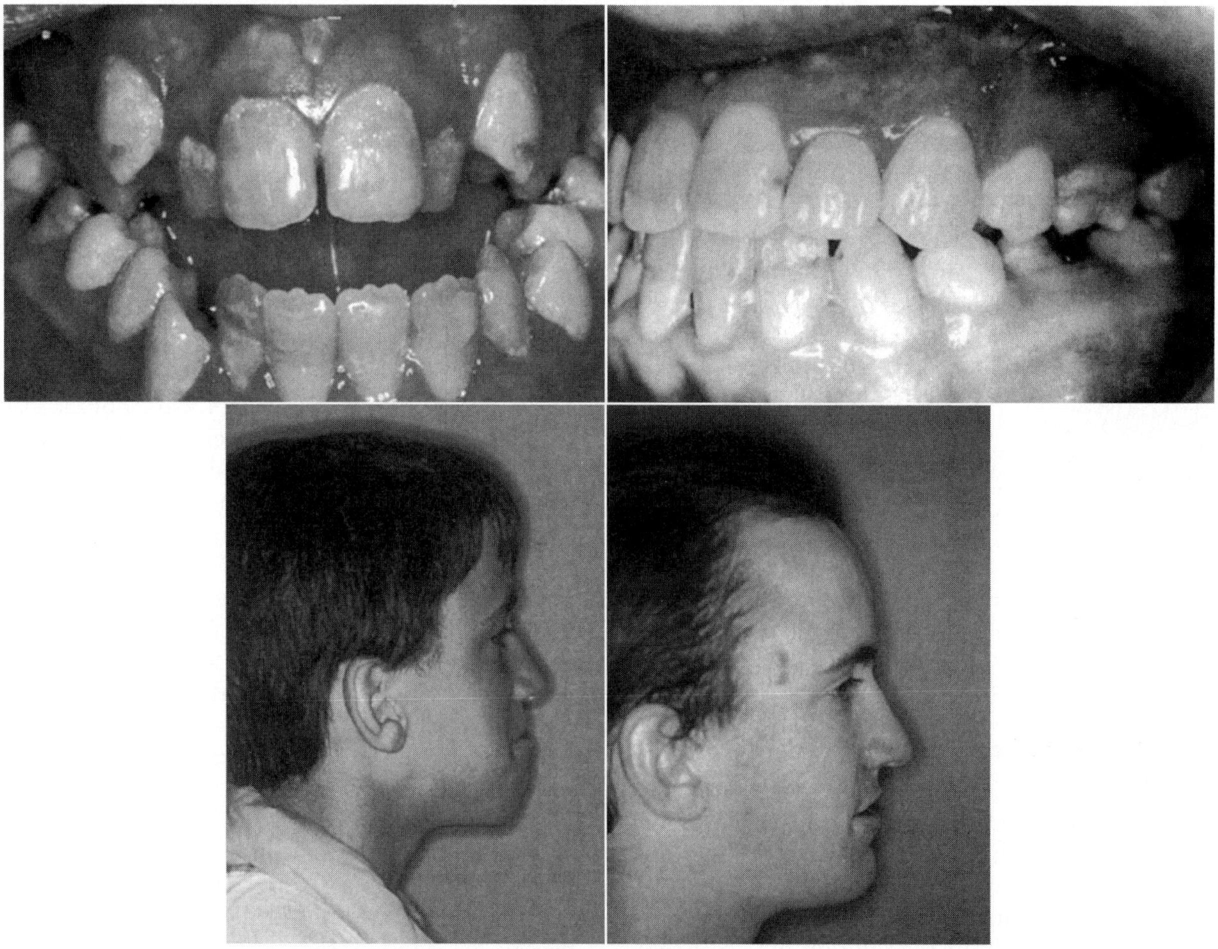

Figure 5-33 Pretreatment and posttreatment photographs of a young man with a prognathic mandible and Class III malocclusion. The dark spots on the teeth are due to fluoride. *(From Graber TM, and Vanarsdall RL Jr:* Orthodontics: current principles and techniques. *2nd ed. St. Louis: Mosby, 1994, pp. 896-897.)*

PROSTHETIC TREATMENT

Obturation of Fistulae

You will recall from Chapter 4 that some fistulae are left intentionally (e.g., alveolar defects before bone grafting). Fistulae in the palatal vault (Fig. 5-34) or at the junction of the hard and soft palate (Fig. 5-35) may be obturated with an acrylic palatal plate. Obturation is usually short term, although there are some postoperative fistulae so large that successful surgical closure is deemed to be impossible, and obturation is essentially permanent. In these cases the plates may be combination devices, obturating unclosed sections of a cleft and also carrying prosthetic teeth (Adisman, 1971; Duthie, 1983; Mazaheri, 1979; Milenkovich, Gold, and Pruzansky, 1981; Morikawa, Toyoda, and Toyoda, 1987; Rosen and Bzoch, 1997; von Schwanewede and Schuberth, 1989). Many clinicians have described the fabrication and use of plates for the obturation of fistulae; the main changes in the past several decades have been technical (e.g., specific materials used) (Adisman, 1971; Delgado, Schaaf, and Emrich, 1992; Moore, 1976; Rosen and Bzoch, 1997; Thompson, Ferguson, and Barton, 1985; von Schwanewede and Schuberth, 1989).

If the defect is in the hard palate, an alternative to an acrylic plate is an oral adhesive or skin barrier material, as discussed in Chapter 4. There are several brand names of such materials; they are usually marketed as adhesives for temporary closure of stomas. Use of such material is relatively easy, but the child must be old enough (1) to remember to remove it before he eats and (2) to cut a new piece of the material to the right size and hold it in place until it adheres. Use of such material is not recommended if the fistula is in the soft palate and the soft palate has mobility because it will be harder to avoid unintentional dislodging and possible subsequent digestion of the patch.

The most difficult fistulae to obturate are those that are essentially labial-oral-nasal, that is, an open pathway from the labial surface of the alveolus, through the alveolus, and up into the nasal cavity (Figs. 5-18, *A*, and 5-36). Successful obturation requires an acrylic plate with an anterior upward extension to "plug" the alveolar defect (Fig. 5-37).

Patients who are fitted with acrylic plates to cover palatal fistulae require regular monitoring by the dentist, prosthodontist, or cleft palate-craniofacial team because the oral tissues may not react favorably to the presence of the plate. The patient (or parents) must be instructed to carefully clean the plate at least twice a day. Oral secretions, food particles, and other debris will accumulate on the upper surface of the plate, next to the oral mucosa, and cause irritation and tissue damage if the cleaning is not regular. In addition, in children and teenagers whose dental situation is changing as a result of natural dental development or orthodontic treatment, the plates must be remade periodically to fit the changing dental status.

Obturators for Unrepaired Palatal Clefts

About 50 years ago the care and habilitation of individuals with clefts was considered to be nearly the exclusive territory of prosthodontists: Although the first known surgical repair

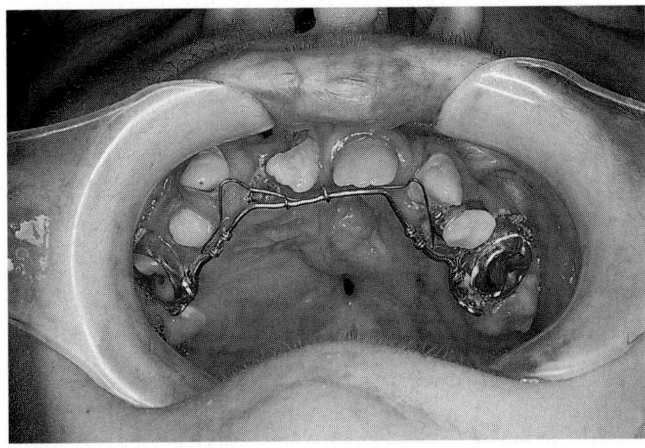

Figure 5-35 A small fistula at the junction of the hard and soft palate.

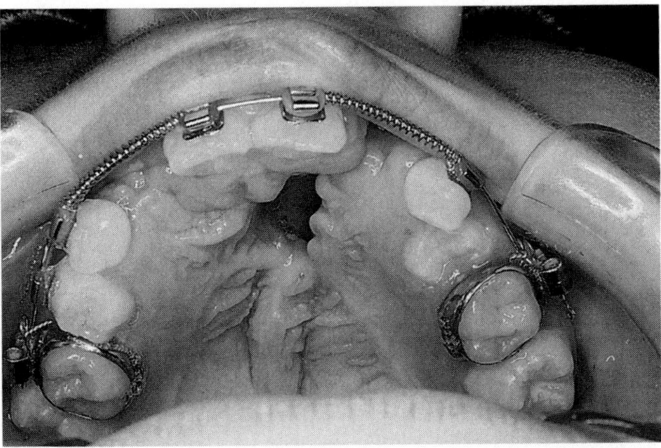

Figure 5-34 A palatal fistula that has opened up as the child progressed through orthodontic expansion of the maxillary arch.

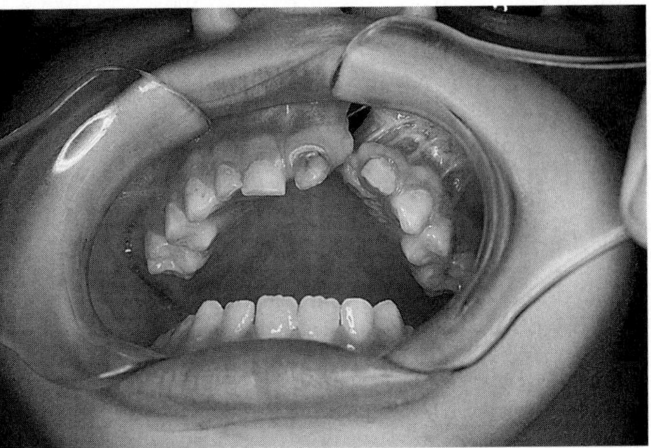

Figure 5-36 A labio-oral-nasal fistula, before bone grafting of the alveolar cleft.

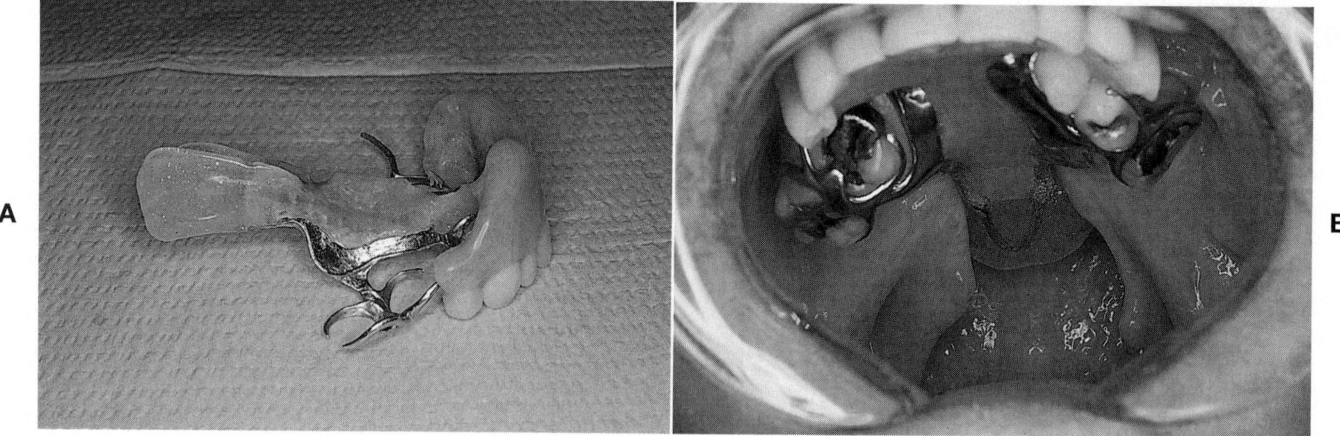

Figure 5-37 A combination appliance for obturating an unrepaired palatal cleft and replacing some missing teeth, with upward extensions anteriorly to obturate alveolar defects.

of a cleft had taken place hundreds of years previously, the functional results were still poor for many patients, so the attainment of usable speech was routinely thought to be dependent on a speech bulb to fill the velopharyngeal space.[15] There are still occasional patients for whom surgical closure of the lip was accomplished but surgical closure of the palate was (or is) an ill-advised or unattainable goal because of (1) co-existing medical concerns, (2) patient or parental preference, or (3) poor results from earlier attempts to obtain structural integrity of the palate.[16] The clinical literature on obturators for unrepaired palatal clefts is lengthy and full of details on the technical aspects of design, fabrication, and modifications of appliances (Adisman, 1971; Hotz and Gnoinski, 1979; Mazaheri, 1971, 1979; Moore, 1976; Posnick, 1977; Rosen and Bzoch, 1997; Walter, 1990). Many such devices, especially when made for older children and adult patients, include prosthetic teeth (see Fig. 5-37, *B*). (Adisman, 1971; Mazaheri, 1979; Rosen and Bzoch, 1997;).[17] Although it is easier for a clinician to see most of the velopharyngeal sphincter in patients with unrepaired clefts compared with patients with repaired clefts (Fig. 5-38), adequate fitting of the pharyngeal portion of the obturator may still be best accomplished with the use of imaging studies such as nasopharyngoscopy or videofluoroscopy to examine changes in the circumferential appearance of the velopharyngeal port in speech tasks other than the simple "ah."

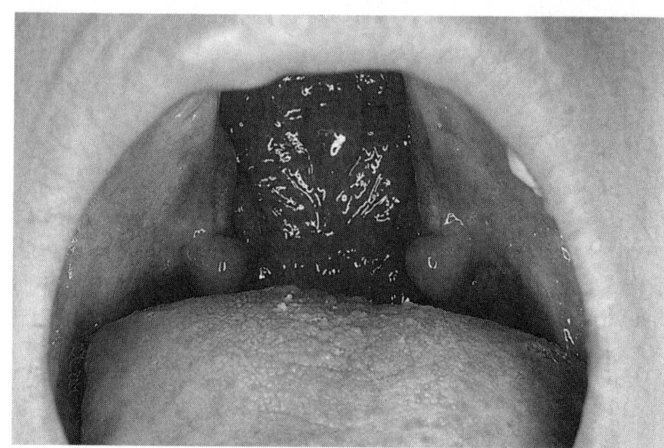

Figure 5-38 In a patient with a wide unrepaired cleft, the clinician can see a substantial portion of the velopharyngeal port on the direct intraoral view, but adequate fitting of the pharyngeal portion of an obturator will still require imaging studies such as nasopharyngoscopy.

When an individual with a cleft is essentially a "permanent prosthetic" patient, optimum care depends on long-term, regular visits with the team. During the child's growing years there will obviously be many changes in the oral structures necessitating changes in the appliance. However, even in the adult years the patient requires routine check-ups with the prosthodontist to be certain that the health of the teeth and oral tissues is being adequately maintained. Obturators for unrepaired clefts, speech bulbs, and palatal lifts (discussed in Chapter 13) have deleterious effects on the teeth and the oral mucosa if not monitored at regular intervals.

Prosthetic Replacement of Missing Teeth

As in noncleft patients, replacement of missing teeth by full dentures or removable or fixed partial bridges is relatively routine. Rather ingenious combination appliances for

[15]The American Cleft Palate–Craniofacial Association was founded in the late 1940s as the "American Association for Cleft Palate Prosthetic Rehabilitation," a fact that signaled both the critical role of prosthodontic care in the habilitation of individuals with clefts and the relatively immature status of surgical care at that time.

[16]You will remember from Chapter 4 that it can be very difficult to obtain structural integrity of tissues and a successful functional result (that is, speech) when the patient has already had several previous procedures.

[17]Obturators for unoperated clefts, plates to cover fistulae, and speech bulbs may also be combined with "overdentures," discussed later in this chapter.

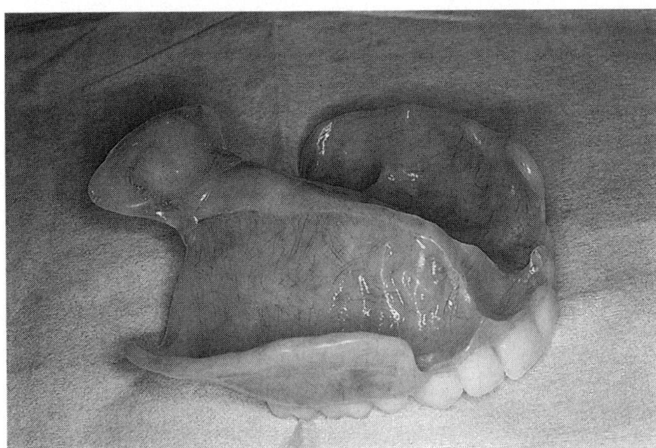

Figure 5-39 A combination appliance for replacing missing teeth and obturating an unrepaired cleft.

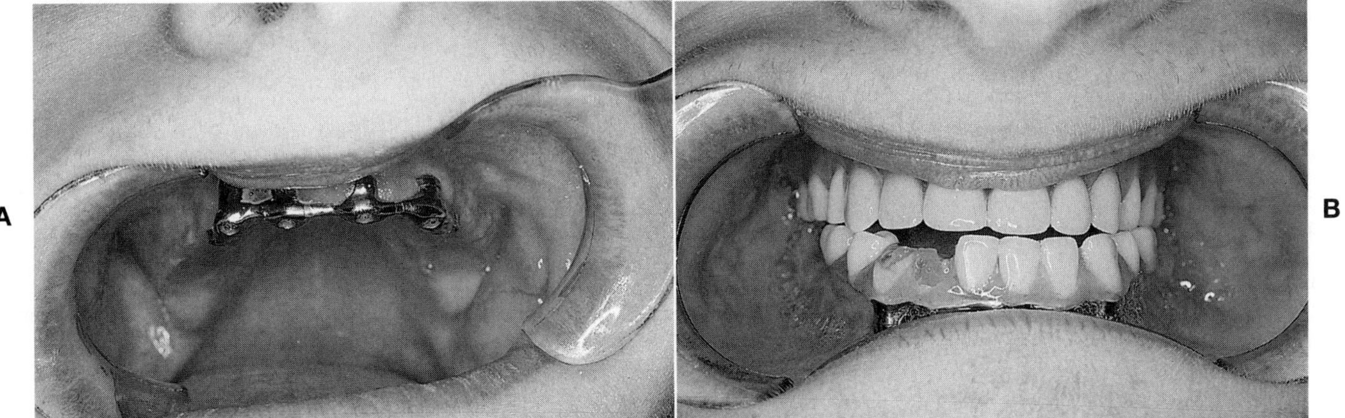

Figure 5-40 Stages in treatment of a patient receiving osseointegrated implants to replace missing teeth. **A,** The posts have been implanted into the maxillary bone. **B,** The posts serve as anchors for the replacement teeth in the maxilla. Treatment in the mandibular arch is in progress.

obturation of unrepaired clefts + replacement of missing teeth, plates to obturate fistulae + provide missing teeth, and so on are illustrated in many texts (Fig. 5-39). You may occasionally see a patient with "overdentures," designed to fit over existing teeth that are poorly formed (Abadi and Johnson, 1982; Mazaheri, 1979; Rosen and Bzoch, 1997). This approach is not used as frequently as once was the case because more patients with poorly formed and missing teeth are now treated with osseointegrated (or "osteointegrated" or "endosseus") implants (Kearns et al., 1997; Lilja et al., 1998; Takahashi et al., 1997). Placement of implants consists of two steps. First, a small metal post (or multiple posts for multiple implants) is placed into the alveolar bone. After a period of healing, the upper portion of the post is surgically exposed and a prosthetic tooth is anchored to it. The post + prosthetic tooth remain firmly embedded in the alveolar bone, thus the term "osseointegrated (or osteointegrated) implants." Osseointegrated implants (Fig. 5-40) are growing in popularity. In congenital craniofacial anomalies, they offer a particularly pleasing alternative for children with multiple missing teeth, for example, various forms of ectodermal dysplasia in which even the teeth that are present are poorly formed and esthetically embarrassing to the patient (Kearns et al., 1997).

Some Final Notes about Prosthetic Treatment

In an article focused on prosthetic treatment for problems in velopharyngeal function (discussed in Chapter 13), Marsh and Wray (1980) made one point that may bear consideration in the treatment of nearly all patients who undergo various forms of prosthetic treatment. Although the authors offered no empirical evidence to support their statement, they voiced concern over patients having "a persistent sense of impairment" if treatment involved long-term prosthetic treatment, supposedly in comparison to surgical treatment (i.e., "the problem is taken care of so long as I wear this thing," versus "the problem has been fixed"). Prosthetic treatment is often preferred by clinicians and patients/families alike because it does not involve all the frightening aspects of surgery (hospitalization, pain, general anesthesia, time off from work for patient or family, and the expenses attendant on frequent clinical or office visits). But the financial and emotional costs of prosthetic treatment (whether for replacement of teeth or obturation of a velopharyngeal defect) are not negligible, and figuring the "bottom line" for families requires consideration of many factors. As in every other area of treatment, one of the most important factors in success of the outcome is the amount of attention that clinicians give to what the patients and families have to say.

REFERENCES

Abadi B, and Johnson J: The prosthodontic management of cleft palate patients. *Journal of Prosthetic Dentistry* 48:297-302, 1982.

Adisman IK: Cleft palate prosthetics. In Grabb WC, Rosenstein SW, and Bzoch KR (eds.): *Cleft lip and palate: surgical, dental and speech aspects.* Boston: Little, Brown, 1971, pp. 617-642.

Aduss H: Management of the maxillary segments in complete unilateral cleft lip and palate: maxillary orthopedics. In Georgiade NG (ed.): *Symposium on management of cleft lip and palate and associated deformities.* St. Louis: Mosby, 1974, pp. 47-57.

Aduss H: Commentary on Enemark H, Bolund J and Jorgensen I: Evaluation of unilateral cleft lip and palate treatment: Long-term results. *Cleft Palate Journal* 37:361, 1990.

Aduss H, and Pruzansky S: The nasal cavity in complete unilateral cleft lip and palate. *Archives of Otolaryngology* 85:53-61, 1967.

Aduss H, and Pruzansky S: The width of the cleft at the level of the tuberosities in complete unilateral cleft lip and palate. *Plastic and Reconstructive Surgery* 41:113-123, 1968.

Aduss H, Friede H, and Pruzansky S: Management of the protruding premaxilla. In Georgiade NG (ed.): *Symposium on management of cleft lip and palate and associated deformities.* St. Louis: Mosby, 1974, pp. 111-117.

American Cleft Palate–Craniofacial Association: *Parameters for the evaluation and treatment of patients with cleft lip and palate and/or other craniofacial anomalies.* Pittsburgh: The Association, 1993.

Asher C: Neonatal care of infants with clefts of the lip and palate. *British Dental Journal* 160:438-439, 1986.

Asher-McDade C, and Shaw WC: Current cleft lip and palate management in the United Kingdom. *British Journal of Plastic Surgery* 43:318-321, 1990.

Balluff MA, and Udin RD: Using a feeding appliance to aid the infant with a cleft palate. *Ear, Nose, and Throat Journal* 65:50-55, 1986.

Bergland O: Changes in cleft palate malocclusion after the introduction of improved surgery. *Transactions of the European Orthodontics Society* 43:383-397, 1967.

Bergland O, and Sidhu SS: Occlusal changes from the deciduous to the early mixed dentition in unilateral complete clefts. *Cleft Palate Journal* 11:317-326, 1974.

Berkowitz S: State of the art in cleft palate orofacial growth and dentistry: a historical perspective. *American Journal of Orthodontics* 74:564-576, 1978.

Berkowitz S: *Cleft lip and palate: perspectives in management.* Volume I. San Diego: Singular, 1996.

Berkowitz S, and Pruzansky S: Stereophotogrammetry of serial casts of cleft palate. *Angle Orthodontist* 38:136-149, 1968.

Boekelheide A, Curtin G, Muraoka V, and Ursich C: Comparison of the effects of postsurgical feeding techniques following cleft lip repair on suture line integrity, volume of oral fluid intake, and length of hospital stay: a multi-center study. Presented before the 49th annual meeting of the American Cleft Palate–Craniofacial Association (premeeting symposium), Portland, OR, May 12, 1992.

Choi BH, Kleinheinz J, Joos U, and Komposch G: Sucking efficiency of early orthopaedic plate and teats in infants with cleft lip and palate. *International Journal of Oral and Maxillofacial Surgery* 20:167-169, 1991.

Clarren SK, Anderson B, and Wolf LS: Feeding infants with cleft lip, cleft palate, or cleft lip and palate. *Cleft Palate Journal* 24:244-249, 1987.

Collito MB: Management of the maxillary segments in complete unilateral cleft lip patients. In Georgiade NG (ed.): *Symposium on management of cleft lip and palate and associated deformities.* St. Louis: Mosby, 1974, pp. 58-61.

Cooper HK, Long RE Sr, Long RE Jr, and Pepek JM: Orthodontics and oral orthopedics. In Cooper HK, Harding R, Krogman W, Mazaheri M, and Millard R (eds.): *Cleft palate and cleft lip: a team approach to clinical management and rehabilitation of the patient.* Philadelphia: WB Saunders, 1979, pp. 358-429.

Cunningham ML, and Jerome JT: Linear growth characteristics of children with cleft lip and palate. *Journal of Pediatrics* 131:707-711, 1997.

Delgado AA, Schaaf NG, and Emrich L: Trends in prosthodontic treatment of cleft palate patients at one institution: a twenty-one year review. *Cleft Palate–Craniofacial Journal* 29:425-428, 1992.

DiBiase DD, and Hunter SB: A method of pre-surgical oral orthopaedics. *British Journal of Orthodontics* 10:25-31, 1983.

Dorf DS, Reisberg D, and Gold HO: Early prosthetic management of cleft plate. Articulation development prosthesis: a preliminary report. *Journal of Prosthetic Dentistry* 3:222-226, 1985.

Duncan PA, Shapiro LF, Soley RL, and Turet SE: Linear growth patterns in patients with cleft lip or palate or both. *American Journal of Diseases in Childhood* 137:159-163, 1983.

Dunning Y: Feeding babies with cleft lip and palate. *Nursing Times* January 29:46-47, 1986.

Duthie N: Prosthetic treatment of a cleft palate. *British Dental Journal* pp. 57–58, July 23, 1983.

Enemark H, Bolund S, and Jorgensen I: Evaluation of unilateral cleft lip and palate treatment: long term results. *Cleft Palate Journal* 27:354-361, 1990.

Fara M, Mullerova Z, and Smahe Z: Presurgical orthopedic treatment in unilateral cleft lip and palate. In Bardach J, and Morris HL (eds.): *Multidisciplinary management of cleft lip and palate.* Philadelphia: WB Saunders, 1990, pp. 586-592.

Figueroa AA, Reisberg DJ, Polley JW, and Cohen M: Intraoral-appliance modification to retract the premaxilla in patients with bilateral cleft lip. *Cleft Palate–Craniofacial Journal* 33:497-500, 1996.

Fleming P, Pielou WD, and Saunders IDF: A modified feeding plate for use in cleft palate infants. *Journal of Paediatric Dentistry* 1:61-64, 1985.

Frances JM, Knorr D, Martinez R, and Neuhauser G: Hypophysarer Zwergwuchs bei Lippen-Kiefer-Spalte. *Helvetica Paediatrica Acta* 21:315-322, 1966.

Friede H, and Lennartsson B: Forward traction of the maxilla in cleft lip and palate patients. *European Journal of Orthodontics* 3:21-39, 1981.

Georgiade NG: The management of premaxillary and maxillary segments in the newborn cleft patient. *Cleft Palate Journal* 7:411-418, 1970.

Georgiade NG, and Latham RA: Intraoral traction for positioning the premaxilla in the bilateral cleft lip. In Georgiade NG (ed.): *Symposium on management of cleft lip and palate and associated deformities.* St. Louis: Mosby, 1974, pp. 123-127.

Georgiade NG, and Latham RA: Maxillary arch alignment in bilateral cleft lip and palate infant, using pinned coaxial screw appliance. *Plastic and Reconstructive Surgery* 56:52-60, 1975.

Georgiade NG, Mason R, Riefkohl R, Georgiade G, and Barwick W: Preoperative positioning of the protruding premaxilla in the bilateral cleft lip patient. *Plastic and Reconstructive Surgery* 83:32-38, 1989.

Gnoinski WM: Early maxillary orthopaedics as a supplement to conventional primary surgery in complete cleft lip and palate cases—long-term results. *Journal of Maxillo-Facial Surgery* 10:165-172, 1982.

Gnoinski WM: Infant orthopedics and later orthodontic monitoring for unilateral cleft lip and palate patients in Zurich. In Bardach J, and Morris HL (eds.): *Multidisciplinary management of cleft lip and palate.* Philadelphia: WB Saunders, 1990, pp. 578-585.

Goumy F, Dalens B, and Malpuech G: Association d'une dysraphia de la ligne mediane et d'une insuffisance antehypophysaire congenitale avec micropenis et hypoclydemie neonate. *Pediatrie* 33:551-559, 1978.

Graf-Pinthus B, and Bettex M: Long term observation following presurgical orthopedic treatment in complete clefts of the lip and palate. *Cleft Palate Journal* 11:253-260, 1974.

Gruber H: Presurgical maxillary orthopedics. In Bardach J, and Morris HL (eds.): *Multidisciplinary management of cleft lip and palate.* Philadelphia: WB Saunders, 1990, pp. 592-600.

Habel A, Sell D, and Mars M: Management of cleft lip and palate. *Archives of Disease in Childhood* 74:360-366, 1996.

Hayward JR: Management of the premaxilla in bilateral clefts. *Journal of Oral and Maxillofacial Surgery* 41:518-524, 1983.

Hotz M: Aims and possibilities of pre- and post-surgical orthopedic treatment in uni- and bilateral clefts. *Transactions of the European Orthodontic Society* 1973, pp. 553-558.

Hotz M: Orofaziale Entwicklung unter erschwerten Bedingungen. *Fortschritte der Kieferorthopadie* 44:257-271, 1983.

Hotz M, and Gnoinski W: Comprehensive care of cleft lip and palate children at Zurich University: a preliminary report. *American Journal of Orthodontics* 70:481-504, 1976.

Hotz M, and Gnoinski W: Effects of early maxillary orthopaedics in coordination with delayed surgery for cleft lip and palate. *Journal of Maxillofacial Surgery* 7:201-210, 1979.

Hotz M, and Perko M: Early management of bilateral total cleft lip and palate. *Scandinavian Journal of Plastic and Reconstructive Surgery* 8:104-108, 1974.

Hotz M, Gnoinski WM, Nussbaumer H, and Kistler E: Early maxillary orthopedics in CLP cases: guidelines for surgery. *Cleft Palate Journal* 15:405-411, 1978.

Huddart AG: An analysis of the maxillary changes following presurgical dental orthopaedic treatment in unilateral cleft lip and palate cases. *Transactions of the European Orthodontic Society* 1967, pp. 299-314.

Huddart AG: An evaluation of pre-surgical treatment. *British Journal of Orthodontics* 1:21-25, 1974.

Huddart AG: Presurgical orthopedic treatment in unilateral cleft lip and palate. In Bardach J, and Morris HL (eds.): *Multidisciplinary management of cleft lip and palate.* Philadelphia: WB Saunders, 1990, pp. 574-578.

Huddart AG, and Bodenham RS: The evaluation of arch form and occlusion in unilateral cleft palate subjects. *Cleft Palate Journal* 9:194-209, 1972.

Huebener DV, and Marsh JL: Alveolar molding appliances in the treatment of cleft lip and palate infants. In Bardach J, and Morris HL (eds.): *Multidisciplinary management of cleft lip and palate.* Philadelphia: WB Saunders, 1990, pp. 601-607.

Hummel S: Eine Saughilfe fur Saeuglinge mit Lippen-Kiefer-Gaumen-Spalte. *Fortschritte der Kieferorthopadie* 48:26-33, 1987.

Jacobson BN, and Rosenstein SW: Early maxillary orthopedics: a combination appliance. *Cleft Palate Journal* 2:369-376, 1965.

Jacobson BN, and Rosenstein SW: Early maxillary orthopedics for the newborn cleft lip and palate patient. *Angle Orthodontist* 54:247-263, 1984.

Jensen BL, Dahl E, and Kreiborg S: Longitudinal study of body height, radius length and skeletal maturity in Danish boys with cleft lip and palate. *Scandinavian Journal of Dental Research* 91:473-481, 1983.

Jolleys A, and Robertson NRE: A study of the effects of early bone-grafting in complete clefts of the lip and palate—five year study. *British Journal of Plastic Surgery* 25:229-237, 1972.

Jones JE: Early management of severe bilateral cleft lip and palate in an infant. *ASDC Journal of Dentistry for Children* 48:50-54, 1981.

Jones JE, and Kerkhof RL: Obturator construction for maxillary orthopedics in cleft lip and palate infants. *Quintessence of Dental Technology* 8:583-586, 1984.

Jones JE, Henderson L, and Avery DR: Use of a feeding obturator for infants with severe cleft lip and palate. *Special Care in Dentistry* 2:116-120, 1982.

Jones WB: Weight gain and feeding in the neonate with cleft: a three-center study. *Cleft Palate Journal* 25:379-384, 1988.

Jordon RE, Kraus BSD, and Neptune CM: Dental abnormalities associated with cleft lip and/or palate. *Cleft Palate Journal* 3:22-55, 1966.

Kearns G, Perott DH, Sharma A, Kaban LB, and Vargervik K: Placement of endosseous implants in grafted alveolar clefts. *Cleft Palate–Craniofacial Journal* 34:520-525, 1997.

Kelly EE: Feeding cleft palate babies—today's babies, today's methods. *Cleft Palate Journal* 8:61-64, 1971.

Kelly JR, Sorenson HW, and Turner EG: Prosthodontic treatment for Pierre Robin syndrome. *Journal of Prosthetic Dentistry* 39:554-560, 1978.

Komposch G: Die praechirurgische kieferorthopaedische Behandlung von Saeuglingen mit Lippen-Kiefer-Gaumen-Spalten. *Fortschritte der Kieferorthopadie* 47:362-369, 1986.

Laron Z, Taube E, and Kaplan I: Pituitary growth hormone insufficiency associated with cleft lip and palate: an embryonal developmental defect. *Helvetica Paediatrica Acta* 24:576-581, 1969.

Larson M, Hellquist R, and Jacobsson OP: Dental abnormalities and ectopic eruption in patients with isolated cleft palate. *Scandinavian Journal of Plastic and Reconstructive and Hand Surgery* 32:203-212, 1998.

Larson M, Sallstrom K-O, Larson L, McWilliam J, and Ideberg M: Morphologic effect of preoperative maxillofacial orthopedics (T-traction) on the maxilla in unilateral cleft lip and palate patients. *Cleft Palate–Craniofacial Journal* 30:29-34, 1993.

Larson O, and Nilsson B: Early bone grafting in complete cleft lip and palate cases following maxillofacial orthopedics. VI: Assessments from photographs and anthropometric measurements. *Scandinavian Journal of Plastic and Reconstructive Surgery* 17:209-223, 1983.

Latham RA: Orthopedic advancement of the cleft maxillary segment: a preliminary report. *Cleft Palate Journal* 17:227-233, 1980.

Latham RA, Kusy RP, and Georgiade NG: An extraorally activated expansion appliance for cleft palate infants. *Cleft Palate Journal* 13:253-261, 1976.

LaVelle WE, and Van Demark DR: Construction of a maxillary orthopedic prosthesis for simultaneous maxillary expansion and obturation. *Journal of Prosthetic Dentistry* 35:665-670, 1976.

Lennartsson B, Friede H, and Johanson B: Effect of post-surgical jaw-orthopaedic treatment in unilateral cleft lip and palate patients. *Scandinavian Journal of Plastic and Reconstructive Surgery* 18:227-231, 1984.

Lilja J, Yontchev E, Friede H, and Elander A: Use of Titanium implants as an integrated part of a CLP protocol. *Scandinavian Journal of Plastic and Reconstructive and Hand Surgery* 32:213-219, 1998.

Loevy HT, and Aduss H: Tooth maturation in cleft lip, cleft palate, or both. *Cleft Palate Journal* 25:343-347, 1988.

Markowitz JA, Gerry RG, and Fleishner R: Immediate obturation of neonatal cleft palates. *Mt. Sinai Journal of Medicine* 46:123-129, 1979.

Marsh J, and Wray R: Speech prosthesis versus pharyngeal flap: a randomized evaluation of the management of velopharyngeal incompetency. *Plastic and Reconstructive Surgery* 5:592-594, 1980.

Martin LW: A new "gravity-flow" nipple for feeding infants with congenital cleft palate. *Pediatrics* 72:244, 1983.

Mazaheri M: Prosthodontic care. In Cooper HK, Harding R, Krogman W, Mazaheri M, and Millard R (eds.): *Cleft palate and cleft lip: a team approach to clinical management and rehabilitation of the patient.* Philadelphia: WB Saunders, 1979, pp. 268-357.

McNeil CK: *Oral and facial deformity.* New York: Pitman, 1954.

Milenkovich PM, Gold HO, and Pruzansky S: Orthodontic-prosthodontic collaboration in the treatment of craniofacial anomalies. *International Journal of Orthodontics* 19:9-18, 1981.

Mishima K, Sugahara T, Mori Y, Minami K, and Sakuda M: Effects of presurgical orthopedic treatment in infants with complete bilateral cleft lip and palate. *Cleft Palate–Craniofacial Journal* 35:227-232, 1998.

Mishima K, Sugahara T, Mori Y, and Sakuda M: A three-dimensional comparison between the palatal forms in complete unilateral cleft lip, alveolus, and palate (UCLP) infants with and without Hotz's plate. *Cleft Palate–Craniofacial Journal* 33:77-83, 1996a.

Mishima K, Sugahara T, Mori Y, and Sakuda M: Three-dimensional comparison between the palatal forms in complete unilateral cleft lip and palate with and without Hotz plate from cheiloplasty to palatoplasty. *Cleft Palate–Craniofacial Journal* 33:312-317, 1996b.

Monroe CW: Use of bone grafts in complete clefts of the alveolar ridge. In Georgiade NG (ed.): *Symposium on management of cleft lip and palate and associated deformities.* St. Louis: Mosby, 1974, pp. 242-247.

Monroe CW, and Rosenstein SW: Maxillary orthopedics and bone grafting in cleft palate. In Grabb WC, Rosenstein SW, and Bzoch KR (eds.): *Cleft lip and palate: surgical, dental and speech aspects.* Boston: Little, Brown, 1971, pp. 573-582.

Moore DJ: The continuing role of the prosthodontist in the treatment of patients with cleft lip and palate. *Journal of Prosthetic Dentistry* 36:186-192, 1976.

Moore RB: Orthodontic management of the patient with cleft lip and palate. *Ear, Nose and Throat Journal* 65:46-58, 1986.

Morikawa M, Toyoda M, and Toyoda S: Prosthetic management of postsurgical fistulas in patients with cleft lip and palate. *Journal of Prosthetic Dentistry* 58:614-616, 1987.

Nordin E-E, Larson O, Nylen B, and Eklund G: Early bone grafting in complete cleft lip and palate cases following maxillofacial orthopedics. I: The method and skeletal development from seven to thirteen years of age. *Scandinavian Journal of Plastic and Reconstructive Surgery* 17:33-50, 1983.

O'Donnell JP, Krischer JP, and Shiere FR: An analysis of presurgical orthopedics in the treatment of unilateral cleft lip and palate. *Cleft Palate Journal* 11:374-393, 1974.

Oliver HT: Construction of orthodontic appliances for the treatment of newborn infants. *American Journal of Orthodontics* 56:468-473, 1969.

Paradise JL, and McWilliams BJ: Simplified feeder for infants with cleft palate. *Pediatrics* 53:566-568, 1974.

Pashayan HM, and McNab M: Simplified method of feeding infants born with cleft palate with or without cleft lip. *American Journal of Diseases of Children* 133:145-147, 1979.

Peat JH: Effects of presurgical oral orthopedics on bilateral complete clefts of the lip and palate. *Cleft Palate Journal* 19:100-103, 1982.

Peterson-Falzone SJ: Speech disorders associated with dentofacial anomalies. In Kaban LB (ed.): *Pediatric oral and maxillofacial surgery.* Philadelphia: WB Saunders, 1990, pp. 63-70.

Plint DA, and Mars M: Letter to the editor. *British Journal of Orthodontics* 10:219, 1983.

Posnick JC: The treatment of secondary and residual dentofacial deformities in the cleft patient: surgical and orthodontic therapy. *Clinics in Plastic Surgery: Secondary Management of Craniofacial Disorders* 24:583-597, 1997.

Posnick W: Prosthetic management of palatopharyngeal incompetency for the pediatric patient. *Journal of Dentistry for Children* March-April: 117-121, 1977.

Prahl-Anderson B: The dental development in patients with cleft lip and palate. *European Orthodontic Society: Transactions of the 52nd Congress* 52:155-161, 1976.

Pruzansky S: Pre-surgical orthopedics and bone grafting for infants with cleft lip and palate: a dissent. *Cleft Palate Journal* 1:164-187, 1964.

Pruzansky S, and Aduss H: Arch form and the deciduous occlusion in complete unilateral clefts. *Cleft Palate Journal* 1:411-418, 1964.

Pruzansky S, and Aduss H: Prevalence of arch collapse and malocclusion in complete unilateral cleft lip and palate. *European Orthodontic Society Report of Congress* 1967, pp. 365-382.

Raggazzini F, La Causa C, and Marianelli L: Il nanisimo ipofisario da labio-gnato-palatoschisi. *Minerva Pediatrica* 30:1163-1166, 1978.

Ranalli D, and Mazaheri M: Height-weight growth of cleft children, birth to six years. *Cleft Palate Journal* 12:400-404, 1975.

Ranta R: Eruption of the premolars and canines and factors affecting it in unilateral cleft lip and palate cases: an orthopantomographic study. *Suomen Hammaslaakariseuran Toimituksia* 67:350-355, 1971.

Ranta R: The development of the permanent dentition in children with complete cleft lip and palate. *Proceedings of the Finnish Dental Society* 68(Suppl 3), 1972.

Razek MKA: Prosthetic feeding aids for infants with cleft lip and palate. *Journal of Prosthetic Dentistry* 44:556-561, 1980.

Reisberg DJ, Figueroa AA, and Gold HO: An intraoral appliance for management of the protrusive premaxilla in bilateral cleft lip. *Cleft Palate–Craniofacial Journal* 25:53-57, 1988.

Rintala AE, and Gylling UO: Birth weight of infants with cleft lip and palate. *Scandinavian Journal of Plastic and Reconstructive Surgery* 1:109-112, 1967.

Robertson NRE: Facial form of patients with cleft lip and palate: the long-term influence of presurgical oral orthopaedics. *British Dental Journal* 155:59-61, 1983.

Robertson NRE, and Hilton R: The changes produced by presurgical oral orthopedics. *British Journal of Plastic Surgery* 24:57-68, 1971.

Robertson NRE, Shaw WC, and Volp C: The changes produced by presurgical orthopedic treatment of bilateral cleft lip and palate. *Plastic and Reconstructive Surgery* 59:86-93, 1977.

Rosen MS, and Bzoch KR: Prosthodontic management of the individual with cleft lip and palate for speech habilitation needs. In Bzoch KR (ed.): *Communicative disorders related to cleft lip and palate.* Austin: Pro-ed, 1997, pp. 153-167.

Rosenstein SW: A new concept in the early orthopedic treatment of cleft lip and palate. *American Journal of Orthodontics* 55:765-775, 1969.

Rosenstein SW: Management of the maxillary segments in complete unilateral cleft lip patients. In Georgiade NG (ed.): *Symposium on management of cleft lip and palate and associated deformities.* St. Louis: Mosby, 1974a, pp. 43-46.

Rosenstein SW: Management of the protruding premaxilla: maxillary orthopedics. In Georgiade NG (ed.): *Symposium on management of cleft lip and palate and associated deformities.* St. Louis: Mosby, 1974b, pp. 118-122.

Ross RB: The management of dental arch deformity in cleft lip and palate. *Clinics in Plastic Surgery* 2:325-342, 1975.

Ross RB: Treatment variables affecting facial growth in complete unilateral cleft lip and palate. *Cleft Palate Journal* 24:54-77, 1987.

Ross RB: Discussion of Georgiade NG, Mason R, Riefkohl R, Georgiade G, and Barwick W: Preoperative positioning of the protruding premaxilla in the bilateral cleft lip patient. *Plastic and Reconstructive Surgery* 83:39-40, 1989.

Ross RB, and Johnston MC: The effect of early orthodontic treatment on facial growth in cleft lip and palate. *Cleft Palate Journal* 4:157-164, 1967.

Rudman D, Davis G, Priest J, Patterson J, Kutner M, Heymsfield S, and Bethel R: Prevalence of growth hormone deficiency in children with cleft lip or palate. *Journal of Pediatrics* 93:378-382, 1978.

Rutrick R, Black PW, and Jurkiewicz MJ: Bilateral cleft lip and palate: presurgical treatment. *Annals of Plastic Surgery* 12:105-117, 1984.

Rygh P, and Tindlund R: Orthopedic expansion and protraction of the maxilla in cleft palate patients—a new treatment rationale. *Cleft Palate Journal* 19:104-112, 1982.

Samant A: A one-visit obturator technique for infants with cleft palate. *Journal of Oral and Maxillofacial Surgery* 47:539-540, 1989.

Seth AK, and McWilliams BG: Weight gain in children with cleft palate from birth to two years. *Cleft Palate Journal* 25:146-150, 1988.

Severens JL, Prahl C, Kuijpers-Jagtman AM, and Prahl-Andersen B: Short-term cost-effectiveness analysis of presurgical orthopedic treatment in children with complete unilateral cleft lip and palate. *Cleft Palate–Craniofacial Journal* 35:222-226, 1998.

Shaw WC: Early orthopaedic treatment of unilateral cleft lip and palate. *British Journal of Orthodontics* 5:119-132, 1978.

Sierra FJ, and Turner C: Maxillary orthopedics in the presurgical management of infants with cleft lip and palate. *Pediatric Dentistry* 17:419-423, 1995.

Smahel Z: Treatment effect on facial development in patients with unilateral cleft lip and palate. *Cleft Palate–Craniofacial Journal* 31:431-445, 1994.

Solis A, Figueroa AA, Cohen M, Polley JW, and Evans CA: Maxillary dental development in complete unilateral alveolar clefts. *Cleft Palate–Craniofacial Journal* 35:320-328, 1998.

Spira M, Findley S, Hardy SB, and Gerow FJ: Early maxillary orthopedics in cleft palate patients: a clinical report. *Cleft Palate Journal* 6:461-470, 1969.

Takahashi T, Fukuda M, Yamaguchi T, and Kochi S: Use of endosseous implants for dental reconstruction of patients with grafted alveolar clefts. *Journal of Oral and Maxillofacial Surgery* 55:576-583, 1997.

Thompson RPJ, Ferguson JW, and Barton M: The role of removable orthodontic appliances in the investigation and management of patients with hypernasal speech. *British Journal of Orthodontics* 12:70-77, 1985.

Trankmann J: Postnatale prae- und post-operative kieferorthopaedische Behandlung bei Lippen-Kiefer-Gaumen-Spalten. *Quintessenz* 1:69-78, 1986.

Troutman KC: Maxillary arch control in infants with unilateral clefts of the lip and palate. *American Journal of Orthodontics* 66:198-208, 1974.

Vargervik K: Orthodontic management of unilateral cleft lip and palate. *Cleft Palate Journal* 18:256-270, 1981.

Vargervik K: Growth characteristics of the premaxilla and orthodontic treatment principles in bilateral cleft lip and palate. *Cleft Palate Journal* 20:289-302, 1983.

Vargervik K: Orthodontic treatment of cleft patients: characteristics of growth and development/treatment principles. In Bardach J, and Morris HL (eds.): *Multidisciplinary management of cleft lip and palate.* Philadelphia: WB Saunders, 1990, pp. 642-649.

Vargervik K: Orthodontic treatment of children with cleft lip and palate. In Bardach J, and Shprintzen RJ (eds.): *Cleft palate speech management.* St. Louis: Mosby, 1995, pp. 295-304.

von Schwanwede H, and Schuberth H: Long-term results of prosthetic therapy in adult cleft lip alveolus and palate patients. *Journal of Cranio-Maxillo-Facial Surgery* 17:52-54, 1989.

Walter JD: Palatopharyngeal activity in cleft palate subjects. *Journal of Prosthetic Dentistry* 63:187-192, 1990.

Williams AC, Rothman BN, and Sedman IH: Management of a feeding problem in an infant with cleft palate. *Journal of the American Dental Association* 77:81-83, 1968.

Chapter 6

Hearing Disorders in Cleft Palate and Other Craniofacial Anomalies

Ear disease and hearing loss constitute a major potential threat to communication in individuals with cleft palate and many of the multi-anomaly craniofacial disorders (Fig. 6-1). More than 90% of infants with cleft palate are born with fluid already present in the middle ear cavity (Paradise, Bluestone, and Felder, 1969), and youngsters with clefts are vulnerable to middle ear disease until their later childhood or teenage years. As you learned in Chapter 2, many of the multi-anomaly disorders involve structural anomalies of the outer or middle ear, with a high likelihood of conductive hearing loss. Furthermore, in some associations or syndromes there is a known risk of sensorineural or mixed hearing loss. The aggregate effect of all these factors produces a high probability of hearing problems, either on a temporary or long-term basis.

The basics of otologic anatomy and function, as well as audiologic testing, are covered in other undergraduate and graduate courses and will not be repeated here. However, we will briefly review the relationship between the velopharyngeal system and the auditory system before going on to discuss hearing loss in cleft and other craniofacial anomalies.

RELATIONSHIP BETWEEN THE VELOPHARYNGEAL SYSTEM AND THE MIDDLE EAR

The musculature of the velopharyngeal system is intimately tied to that of the eustachian tube. As you know, the tube provides for (1) aeration of the middle ear cavity, (2) equalization of pressure between the middle ear cavity and the ambient or atmospheric pressure, and (3) drainage of middle ear fluid and secretions into the nasopharynx. The primary muscle responsible for opening the eustachian tube is the tensor veli palatini, the inferior bundle of which is termed the "dilator tubae."[1]

[1]See Chapter 3 for a detailed description of the anatomy and physiologic features of the tensor as well as the other palatal and pharyngeal muscles.

The traditionally accepted explanation of the high susceptibility of children with clefts to middle ear disease is that the cleft interferes with the ability of the tensor to open the eustachian tube (Fig. 6-2) (Bluestone, 1971; Bluestone et al., 1975; Doyle, Cantekin, and Bluestone, 1980; Moore, Moore, and Yonkers, 1986; Paradise, Bluestone, and Felder, 1969). The dilator tubae attaches to the fibroelastic layer that separates the two bundles of the tensor and runs to a supermedial attachment on the lateral wall of the eustachian tube. A tendinous segment travels downward around the hamulus of the pterygoid bone and inserts into the palatine aponeurosis (a firm plate of fibrous connective tissue), where it joins the tensor from the opposite side. Tensor fibers also insert into the hard palate. When there is a cleft of the secondary palate, the normal "anchor" for the palatal end of the tensor is missing, meaning that the muscle cannot contract to efficiently open the pharyngeal orifice of the eustachian tube. Another factor disrupting this function is abnormal anatomic relationships between the cartilage of the tube and the tensor muscle (Shibahara and Sando, 1988).

Clinicians as well as anatomists and physiologists have argued for years about whether the levator veli palatini plays any role in opening the eustachian tube. In 1978 Seif and Dellon concluded from anatomical dissections of normal specimens that the levator, rather than the tensor, is primarily responsible for tubal function. They concluded that no muscle actively opens the tube in the sense of pulling open a lumen. Rather, they viewed the drainage of secretions from the tube as a function of gravity, assisted by contraction of the levator because such action elevates the central portion of the tube (Fig. 6-3). Secondarily, they proposed that contraction of the tensor pushes the membranous covering of the tube medially during swallowing and perhaps during speech, performing a sort of "milking" action. Their report provoked a vehement letter to the editor from Rood and Doyle (1979), which in turn provoked an equally vehement answer from Dellon (1979).

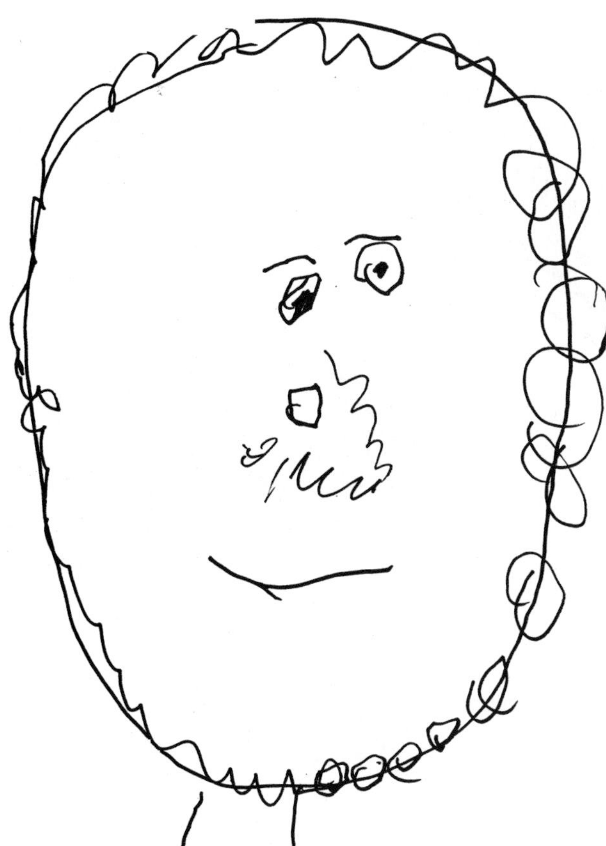

Figure 6-1 Self-portrait drawn by a 3½-year-old boy who has a bilateral cleft lip and palate (not clearly portrayed in his representation). His mother asked him if all the circles around his head were curls. He replied no, they were extra ears so that he could hear better and then his speech would be better.

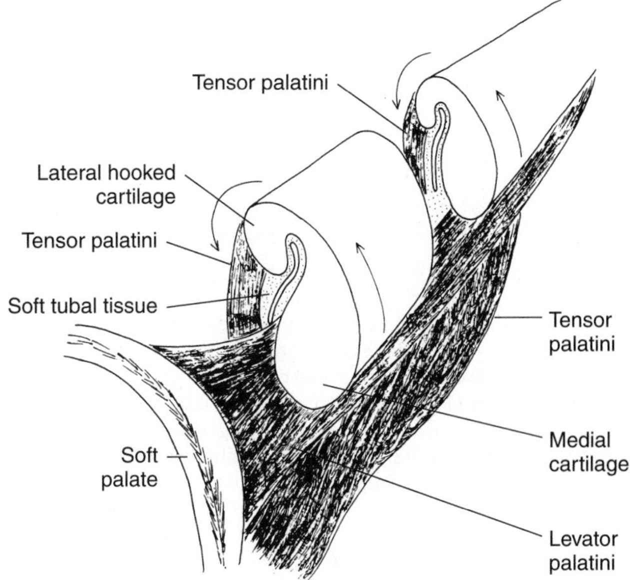

Figure 6-2 The traditional explanation of how the tensor veli palatini opens the eustachian tube is that the dilator tubae portion of the muscle pulls the lateral hooked cartilage away from the membranous wall of the tube. *(From Zemlin WR:* Speech and hearing: anatomy and physiology. *4th ed. Boston: Allyn and Bacon, 1998.)*

Each set of authors accused the other of drawing conclusions from extremely small samples (four adult and three fetal specimens in the Seif and Dellon work, a total of six adult heads and four fetal heads in two reports by Rood and Doyle). Perhaps the strongest point made in Rood and Doyle's (1979) criticism of the article by Seif and Dellon was that the latter authors had not dealt with the fact that the tensor veli palatini consists of two bundles with two different bony attachments. The superior bundle attaches to the cranial base, but the dilator tubae originates from the lateral membranous wall. Seif and Dellon had essentially ignored the dilator tubae in making their interpretations and reaching their conclusions.

Just before the report of Seif and Dellon (1979) and response from Rood and Doyle (1979), Cantekin et al. (1977) reported that excision or transection of the tensor veli palatini muscle in monkeys consistently resulted in negative middle ear pressure and middle ear effusion. In an electromyographic and electrical stimulation study on dogs, Honjo, Okazaki, and Kumazawa (1979) concluded that the sole muscle responsible for tubal opening is the tensor veli palatini and that the levator does not participate in the functioning of the tube. Because the cranial base in dogs is considerably different from that in humans, there is a question as to how applicable these results are to eustachian tube physiology in humans. The study of Cantekin et al. (1977) is perhaps more applicable.

Finkelstein et al. (1990) examined two patients with unilateral paralysis of the levator (as well as 28 other patients with a variety of palatal anomalies) and found no history of serous otitis media nor current disease. They took this to mean that the levator played no role in the function of the eustachian tube. However, as pointed out in the commentaries on the article by Edgerton (1990) and Shprintzen and Gereau (1990), this "study" was fraught with methodological errors and questionable conclusions. Edgerton (1990) recalled that early German anatomists had demonstrated that contraction and fattening of the muscle belly of the levator would passively lift the eustachian tube cartilage and open the lumen. He also recalled his own work with Dellon (1971) in which they found that retrodisplacement of the levator as a part of palatal repair provided substantial improvement in hearing. Shprintzen and Gereau (1990) pointed out that Finkelstein et al. had used subjects well above the age at which serous otitis media tends to resolve naturally, that they failed to control for other variables that might have bearing on presence or absence of ear disease (climate, exposure to pathogens, etc.), and that they assumed a cause-and-effect relationship (or lack of one) between two observable events (abnormal levator, lack of ear disease).

The general impression gained from reviewing articles on this topic of "tensor veli palatini (only)" versus

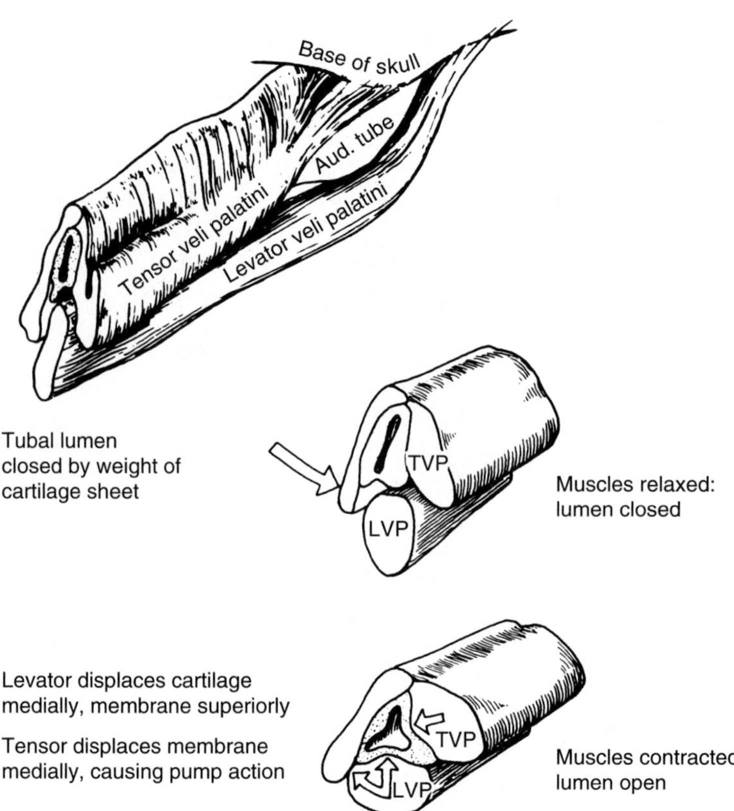

Figure 6-3 Seif and Dellon (1978) proposed a different explanation of how the eustachian tube is opened: during swallowing and speech a "milking" or pumping action is created by contraction of the levator *(LVP)* and tensor *(TVP)* muscles. *(From Zemlin WR:* Speech and hearing: anatomy and physiology. *4th ed. Boston: Allyn and Bacon, 1998.)*

importance of the levator veli palatini remains that the tensor is the primary muscle important for eustachian tube function, with a secondary role for the levator.

In your anatomy courses, you also learned that the eustachian tube is essentially positioned horizontally in the infant and assumes a more tilted position as the child matures (Fig. 6-4). The horizontal position of the tube in the infant is a disadvantage because it decreases the ability of the tensor to open the tube and also permits retrograde passage of nasopharyngeal bacteria into the middle ear.

When the eustachian cannot open efficiently and the middle ear cannot be ventilated, the tympanic membrane retracts and an effusion from the middle ear mucosa develops as the negative pressure increases within the middle ear cavity. The negative middle ear pressure also draws bacteria up through the tube (Fig. 6-5). Eustachian tube "obstruction" is seen as the primary cause for the ear disease in children with clefts, but abnormal compliance or "floppiness" of the tube is also a factor (Bluestone, 1971; Bluestone et al., 1972, 1975; Bluestone, Klein, and Kenna, 1990a; Bluestone, Wittel, and Paradise, 1972; Moore, Moore, and Yonkers, 1986). Bluestone (1971) suggested that the tube may be floppy or hypercompliant because of the quality of the cartilage, muscular dysfunction, or other factors. Shibahara and Sando (1988) documented abnormal tube cartilage in cleft palate specimens. However, Takahashi, Honjo, and Fujita (1994) reported that the eustachian tubes of patients with otitis media with effusion were more collapsible both in subjects with clefts and subjects without clefts, leading them to speculate that the abnormal compliance of the tube could be due to an inflammatory condition of the tubal mucosa rather than to abnormal anatomy or inherently abnormal cartilage. In other words, the floppiness of the tube may be the result of inflammation, not the presence of the cleft. However, this suggestion does not negate the anatomic abnormalities of the tube and the abnormal relationship between the tube and the tensor veli palatini reported by other investigators.

Another consequence of middle ear disease is decreased pneumatization of the temporal bone, a finding that has been reported in children with cleft palate (Stool and Winn, 1969) and in subjects without cleft palate (Stool, 1989). In fact, the list of reported complications of otitis media that persist or go undertreated is quite extensive: tympanic membrane perforations, cholesteatoma, ossicular chain discontinuity and fixation, mastoiditis, labyrinthitis, and infections of the auditory canal (Bluestone, Klein, and Kenna, 1990b; Severeid, 1977).

TYPE AND EXTENT OF HEARING LOSS ASSOCIATED WITH CLEFT PALATE

According to Dhillon (1988), the first published report of the association of hearing loss with cleft palate appeared in 1878. For more than five decades there have been repeated reports of a typically conductive bilateral loss, usually mild to moderate in degree (Drettner, 1952; Gaines, 1940;

Infant ear

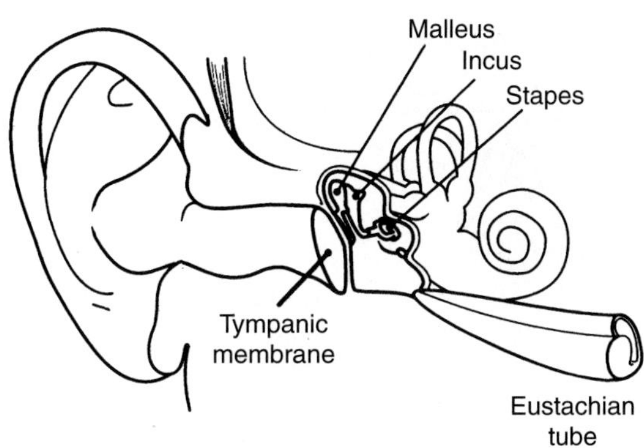

Adult ear

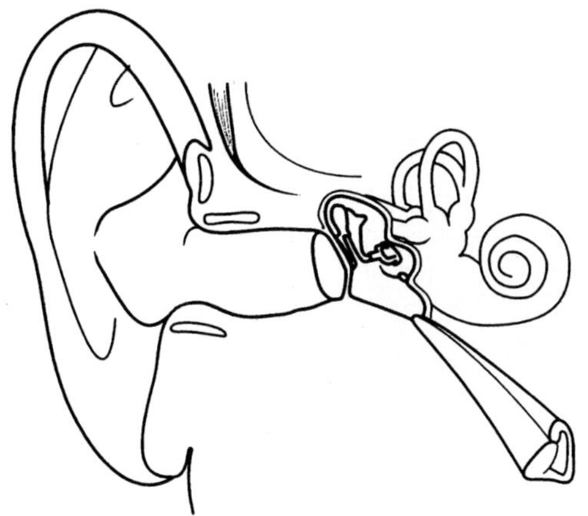

Figure 6-4 The eustachian tube of an infant lies on a more horizontal plane than in the adult, which can contribute to retrograde flow of fluid and bacteria into the middle ear cavity. *(From Bess FH, and Humes LE:* Audiology: the fundamentals. *2nd ed. Baltimore: Williams & Wilkins, 1995.)*

Halfond and Ballenger, 1956; Handzic et al., 1989; Heller, Hochberg, and Milano, 1970; Holborow, 1962; Holmes and Reed, 1955; Masters, Bingham, and Robinson, 1960; Paradise, Bluestone, and Felder, 1969; Sataloff and Fraser, 1952; Skolnik, 1958; Yules, 1975). Historically, findings with regard to severity have varied in accordance with the testing methods and the definitions used by investigators to delimit each category of loss. As in any area of clinical investigation, variations in these standards must be borne in mind as one attempts to compare results of one study with another, especially if there was a substantial time gap between the two, because clinical standards, by nature, change as science matures.

The hearing loss associated with chronic otitis media is not always exclusively conductive in nature. There have been reports of high-frequency loss (Ahonen and McDermott, 1984; Bennett, 1972; Manning et al., 1994; McDermott, Fausti, and Frey, 1986). Bennett (1972) found either mixed or sensorineural hearing loss in 31 of 58 (53%) teenagers and adults with clefts who were too young for presbycusis to be an explanation for the sensorineural loss. In many cases the drop was seen only at 6000 Hz (the highest frequency tested in this study). Bennett wondered, "Is there a progressive sensorineural hearing impairment in congenital cleft disease?" (p. 1223). Her published report did not indicate whether the cases had been screened for possible syndromic involvement. Ahonen and McDermott (1984) tested the frequency range of 250 through 20,000 Hz in children with repaired cleft palate and a history of otitis media compared with control subjects without clefts or a history of ear disease. The children in the cleft group had poorer hearing throughout the tested range, but statistically significant differences were found only in the range above 9000 Hz. A later study (McDermott, Fausti, and Frey, 1986) compared children with clefts and a history of ear disease with control subjects without clefts but a high incidence of middle ear disease and found that both groups showed losses in the 8000 to 20,000 Hz range that were not found in controls. They concluded that middle ear disease alone is a "sufficient condition" for loss of auditory sensitivity in the high frequencies.

There have been differing opinions about the cause for high-frequency loss in individuals (cleft or noncleft) with a history of otitis media. Paparella and associates (Goycoolea et al., 1980; Paparella et al., 1972, 1984) felt that sensorineural hearing loss in patients with otitis media could be the result of toxic metabolites passing across the round window membrane into the inner ear. Others (Strohm, 1986; Tonndorf, 1966; Tonndorf and Pastaci, 1986) argued that conductive high-frequency losses could result from anatomical changes in inner ear spaces. Manning et al. (1994) interpreted elevated thresholds by ABR testing at 2000 Hz and above as evidence of sensorineural loss in two infants with clefts. In a relatively recent report (Handzic-Cuk et al., 1996, p. 241), the authors stated, "Children with bilateral or unilateral cleft lip and palate and isolated cleft palate mostly suffer from moderate (21-40 dB) and severe (>40 dB) conductive, bilateral hearing loss by the age of 6 years, accompanied by sensorineural hearing loss of 30 dB on average." However, the extensive tabular data presented within the article do not support this statement: The tables do not specify how many of the patients in any given age group (or how many in the entire study) actually showed *any* sensorineural loss.

OTITIS MEDIA ASSOCIATED WITH CLEFT PALATE

Studies in Infants and Young Children

Although clinicians had long known that individuals with cleft palate were particularly prone to ear disease and hearing loss, the extent to which otitis media predominated in babies with clefts was not fully appreciated until the late 1960s. In the reports of Paradise, Bluestone, and Felder (1969) and Stool and Randall (1967) the percentage of

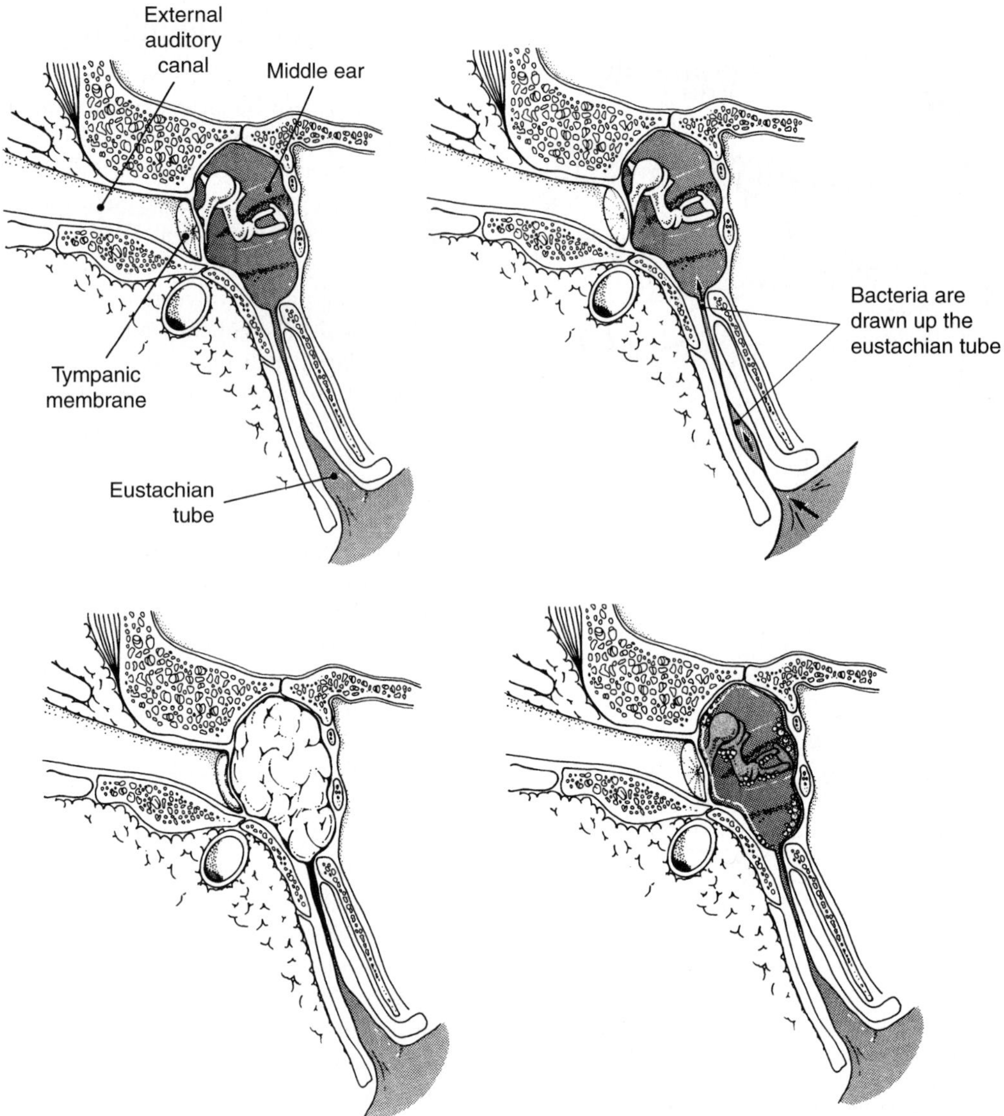

Figure 6-5 Negative pressure in the middle ear can draw bacteria from the pharyngeal opening of the eustachian tube upward through the tube and into the middle ear cavity. *(From Bess FH, and Humes LE:* Audiology: the fundamentals. *2nd ed. Baltimore: Williams & Wilkins, 1995.)*

children with fluid present in the middle ear was more than 95%. These findings motivated a major campaign for myringotomies and placement of ventilating tubes in babies with clefts (Fig. 6-6) (Bluestone et al., 1972; Fria et al., 1987; Hubbard et al., 1985; Paradise, 1976; Stool, 1989). Interestingly, in a relatively recent study (Paradise, Elster, and Tan, 1994) it was demonstrated that breast milk helps to decrease the incidence of otitis media in infants with clefts.

In 1985 Hubbard et al. looked at hearing acuity in two groups of babies with cleft palate; one group had early myringotomy and the other did not. At the time of the assessment that formed the basis for the study, the children were distributed into three age groups: 5 to 6 years, 7 to 8 years, and 9 to 11 years. Both groups had about equal numbers of tympanic membrane perforations. The pure-tone averages for the early-tube group were a few decibels less than those for the later myringotomy group (6.1 dB left, 5.8 dB right in the early tubes group, 11.7 dB left, 9.4 dB right in the later tubes group). This study was followed by others that indicated better results from earlier rather than later intervention.

Broen et al. (1996) reported the hearing histories of 28 children with clefts and 29 noncleft children who were seen at 3-month intervals from 9 to 30 months of age. Information on placement of ventilating tubes from birth to enrollment in the study was obtained from parents and medical records. As you would expect, ventilation tubes were placed earlier and more often in the children with clefts. Also, there was a significant correlation between the

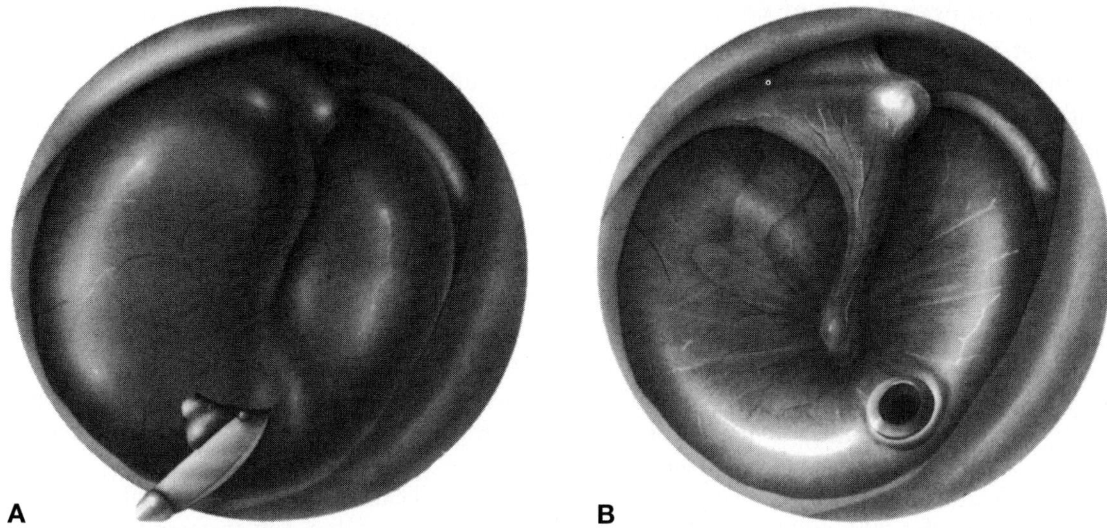

Figure 6-6 Myringotomy **(A)** and a ventilating tube or "grommet" **(B)** in the tympanic membrane. Note the bulging appearance of the membrane before the pressure-equalization tube is placed. *(From Bess FH, and Humes LE:* Audiology: the fundamentals. *2nd ed. Baltimore: Williams & Wilkins, 1995.)*

age at first tube placement and the frequency of hearing screening failures: the later the tubes were placed, the poorer the child's hearing.

In a cross-sectional study of the ear status of 3-year-old children with repaired clefts who had not all had aggressive ear care, Rynnel-Dagoo et al. (1992) reported that one third had long-standing secretory otitis media and that 12 of the 44 children (27%) had had two of more episodes of acute otitis media. About one third had had placement of ventilating tubes, but by the age of 3 years only one child still had tubes. Hearing was "normal" (pure tone average of 20 dB or less for 500 to 3000 Hz) in 82% of the children, and the specific antipneumococcal antibody activity was compatible with the activity found in healthy age-matched controls. The authors felt that these data supported a more conservative approach to otologic care in children with clefts, with careful monitoring rather than universal use of ventilating tubes.

In 1993 Muntz reported the results of a retrospective survey of 132 children with clefts. He did not specify the ages of the children at the times of team visits (clinical evaluations), but the impression gained from the article is that most, if not all, were seen initially as infants. A total of 96.2% had significant middle ear disease, defined as three or more episodes of acute otitis media in a 6-month period or chronic otitis media with effusion for longer than 3 months. This percentage coincides well with the percentage of infants with middle ear fluid reported by Paradise, Bluestone, and Felder (1969) and by Stool and Randall (1967). Muntz (1993) also reported that, at the 3-year team visit, the mean pure tone average was about 17 dB (17.7 dB right ear, 17.0 dB left ear) in these children. Because this level is greater than the 15 dB suggested by Northern and Downs (1974) as a demarcation for hearing levels that could lead to problems in speech and language development, Muntz (1993, pp. 179-180) decided that, although "[the cleft palate population] as a whole was considered to be relatively well served by annual cleft palate team visits and suggested primary care by local physicians . . . more aggressive and frequent monitoring of this high-risk patient population is indicated."

In an older retrospective study on the prevalence of ear disease in 5-year-olds with repaired clefts, Potsic et al. (1979) compared three groups of subjects: one with no myringotomies, one with myringotomies performed after initial palate repair and only when deemed necessary, and one with myringotomies performed simultaneously with palate repair. The standards for "hearing impairment" in this study were stricter than those in the study of Rynnel-Dagoo et al. (1992), in that a pure tone average of 10 to 20 dB for the frequencies of 500 to 2000 Hz was termed a mild loss rather than normal hearing. A conductive hearing loss of 10 dB or greater was found in 57% of the nonmyringotomy group, 37% of the myringotomy-as-needed group, and 43% of the simultaneous myringotomy-palatoplasty group. Serous otitis media was present in 67%, 33%, and 41% of each group, respectively. There were no statistically significant differences among the groups with regard to prevalence of otologic abnormalities or conductive hearing loss. The authors concluded simply that the prevalence of hearing impairment and secretory otitis media at age 5 years in these three groups was consistent with what had been previously reported in children with clefts, and that, "Formulas or schedules for myringotomies and tube placements are not likely to be the answer to maximize the auditory capabilities of cleft palate patients. Identification of hearing impairment, treatment and continued monitoring will have to be based on clinical judgment. . . ." (p. 58).

Variables Affecting Prevalence of Ear Disease

Types of clefts. Paradise, Bluestone, and Felder (1969) found that the prevalence of otitis media was 96% in infants with cleft lip and palate or cleft palate only compared with only 22% in babies with cleft lip only and 19.5% in noncleft babies. This same pattern has held in other studies, so long as the authors or investigators have been careful not to classify babies as "cleft lip only" when they might at the same time have a submucous cleft of the secondary palate.[2] Spauwen et al. (1988) reported that bilateral chronic otitis media with effusion occurred just as frequently in isolated clefts of the secondary palate as in cleft lip and palate. In the study conducted by Handzic-Cuk et al. (1996) in Croatia a total of 59.7% of 243 patients from the ages of 1 year to 22+ years showed a conductive hearing loss in the speech frequencies (greater than 10 dB hearing level for 500, 1000, and 2000 Hz), and patients with isolated cleft palate showed greater improvement in hearing level with age than patients with either unilateral or bilateral clefts. To date, there have been no *infant* studies on differences in the occurrence of otitis media across patients with cleft palate only, unilateral cleft lip and palate, or bilateral cleft lip and palate (Gould, 1990).

Patients with submucous clefts and *perhaps* some other types of congenital velopharyngeal inadequacy may also be subject to a high prevalence of otitis media. Caldarelli (1978) found evidence of serous otitis media in 50% of patients (age range 4 to 37 years) with one or more of the classic visible stigmata of a submucous cleft, that is, bifid uvula, muscular dehiscence in the velum, or bony defect in the hard palate. The prevalence in individuals with "congenital palatopharyngeal incompetency type 2" (no visible stigmata) was 42%.[3] Durr and Shapiro (1989) used a slightly different classification of patients, adding "congenital palatopharyngeal neuromuscular dysfunction" to the categories used by Caldarelli. (The latter group, "CPND," would have been included under "CPI 2" in Caldarelli's study.) The age range in the Durr and Shapiro study was 3.5 to 23 years, mean 10.1 years. They found middle ear disease in 9 of 15 (60%) of patients with "CPI 1," 17 of 50 (34%) of patients with "CPI 2," and 4 of 15 (26.7%) of patients with "CPND." Spauwen et al. (1988) reported that chronic otitis media occurred in only two of the 17 patients aged 3 to 12 years with congenitally short palate as opposed to 24 of 34 of their patients with overt clefts. In two studies investigating the prevalence of ear disease in children with bifid uvula *only,* there was only a slightly higher (nonsignificant) prevalence of otitis media than in children with normal uvulae, and in both studies the authors concluded that bifid uvula alone was not really a marker for ear disease (Rivron, 1989; Schwartz et al., 1985).[4]

Heller et al. (1978) studied the prevalence of hearing loss in 77 patients with "velopharyngeal insufficiency." The patient population included seven with submucous clefts, 10 with palatal paresis, and 22 with palatopharyngeal disproportion. Hearing loss was present in 22% of each of the first two groups and in 56% of the latter group. The ages of the subjects were not specified. Of those who had hearing loss, the loss was conductive in 74%, sensorineural in 16%, and mixed in 10.

Age. There is some evidence that middle ear problems in the infant with a cleft increase in the first few months of life, as they tend to do in infants without clefts. Too-Chung (1983) documented normal middle ear function by tympanometry in 84 babies with clefts at birth but middle ear "complications" by the age of 17 weeks.[5] Age continues to be an important variable as the child matures, with a decrease in otologic problems both in cleft and noncleft children as age increases. The literature on ear disease and hearing loss in cleft palate includes multiple studies, and some reports apparently based on clinical insight, which support this observation (Bennett, 1972; Caldarelli, 1975; Heller, Hochberg, and Milano, 1970; Moller, 1975, 1981; Severeid, 1972). Obviously, this is a difficult relationship to establish. The older a child gets, the more likely that a variety of physical interventions (palatoplasty, myringotomies and tubes, perhaps secondary palatal procedures) have taken place and influenced results. However, there appears to be an underlying natural tendency for the occurrence of otitis media to decrease as *either* noncleft or cleft palate children mature. Perhaps this is related to the plane of the eustachian tube becoming more vertical than horizontal as the child grows, improving the muscle vectors for function of the tensor veli palatini, or to an increase in cartilage support of the tube (Bluestone et al., 1975; Severeid, 1972).

In the 1988 study by Gordon, Jean-Louis, and Morton, more than 80% of 50 children with clefts between the ages of 9 and 17 years had normal middle ear pressures and normal hearing. Only half of these 50 children had had

[2]Hayes (1994) included 34 infants with an isolated cleft lip or palate or both in her study of hearing loss in infants with craniofacial anomalies but did not differentiate among those with cleft lip only, cleft lip and palate, or cleft palate only, rendering her data and conclusions useless.

[3]None of the children in this study were examined by nasopharyngoscopy, so "occult" submucous clefts (see Chapter 8) could easily have been missed.

[4]In a histologic study of 35 adult human cadaver heads, Todd and Krueger (1992) found 7 with what they termed "minuscule submucous cleft palate" (haphazardly organized fibers of the levator palatini, midsagittal paucity of the musculus uvulae) and a "trend" for evidence of prior otitis media (abnormal pneumatization of the mastoid, scarred tympanic membranes) as opposed to the findings in cadavers with histologically normal uvulae. However, the findings were not statistically significant.

[5]However, 16 of these children had cleft lip only and four had Robin sequence.

placement of "grommets" (a synonym for ventilating tubes), which suggests that the ear problems had spontaneously resolved without the use of tubes in about 30%. Unfortunately, the article did not specify the ages at which the tubes had been placed.

In a 1990 study of the longitudinal audiologic records of 480 individuals with clefts, Gould found that after the age of 10 years of age most of these patients had "demonstrated normal hearing for a sufficient time to allow them to be released from routine follow-up." This is not to suggest that 10 years is somehow a magic threshold age for a decrease in otologic problems. Rather, Gould noted that the only patients on whom he had records after the age of 10 years were those with a continuing problem. He also noted that those children born after 1969 had better improvement in hearing than those born before that year, which was the year that brought an increase in the routine use of ventilating tubes.

Effects of palatoplasty. If the high prevalence of otitis media in individuals with clefts is in fact due to the presence of the cleft itself, the obvious conclusion is that repairing the cleft should help to eliminate ear disease. Clinicians have been looking into this question for at least two decades, but the results have varied, making the task of counseling families and predicting future problems very difficult. Three obvious problems in investigating the effect of palatoplasty on ear disease are (1) variation in the type of palatoplasty carried out, (2) variation in the age at which surgical repair was performed, to say nothing of the variation in amount of time elapsed between palatoplasty and follow-up for otologic and audiologic testing, and (3) inconsistency in whether (and when) tubes were placed in the ears. Most studies, but not all, have taken into account the possibility that a decrease in otitis media after palatoplasty could be at least partially attributable to the passage of time and thus the increased age of the child.

A series of studies of the ventilatory function of the middle ear and the radiographic evidence of the protective and drainage functions of the eustachian tube, conducted at the Cleft Palate Center in Pittsburgh in the 1970s, documented improvement in these functions in children with repaired palates in comparison to infants and children whose palates had not been repaired (Bluestone, 1971; Bluestone, Wittel, and Paradise, 1972; Bluestone et al., 1972, 1975; Paradise and Bluestone, 1974). Bluestone (1971) conjectured that persistent hearing losses in patients with repaired clefts were due to postoperative scarring and poor mobility of the palate. These studies were cross-sectional. In a longitudinal study of eustachian tube function in 24 children with clefts (Doyle et al., 1986), also done at the University of Pittsburgh, passive opening of the tube (opening forced by the application of positive pressure in the middle ear cavity) improved after palatoplasty, but active tubal opening (opening by muscle forces during swallowing) did not. That is, in children with a history of otitis media and repaired clefts, 70% showed defectiveness in tubal opening on swallow despite the surgical closure of the cleft.[6]

There are many surgical techniques for closing the palate, and investigators have tried for years to ascertain whether one technique produces better results in terms of eliminating or reducing further ear disease. To date, no single technique has proven universally advantageous. One area of specific concern has been whether surgery includes fracturing of the hamulus to obtain more medial "relocation" of the tensor veli palatini and thus facilitate closure of the palate. Fracturing the hamulus was a frequent part of palatoplasty in the 1950s and 1960s (Holborow, 1962; Skolnik, 1958), coming into controversy when otologists became more routinely involved in the care of babies with cleft palates and voiced their concern about the possible effects of this procedure on the ability of the tensor to open the eustachian tube (Moore, Moore, and Yonkers, 1986; Stool, 1989). Today, most techniques for palatoplasty do not include hamulotomy.

As noted earlier, Edgerton and Dellon reported in 1971 that retrodisplacement of the levator (into a more normal position) as a part of palatal repair provided substantial improvement in hearing. In 1983 Morgan, Dellon, and Hoopes conducted another investigation of this question, comparing the hearing loss in 34 patients who had had levator retrodisplacement with that in eight patients whose palatoplasties did not include retrodisplacement. All patients were operated on between the ages of 12 and 21 months. Apparently none had preoperative audiograms or any other type of functional or medical assessment of the ears. This was simply a comparison of the cross-sectional audiologic results. A total of 73.5% of those in the levator retrodisplacement group had normal hearing postoperatively in contrast to 37.5% in the nondisplacement group. Abnormal hearing was defined as a loss of 20 dB or more in the worse ear at 500, 1000, and 2000 Hz. Each patient had at least two postoperative audiograms, and follow-up ranged from 3 to 9 years. If one assumes that that the two groups of children were comparable in the mean age at the time of surgery and in the length of follow-up, so that increasing age itself was not a differentiating factor and thus a possible cause for improved auditory function, then the data do seem to support levator retrodisplacement as a possible means for improving the chances for otologic health and normal hearing after palatoplasty. However, it should be noted that this study was done long after myringotomies and

[6]Lauffer et al. (1993) used brainstem-evoked potentials to assess hearing in 37 infants with clefts and also reported that surgical closure of the cleft did not produce improvement in conductive hearing loss. However, recent years have seen the development for improved means of assessing hearing thresholds in infants, so that audiologists no longer rely exclusively on brainstem-evoked potentials (the technique also used in the study by Fria et al. [1987] for assessment of children once considered too young for "behavioral" audiometric testing).

tubes became routine treatment for infants with clefts, yet the infants in the study did not even have preoperative assessment of their ears, let alone state-of-the-art treatment.

In another study that confused the effects of age with the effects of surgery, Gopalakrishna, Goleria, and Raje (1984) reported that "... when the cleft palate had been repaired before the age of 6 years, eustachian tube function improved significantly ... as shown by the lower incidence of negative middle ear pressure and eustachian tube block" (p. 558). These authors did not specify the age at surgery except to say that all were operated on before the age of 6 years. They looked at 20 patients with unoperated clefts, 28 normal control subjects, and 20 with repaired clefts. Each group was divided into "under the age of 6 years" and "over the age of 6 years" at the time of examination. Some improvement in middle ear function was found in both groups with clefts over the age of 6 years, but more so in those with repaired clefts. However, the data were not subjected to statistical analysis and thus we do not know to what extent age itself might have played a role in the improvement. Similar problems affected the study by Garabedian et al. (1988). They combined the data obtained on children with clefts of the soft palate only, clefts of the hard and soft palate, and unilateral and bilateral clefts of the lip and palate; the babies in the first two groups had surgical closure of their palates earlier than those in the last two groups, and the ages at the time of impedance testing and audiologic assessment were not specified.

There are still some surgeons and treatment centers following the regimen of closing the velum first ("primary veloplasty") and waiting to close the hard palate until the child is 5 or 6 years of age or even older (see Chapter 4). In a study that was essentially outdated even before it was performed, Frable, Brandon, and Theogaraj (1985) reviewed 36 patients who had had primary veloplasty between 12 and 15 months of age, with simultaneous placement of ear tubes. The prevalence of subsequent ear disease was 17%. However, the age at surgery was much later than even other practitioners of primary veloplasty would recommend and certainly later than most treatment centers recommend placement of ventilating tubes in babies with clefts. Braganza, Kearns, Burton, Seid, and Pransky (1991) reported changes in ear status in four infants in whom primary veloplasty was performed several weeks or months after placement of ventilating tubes. In each case the otorrhea was refractory to other types of treatment (antibiotics, otic drops). The veloplasty apparently represented a last resort in the battle against the otorrhea, which was in fact greatly reduced or eliminated postoperatively.[7]

[7]The age of soft palate repair was 4 months in one infant, 6 months in two infants, and 9 months in one infant. It is worth noting that there are many treatment centers in the United States and Europe that perform *complete* repairs of the hard and soft palate at 9 months of age, and a few in which palatal repairs are done within the first few months of life (see Chapter 4).

Freeland and Evans (1981) reported a prevalence of otitis media with effusion of 56% in 6-month-old infants who were being hospitalized for palatal repair and who had not had prior treatment for middle ear effusions. After palate repair the prevalence fell to 41% "either spontaneously or as a result of palatal surgery," as the authors put it. This drop is not very impressive, whatever the cause, and the authors endorsed use of myringotomy and tubes in infants. Dhillon (1988) found little improvement in the incidence of otitis media with effusion after palatoplasty in a series of 50 patients operated on between the ages of 6 and 19 months. The type of palatoplasty was not specified; all the babies had bilateral myringotomies performed simultaneously with palatal closure, but a tube was placed in only one ear. Preoperatively, the incidence of otitis media with effusion in these babies was 97%. Postoperatively, otitis media with effusion was present up to 24 months later in approximately 80% of the "nontubed" ears. A few years later, Robinson et al. (1992) similarly reported little impact of palatal surgery on middle ear status. In their study otitis media with effusion persisted in more than 70% of 150 children for up to 3 years after palate repair. The range of ages at surgery—5 to 18 months—was similar to those in the Dhillon study, and there was apparently a wide variety in the surgical techniques used. In both of these studies the conclusion was that ventilating tubes are a necessity for infants with clefts because palatoplasty alone will not be a sufficient deterrent to middle ear disease.

One study in 1994 (Smith, DiRuggiero, and Jones, 1994) provided data that the improvement in eustachian tube function seen in children with clefts after palate repair may take several years to show up, which immediately raises the question of whether the improvement they found was simply a function of increased age of the child. In this study the average time to recovery of eustachian tube function was 6 years (range 1 to slightly more than 10 years). Furthermore, the hearing loss before tube placement and palatoplasty largely resolved after tube placement, without "significant permanent hearing deficit" (p. 423). This study had such a wide range of poorly controlled variables that it is difficult to sift out the pertinent information. The range of ages at palatal surgery was 3 to 60 months, with a mean of 19.5 months (late for palatal surgery by current practices, but many times this factor is out of the control of the treating cleft palate or craniofacial team because of age at referral, interfering illnesses, etc.). Age at insertion of tympanostomy tubes was not specified. Although the authors wished to make the point that normalization of eustachian tube function may take several years after palatoplasty, it is possible that at least in some cases the improvement may have been as much a function of age as tube placement.

In most studies of this question there has been a rather wide range of ages at which the palate was repaired. For example, in the 1987 study of Bellis and Passy, in which palatoplasty was also found to have a beneficial effect on ear disease, the age of palate repair for their 54 patients ranged from 2.5 months to 25 years, although most (86%) were under the age of 1 year at the time of surgery. In the somewhat older Pittsburgh studies the age at palatal closure tended to fall around 18 to 24 months. In one recent study in which the palatal clefts were closed within the first month of life in 18 children, 13 (72%) still required placement of ventilating tubes sometime during their first 3 years of life because of persistent or recurrent perfusion (Nunn et al., 1995). The surgical technique in this study was a pushback palatoplasty (see Chapter 4). The authors concluded that early palate closure did not significantly alter the need for myringotomy and tubes in children with clefts.

The impression gained in reviewing the studies of the effects of palatal closure on subsequent ear disease is that surgical closure alone is not enough to optimize otologic health and that ventilating tubes are required. However, there are complications to those tubes, such as regurgitation of fluids through them into the outer ear canal if the palate has not yet been closed, permanent tympanic membrane perforations, and scarring (Braganza et al., 1991; Paradise and Bluestone, 1974; Rynnel-Dagoo et al., 1992).

Effects of other types of physical management. Many patients with cleft lip and palate undergo advancement of the midface in their teenage or adult years to improve facial appearance and the occlusion (see Chapter 4). Barker (1987) reported the apparent influence of maxillary advancement on eustachian tube function and hearing sensitivity in five subjects with unilateral cleft lip and palate plus five noncleft subjects who underwent mandibular set-backs and 10 noncleft subjects who had both maxillary advancement and mandibular set-backs. The patients were teenagers and adults (aged 14 to 39 years), and none had a history of previous otologic surgery. All subjects had audiologic examinations plus tubal function tests and middle ear pressure measurements (tympanometry) immediately before surgery, 48 hours after surgery, and again 6 to 8 weeks postoperatively. In the patients with cleft palate, 10% actually showed improvement in tubal function 6 to 8 weeks postoperatively. There was no loss in hearing sensitivity for these patients. In the non-cleft patients, 65% showed poor tubal function immediately postoperatively and 48% still had problems six to eight weeks later. The authors concluded that careful audiologic/otologic monitoring was necessary for all patients undergoing maxillary or mandibular surgery. Gotzfried and Thumfart (1988) studied the function of both the levator palatini and the tensor veli palatini, together with audiometric and tympanometric data, on 26 patients before and after Le Fort I osteotomy. They found a temporary functional impairment in palatal muscle tissue and also in "sound transmission ability" of the middle ear, which they attributed to postoperative edema. In two cases a mild preoperative hearing loss (20 dB range) and flat tympanograms improved to 0 to 10 dB thresholds and normal tympanograms once the postoperative edema had subsided. The authors attributed the positive changes to a change in the muscle tension in the palate, caused by a change in the vectors of motion once the maxilla was advanced, and recommended routine preoperative audiometric and tympanometric studies for all patients undergoing midface advancement. The results of these two studies seem roughly comparable, providing some evidence of possible improvement in eustachian tube function in persons with clefts who undergo maxillary advancement as teenagers or adults, but also warning us that all patients (cleft or noncleft) who undergo maxillary advancement or mandibular set-back procedures should receive careful audiologic and otologic monitoring both preoperatively and postoperatively.

Many patients with clefts require secondary surgery on the palate or velopharyngeal system to provide them with adequate velopharyngeal closure. Thankfully the percentage of patients requiring such secondary surgery has dropped steadily over the last several decades because of the increased ability of surgeons to produce a closed, physiologically normal palate with the initial palatal surgery (see Chapter 4). In the 1960s through the 1980s there was concern about how various types of secondary velopharyngeal procedures affected middle ear disease in patients, in addition to how these procedures changed speech. As in most questions in this field, tracking the results of intervention has been difficult because of variation in the initial state (the patient before treatment), the "maneuver" (treatment), and the subsequent state (posttreatment, but how long and with what intervening variables?).

There were several studies in the 1960s and 1970s attempting to determine whether pharyngeal flap surgery had a positive or negative effect on ear disease. Most of the patients included in these studies had overt clefts, although some did not. The authors did not always specify the age at which patients were operated on, often giving only a wide range. Similarly, the specific type of pharyngeal flap was not always identified. The reports by Graham and Lierle (1962), Aschan (1966), LeWorthy and Schliesser (1975), and Yules (1975) lack key information on operative technique or the exact ages at surgery.[8]

The bulk of the information contained in these reports seemed to indicate that a pharyngeal flap did no permanent harm to otologic health or hearing and that improvement in the ears was seen in a varying number of cases. Graham and Lierle (1962) simply reported that pharyngeal flap surgery did not aggravate existing hearing loss. Aschan (1966) reported an improvement in hearing in 7% of his 82 cases, but in the remaining 93% there was no change. Two of the 53 patients reported by LeWorthy and Schliesser (1975) demonstrated a slight decrease in hearing after surgery; 14 (26%) showed improvement to normal hearing, and the

[8]However, in fairness, it must be pointed out that variations in *types* of pharyngeal flaps evolved gradually during these years, so that at one time the designation "pharyngeal flap" may have been considered sufficient.

remaining patients showed no change in hearing status. Yules (1975) reported that 12% of his 69 patients who underwent a palatal pushback and superiorly based pharyngeal flap as a secondary procedure after earlier palatoplasty had improvement in hearing. The range of patient ages was 5 to 48 years; no information was given on improvement in hearing in relation to age of the patient. Heller et al. (1978) reported improved hearing only in some cases of their 51 patients with velopharyngeal inadequacy (of various types), 41 of whom had pharyngeal flaps, four of whom had a Hynes pharyngoplasty, and six of whom had other types of palate surgery.

Lendrum and Dhar (1984) reported improvement in hearing in 40% of cases after an Orticochea pharyngoplasty (see Chapter 4 for an explanation of this procedure), but the report is fraught with methodological errors. The patients included 33 with a prior unsatisfactory cleft palate repair, 12 with submucous clefts (five of whom had had a prior unsatisfactory repair), and eight cases of noncleft velopharyngeal inadequacy. They ranged in age from 3 to 40 years at the time the procedure was performed. Each had a preoperative and postoperative audiogram, but the amount of time that had elapsed after the surgical procedure was not specified. Hearing was normal preoperatively in 22 of the 53 patients. Hearing loss before surgery ranged from 20 to 30 dB in seven, 31 to 50 dB in 20, and 51 to 70 dB in four patients. Postoperatively, hearing improved in 19 of the patients. However, each who had pre-existing hearing loss received a myringotomy at the time of the pharyngoplasty, making it impossible to say that the improvement in hearing was actually a function of the pharyngoplasty.

Spauwen et al. (1988) reported on the effects of an inferiorly based pharyngeal flap (see Chapter 4 for an illustration) on 51 children between the ages of 3 and 12 years. A major strength of this study was the fact that the children had multiple otologic-tympanometric-audiologic assessments, with a minimum of two assessments before surgery and two postoperatively. Thirty-four of them had overt clefts, and 17 had congenitally short palates. The children with clefts had had prior surgical closure "including levator sling reconstruction" (p. 27), but the report does not specify that *all* repairs included levator reconstruction, nor does it specify the timing of surgery. Bilateral chronic otitis media with effusion was present in 24 of the 34 children with clefts, as opposed to only two of the 17 with congenitally short palates. The authors divided the subjects into those under the age of 6 years versus those aged 6 years or older at the time of the pharyngeal flap. The younger group showed a significantly higher prevalence of bilateral chronic otitis media with effusion than the older group did. Interestingly, the apparent decrease in the prevalence of otitis media with effusion with age did not depend on previous otologic treatment. Ten patients were excluded from the study because they had either ventilating tubes or tympanic membrane perforations. Of the remaining 41, 17 had bilateral chronic otitis media with effusion and in 10 of these it reverted to normal. The authors stated (p. 27), "This means that in 60% of patients with bilateral chronic otitis media with effusion, the continuance of chronic ear disease was broken within 3 months after pharyngoplasty." Three of the patients with normal hearing before pharyngoplasty had a transient deterioration from edema. Children more than 6 years old showed the most benefit, whereas the younger children, preoperatively more frequently affected, appeared to be more resistant to postoperative improvement. The authors concluded that the "immediate" effects of pharyngoplasty seemed to accelerate the natural course of bilateral chronic otitis media with effusion, that is, the surgery facilitated earlier resolution of the disease in comparison to simply letting the disease resolve with increasing age. They conjectured that the inferiorly based pharyngeal flap may help to correct the forward-directed vector of the levator in patients with clefts, pulling the soft palate and levator sling backward "across a mechanical dead-point, realizing a better point of impact on the eustachian tube cartilage" (p. 30). They did not claim to have verified this interpretation through actual muscle studies (e.g., anatomic dissections, electromyography).

CONGENITAL ANOMALIES OF THE HEARING MECHANISM

In Chapter 2, you learned about some of the multi-anomaly disorders likely to be seen in cleft palate/craniofacial clinics. Ear disease, hearing loss, and congenital malformations of the auditory system were listed in the clinical details about these disorders. There are several comprehensive texts and references dealing with congenital disorders of the hearing mechanism, most notably Gorlin, Toriello, and Cohen (1995), and you are advised to check updated on-line references.

Table 6-1 summarizes the otologic problems in those multi-anomaly disorders discussed in Chapter 2. The references from which this information was drawn are given in that chapter.

CURRENT TRENDS IN TREATMENT

As of this writing, the otologists and audiologists who take responsibility for providing optimal ear care for children and adults with clefts are still advocating early and continuous otologic surveillance of these patients. There continues to be some level of controversy about whether the blanket recommendation for early myringotomies and placement of ventilation tubes may have, in the aggregate, enough drawbacks to warrant reconsideration and perhaps a return to a less aggressive (or less universally aggressive) approach to care. In 1986 Moore, Moore, and Yonkers concluded from their review of the literature, "If the lip and palate cannot be repaired by the age of six months, tubes should be placed while waiting for the infant to reach acceptable criteria to allow cleft repair." In 1989 Stool reflected on the history of both what was known about ear disease clefts and what interventional steps could be taken.

Table 6-1 **Summary of Ear Malformations, Ear Disease, and Hearing Loss in the Multi-Anomaly Disorders Described in Chapter 2**

Disorder	*Ear Malformations*	*Otologic Disease*	*Hearing Loss*
Robin sequence	None known in "pure" Robin cases unassociated with other syndromes	Prevalence of ear disease at least as high as in other cases of cleft palate, perhaps higher	Typically bilateral, conductive
Stickler syndrome	None known	Subject to ear disease if a cleft is present	Progressive sensorineural loss in about 80% of cases; conductive loss as in other cases of clefts of the secondary palate
Velocardiofacial syndrome	Minor auricular malformations in about 70% of cases; low-set, somewhat posteriorly rotated ears	Vulnerable to otitis media because of presence of cleft or other form of velopharyngeal inadequacy	Conductive hearing loss when otitis media is present. Some sporadic reports of sensorineural loss
Hemifacial microsomia (oculoauriculo-vertebral spectrum)	Ear deformities ranging from minor auricular malformations and preauricular pits to complete absence of the auricle, stenosis or atresia of the external auditory canal, variable ossicular malformations and other deformities of the middle ear, incomplete pneumatization of the temporal bone	No known tendency toward otitis media unless a cleft palate is also present	Usually conductive, ranging from mild to severe. Typical loss is 50-60 dB, flat or rising in pattern. Some reported cases of cochlear involvement and sensorineural loss. Loss may be bilateral even if the externally visible deformities of the ear are only unilateral.
Mandibulofacial dysostosis	Typically bilateral malformations of the auricle, external auditory canal, and middle ear. Range from mild to severe. Hypoplastic tympanic and epitympanic cavities, ossicular malformations ranging from mild to complete absence	No known tendency toward otitis media unless a cleft palate is also present	Usually bilateral conductive loss, often maximum in degree, flat or rising in pattern. A few reported cases of mixed loss
Nager syndrome	Same as in mandibulofacial dysostosis	Complete agenesis of the soft palate may contribute to ear middle ear disease if the structures of the middle ear are in fact present	Same as in mandibulofacial dysostosis
EEC syndrome	None known	Middle ear disease resulting from presence of cleft palate. Sloughing off of squamous cells in the external auditory canal may contribute to external otitis	Conductive hearing loss as in other cases of cleft palate
Apert syndrome	Some reports of malformations of the middle ear	Many patients have nearly constant middle ear disease, even if cleft palate is not present. Apparently related to nasopharyngeal dysmorphology (obstruction)	Frequent conductive loss, variable in degree
Crouzon syndrome	Some reports of malformations of the external and/or middle ear	Nasopharyngeal dysmorphology seems to foster middle ear disease	Frequent conductive loss, variable in degree
Pfeiffer syndrome	High prevalence of stenosis or atresia of the auditory canal, middle ear hypoplasia, and ossicular hypoplasia	Recurrent middle ear disease as in Apert and Crouzon syndromes	Frequent conductive loss, variable in degree
Saethre-Chotzen syndrome	Ears may be low set and posteriorly rotated; other minor external ear anomalies	Tendency toward middle ear disease when the nasopharynx is severely crowded	Frequent conductive loss, variable in degree

He concluded, ". . . even though we ventilate the ears, we have not completely eliminated middle ear disease in this population" (p. 345). Perhaps we will never reach complete elimination of the problem, but it seems clear that aggressive planning for monitoring and management has brought the experience of ear disease in patients with clefts more into line with what is experienced by other children and adults.

REFERENCES

Ahonen JE, and McDermott JC: Extended high-frequency hearing loss in children with cleft palate. *Audiology* 23:467-476, 1984.

Aschan G: Hearing and nasal function correlated to postoperative speech in cleft palate patients with velopharyngoplasty. *Acta Otolaryngologica* 61:371-379, 1966.

Barker GR: Auditory tube function and audiogram changes following corrective orthognathic maxillary and mandibular surgery in cleft and non-cleft patients. *Scandinavian Journal of Plastic and Reconstructive Surgery* 23:133-138, 1987.

Bellis ME, and Passy V: Long-term hearing effects in cleft palate patients. *Ear, Nose, and Throat Journal* 66:49-55, 1987.

Bennett M: The older cleft palate patient (a clinical otologic-audiologic study). *Laryngoscope* 82:1217-1225, 1972.

Bluestone CD: Eustachian tube obstruction in the infant with cleft palate. *Annals of Otology, Rhinology and Laryngology* 80(Supplement 2):1-30, 1971.

Bluestone CD, Klein JO, and Kenna MA: Otitis media with effusion, atelectasis, and eustachian tube dysfunction. In Bluestone CD, and Stool SE (eds.): *Pediatric otolaryngology.* 2nd ed. Volume 1. Philadelphia: WB Saunders, 1990a, pp. 330-331.

Bluestone CD, Klein JO, and Kenna MA: Intratemporal complications and sequelae of otitis media. In Bluestone CD, and Stool SE (eds.): *Pediatric otolaryngology.* 2nd ed. Volume 1. Philadelphia: WB Saunders, 1990b, pp. 583-636.

Bluestone CD, Wittel RA, and Paradise JL: Roentgenographic evaluation of eustachian tube function in infants with cleft and normal palates. *Cleft Palate Journal* 9:93-100, 1972.

Bluestone CD, Beery QC, Cantekin EI, and Paradise JL: Eustachian tube ventilatory function in relation to cleft palate. *Annals of Otology* 84:333-338, 1975.

Bluestone CD, Paradise JL, Beery QC, and Wittel RA: Certain effects of cleft palate repair on eustachian tube function. *Cleft Palate Journal* 9:183-193, 1972.

Braganza RA, Kearns DB, Burton DM, Seid AB, and Pransky SM: Closure of the soft palate for persistent otorrhea after placement of pressure equalization tubes in cleft palate infants. *Cleft Palate–Craniofacial Journal* 28:305-307, 1991.

Broen PA, Moller MT, Carlstrom J, Doyle SS, Devers M, and Keenan KM: Comparison of the hearing histories of children with and without cleft palate. *Cleft Palate–Craniofacial Journal* 33:127-133, 1996.

Caldarelli DD: Incidence and type of otopathologic disease in the older cleft-palate patient. *Cleft Palate Journal* 12:311-314, 1975.

Caldarelli DD: Incidence and type of otopathology associated with congenital palatopharyngeal incompetence. *Laryngoscope* 87:1979-1984, 1978.

Cantekin EI, Bluestone CD, Saez CA, Doyle WJ, and Phillips DC: Normal and abnormal middle ear ventilation. *Annals of Otology, Rhinology, and Laryngology* 86(Supplement 41):1-15, 1977.

Dellon AL: Response to Rood and Doyle. *Cleft Palate Journal* 16:442-443, 1979.

Dhillon RS: The middle ear in cleft palate children pre and post palatal closure. *Journal of the Royal Society of Medicine* 81:710-712, 1988.

Doyle WJ, Cantekin EI, and Bluestone CD: Eustachian tube function in cleft palate children. *Annals of Otology, Rhinology and Laryngology* 89(Supplement 68):34-40, 1980.

Doyle WJ, Reilly JS, Jardini L, and Rovnak S: Effect of palatoplasty on the function of the eustachian tube in children with cleft palate. *Cleft Palate Journal* 23:63-68, 1986.

Drettner B: The nasal airway and hearing in patients with cleft palate. *Acta Otolaryngologica* 42:131-142, 1952.

Durr DG, and Shapiro RS: Otologic manifestations in congenital velopharyngeal insufficiency. *Archives of Adolescent and Pediatric Medicine* 43:75-77, 1989.

Edgerton MT: Commentary on Finkelstein et al. *Plastic and Reconstructive Surgery* 85:693-694, 1990.

Edgerton MT, and Dellon AL: Surgical retrodisplacement of the levator veli palatini muscle: preliminary report. *Plastic and Reconstructive Surgery* 47:154-167, 1971.

Finkelstein Y, Talmi YP, Nachmani A, Hauben DJ, and Zohar Y: Levator veli palatini muscle and eustachian tube function. *Plastic and Reconstructive Surgery* 85:684-692, 1990.

Frable MA, Brandon GT, and Theogaraj SD: Velar closure and ear tubings as a primary procedure in the repair of cleft palates. *Laryngoscope* 95:1044-1046, 1985.

Freeland AP, and Evans DM: Middle ear disease in the cleft palate infant: its effect on speech and language development. *British Journal of Plastic Surgery* 34:142-143, 1981.

Fria TJ, Paradise JL, Sabo DL, and Elster BA: Conductive hearing loss in infants and young children with cleft palate. *Pediatrics* 111:84-87, 1987.

Gaines FP: Frequency and effect of hearing losses in cleft palate cases. *Journal of Speech and Hearing Disorders* 5:1-9, 1940.

Garabedian EN, Polonovski JM, Cotin G, and LaCombe H: Influence du traitement chirurgical des fentes velo-palatines sur la pathologie de l'oreille moyenne. *Annales des Otolaryngologie* (Paris) 105:159-163, 1988.

Gopalakrishna A, Goleria KS, and Raje A: Middle ear function in cleft palate. *British Journal of Plastic Surgery* 37:558-565, 1984.

Gordon ASD, Jean-Louis F, and Morton RP: Late ear sequelae in cleft palate patients. *International Journal of Pediatric Otorhinolaryngology* 15:149-156, 1988.

Gorlin RJ, Toriello HV, and Cohen MM Jr: *Hereditary hearing loss and its syndromes.* Oxford Monographs on Medical Genetics No. 28. New York: Oxford University Press, 1995.

Gotzfried HF, and Thumfart WF: Pre- and postoperative middle ear function and muscle activity of the soft palate after total maxillary osteotomy in cleft patients. *Journal of Cranio-Maxillo-Facial Surgery* 16:64-68, 1988.

Gould HJ: Hearing loss and cleft palate: the perspective of time. *Cleft Palate–Craniofacial Journal* 27:36-39, 1990.

Goycoolea MV, Paparella MM, Goldberg B, and Carpenter AM: Permeability of the round window membrane in otitis media. *Archives of Otolaryngology* 106:430-433, 1980.

Graham MD, and Lierle DM: Posterior pharyngeal flap palatoplasty and its relationship to ear disease and hearing loss. *Laryngoscope* 72:1750-1755, 1962.

Halfond MM, and Ballenger JJ: An audiologic and otorhinologic study of cleft lip and palate cases. 1. Audiological evaluation. *Archives of Otolaryngology* 64:58-62, 1956.

Handzic J, Subotic R, Sprem N, and Bagatin M: Hearing thresholds in cleft lip or palate patients. *Chirurgiae Maxillofaciale Plasticae* 19:19-23, 1989.

Handzic-Cuk J, Cuk V, Risavi R, Katusic D, and Stajner-Katusic S: Hearing levels and age in cleft palate patients. *International Journal of Pediatric Otorhinolaryngology* 37:227-242, 1996.

Hayes D: Hearing loss in infants with craniofacial anomalies. *Otolaryngology–Head and Neck Surgery* 110:39-45, 1994.

Heller JC, Hochberg I, and Milano G: Audiologic and otologic evaluation of cleft palate children. *Cleft Palate Journal* 7:774-783, 1970.

Heller JC, Gens GW, Croft CB, and Moe DG: Conductive hearing loss in patients with velopharyngeal insufficiency. *Cleft Palate Journal* 15:246-253, 1978.

Holborow CA: Deafness associated with cleft palate. *Journal of Laryngology and Otology* 76:762-773, 1962.

Holmes EM, and Reed GF: Hearing and deafness in cleft-palate patients. A.M.A. *Archives of Otolaryngology* 62:620-624, 1955.

Honjo I, Okazaki N, and Kumazawa T: Experimental study of the eustachian tube function with regard to its related muscles. *Acta Otolaryngologica* 87:84-89, 1979.

Hubbard TW, Paradise JL, McWilliams BJ, Elster BA, and Taylor FH: Consequences of unremitting middle-ear disease in early life: otologic, audiologic and developmental findings in children with cleft palate. *New England Journal of Medicine* 312:1529-1534, 1985.

Lauffer H, Proschel U, Spitzer D, and Wenzel D: Akustisch evozierte Hirnstammpotentiale bei Sauglingen mit Velumspalten. [Acoustically evoked brain potentials in infants with velum clefts.] *Klinische Padiatrie* 205:30-33, 1993.

Lendrum J, and Dhar BK: The Orticochea dynamic pharyngoplasty. *British Journal of Plastic Surgery* 37:160-168, 1984.

LeWorthy GW, and Schliesser H: Hearing acuity before and after pharyngeal flap procedure. *Plastic and Reconstructive Surgery* 56:49-51, 1975.

Manning SC, Brown OE, Roland PS, and Phillips DL: Incidence of sensorineural hearing loss in patients evaluated for tympanostomy tubes. *Archives of Otolaryngology–Head and Neck Surgery* 120:881-884, 1994.

Masters FW, Bingham HG, and Robinson DW: The prevention and treatment of hearing loss in the cleft palate child. *Plastic and Reconstructive Surgery* 26:503-509, 1960.

McDermott JC, Fausti SA, and Frey RH: Effects of middle-ear disease and cleft palate on high-frequency hearing in children. *Audiology* 25:136-148, 1986.

Moller P: Long-term otologic features of cleft palate patients. *Archives of Otolaryngology* 101:605-607, 1975.

Moller P: Hearing, middle ear pressure and otopathology in a cleft palate population. *Acta Otolaryngologica* 92:521-528, 1981.

Moore IJ, Moore GF, and Yonkers AJ: Otitis media in the cleft palate patient. *Ear, Nose, and Throat Journal* 65:15-23, 1986.

Morgan RF, Dellon AL, and Hoopes JE: Effects of levator retrodisplacement on conductive hearing loss in the cleft palate patient. *Annals of Plastic Surgery* 10:306-308, 1983.

Muntz HR: Middle ear disease and cleft palate. *Facial Plastic Surgery* 9:177-180, 1993.

Northern JL, and Downs MP: *Hearing in children.* Baltimore: Williams & Wilkins, 1974.

Nunn DR, Derkay CS, Darrow DH, Magee W, and Strasnick B: The effect of very early cleft palate closure on the need for ventilation tubes in the first years of life. *Laryngoscope* 105:905-908, 1995.

Paparella MM, Morizono T, Le CT, Mancini F, Siplia P, Choo YB, Liden G, and Kim CS: Sensorineural hearing loss in otitis media. *Annals of Otology, Rhinology, and Laryngology* 93:623-629, 1984.

Paparella MM, Oda M, Hiraide F, and Brady D: Pathology of sensorineural hearing loss in otitis media. *Annals of Otology, Rhinology, and Laryngology* 81:632-647, 1972.

Paradise JL: Management of middle ear effusion in infants with cleft palate. *Annals of Otology, Rhinology, and Laryngology* 25(Suppl):285-288, 1976.

Paradise JL, and Bluestone CD: Early treatment of the universal otitis media of infants with cleft palate. *Pediatrics* 53:48-53, 1974.

Paradise JL, Bluestone CD, and Felder H: The universality of otitis media in 50 infants with cleft palate. *Pediatrics* 44:35-42, 1969.

Paradise JL, Elster BA, and Tan L: Evidence in infants with cleft palate that breast milk protects against otitis media. *Pediatrics* 94:853-860, 1994.

Parnes LS, Gagne JP, and Hassan R: Cochlear implants and otitis media: considerations in two cleft palate patients. *Journal of Otolaryngology* 22:345-348, 1993.

Potsic WP, Cohen M, Randall P, and Winchester R: A retrospective study of hearing impairment in three groups of cleft palate patients. *Cleft Palate Journal* 16:56-58, 1979.

Rivron RP: Bifid uvula: prevalence and association in otitis media with effusion in children admitted for routine otolaryngological operations. *Archives of Laryngology and Otology* 103:249-252, 1989.

Robinson PJ, Lodge S, Jones BM, Walker CC, and Grant HR: The effect of palate repair on otitis media with effusion. *Plastic and Reconstructive Surgery* 89:640-645, 1992.

Rood SR, and Doyle WJ: Letter to the editor. *Cleft Palate Journal* 16:441-442, 1979.

Rynnel-Dagoo B, Lindberg K, Bagger-Sjoback D, and Larson O: Middle ear disease in cleft palate children at three years of age. *International Journal of Pediatric Otorhinolaryngology* 23:201-209, 1992.

Sataloff J, and Fraser J: Hearing loss in children with cleft palate. *Archives of Otolaryngology* 55:61-64, 1952.

Schwartz RH, Hayden GF, Shprintzen RJ, Rodriquez WJ, and Cassidy JW: The bifid uvula: is it a marker for an otitis prone child? *Laryngoscope* 95:1100-1102, 1985.

Seif S, and Dellon AL: Anatomic relationships between the human levator and tensor veli palatini and the eustachian tube. *Cleft Palate Journal* 15:329-336, 1978.

Severeid LR: A longitudinal study of the efficacy of adenoidectomy in children with cleft palate and secretory otitis media. *Transactions of the American Academy of Ophthalmology and Otolaryngology* 76:1319-1324, 1972.

Severeid LR: Development of cholesteatoma in children with cleft palate: a longitudinal study. In McCabe BF, Sade J, and Abramson M (eds.): *Cholesteatoma.* Birmingham (AL): Aesculapius Publishing, 1977, pp. 287-289.

Shibahara Y, and Sando I: Histopathologic study of eustachian tube in cleft palate patients. *Annals of Otology, Rhinology, and Laryngology* 97:403-408, 1988.

Shprintzen RJ, and Gereau SA: Commentary on Finkelstein et al. *Plastic and Reconstructive Surgery* 85:695-697, 1990.

Skolnik EM: Otologic evaluation in cleft palate patients. *Laryngoscope* 68:1908-1949, 1958.

Smith TL, DiRuggiero DC, and Jones KR: Recovery of eustachian tube function and hearing outcome in patients with cleft palate. *Otolaryngology–Head and Neck Surgery* 111:423-429, 1994.

Spauwen PHM, Ritsma RJ, Huffstadt BJC, Schutte HK, and Brown IF: The inferiorly based pharyngoplasty: effects on chronic otitis media with effusion. *Cleft Palate Journal* 25:26-32, 1988.

Stool SE: Research revisited. *Cleft Palate Journal* 26:344-345, 1989.

Stool SE, and Randall P: Unexpected ear disease in infants with cleft palate. *Cleft Palate Journal* 4:99-103, 1967.

Stool SE, and Winn R: Pneumatization of the temporal bone in children with cleft palate. *Cleft Palate Journal* 6:154-159, 1969.

Strohm M: Trauma of the middle ear. *Advances in Oto-Rhino-Laryngology.* Basel: Karger, 1986.

Takahashi H, Honjo I, and Fujita A: Eustachian tube compliance in cleft palate—a preliminary study. *Laryngoscope* 104:83-86, 1994.

Todd NW, and Krueger BL: Minuscule submucous cleft palate: cadaver study. *Annals of Otology, Rhinology, and Laryngology* 101:417-422, 1992.

Tonndorf J: Bone conduction: studies in experimental animals. *Acta Oto-Laryngologica* 213(Supplement): 1966.

Tonndorf J, and Pastaci H: Middle ear sound transmission, a field of early interest of Merle Lawrence. *American Journal of Otolaryngology* 7:120-129, 1986.

Too-Chung MA: The assessment of middle ear function and hearing by tympanometry in children before and after early cleft palate repair. *British Journal of Plastic Surgery* 36:295-299, 1983.

Yules RB: Hearing in cleft palate patients. *Archives of Otolaryngology* 91:319-323, 1975.

Chapter 7

Communication Disorders Associated with Cleft Palate

Children born with cleft lip and palate are at risk for resonance, articulation, and expressive language problems that may impair communication for many years. The impact of a palatal cleft may be evident during the early vocalizations of babies before surgical management and may persist long after an adequate oral-pharyngeal mechanism has been established. The most remarkable speech production problems demonstrated by children with cleft palate are those related to velopharyngeal inadequacy, including hypernasality, audible nasal emission, weak pressure consonants, and compensatory articulation patterns. Despite the attention typically given to these distinctive characteristics, the clinician must bear in mind that most children with cleft palate evidence adequate velopharyngeal function after palatal surgery and do not demonstrate these problems. Indeed, many of these children produce only developmental speech sound errors, whereas others produce sound distortions as a result of their dental or occlusal status. Still others demonstrate normal speech production.

To fully understand the communication problems associated with cleft palate, the clinician must first recognize and appreciate the heterogeneity that is evident within this population. A palatal cleft can and does influence children in different ways. This chapter will describe the speech and language problems associated with cleft palate. The major etiological factors associated with these problems will also be discussed.

SPEECH PRODUCTION PROBLEMS ASSOCIATED WITH CLEFT PALATE

Resonance

Resonance, an acoustical phenomenon, is a complex attribute of speech that is not completely understood. Simply, it may be defined as "the vibratory response of a body or air-filled cavity to a frequency imposed upon it" (Wood, 1971). Thus resonance is a physical rather than a perceptual phenomenon. Unfortunately, there is no completely acceptable general term that can be used to identify the perceptual aspects of the speech signal because it varies under a variety of resonating conditions. For this reason, "resonance" is used here to describe the perceptual as well as the physical attributes of speech. The student should realize, however, that we would prefer to use a different word if we had one.[1]

Speakers do not have speech patterns that are either normal or abnormal with respect to resonance. Rather, like all other attributes of speech, resonance characteristics fall along a continuum. Normal resonance is marked by some nasal resonance. One person may sound slightly more hypernasal than another in paired-comparison judgments, but both may be considered by the majority of listeners to be normal speakers. Given just a bit more nasality, one might well fall into a borderline classification, where some listeners would consider the speech to be normal and others would think that it was disordered. As nasal quality increases, speech moves further from the mean in the direction of a greater degree of deficiency. Those with hypernasality may be placed along a continuum from least to most defective, and so it is with all of the other disorders of resonance as it is with other speech attributes as well.

Hypernasality. Hypernasality is a resonance alteration of vowels and vocalic consonants that occurs when the oral and nasal cavities are abnormally coupled. The result is that the sound wave is diverted into the nasal airways, and speech sounds as if it is coming through the nose. Hypernasality problems should not be confused with atypical air flow, although the two conditions usually occur together. When the velopharyngeal port cannot be closed, high-pressure consonants are likely to be accompanied by visible (e.g., on a mirror) and, in more serious cases, audible nasal escape unless, of course, the air stream is prevented

[1]Some writers have suggested a way around this semantic dilemma by using the designation "oral-nasal balance" (McDonald and Baker, 1951) when referring to problems of resonance. That is a satisfactory solution so long as its meaning is clarified to permit definitions of nasal characteristics that are either increased or decreased.

from moving freely through the nasal passages by nasal obstruction. The nasal emission referred to throughout this book is evidence of velopharyngeal inadequacy, but it is not synonymous with hypernasality.

In considering the speech of individuals with palatal clefts, it is important to remember that many do not have hypernasality because they do not have defective velopharyngeal valving. The achievement of adequate velopharyngeal closure is the goal of all surgical management of the soft palate, and valving integrity is accomplished for most children. The speech pathologist should not start with the false assumption that people with repaired palatal clefts are hypernasal. Many are free of hypernasality entirely; some have only mild hypernasality; a few are moderately affected; and fewer still have severe hypernasality. Our clinical expectation should be that speech after palatal repair will be normal or nearly so. If that is not the outcome, explanations should be sought.

Hyponasality and denasality. Hyponasality refers to a reduction in nasal resonance that is heard when the nasal airway itself is partially blocked or the entrance to the nasal passages is partially occluded, as might occur if a moderately large adenoid pad were present. If the nasal airways were completely occluded, speech would be denasal, meaning that nasal air flow associated with /m/, /n/, and /ŋ/ would be eliminated and the sound wave altered; the nasal consonants would approach but not match /b/, /d/, and /g/. When either hyponasality or denasality is heard, speech pathologists may be lulled into thinking that the velopharyngeal valve is intact. In reality, the valve may be faulty, but the increased nasal resistance minimizes its effects. In cases such as this, the role of the velopharyngeal valve is obscured until the nasal airway is corrected, at which time the defective valve becomes apparent as the speech takes on the characteristics of velopharyngeal inadequacy (i.e., visible or audible nasal escape, hypernasality, and reduced intraoral pressure).

Mixed nasality. A number of authors (McWilliams and Philips, 1990; Peterson-Falzone, 1982) have described resonance characterized by elements of both hyponasality and hypernasality. Hypernasality and hyponasality may co-occur in patients with velopharyngeal inadequacy who evidence increased nasal resistance that is not great enough to eliminate nasal resonance entirely but is too great to permit nasal consonants to maintain their integrity. This resonance pattern is more frequently perceived in patients with a pharyngeal flap or prosthetic devices, but it has also been described in patients with dyspraxia (Peterson-Falzone, 1982) and in patients with incongruous movements of the velum and pharyngeal walls (Shprintzen et al., 1977). Instrumental assessment of this problem is long overdue.

Cul-de-sac resonance. Cul-de-sac resonance is a variation of hyponasality. It differs only in the place of obstruction and in the way the speech sounds. A cul-de-sac is defined as a blind pouch or a passage with only one outlet. The speech has a muffled characteristic, which you can hear in your own speech if you repeat the consonant-vowel (CV) chain "mi, mi, mi" and then, continuing to produce the chain, pinch your nostrils tightly together. You will hear and feel the air stream necessary for the nasals as it enters the open airway, but you will trap it by the tight anterior constriction. The resonating cavity, normally an open tube, thus becomes a cul-de-sac with concomitant changes in its resonating properties.

Speech pathologists should be aware that people with complete clefts of the lip and palate are at high risk for intranasal conditions capable of changing the architecture of the airways and, thus, their acoustical properties. To the extent that these problems alter the nasal cavities, speech will be influenced. In addition, nasal emission may be minimized or eliminated.

Articulation

Numerous investigations have been conducted to describe the articulation skills of children with cleft palate (Bzoch, 1965; Fletcher, 1978; McWilliams, 1960; McWilliams and Musgrave, 1977; Philips and Harrison, 1969; Riski, 1979; Van Demark, Morris, and Vandehaar, 1979). The findings are similar across studies despite differences in research methods and physical management regimens for the subjects studied. As a group, individuals with cleft palate demonstrate remarkable variability in articulation performance. Some young children with clefts have normal articulation (Dalston, 1990; McWilliams, 1960). As a group, however, these children achieve articulation test scores below available norms or demonstrate poorer articulation than age-matched controls (Bzoch, 1965; McWilliams and Musgrave, 1977; Morris, 1962; Philips and Harrison, 1969; Van Demark, Morris, and Vandehaar, 1979). Even children and adolescents with adequate velopharyngeal function often demonstrate poorer articulation skills than their noncleft peers (Fletcher, 1978).

Prevalence. Definitive information regarding the prevalence of articulation problems in children with cleft palate has historically been difficult to obtain. The majority of investigations that have examined articulation proficiency in large groups of subjects have had a common yet unavoidable methodological constraint—children who return for routine follow-up by cleft palate teams are not necessarily similar to those who do not receive such care. Thus, the group of children available for study at any one treatment center may be heavily weighted with children who demonstrate problems of one kind or another and need additional care. Prevalence data that are available must be interpreted cautiously because patients with essentially normal speech may have been underrepresented in many of the studies reported to date.

Other problems have also confounded efforts to compare prevalence data across various published reports. The use of different subject selection criteria often limits meaningful comparisons. In addition, differences in management of the palatal cleft has likely influenced the findings reported by different centers, so the prevalence of articulation problems noted in patients at one center may not be representative of that seen in other centers.

The clinical findings in several recent reports illustrate the difficulty encountered when attempting to compare data obtained at different treatment centers. Dalston (1990) described the communication skills of 63 children (aged 4 years to 5 years 11 months) and 36 adolescents (aged 14 years to 15 years 11 months) with repaired cleft palate. Seventy-five percent of the younger patients in his study and 25% of the older patients demonstrated some type of communicative disorder. Articulation deficits were noted in 74% of the 4- to 5-year-old children and in 14% of the adolescents. Broen et al. (1996) reported a much larger percentage of normal speech in the 28 young children with repaired cleft palate that they studied longitudinally. According to the authors, data obtained when the children were at least 5 years old suggested that only 50% required treatment for speech after primary palatal surgery (four had secondary management for velopharyngeal inadequacy and 14 were enrolled in speech therapy). Because the children studied by Broen et al. were participants in a longitudinal investigation, it seems possible that their parents may have received more guidance regarding home stimulation of speech and language than would have been available to the children studied by Dalston.

Peterson-Falzone (1990) conducted a cross-sectional analysis of speech for 240 children (ages 4 years to 10 years 11 months) with repaired cleft palate. More than 90% of the young schoolaged children she studied demonstrated articulation problems related to place or manner of production. Approximately 17% exhibited consistent audible nasal emission with associative hypernasality. According to Peterson-Falzone, only 3% of the children she studied demonstrated speech that was "entirely asymptomatic." It is pertinent to note that potential patients who had received secondary surgical/ prosthetic management for velopharyngeal inadequacy were excluded from this study during subject selection. Had these patients been included, it is likely that the overall prevalence of articulation problems would have been higher than that reported. It should also be noted that many of the patients studied by Peterson-Falzone had received primary palatal surgery outside the United States and had not received routine team management. This latter finding probably accounts, at least in part, for the high prevalence of articulation problems observed in her schoolaged group. Cautious interpretation of her findings is warranted, since the patients who returned for follow-up assessment may have been those who continued to have problems.

Despite the limitations associated with prevalence reports, several tentative conclusions can be drawn from the reports described above. First, normal articulation can probably be expected in at least 25% of all preschoolers with repaired cleft palate (+/– cleft lip) who receive routine care by a cleft palate–craniofacial team. Second, a significant number of individuals will continue to demonstrate problems with articulation in adolescence. Finally, the prevalence of articulation problems in the cleft palate population is probably greater for those children and adolescents who do not receive continuing management by a cleft palate team.

Nasal emission. Hypernasality and nasal emission are both speech characteristics associated with poor velopharyngeal structure and function. Although hypernasality is a resonance disorder that influences the character of vowels, nasal emission is an articulation disorder that affects high-pressure consonants. Nasal emission of air may be associated with reduced oral air pressure for pressure consonants, and the combination of hypernasality and reduced oral breath pressure may mask place and manner of articulation.

Inaudible nasal emission. Normally, most speakers produce connected discourse without evidence of nasal air escape. Speakers who do not achieve sufficient velopharyngeal closure for production of the pressure sounds may demonstrate visible nasal escape from one or both nostrils for obstruents. This escape, although inaudible, may fog a cold mirror held at the nose and thus is sometimes referred to as "visible" nasal emission. The context in which this inappropriate nasal emission occurs should be carefully noted because this is one of the indicators of either a velopharyngeal valve that is not completely competent or of a symptomatic oronasal fistulae.

Audible nasal emission. Audible nasal emission can be defined as the sound that is heard when air passes through the nasal passages. You can create audible nasal emission by exhaling forcibly through your nose. This rush of air creates a noise that becomes a part of the speech signal generated and influences how it is perceived by listeners. When marked intranasal resistance to air flow is present, the speech sound may be accompanied by extraturbulent noises, which we refer to as nasal turbulence (McWilliams, 1982). In these cases, clearing the nasal airway, sometimes simply by blowing the nose, may eliminate the noise, but it will not eliminate the air flow through the faulty valve, and the resulting emission may still be audible. It must be stressed that nasal turbulence is a severe form of audible nasal escape and that the noise generated is distracting to listeners. It points to a faulty velopharyngeal valve and to increased resistance in the nasal airway.

We should point out that the extent of the velopharyngeal opening associated with audible nasal emission may vary from less than 5 mm^2 (McWilliams and Philips, 1989) to completely open. Kummer and Neale (1989) hypothesized that nasal turbulence (referred to as a nasal rustle) results when frication is produced by air forced through a small velopharyngeal gap. In a more recent study, Kummer et al. (1992) examined that hypothesis by comparing velopharyngeal gap size in 8 patients with hypernasality, 10 patients with hypernasality and audible nasal emission, and

10 patients with nasal rustle (turbulence). No differences in videofluoroscopic measures of velopharyngeal function were evident between the two hypernasality groups. Patients in the nasal turbulence group, however, demonstrated closer velopharyngeal contact and better lateral pharyngeal wall movement than did the subjects in the other groups. The authors cautioned that although nasal turbulence may be perceived as a more severe form of nasal emission, it may actually be associated with mild velopharyngeal inadequacy or represent phoneme-specific velopharyngeal inadequacy.

Other terminology has been used to describe the characteristics of audible nasal turbulence. Morley (1970) referred to a "nasopharyngeal snort" that results from the passage of air through a sphincter that is closed but not tightly so. Although velopharyngeal closure may be sufficient for impounding intraoral air pressure for obstruents, these consonants may be released nasally rather than orally. This may reflect weak closure of the velopharyngeal port. Morley stated that these snorts often accompany /s/ sounds and other fricatives but can be associated with other sounds as well. The posterior nasal fricative described by Trost (1981) and discussed later in this chapter, closely resembles Morley's description of the nasopharyngeal snort.

McWilliams and Musgrave (1977) warned that other speech disorders, such as lateralized /s/ associated with dental anomalies, may easily be confused with audible nasal emission and attributed mistakenly to a faulty valve. This occurs because both types of errors are associated with an alteration in the direction of the air stream for speech but for different reasons. The speech pathologist should be alert to the need for careful study when nasal escape is audible.

Compensatory articulation patterns. Atypical patterns of articulation have often been observed in the speech of individuals with cleft palate. Some of these patterns appear to develop in compensation for velopharyngeal inadequacy, whereas others develop in compensation for palatal fistulae or malocclusion. Children with cleft palate who demonstrate velopharyngeal inadequacy respond differently to the perceptual consequences associated with the disorder. Hutters and Bronsted (1987) described three strategies that speakers with cleft palate and associated velopharyngeal inadequacy adopt. The first is a *passive* or do-nothing strategy. With this strategy, the speaker makes no attempt to modify the consequences of velopharyngeal inadequacy. Nasalization and nasal frication are simply allowed to occur. The other two strategies described by Hutters and Bronsted, compensation and camouflage, are active strategies that the speaker uses to reduce the consequences of velopharyngeal inadequacy.[2]

[2]Despite the use of terms such as "passive" and "active," these strategies are developed at an unconscious level.

Compensation involves substituting sounds produced with constrictions inferior to the velopharyngeal valve (i.e., glottal and pharyngeal articulations) for pressure consonants. *Camouflage* occurs when a speaker attempts to mask the perceptual consequences of velopharyngeal inadequacy through the use of weak articulation—including breathy phonation or the frequent substitution of /h/ for pressure consonants. The speech characteristics associated with these latter two active strategies will be further described below.

Historical accounts of compensatory articulation errors in children with cleft palate typically included descriptions of only glottal stops and pharyngeal fricatives (Morley, 1970; Morris, 1972). *Glottal stops* are the most common compensatory articulations produced by individuals with cleft palate (Peterson-Falzone, 1989; Trost-Cardamone, 1990b). These laryngeal productions typically occur as substitutions for oral stop consonants but are also frequently substituted for fricatives and affricates (Table 7-1). Although less commonly seen, children with severely disordered articulation may also substitute glottal stops for liquids and glides (Bzoch, 1965). Glottal stops may be co-articulated with oral stops (Henningsson and Isberg, 1986; Morley, 1970; Trost, 1981) or occur as prevocalic, intrusive productions (Sherman, Spriestersbach, and Noll, 1959). Although not a phoneme of English, glottal stops may also occur as an allophone of /t/ or /d/ and are produced as substitutions for final consonants by children with delayed speech (Peterson-Falzone, 1986; Shriberg and Kent, 1995; Stoel-Gammon and Dunn, 1985).

Pharyngeal fricatives are produced as turbulent air passes through a constriction created by the tongue dorsum and posterior pharyngeal wall (Morley, 1970; Trost, 1981). These linguopharyngeal productions are typically substituted for oral fricatives and affricates but may also occur as co-articulations (Henningsson and Isberg, 1986; Trost, 1981). Morley (1970) distinguished between pharyngeal and glottal fricatives. The former involved use of frication between the tongue dorsum and the pharyngeal wall, whereas the latter is "made with increased frication between overtense vocal cords" (Fig. 7-1). Pharyngeal fricatives are rare other than in the speech of persons with cleft palate or related conditions.

Kawano et al. (1985) described a 20-year-old patient with cleft lip and palate who replaced /s/ and /f/ with an unusual *laryngeal fricative.* Nasopharyngoscopic and videofluoroscopic recordings demonstrated that the laryngeal fricative was produced with a constriction formed by the depressed epiglottis and the elevated arytenoid cartilages. Trost-Cardamone (1997a) asserted that the laryngeal fricative is probably not a "categorically distinct" compensatory articulation but instead appears to be a variant of the pharyngeal fricative.

Additional compensatory patterns of articulation have been described in recent years, including the pharyngeal

Table 7-1 **Compensatory Articulations**

Compensatory Articulations	*Phonetic Symbol*		*Target Phone Class*	
	Unvoiced	*Voiced*	*Substitutions*	*Co-articulations*
Glottal stop		/ʔ/	Any pressure consonant (typically stops)	Any pressure consonant (typically stops)
Pharyngeal affricate	/ʔʢ/	/ʔʕ/	Oral affricates	None
Pharyngeal fricative	/ʢ/	/ʕ/	Sibilant fricatives ± oral affricates	Sibilant fricatives
Pharyngeal stop	/ʡ̥/	/ʡ/	k, g	None
Posterior nasal fricative	/Δ/		Any pressure consonant	Any pressure consonant
Velar fricative	/X/	/Y/	Sibilant fricatives	None
Middorsum palatal stop	/ɟ̥/	/ɟ/	/t/, /d/, /k/, /g/	None

Modified from Trost-Cardamone JE: Diagnosis of specific cleft palate speech error patterns for planning therapy or physical management needs. In Bzoch KR (ed.): *Communicative disorders related to cleft lip and palate.* Austin: Pro-Ed, 1997a.

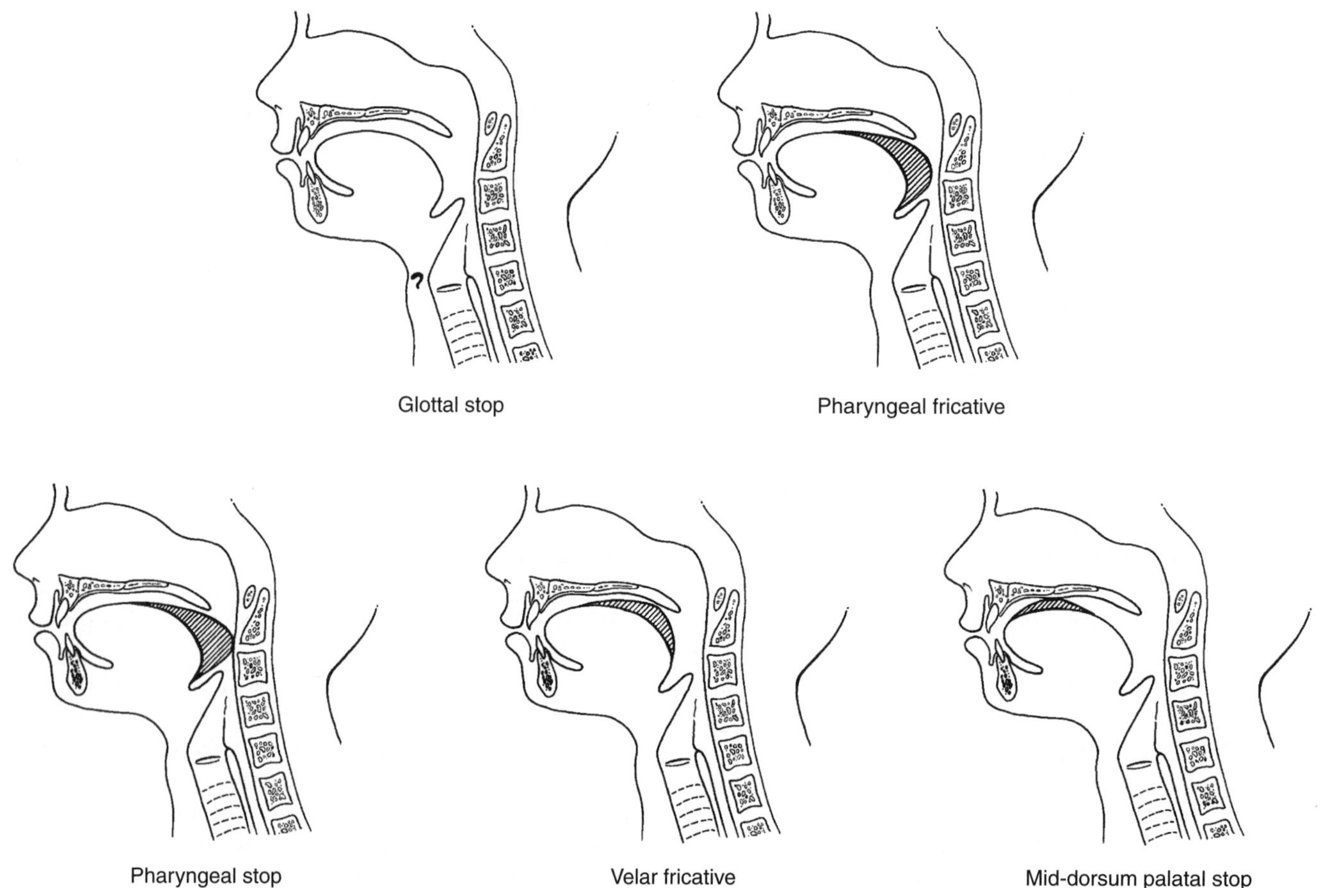

Figure 7-1 Compensatory articulations. *(Modified from Trost JE: Articulatory additions to the classical description of the speech of persons with cleft palate.* Cleft Palate Journal *18:193-203, 1981; Trost-Cardamone JE: Speech compensatory misarticulations. Proceedings of the American Cleft Palate–Craniofacial Association preconference symposium, New Orleans, 1997b.)*

stop, pharyngeal affricate, posterior nasal fricative, velar fricative, palatal fricative, and the middorsum palatal stop (see Fig. 7-1 and Table 7-1).

Trost (1981) provided perceptual and radiographic descriptions of the pharyngeal stop, posterior nasal fricative, and middorsum palatal stop. The pharyngeal stop was described as a linguapharyngeal stop substitution for /k/ and /g/. Trost noted that the location of this stop is influenced by the phonetic context in which it occurs. Similar radiographic findings were reported in several previous studies (Brooks, Shelton, and Youngstrom, 1965, 1966; Honjow and Isshiki, 1971). Although not included in her original report, Trost-Cardamone (1990a) has since described the *pharyngeal affricate*—an articulatory gesture that consists of both a glottal stop and a pharyngeal affricate.

The *posterior nasal fricative* is produced as the velum approximates the posterior pharyngeal wall but leaves an incompletely closed velopharyngeal port (Fig. 7-2). Radiographically a blurring of movement or a velar flutter is seen. According to Trost (1981) the posterior nasal fricative is distinctive because of audible frication. It is typically substituted for /s/, /z/, /ʃ/, /ʒ/ and may occur as a co-articulation with fricatives, affricates, or stop consonants. In some cases a linguavelar articulation occurs and appears to represent the tongue's efforts to provide *lingual assistance* to an impaired velum. Trost (1981) noted this particular type of gesture in patients with submucous clefts and neurogenic disorders. Posterior nasal fricatives are frequently the predominant misarticulation observed in patients with phoneme-specific nasal emission and have also been observed in patients after pharyngeal flap surgery. In the latter case, these productions persist as a learned behavior or occur as a result of pharyngeal flap inadequacy. Posterior nasal fricatives may be perceived as a nasal snort.

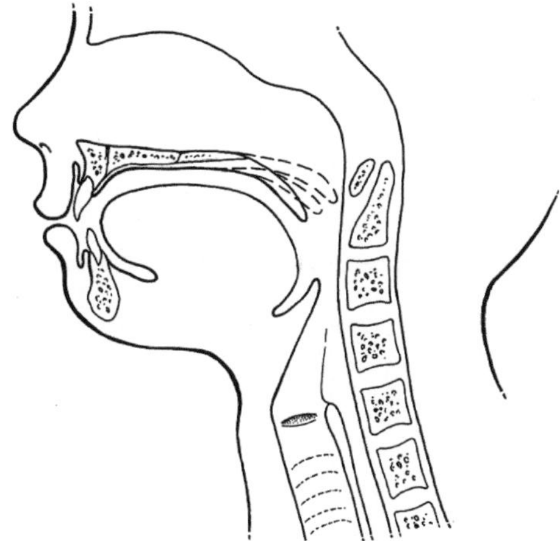

Figure 7-2 Posterior nasal fricative. *(Modified from Trost JE: Articulatory additions to the classical description of the speech of persons with cleft palate.* Cleft Palate Journal *18:193-203, 1981.)*

The third type of articulation described by Trost (1981) was a *middorsum palatal stop*. The place of articulation for this stop production is similar in vocal tract location to that used for /j/ (Fig. 7-1). When used, it occurs as a substitution for /t/, /d/, /k/, or /g/. According to Trost, the phoneme boundaries between /t/ and /k/ as well as /d/ and /g/ are lost during production of this palatal stop. Perceptually, a voiceless middorsum palatal stop sounds equally like /t/ and /k/, whereas a voiced production sounds equally like /d/ and /g/.

Some authors have argued that the middorsum palatal stop cannot represent a compensation for velopharyngeal inadequacy because the place of articulation associated with this gesture is anterior to the velopharyngeal valve (Hoch et al., 1986). Others have argued that the middorsum palatal stop can be considered compensatory for velopharyngeal inadequacy only when substituted for tip-alveolar stops. According to Peterson-Falzone (1986, p. 273), ". . . when the speaker substitutes this gesture for the tip-alveolar stops, this compensatory articulation fits the general patterns of 'backing.' " When substituted for velar stops, however, there is no apparent attempt to compensate for velopharyngeal inadequacy because the place of articulation has moved anterior in the vocal tract. Several authors have reported that this particular type of compensatory gesture may occur as a result of anterior palatal fistulae (Hoch et al., 1986) or dental/occlusal anomalies (Golding-Kushner, 1995). Regardless of the compensatory function assigned to this articulatory gesture, it is important to point out that middorsum palatal stops have been identified in children without palatal clefts/fistulae who have normal velopharyngeal function (Chapman and Hardin, 1992). "In such cases, it is likely that the middorsum palatal stop simply represents a placement error that might occur in any child developing articulatory precision" (Chapman and Hardin, 1992, p. 441).

Yamashita and Michi (1991) described the misarticulations of three preschoolers with repaired cleft palate and a normal palatal vault who demonstrated velopharyngeal adequacy. Electropalatographic and spectrographic measurements were made. Three types of sound distortions created by abnormal lingual-palatal contact were described: lateral misarticulations, nasopharyngeal misarticulations, and palatized misarticulations. Yamashita and Michi likened the nasopharyngeal misarticulation they observed to the posterior nasal fricative previously described by Trost (1981) but stated that this gesture was observed in affricates and plosives as well as fricatives. They also reported that the same articulatory movements used to produce the middorsum palatal stop were used by their subjects to produce *palatal fricatives* and *affricates*. The production of palatal misarticulations in the absence of palatal fistulae or significant dental/occlusal anomalies was an interesting finding.

The *velar fricative* has been described as a compensatory gesture produced when air flows through a constriction created between the tongue dorsum and velum. It can be thought of as a /k/ produced as a fricative. It typically occurs as a substitution for oral fricatives or velar stops (Bzoch, 1956; Lynch, Fox, and Brookshire, 1983; Trost, 1981), and is most often associated with lingual dysarthia (Trost, 1981). Both velar and palatal fricatives are phonemic in some languages.

Prevalence. The prevalence of compensatory articulations has long been linked to age of palatal surgery. Dorf and Curtin (1990) examined the impact of age at time of palatal surgery on speech development for 131 children with cleft palate. Forty-nine children who received surgery before 12½ months of age comprised the early surgery group. The late surgery group consisted of 82 children who had received surgery at or beyond 12½ months of age. Approximately 90% of the children who received surgery after 11 months of age produced at least one compensatory articulation; only 5% of the children who had received early palatal closure demonstrated these error types. According to the authors, the subjects' stage of phonemic development ("articulation age") at the time of surgery appeared more highly related to postoperative articulation status than did chronological age per se. Subjects in the late closure group who did not have compensatory articulations had a delay in the onset of phonemic development. The authors speculated that this delay may have been advantageous because it precluded development of compensatory articulation errors before surgery. Children in the early closure group who had these maladaptive patterns had demonstrated an early onset of phonemic development and had acquired these patterns before surgery. Dorf and Curtin concluded that phonemic development was a more important consideration than chronological age when determining the optimal age of palatal surgery. They recommended that surgery be performed before the onset of meaningful speech to circumvent the development of compensatory articulation patterns.[3]

Cohn and McWilliams (1983) reported articulation data on 204 children with clefts who had received palatal closure by 18 months of age. None of the 105 children with unilateral clefts and only 7 of the 109 children (6%) with isolated cleft palate had pharyngeal misarticulations. Glottal stops were produced by only one of the children with unilateral cleft lip and palate (<1%) and five children with isolated cleft palate (4.5%). Only one child in the group produced a nasal snort.

Data provided in recent reports have suggested that the relationship between age of surgery and development of compensatory articulations is not as definitive as Dorf and Curtin suggested (Table 7-2). Peterson-Falzone (1990) examined the speech of 240 children with repaired cleft palate at ages 4 to 11 years. None of the children had received secondary surgical or prosthetic management for velopharyngeal inadequacy nor did any child have a patent oronasal fistula. Fifty-two of the 240 subjects (22%) demonstrated compensatory articulations. When children from this group who had middorsum palatal stops only were excluded, the total number of subjects exhibiting compensatory articulations was reduced to 30 (12.5%). These errors were more frequently recorded for children with bilateral cleft lip and palate than for children with

[3]We recommend that the data reported by Dorf and Curtin be interpreted cautiously because the authors did not provide information about (1) the age of the children at the time a compensatory articulation was recorded or (2) the number of compensatory articulations a child would have to produce to be categorized in the compensatory group. The presence of glottal stops would not be an unusual finding in a young toddler, nor would the presence of a single glottal stop necessarily be a significant finding in older children. If the children were categorized at a very young age, it seems likely that these data represent a gross overestimate of the number of children for whom compensatory articulations are productive.

Table 7-2 **Prevalence of Compensatory Articulations**

	Dorf and Curtin (1990)		*Peterson-Falzone (1990)*		*Dalston (1990)*	
	No.	%	No.	%	No.	%
Unilateral cleft lip and palate	25/29	86	20/132	15	13/53	24
Bilateral cleft lip and palate	23/24	95	24/63	38	12/29	41
Cleft palate only	24/29	83	8/45	18	20/77	26
Total	72/82	88	52/240	22	45/159	28

Modified from Dalston RM: Timing of cleft palate repair: a speech pathologist's viewpoint. *Cleft palate surgery: problems in plastic and reconstructive surgery* 2:30-38, 1992.

other cleft types. Prevalence trends as a function of age were not evident in these cross-sectional data.

Dalston (1992) also examined the prevalence of compensatory articulation errors in his clinical population. He used patient selection criteria similar to those reported by Peterson-Falzone (1990) but included children as young as 3 years old in his study. Of the 159 patients who met his selection criteria, only 28% had compensatory articulations. Only 21% of the subjects manifested these errors when subjects with middorsum palatal stops only were eliminated. As was true in Peterson-Falzone's data, compensatory articulations were evident almost twice as frequently among patients with bilateral cleft lip and palate as among patients with other cleft types.

In contrast to Dorf and Curtin's findings, however, Dalston noted "a *tendency* for patients who underwent early surgery to be at greater risk of developing compensatory articulations than patients who underwent surgery at a later age" (1992, p. 35). Peterson-Falzone also reported slightly fewer compensatory articulations in her later surgery group than her early surgery group. As Dalston pointed out, however, only a limited number of patients had received surgery before 12 months of age in both his study (n = 13) and Peterson-Falzone's study (n = 17).

As early as the 1960s, clinical investigators were noting a decrease in the frequency of glottal stop and pharyngeal fricative substitutions (Morley, 1962; Renfrew, 1960). If fewer patients with cleft palate are demonstrating compensatory articulations, it is likely that this trend is related to the increasingly younger age of patients at the time of palatal surgery as well as to more aggressive management of velopharyngeal inadequacy.

In summary, there is a growing body of evidence to indicate that compensatory articulation patterns are not produced by the majority of children with cleft palate in the United States today. Recent clinical findings suggest that only an estimated 25% of these children will have these atypical patterns of articulation (Dalston, 1992; Peterson-Falzone, 1990). It should be noted, however, that the prevalence of compensatory articulation errors among children with cleft palate may have been underestimated in recent reports. A number of subjects in both the Peterson-Falzone and Dalston studies had been seen for multiple examinations. However, only information obtained during the last patient visit was examined in these studies. One cannot discount the possibility that some of the older children had manifested these errors at one time and had eliminated them with therapy. Little is known at this time about the spontaneous changes that may occur in these patterns over time. Obtaining these data would be difficult and would likely pose ethical problems because, as Peterson-Falzone pointed out, any child who has these maladaptive articulation patterns should receive therapy.

Only one study to date has examined the relative prevalence of compensatory articulations by type. Peterson-Falzone (1989) examined the articulation of 112 patients with repaired cleft palate at a mean age of 9 years 6 months (age range: 1 year 6 months to 56 years 11 months). Fifty-seven percent of the total subject group had glottal stops. Middorsum palatal stops were the next most common compensatory error (39%), followed by pharyngeal fricatives (15%), velar stops (14%), pharyngeal affricates (12.5%), palatal fricatives (10%), pharyngeal stops (8%), and velar fricatives (4.5%). Peterson-Falzone reported that 59% of her subjects produced glottal stops or middorsum palatal stops exclusively. She cautioned that the number of different types of compensatory errors produced by a speaker was not always indicative of the severity of the articulation disorder.

Peterson-Falzone further examined the distribution of compensatory articulations among her subjects according to cleft type and perceptual evidence of velopharyngeal adequacy. Although more frequent use of glottal stops was evident among patients with velopharyngeal inadequacy regardless of cleft type, they were pervasive in the cleft palate only group. Peterson-Falzone noted that the majority of patients in this cleft-type group had velopharyngeal inadequacy and tended to use glottal stops exclusive of other compensatory articulations. She questioned whether the predominance of glottal stops in this group reflected the high prevalence of velopharyngeal inadequacy or whether the lack of other atypical patterns of articulation was indicative of the absence of dental or occlusal hazards to speech.

A greater percentage of adults (75% of 16) than children (45% of 96) in Peterson-Falzone's study demonstrated perceptual evidence of velopharyngeal inadequacy. Although a comparable percentage of adults and children produced glottal stops as their only compensatory articulation, pharyngeal articulations (+/– glottal stops) were more frequently evident among adult patients (44%) than child patients (15%).

None of the studies cited above examined the extent to which compensatory articulations characterized the speech of the subjects included for study. The prevalence figures cited reflect the number of children in the authors' caseloads who demonstrated at least one compensatory production. It seems likely that substantially fewer individuals would be categorized in the compensatory articulation group if group enrollment were restricted to those children who had clear patterns of these productions. Chapman and Hardin (1992) reported that although nine of the ten 2-year-old toddlers with repaired cleft palate that they studied produced at least one compensatory articulation, their overall frequency of occurrence was quite small (median 5). Eight of the nine children who had these patterns produced glottal stops, middorsum palatal stops, or a combination of both. Of particular interest, however, was the finding that two of the five noncleft subjects demonstrated use of these "compensatory" error patterns as well.

Validity and reliability issues. A number of authors have questioned the use of the term "compensatory" when describing some of the atypical patterns of articulation described above. Peterson-Falzone (1986) argued that the use of this term may be presumptive because data regarding the occurrence of these patterns in the speech of individuals without velopharyngeal inadequacy is limited in some cases and nonexistent in others. In addition, as indicated earlier, some of the articulatory patterns described are produced with a constriction anterior to the velopharyngeal valve and therefore do not appear to serve a compensatory function (Hoch et al., 1986).

Transcription of compensatory articulation patterns is a difficult task that deserves some commentary here. Although a number of investigators have described these atypical patterns of articulation in their clinical population, few have attended to or reported information regarding reliability of their clinical judgments. In her original report describing compensatory patterns, Trost (1981) provided some information about clinicians' ability to distinguish between different patterns. After a 1-hour training session, she asked six speech-language pathologists (three experienced and three inexperienced in craniofacial disorders) to listen to audiorecordings of 24 patients producing sentence pairs. Each listener was instructed to identify the particular type of compensatory articulation produced by each speaker "in underlined segments of the sentence." Trost reported percentages of agreement above 85% for five of her six judges. Although these data provided preliminary support for the "perceptual distinctiveness" of these compensatory articulations, they were derived from a task far more simplistic than the one a clinician faces each time compensatory articulations are transcribed during articulation testing.

Van Demark et al. (1993) examined the extent to which speech pathologists and parents could perceive differences between the vocalizations and speech of babies and young children with and without cleft palate. Listeners were asked to listen to 90 samples of vocalization or speech obtained from both cleft and noncleft babies and indicate whether each sample was normal or abnormal. Despite the simplicity of the task, poor interjudge agreement was evident across all listener groups. According to the authors, differences in interpretation of the perceptual data rather than an inability to hear salient information appeared to account for some of the disagreements observed between the speech pathologists. For example, judges agreed on the presence of glottal stops in some samples but disagreed on whether the sample should be considered "normal" or "abnormal."

Only one study to date has examined the reliability of speech-language pathologists transcribing compensatory articulation patterns. Gooch et al. (unpublished data) presented audiorecordings of 110 target words embedded in the carrier phrase "I have _____ here" to two groups of speech-language pathologists (10 experienced and 10 inexperienced in transcribing the speech of children with cleft palate). Some of the target words were error free, whereas others contained compensatory articulations or conventional speech sound errors. Judges were instructed to phonetically transcribe only the target word in this task. Before the transcription task, both groups of judges viewed the compensatory articulation training videotape developed by Trost-Cardamone (1987). After the transcription task, their transcriptions were compared with those provided by Trost-Cardamone. The results of the study indicated poor interjudge and intrajudge agreement. The average percentage of compensatory articulations transcribed identically to Trost-Cardamone's by the experienced judges was 54% (range 41% to 71%). The inexperienced judges performed even poorer on the task, agreeing on an average of only 29% (range 19% to 38%) of the compensatory articulations. The average percentage of agreement among the experienced listeners ranged from 25% to 47% (mean 39%) and from 21% to 47% (mean 30%) for the inexperienced listeners. Intrajudge agreement for the experienced and inexperienced judges averaged 76% (range 62% to 92%) and 57% (range 42% to 62%), respectively. The authors attributed the judges' poor reliability to a number of factors, including limited training and clinical exposure to these patterns.

The data reported by Gooch et al. underscore the importance of obtaining reliability data for clinicians when clinical judgments of compensatory articulation are reported. These data are sorely lacking at the present time and, without them, our efforts to examine the prevalence of compensatory articulation errors in children with cleft palate are severely compromised.

Other adaptive and maladaptive behaviors. Other remarkable strategies have been adopted by speakers with cleft palate to cope with velopharyngeal inadequacy. We have on rare occasion observed click substitutions of stop consonants in children with velopharyngeal inadequacy. In addition, several authors have described sibilants produced with ingressive airflow (McWilliams and Philips, 1979; Peterson-Falzone, 1986). According to Peterson-Falzone, the perceptual characteristic is one of a "short sucking sound." Although our knowledge of these gestures is limited to anecdotal clinical reports, both apparently represent the speaker's effort to capitalize on negative pressure for the production of plosion and frication.

We have also observed children with cleft lip and palate who demonstrate a distinctive lateral excursion of the mandible during production of sibilants, particularly /s/. Clinically, these children present with anterior dental/occlusal anomalies and oral distortion of sibilants. Lateral mandibular displacement appears to enhance the perceptual quality of /s/ by providing the child with an adequate dental cutting. Vallino and Tompson (1993) reported a similar phenomenon in noncleft patients with malocclusion whom they studied just before orthognathic surgery. The authors observed both lateral and anterior shifting of the mandible, particularly during production of /ʃ/, /ʧ/, and /ʤ/.

Finally, a number of authors have described a nasal grimace in children with cleft palate who have evidence of velopharyngeal inadequacy (e.g., Bzoch, 1997a; Golding-Kusher, 1995, Van Demark and Hardin, 1990). In most cases, constriction of the anterior nares probably reflects the speaker's attempt to valve air anteriorly that was lost through the velopharyngeal port. This compensatory behavior may persist as a learned behavior in some patients for whom velopharyngeal adequacy has been established. Bzoch (1997b) reported that although 4% of the patients he studied in the 1960s demonstrated nasal grimacing, none of patients in his 1980s series demonstrated this behavior.

Patterns of misarticulation. Patterns of articulation have been studied extensively in children with cleft palate. Some of the trends that will be reviewed in this chapter are strong, presumably trustworthy, and have face validity. Others, however, are weak and must be regarded with caution although their recurrence suggests reliability of observation (Gilbert, McPeek, and Mosteller, 1977). Interpretation of trends from one study to another is sometimes difficult because different procedures have been used to study similar problems. For example, a variety of criteria has been used in the selection of subjects. In some studies, patients with different types of clefts were grouped together; in others, more homogeneous subject groups were used. Studies differ also in the quality of techniques used to measure velopharyngeal valving. Some investigators studied only misarticulating subjects; others lumped together speakers with normal articulation and those with articulation errors. Studies have differed in the techniques used to measure articulation so that there are variations in the sounds and contexts studied. Different stimuli have been used to elicit responses and different criteria to score the responses. The studies have differed on many other important variables as well, including research design. Thus it is not always possible to equate one investigation with another. However, in spite of these understandable variations and limitations in methods, patterns do emerge that should be understood and used clinically.

Error types. Descriptive accounts of articulation in speakers with cleft palate have demonstrated that omissions and substitutions occur more frequently than other error types in young children (Bzoch, 1956; Spriestersbach, Darley, and Rouse, 1956), although errors related to distortion occur most frequently in older children and adults (Bardach et al., 1984; Counihan, 1956; McWilliams, 1953, 1958; Van Demark, 1966). The omissions observed in young children with cleft palate often reflect normal developmental processes (i.e., final consonant deletion, weak syllable deletion) that might be expected in any child. The clinician should recognize, however, that speakers with velopharyngeal insufficiency could delete final consonants as a means of avoiding nasal emission because the available air pressure has been depleted. Sounds lacking normal oral air pressure could also be interpreted as omissions although some energy marks the final consonant. Bernthal and Weiner (1976) demonstrated that acoustic energy is often present where articulation evaluators have reported speech sound omission.

The prevalence of sound distortions in the cleft palate population is not unexpected given the velopharyngeal dysfunction and dental/occlusal problems that many of these individuals face. Although nasal distortion is probably one of the most salient characteristics of speech associated with cleft palate, research findings indicate that misarticulations related to oral distortion occur far more frequently than those attributed to nasal distortion (Bzoch, 1956; Van Demark, 1964). Bzoch (1956) observed that nasal distortions persist with age, whereas other distortions tend to decrease in frequency of occurrence.

Manner and place of articulation. Numerous investigations have demonstrated that children with cleft palate have more difficulty producing pressure consonants than other classes of consonants (McWilliams, 1953; Philips and Harrison, 1969; Spriestersbach, Darley, and Rouse, 1956; Van Demark, 1969; Van Demark, Morris, and Vandehaar, 1979). They typically misarticulate fricatives and affricates most frequently, followed by plosives, glides, and then nasals. Velopharyngeal inadequacy is generally considered to be a major factor responsible for errors on the former three classes of sounds because each require high intraoral air pressure.

Using factor analysis, Fletcher (1978) analyzed articulation data from 70 subjects with cleft palates and identified a sibilant-nonsibilant contrast. He sorted the sounds studied into three categories—(1) sibilants: /s/, /z/, /ʃ/, /ʧ/, /ʤ/, (2) nonsibilant fricatives: /θ/, /ð/, /v/, /f/, and (3) plosives: /p/, /b/, /t/, /d/, /k/, /g/. According to Fletcher, this classification resulted in more homogeneous groupings of sounds than the more traditional assignment of sounds to fricative and affricative categories. He reported mean error percentages of 47 for sibilants, 24 for nonsibilant fricatives, and 17 for plosives, findings consistent with those of McWilliams (1953, 1958) and Spriestersbach, Darley, and Rouse (1956). His subjects misarticulated over 40% of the /s/ sounds studied in the initial, medial, and final position of words. This latter finding was consistent with previous reports that have identified /s/ as the sound most frequently and consistently misarticulated by children with cleft palate (Byrne, Shelton, and Diedrich, 1961; McWilliams, 1958; Van Demark, 1979).

Several investigators have studied whether persons with cleft palate are more likely than noncleft individuals to misarticulate /r/ and /l/. A higher prevalence of misarticulation of /r/ and /l/ would not be expected in individuals with clefts, compared with noncleft individuals, because these are not consonants that require high intraoral air pressure. However, the prevalence of these errors in the cleft palate population is noteworthy. Philips and Harrison (1969) found a high percentage of glide errors in their preschool children with cleft palate. Indeed, percentages of errors on glides and plosives were similar in the three age groups they studied. An unexpectedly high prevalence of these errors has also been observed in adults. McWilliams (1958) studied the speech of 48 adults with cleft palate and found that 13 of them misarticulated /r/. Finally, the findings of at least two early studies (Pitzner and Morris, 1966; Van Demark, 1969) found that individuals with cleft palate who had poor velopharyngeal closure were more likely to misarticulate these sounds than were those with palatal clefts who had good velopharyngeal function. Van Demark and Van Demark (1967) compared the articulation of children with cleft palate who had good velopharyngeal function and children with functional articulation disorders. The latter group more frequently misarticulated glides and also used more sound substitutions. Although some authors (Van Demark, Morris, and Vandehaar, 1979) have reported that speakers with cleft palate misarticulate /r/ and /l/ more often than do noncleft individuals, these assertions are based largely on comparisons to normative data—few investigators have included noncleft subjects in their study for comparative purposes.

Defects associated with cleft palate may influence place as well as manner of articulation. For example, nasal emission associated with velopharyngeal inadequacy may particularly impair frication while also encouraging articulation placement posterior to a fistulae or to an opening of the velopharyngeal valve. Thus manner requirements that are difficult for the speaker with velopharyngeal inadequacy to achieve may be associated with articulation errors that involve a shift in place of articulation.

Counihan (1956) examined place of articulation differences and rank-ordered sounds from least to most frequently misarticulated as follows: lip sounds, tongue-tip simple sounds, tongue-tip complex sounds, and back-of-tongue sounds. Logemann (1983) stated that children with cleft palate who are between 24 months and 5 years old tend to have articulatory placement errors but correct manner of articulation. They maintain manner by placing articulation posterior to fistulas or velopharyngeal opening. Older children present accurate articulatory placement but manner errors in the form of faulty release of stops, fricatives, and affricates.

Moll (1968) asserted that findings related to place of consonant articulation were confounded by manner of consonant production in early studies. He combined the results of five early investigations and examined place of articulation classes separately for each manner of production category. Consonants involving lingual contacts were found to be more defective than those involving only the lips across all manner of production categories. Moll stated that, except for this latter finding, place of articulation data contribute little to descriptions of articulation in children with cleft palate.

Voicing. Individuals with clefts appear to misarticulate voiceless sounds more frequently than the voiced cognates (McWilliams, 1953, 1958; Spriestersbach, Darley, and Rouse, 1956). Spriestersbach, Moll, and Morris (1961) found that voiced stops and affricates were articulated better than their voiceless counterparts but that the reverse was true for fricatives. They stated that these differences could be related to the age of the subjects studied because voiceless fricatives are learned earlier than voiced fricatives, whereas voiceless plosives are learned later than their voiced cognates. The authors subsequently re-examined earlier data reported by Counihan (1956) and McWilliams (1958) for adolescents and adults ". . . for whom the period of articulation development was presumably completed" (p. 370). They found that voiceless stops and fricatives were misarticulated more frequently than their voiced counterparts. Moll (1968) concluded that the relative difficulty of voiced and voiceless consonants may change with age, and that voicing and manner of production may interact to influence articulation. It is also possible that voicing masks placement errors that are evident to the ear when they occur in voiceless members of cognate pairs (Kent, 1982; Sherman, Spriestersbach, and Noll, 1959).

Vowel articulation. Several authors have examined vowel production in individuals with cleft palate and have suggested that, as a group, they may be less proficient than noncleft speakers (Van Demark, Morris, and Vandehaar, 1979). In an early study, Klinger (1956) reported that listeners correctly identified only 53% of the vowels produced by persons with cleft palate. In contrast, 70% of the vowels produced by normal speakers were identified correctly. Cullinan and Counihan (1971) questioned studies indicating that persons with clefts articulate vowels with few or no errors and noted that these studies may have been confounded by contextual cues to vowel identification. They studied the ability of listeners to identify the vowels /a/, /i/, and /u/. Vowels produced by normal speakers were correctly identified 79% of the time, whereas for subjects with clefts, the vowels were recognized in only 53% of the utterances. The source of this loss of vowel intelligibility in speakers with clefts has not been established. However, Cullinan and Counihan noted that tongue height and mouth opening may be adjusted to compensate for velopharyngeal opening.

Hypernasality may also degrade vowel intelligibility. Philips and Kent (1984) stated that nasalized vowels show low-frequency nasal formants below F1 (the first formant), a weakening and small increase in frequency of F2, a reduction of overall energy, a reduction of F2 amplitude, and an increase in formant band widths. Thus nasalized vowels are characterized by low-frequency energy and reduced intensity. The authors indicated that nasalization makes it difficult to differentiate among vowels.

In spite of these findings, it is significant to note that although hypernasality may affect the perceptual characteristics of vowels, vowels tend to retain enough of their features to be recognizable at least in the context of speech (Moll, 1968). Furthermore, relatively few children with (or without) palatal clefts require articulation training for vowels.

Variability in resonance and articulation

Cleft type. Children with cleft lip and palate typically demonstrate poorer articulation than do children with cleft palate only (Fletcher, 1978; McWilliams and Musgrave, 1977; Moll, 1968; Morley, 1970; Riski and DeLong, 1984). This is because patients with unilateral or bilateral complete clefts are subject to maxillary collapse, dental malalignment, missing teeth, ectopic eruption of teeth, supernumerary teeth, and protrusion of the premaxilla—and these conditions are frequently hazardous to normal articulation. Fletcher (1978) reported the following percentages of correct articulation responses in his patients: soft palate only, 91%; soft and hard palate, 72%; unilateral lip and palate, 64%; and bilateral lip and palate, 9%. As cleft severity increased from the soft palate only, to soft and hard palates, to unilateral complete clefts, to bilateral complete clefts, the severity of speech problems also increased.

Riski and DeLong (1984) examined the influence of gender, cleft type, and age at time of testing on the articulation performance of children aged 3 to 8 years. Differences in articulation performance according to gender were not evident; however, cleft-type differences were reported. As a group, children with cleft lip only demonstrated normal articulation development. The children with cleft palate were more heterogeneous for articulation development, with children in the cleft palate only group demonstrating better articulation than those in the cleft lip and palate group.

In a more recent report, Haapanen (1994) examined the relationship between cleft type and speech proficiency for 113 subjects (30 with cleft lip and palate, 55 with cleft palate only, and 28 with cleft lip only). Clinical judgments of hypernasality, audible nasal emission, weak pressure consonants, and compensatory articulations were assigned by a single, experienced listener during the subjects' sixth year examination. Nasalance scores and information regarding secondary management were also obtained. Hypernasality was evident in 38% of the isolated cleft palate subjects and only 11% of the cleft lip and palate subjects. Audible nasal emission was recorded for 36% of the cleft palate and 28% of the cleft lip and palate groups. The cleft lip only group did not demonstrate either hypernasality or audible nasal emission.

Only one recent report has compared the speech of adolescents with clefts to that of a noncleft age-matched group. Karling, Larson, and Henningsson (1993) reported speech results for 103 patients with cleft lip and palate (84 unilateral cleft lip and palate, 19 bilateral cleft lip and palate) when the patients were 7 to 20 years old. Both groups received palatoplasty at a comparable mean age (20 and 21 months). In general, the bilateral cleft group demonstrated poorer speech than the unilateral group. A substantially greater percentage of patients with bilateral clefts (68%) than unilateral clefts (47%) had received speech therapy. In addition, the speech of patients in the bilateral group was judged significantly less intelligible, and these patients had more misarticulations related to the cleft (e.g., backed articulations). All the cleft patients were judged to have poorer speech than age-matched individuals in a noncleft comparison group.

Some investigators have reported better speech in patients with cleft lip and palate than in patients with cleft palate only (Spriestersbach, Moll, and Morris, 1961). This is compatible with the fact that some patients with cleft palate alone have extensive horseshoe-shaped clefts with significant tissue deficiency and that persons with cleft palate alone are much more likely to have associated congenital deformities than are patients with cleft lip and palate (McWilliams and Matthews, 1979; Ross and Johnston, 1972).

Our clinical experience indicates that cleft lip alone is almost never responsible for articulation problems. When the cleft lip is associated with bilateral alveolar clefts or with a very short, tight upper lip, the individual may be unable to close the lips over the anterior teeth for bilabial consonants. However, this problem is rare and appears to resolve spontaneously with lip growth and as dental and surgical treatment improve the position of the premaxilla. Children with deficient tissue in the middle of the upper lip may substitute labiodental sounds for bilabials. These labiodental productions may be indistinguishable to the ear from their bilabial counterparts, but they are readily apparent to the eye. Finally, young children with lip deficiencies may omit bilabial consonants.

We cannot predict with any accuracy at the time of their birth the future speech of patients with cleft palate. Many variables in addition to the severity of the cleft will influence speech development. If all other variables could be controlled, we would expect the severity of the speech disorder to correlate positively with the severity of cleft. Function of the velopharyngeal mechanism after surgery, however, is logically more important to speech than type of cleft and extent of malformation at birth.

Influence of context. The influence of context on articulation proficiency has been studied by a number of investigators. The results of several early studies (McDermott, 1962; Morris, Spriestersbach, and Darley, 1961; Spriestersbach, Darley, and Rouse, 1956; Spriestersbach, Moll, and Morris, 1961) indicated that individuals with cleft palate are more likely to misarticulate consonants when they occur in clusters than when they occur as a singleton. In addition, they are more likely to misarticulate a consonant in a three-element blend than in a two-element blend (McDermott, 1962). Bzoch (1965) found that two-consonant blends better differentiated children with cleft palate and normal children than did fricatives or plosives. He noted that these results were compatible with those of earlier studies (Counihan, 1956, 1960;

McWilliams, 1953, 1958; Starr, 1956). Information about the nature of the errors produced by patients in these reports was not typically provided. It would be interesting to know to what extent these errors involved distortions as opposed to cluster reduction. Such information would be needed to examine the etiological bases of the errors and fully interpret these findings.

The relationship between consonant position in a word and articulatory proficiency has also been examined in individuals with cleft palate. Counihan (1960) and Bzoch (1965) examined the articulation of consonant sounds in these positions. Bzoch's subjects were between 3 and 6 years old, whereas Counihan's ranged from 13 through 23 years. Each author sampled various consonant sounds. Bzoch found a trend toward more frequent misarticulation of sounds in the medial position than in either of the other positions. Counihan found no relationship between misarticulation and word position. The differences observed between these two studies could simply reflect the difference in subjects ages (i.e., young children frequently misarticulate consonants in the medial position of a word after mastery in the initial and final positions). Without additional information about error type, it is difficult to determine from these and other early studies (Byrne, Shelton, and Diedrich, 1961; Starr, 1956) whether contextual influences operate differently for cleft and noncleft children. Morris, Spriestersbach, and Darley (1961) concluded that the position of sound elements in articulation test words does not relate strongly to the distinction between subjects with good and those with poor velopharyngeal closure. Nor did position in test word influence the discriminatory power of two- and three-element blends.

Additional context variables have also been studied. Bless, Ewanowski, and Paul (1978) commented that individuals with velopharyngeal inadequacy are most likely to misarticulate consonants that are adjacent to nasal sounds, whereas individuals with marginal velopharyngeal inadequacy may nasalize oral consonants adjacent to nasals through assimilatory relationships.

The consonant context in which a given vowel is placed may influence perceived hypernasality, especially in cases in which valving is borderline rather than grossly incompetent. Crosby (1952) found that judges could not effectively select cleft from noncleft speakers when the vowels were embedded only in nasal consonants. The subjects with clefts did not sound unlike normal subjects when they produced vowels adjacent to nasals for which the oral and nasal cavities are normally coupled. Larson and Hamlet (1987) report similar results.

Influence of speech rate. Speech rate in speakers with cleft palate has received relatively little study to date. In an early study, McDermott (1962) found that /s/ was articulated less accurately as the rate of syllable production increased. He inferred that the slow rate afforded the subject greater opportunity to compensate for structural defects. Lass and Noll (1970) compared the speech rates of young adults with palatal clefts with those of normal individuals. The subjects with cleft palate tended to speak more slowly than the normal individuals and to show greater variability on the measures studied.

The relationship between speech rate and nasalization has been the focus of several reports in the literature (D'Antonio, 1982; Jones and Folkins, 1985; Jones, Folkins, and Morris, 1990). The limited amount of attention directed toward this relationship is surprising in view of time-honored clinical philosophies regarding rate manipulation. As indicated by Jones, Folkins, and Morris (1990), some speech-language pathologists believe that speakers who demonstrate inconsistent nasalization can produce more normal speech at a slower speaking rate "because slower rates supposedly do not tax the speech production system motorically or mechanically as much as faster rates do" (p. 458). Rate reduction was recommended as a strategy for reducing perceived hypernasality in early texts and continues to be used despite the lack of evidence supporting a strong relationship between the two.

There is some evidence to suggest that a reduction in speech rate can result in interruptions of velopharyngeal closure. Colton and Cooker (1968) found nasality ratings to be higher in normal and hearing-impaired individuals when reading word by word than when reading at a normal rate. They thought the velopharyngeal seal might be broken at the slower rate. This inference was also drawn by Hutchinson, Robinson, and Nerbonne (1978).

Jones and Folkins (1985) studied the effects of rate on the perception of disordered speech, including hypernasality, in six 7- to 10-year-old children with clefts. They found, in support of D'Antonio's (1982) earlier work, that the perception of disordered speech did not increase as a function of increased rate. It would be of interest to repeat this study with subjects representative of a continuum of valving capabilities because it is possible that the outcome might be different or that some speakers might experience difficulty when attempting to increase rate. This latter problem is observed clinically, but it is not known whether it is related to structure and function, to personality, or to both. Certainly, as mentioned earlier, some speakers with clefts adopt a slower than usual speaking rate.

Influence of fatigue. Clinically, some parents of children with repaired cleft palate report that the severity of hypernasality increases when the child is tired or when the child has engaged in prolonged periods of speaking. Despite such claims, limited research has been conducted to examine the influence of fatigue on perceived nasality. Webb, Starr, and Moller (1992) examined the effect of extended speaking on resonance and voice quality in eight subjects with repaired cleft palate and mild hypernasality and in eight noncleft subjects with normal resonance. (It is pertinent to point out that the subjects were not enrolled on the basis of a complaint of increased nasality with fatigue.) The subjects read a standard passage aloud for 40 minutes.

Before the session, in the middle of the session, and after this session they also read a probe passage and sustained an /ɔ/ in the phrase "Then he saw." The investigators reported that changes in hypernasality were greater for the cleft subjects than for the noncleft subjects; however, the extent of the change was small and not always in the direction of increased hypernasality. The cleft group demonstrated smaller voice quality changes, but again the change was not always in the direction of deteriorating vocal quality. Webb, Starr, and Moller questioned the extent to which the task used in their study actually fatigued the subjects.

Developmental trends

Prelinguistic and early linguistic development in babies with cleft palate. A limited number of investigations have examined the impact of palatal clefting on early speech sound development of babies with cleft palate. Although early anecdotal reports suggested delays in the onset of babbling for these babies (Bzoch, 1956), the prelinguistic period of development was virtually ignored until recent years. Clinical researchers have become increasingly attentive to the emerging phonological characteristics of these babies because of (1) advances in our understanding of normal vocal development that have underscored the risks imposed by the clefting condition and (2) concerns about the impact of age at time of surgery on early speech sound development.

Normally developing babies pass through a series of stages in vocal development during the first year of life that appear to be governed in part by changes in both the musculoskeletal system and the nervous system. Initially the infant's larynx is in an elevated position that results in approximation of the epiglottis and velum. The pharyngeal cavity is short, and the tongue occupies the bulk of the baby's oral cavity. Early vocalizations during the first 2 months of life are typically restricted to vegetative and comfort-state productions characterized by glottal attack and quasivowels. Postural changes that emerge between 2 and 4 months of age, including increased head control and sitting with support, result in changes in the shape of the oral cavity that facilitate greater tongue mobility (Kemp-Fincham, Kuehn, and Trost-Cardamone, 1990). Vocalizations during this time include quasivowels accompanied by velar, uvular, and pharyngeal constrictions. As the larynx descends and the velum and epiglottis begin to disengage at approximately 4 months of age, the infant is capable of producing fully resonant vowellike utterances and generating oral air pressure for the production of consonant-like utterances. The infant's vocal tract more closely resembles that of an adult and it is at this time that vowels, primitive consonant-vowel sequences, and other types of vocalizations (e.g., squeals, growls, whispers, bilabial trills, etc.) begin to emerge. Some authors (Kemp-Fincham, Kuehn, and Trost-Cardamone, 1990; Trost-Cardamone, 1990b) have pointed out that the latter part of this expansion stage and the subsequent canonical babbling stage are sensitive periods for perceptual and motor learning. Indeed, it is during this period of phonetic development that differences begin to emerge between normally developing infants and infants with hearing impairment (Oller and Eilers, 1988) and clefts (Kuehn and Trost-Cardamone, 1988). "If a large oronasal opening (unoperated hard palate) persists beyond this stage of phonetic expansion, compensatory motor control mechanisms may be developed to achieve the resonant nuclei essential to the following canonical stage of babbling. Onset of the expansion stage of babbling may therefore signal an important cut-off period for cleft palate infants, after which their different oronasal structures have a greater impact on later speech development" (Kemp-Fincham, Kuehn, and Trost-Cardamone, 1990, p. 740).

There is a growing body of research that indicates some characteristics of prelinguistic vocalizations in normally developing children are predictive of later speech-language proficiency. There is evidence to suggest that frequency of vocalization in babies 3 to 6 months old is positively correlated with the frequency of verbalization and talking at older ages (Stoel-Gammon, 1992). Delays in the onset of canonical babbling and a reduction in the use of consonants during the prelinguistic period have also been linked to delays in speech and language development (Stoel-Gammon, 1994). In addition, use of supraglottic consonants in babbling is positively correlated with speech onset, phonological performance at age 3 years, and problems in communication and academics at age 5 years (Menyuk, Liebergott, and Schultz, 1986; Stoel-Gammon, 1992; Vihman and Greenlee, 1987). Finally, it is also well established that the sound types and syllable shapes evident during the latter stages of prelinguistic development also characterize a child's early words (Oller, 1976; Stoel-Gammon, 1985; Stoel-Gammon and Cooper, 1984; Vihman, Macken, Miller, Simmons, and Miller, 1985). This continuity between early prelinguistic forms and later linguistic productions is of particular importance for babies with cleft palate because their early vocalizations are typically accomplished in an environment of abnormal oropharyngeal structures and intermittent hearing loss associated with middle ear effusions.

Research examining the early speech sound development of babies with cleft palate indicates both qualitative and quantitative differences in their early prelinguistic productions. Olsen (1965) provided one of the earliest descriptive accounts of speech sound development in these babies. He compared the spontaneous vocalizations of 62 babies with unrepaired cleft palate to those available for a comparable number of age-matched noncleft babies. Although both groups produced a comparable proportion of nasals, glides, and fricatives at each age level, fewer tip-alveolar articulations and a smaller proportion of bilabial stops and fricatives were noted in the cleft group at the majority of ages studied. Velar stop consonants were not evident for the cleft group until the 17- to 18-month age level, and anterior stops /b/ and /d/ were not frequently evident until 29 to 30 months of age. As expected, glottal productions were predominant for both groups at 5 to 6 months of age. Although a gradual reduction in glottal articulation and an increase in use of other place features was evident with age for both groups, these laryngeal productions were prominent in the vocalizations of the cleft group at all ages and were surpassed by other place features only at the 29- to 30-month age level. Pharyngeal fricatives were evident in the 11- to 12-month sample for five of the infants with cleft palate and were produced frequently by all of the babies in this group at the older age levels. These atypical articulations were not evident for any of the noncleft babies in the comparison group.

According to Olsen the majority of babies with cleft palate did not demonstrate an obvious nasal quality until 29 to 30 months of age. This was a particularly interesting finding because none of his subjects had received palatal surgery. Because only six of the babies he studied were producing true words by 30 months of age, it is tempting to speculate that hypernasality does not become a salient feature of a child's early utterances unless it is produced within the context of meaningful speech.

Because it is currently uncommon in the United States for palatoplasty to be delayed beyond 18 months of age, it is questionable as to how pertinent his findings may be to cleft palate babies today. The external validity of his findings might also be questioned because his conclusions were based on a limited language sample (~30 vocalizations or utterances) obtained from each subject. Despite differences in timing of surgical management and methods, however, Olsen's major findings have stood the test of time and have been replicated by other investigators in recent years.

Several investigators have attempted to examine the preoperative speech sound development of babies with cleft palate and its relationship to subsequent development after surgery. O'Gara and Logemann (1988) and O'Gara, Logemann, and Rademaker (1992, 1994) conducted a series of longitudinal investigations to examine the phonetic characteristics of prelinguistic utterances and early words produced by babies with cleft palate. Babies who participated in each study were assigned to one of two groups for purposes of data analysis: children who had palatoplasty before 12 months of age were assigned to the early surgery–greater tissue group and babies who had palatoplasty after 12 months of age were assigned to the later surgery–lesser tissue group. In their earliest report, O'Gara and Logemann (1988) examined the comfort state vocalizations of 23 babies with cleft palate (with or without cleft lip) at nine specified intervals from 3 to 36 months of age. As a group, these babies used oral place features less frequently than is typically reported for noncleft infants and never demonstrated the "alveolar takeover" that has been reported in noncleft infants at or beyond 6 months of age. Glottal stops were produced more frequently than oral stops through 23 to 24 months of age for the total group. The frequency of glottal stops progressively decreased for the early surgery–greater tissue group from 3 to 4 months through 18 to 19 months of age when oral stop predominance occurred. In contrast, glottal stops predominated over oral stops at each age level studied for the later surgery–lesser tissue group.

In a follow-up report, the authors (O'Gara, Logemann, and Rademaker, 1992) examined the phonetic features present in the prelinguistic utterances of 16 babies with nonsyndromic clefts of the secondary palate. The mean age of palatal surgery for the early closure and late closure groups was 8.75 and 16 months, respectively. Both groups demonstrated similar patterns of change over time for place features (glottal, velar, palatal, alveolar, and labial), stop types (glottal, oral, nasal), and fricative types (glottal, oral). However, babies in the early surgery group produced fewer glottals and glottal stops. In addition, palatal consonants and oral stops emerged earlier and were produced with greater frequency by babies in the early surgery group than in the later surgery group. No differences were evident between the groups in frequency of oral fricative productions.

In the third investigation of their series the authors (O'Gara, Logemann, and Rademaker, 1994) studied the phonetic development of 23 babies with unilateral cleft lip and palate. The method they used was similar to that used in their original study; however, the authors pooled their data into three time periods (5 to 11 months, 14 to 18 months, and 30 to 25 months) for purposes of statistical analysis. Only one significant interaction between time period and surgery group was found. A significantly higher frequency of oral stop production was evident for the early surgery group at the last two time periods. When the data were collapsed across surgery groups, a significant decrease in glottal productions was evident with age. In addition, a significant increase in use of nasal fricatives and the palatal place feature was apparent across the first two age groups. Finally, a significant increase in use of the alveolar and velar place features, as well as an increase in the use of oral fricatives was evident between 5 and 11 months and 30 and 35 months. O'Gara, Logemann, and Rademaker (1994) speculated that the age-related increase in nasal fricatives among their babies with cleft palate could represent "... the subjects' playful experimentation of nasal release in learning this more difficult class of oral pressure consonants" (p. 450).

A significant limitation of this type of research that should be emphasized here is the strong association between tissue deficiency and timing of surgery in many clinical populations. Babies with small tissue deficits often receive palatal surgery at an earlier age than do babies with large palatal clefts. Differences between babies stratified by age at time of palatal surgery may actually reflect differences in the original defect rather than age of palatal surgery per se. Support for this argument can be found in O'Gara and Logemann's (1988) original report. Differences in frequency of glottal productions were evident between their surgery groups as early as 5 to 6 months of age—presumably long before the majority of their subjects had undergone palatal repair. Although early surgery likely facilitates the acquisition of desirable phonetic features and may, in fact, enhance the rate of acquisition, the size of the palatal cleft probably accounts for at least some of the variability in early speech sound development frequently attributed to age of surgery.

Other investigators have also reported restricted consonant inventories and a high proportion of glottal articulation in the babbling of children with cleft palate. Chapman (1991) compared the early vocalizations of five toddlers with unrepaired cleft palate and five noncleft toddlers aged 12 to 14 months. Children in each of the groups were matched for age and sex, and none had expressive vocabularies greater than five words. No significant differences were found between the groups in absolute size of consonant inventory. However, differences emerged when frequency and type of consonants produced were examined. The noncleft toddlers produced a substantially greater number of consonants (1026) than their cleft counterparts (529). In addition, although oral stops accounted for more than 70% of the consonants produced by the noncleft group, only 1% of the consonants produced by the toddlers with cleft palate were oral stop productions. Forty-two percent of the consonants present in the cleft groups' inventory were glottal articulations (/h/, 38%; /ʔ/, 4%). The most frequently produced consonant for the cleft group was /h/, followed by /w/, /n/, /m/, and /j/. In contrast, the most frequently occurring consonant for the noncleft group was /d/, followed by /g/, /h/, /w/, /j/, and /b/. Finally, differences were also noted between the groups in frequency of multisyllabic productions. The cleft palate group produced fewer multisyllabic productions than the noncleft group did (16% vs. 33%).

Hardin-Jones, Chapman, Schulte, and Halter (1999) compared the prelinguistic vocalizations of 30 nine-month old babies with unrepaired cleft palate to vocalizations obtained from 15 age-matched peers. They reported that only 50% of the babies in their cleft group had reached the canonical babbling stage compared to 93% in the noncleft group. On average, the noncleft babies produced twice as many different consonants as the babies with cleft palate. The authors noted that the largest consonant inventory observed in the cleft group equaled that of the smallest inventory in the noncleft group. These findings contradicted Chapman's (1991) earlier work that revealed no difference in size of consonant inventory between cleft and noncleft toddlers. Hardin-Jones and her colleagues speculated that Chapman's limited sample size may have accounted for the lack of differences observed between the groups.

The immediate impact of palatal surgery on vocalizations produced by babies with cleft palate was studied by Grunwell and Russell (1987). The vocalizations of three infants with cleft palate who received surgery at 11 to 14 months of age were recorded preoperatively and at four postoperative intervals. A significant reduction in total vocalization time and number of vocalizations was evident for each child during the first postoperative recording. A decrease in the mean length of vocalization was apparent for two of the subjects. A notable decrease in size of consonant inventory and a reduction in the percentage of different polysyllabic utterances was evident during the immediate postoperative recording for two subjects. An increase in the number of different consonants used was apparent for these subjects in the third week after surgery when compared with the preoperative and immediate postoperative recordings. These findings suggest an immediate but short-lived effect of surgery on the vocalizations of babies with cleft palate. A reduction in both quantity and quality of vocalizations can be expected in the early postoperative period; however, a return to preoperative performance can be expected within several weeks.

Lohmander-Agerskov et al. (1994) examined prelinguistic vocalizations of babies with cleft palate in relation to various morphologic and functional factors. Tape-recorded samples of babbling were examined for 35 babies with cleft lip or palate (ages 8 to 15 months) who had received primary veloplasty at a mean age of 8 months. Three babies had a cleft of the soft palate only and so had their palatal cleft completely closed in one operation. The remaining subjects had a residual cleft of the hard palate. Two noncleft controls (ages 9 and 11 months) were also studied. Of the 27 babies with clefts of the lip and palate, 25 had worn an intraoral plate to obturate the hard palate. None of the babies with cleft palate only (n = 8) had worn a plate. The width/extent of the clefts were measured. Approximately 1 minute of babbling was transcribed for each baby and included approximately 15 to 20 utterances with 3 to 10 consonants per utterance.

The investigators reported more frequent use of supraglottal place features than glottal articulations for all of the babies. However, the percentage of supraglottal consonants was lower in the cleft babies than the noncleft controls. A significantly higher frequency of anterior sounds and a lower frequency of posterior sounds were evident in the babies with cleft palate only. Although the correlation was not significant, a higher frequency of posterior consonants (palatal, velar, uvular, pharyngeal) than anterior consonants was evident in the two cleft lip and palate groups. Babies with more extensive clefts of the palate only tended to use more posterior sounds.

The findings of Lohmander-Agerskov et al. were at odds with those previously reported by Grunwell and Russell (1987) and Chapman (1991) who found a predominance of glottal articulations in their babies. The authors speculated that these differences might be attributed to differences in management of the cleft between the various centers. In should be noted, however, that despite the lower than expected frequency of laryngeal productions, the babies studied by Lohmander-Agerskov et al. did produce a high frequency of posterior articulation. In fact, posterior place features were more frequently produced than anterior place features by 21 of the 27 babies with cleft lip and palate. A major limitation of this investigation was its reliance on such a small babbling sample. Despite this methodological problem, however, the interactions studied by the authors were long overdue. The associations noted between cleft type, extent of the cleft, and posterior articulation were particularly intriguing and warrant additional study.

Early lexical development. The early lexical and phonological development of children with cleft palate has been examined in several recent investigations. Estrem and Broen (1989) examined the first 50 words of five children with cleft palate (four had received palatoplasty) and five noncleft children matched for size of expressive vocabulary. They found that the children with cleft palate used more words beginning with sonorants (nasals, vowels, approximates) and fewer words beginning with obstruents (stops, fricatives, affricates) than their noncleft counterparts did. The cleft group also used more words beginning with peripheral place consonants (velars, glottals, and labials). The authors speculated that although word choice may have been affected by the phonological characteristics of the target word, lexical selectivity may also have been influenced by differential parental reinforcement (i.e., parents may understand and reinforce words that begin with sounds the child can most accurately produce). The authors noted that the majority of children with cleft palate did not begin to talk until after palatal surgery and were approximately 3½ months older than the noncleft group when they produced their first word. They were also 3½ months older than the noncleft subjects when their expressive lexicon reached 50 words. Olsen (1965) also reported delayed onset of expressive vocabulary for the subjects in this study. Only five of the infants with unrepaired cleft palate in his study were producing at least one true word at the 17- to 18-month and 23- to 24-month age levels, and only six infants were using words by the 29- to 30-month age level. These findings suggest that although onset of speech may occur later for toddlers with cleft palate, they demonstrate a rate of lexical acquisition that is comparable to that of their noncleft peers.

Chapman and Hardin (1992) compared the phonetic and phonological development of fifteen 2-year-old children with cleft palate who had undergone palatal surgery after the onset of meaningful speech with that of a group of five noncleft children matched for age. Differences in size of consonant inventory were not evident between the groups; however, the cleft group correctly produced significantly fewer consonants. In addition, the cleft group correctly produced significantly fewer nasals and liquids. Although they also correctly produced fewer stop consonants, the difference did not reach statistical significance. Finally, only two differences were evident between the groups when phonological process usage was examined. Nasal assimilation and backing were evident more frequently in the cleft group. The authors concluded that ". . . when attempting to systematize and simplify word production, children with cleft palate predictably substitute sounds within their production repertoire (in this case nasals) for more difficult sounds" (p. 440).

Some authors have reported findings suggesting that abnormal phonetic patterns during prelinguistic development may predispose a child to later use of unusual phonological patterns. Russell and Grunwell (1993) examined the prelinguistic and subsequent speech development of eight children with cleft palate. Glottal and pharyngeal articulation predominated before palatal surgery (at 9 to 14 months), and a limited number of plosives involving the lips and anterior tongue were evident. An increase in lingual articulations and oral plosives as well as a corresponding reduction in the number of glottal and pharyngeal productions were evident 6 to 8 weeks postoperatively. However, glottal productions were still predominant for plosives and fricatives. On 6-month follow-up, the group had more normal phonetic patterns but continued to show delays in phonetic development. Palatal fricatives noted for some children during early speech development appeared related to prelinguistic consonant inventories as opposed to dental/occlusal problems. Russell and Grunwell noted that "the lack of plosives and fricatives involving the lips and front of the tongue" during prelinguistic utterances tended to predispose their subjects "towards using a backing process during their early speech utterances" (p. 37). Practically, these preliminary findings suggest that a child's prelinguistic consonant inventory can provide useful information about the presence and severity of future speech problems. Babies who demonstrate absence of plosives or dominance of glottals in their prespeech productions should be monitored closely during early speech development for evidence of spontaneous recovery.

Summary and implications. Descriptive accounts of early vocalizations indicate both qualitative and quantitative differences in the early prelinguistic productions of cleft and noncleft babies. Compared with their same-age noncleft peers, babies with unrepaired cleft palate vocalize less frequently and demonstrate fewer total consonant productions (Chapman, 1991), fewer multisyllabic productions (Chapman, 1991), and a more restricted consonant inventory during babbling (Hardin-Jones et al., 1999; Olsen, 1965). Examination of their prelinguistic productions typically reveals a clear preference for nasals, glides, and the glottal fricative /h/. This is in contrast to the preponderance of stop consonants typically reported for noncleft babies. Babies with clefts produce glottal articulations more frequently than age-matched noncleft babies. Although the frequency of these productions progressively decreases for both groups during the latter part of the prelinguistic period, they persist at a relatively high rate of production after onset of the expressive lexicon for babies with clefts (O'Gara and Logemann, 1988; Olsen, 1965). The differences evident for babies with palatal clefts persist long after palatoplasty has been performed and appear to influence subsequent phonetic development (O'Gara and Logemann, 1988) and lexical development. Onset of the expressive lexicon may be delayed for many of these children and characterized by words that begin with consonants that are unaffected by the structural constraints imposed by the palatal cleft (Estrem and Broen, 1989). The significance of early delays in vocal development for these babies cannot be overstated since, as pointed out by Dalston (1992), ". . . the presence of these early qualitative differences may help explain the fact that youngsters with palatal clefts typically manifest numerous articulation problems in early childhood" (p. 30).

It is not clear why babies with cleft palate vocalize less frequently than their noncleft peers or why they demonstrate delays in onset of canonical babbling. However, the limited consonant repertoire and reduction in total number of babbles produced by these children is of concern because it limits the opportunities that the child has to establish the feedback system needed to produce and monitor speech. Stoel-Gammon (1992) and others have emphasized the role of feedback and practice on normal vocal development. "Speech has a skill component and, as with any skilled activity, practice increases the control and precision with which a movement is performed. Thus, the more often a baby produces the movements that shape the vocal tract to produce particular sounds and sound sequences, the more automatic those movements become and ultimately the easier it is to execute them in producing meaningful speech" (p. 451). Thus the more "practiced" CV syllables a child has during babbling, the more forms he or she will have to attach meaning to for acquisition of words. Practice producing different CV syllables is also important in providing the babies with feedback regarding their own productions. Repeated productions allows a baby to match his oral-motor movements with the sounds that result from that movement. When that practice does not occur, the auditory and tactile/kinesthetic feedback loops necessary for normal vocal production are not formed.

It seems likely that some of the early delays in speech sound development reported in babies with cleft palate can be traced, at least in part, to both limited oral-motor practice and distorted feedback. The fluctuating nature of conductive hearing loss associated with middle ear infections has long been associated with early phonological delays in the cleft and noncleft population. Babies with unrepaired palatal clefts are obligated to practice sounds with limited articulatory surfaces and, depending on their middle ear status, distortions in the auditory input they receive. The nasal coupling that is present before palatal surgery will also introduce distortion that probably obscures the acoustic contrasts of CV syllables in babbling. As Kemp-Fincham, Kuehn, and Trost-Cardamone (1990, p. 740) pointed out, "This potential lack of perceptual-acoustic differentiation may subsequently impede the expression of semantic contrasts in the oral mode, resulting in a possible delay in the onset of meaningful speech."

A final comment seems warranted regarding this body of research. A disturbing limitation associated with much of the research characterizing the early speech sound development of children with cleft palate today is the lack of noncleft comparison subjects. Although toddlers may pass through the same general stages of phonological development, considerable variability is evident in the strategies they use during acquisition of the expressive lexicon. This normal variability and the limited normative data available should lead researchers to include normally developing babies as matched controls when efforts are made to study the early speech sound development of babies with cleft palates. Without such comparative data, interpretation of early behaviors is limited at best.

Older children and adolescents. Cross-sectional studies have demonstrated that the articulation performance of children with cleft palate improves with age (Van Demark, 1969; Van Demark and Morris, 1983; Van Demark, Morris, and Vandehaar, 1979). Van Demark, Morris, and Vandehaar (1979) reported longitudinal data for 351 patients with cleft palate aged 2½ to 18 years. Systematic improvement in articulation test scores was evident until approximately 10 years of age. Improvement continued beyond that age but at a much slower rate. On average, only 80% of the articulation test items were correctly produced by age 16 years. At that age, their subjects produced 98% of the plosives correctly, but that level of proficiency was not achieved for fricatives and affricates.

Riski and DeLong (1984) examined the articulation performance of children 3 to 8 years old. They noted that their subjects' performance was strikingly similar to that of the Iowa subjects (Van Demark, Morris, and Vandehaar, 1979) at 3 and 4 years of age, but their children articulated better than the Iowa children from ages 5 through 8 years. Their children had received palatal repair at earlier ages than the Iowa children.

Karnell and Van Demark (1986) re-examined the patients described by Van Demark, Morris, and Vandehaar (1979) and reported longitudinal articulation data. Subjects' performance on the Iowa Pressure Articulation Test (IPAT) was reported in terms of the percentage of responses that were correct, oral distortions, nasal distortions, glottal stops, pharyngeal fricatives, omissions, and substitutions. Clinical ratings of articulation defectiveness improved throughout the study but with rate of improvement decreasing markedly after about 10 years of age. The data showed that on average the subjects did not achieve ". . . what speech pathologists may consider perfectly normal speech at age 16 years. However, such deficits probably are not so severe by this age as to require intervention" (p. 287). Errors in each of the articulation test categories studied occurred infrequently during observations made in the older years. Glottal stops and pharyngeal fricatives occurred infrequently at any time in the study. Nasal distortions also occurred infrequently, but their occurrence did increase slightly after age 10 years in one subgroup—the members of which scored below 20% on the IPAT at age 4 years and did not have secondary surgery of the velopharyngeal mechanism before age 8 years. Members of this subgroup tended to become slightly worse at about 12 years of age.

Several investigators have observed better speech in younger children than older children with cleft palate. In an early study, Renfrew (1960) found substantially better speech in schoolaged children with clefts observed from 1953 to 1960 than in children seen between 1946 to 1953. Similarly, Counihan (1956) reported that his subjects more than 16 years old actually articulated less well than younger children with clefts. Perhaps the differences observed by the authors reflected improvement in care that benefited the younger subjects. Van Demark, Morris, and Vandehaar (1979) compared data from 16-year-old patients with data McWilliams reported in 1958 for adults at a mean age of 24.6 years. The articulation tests used in the two studies were different, but the sounds were similarly rank ordered for number of correct responses. The subjects in the Van Demark study correctly produced several sounds at substantially higher percentages than did McWilliams' subjects. Van Demark, Morris, and Vandehaar attributed the differences in percentage of correct responses to improvements in treatment.

Few investigators have examined the late results of multidisciplinary management for individuals with cleft palate. Bardach et al. (1984, 1990, 1992) conducted a series of investigations to study treatment outcome for different cleft type groups. In their initial report, speech outcome was described for 45 adolescents and adults with repaired unilateral cleft lip and palate, ages 14 to 22 years. Only 29 of the patients demonstrated normal (or near normal) oral-nasal resonance. Ten patients had excessive hypernasality and the remaining six (all postpharyngeal flap) demonstrated hyponasality. Four of the patients demonstrated abnormal articulation patterns that clearly warranted therapy; the authors noted that an additional 15 subjects could benefit from therapy. Oral distortions were frequently noted in this group of patients. This latter finding was not particularly surprising because at least 20 of their patients were still receiving orthodontic treatment. The authors did not indicate how many of the patients had normal speech production but did state that 26 (58%) of their patients did not require additional speech therapy.

In their latter three reports, Bardach et al. (1990, 1992; Morris et al., 1993) described the treatment results of young patients (ages 5 to 10 years) with bilateral cleft lip and palate (1992), unilateral cleft lip and palate (1990), and cleft palate only (1993) who had completed the preliminary stages of treatment, as well as adolescents 11 to 19+ years old. Data obtained from children who had received pharyngeal flap surgery were analyzed separately. Oral distortion of fricatives was a frequent finding among the older patients with bilateral and unilateral cleft lip and palate (Bardach et al., 1990, 1992). A high frequency of malocclusion and mild consonant distortions (both oral and nasal) were also observed in the older patients with cleft palate only (Morris et al., 1993). The majority of adolescents in all three studies demonstrated satisfactory velopharyngeal function. Speech was judged to be within normal limits for only 17 of the 30 older patients (57%) with bilateral cleft lip and palate; comparable information was not provided for the patients with unilateral clefts or clefts of the palate only. Although these results would indicate poor overall outcome, the inclusion of young adolescents who had probably not completed orthodontic management confounds interpretation of the data.

Other investigators have also reported the persistence of articulation and resonance problems in their adolescent patients with clefts. Lohmander-Agerskov et al. (1993) described the speech of a consecutive series of 31 patients (aged 10 to 14 years) with isolated cleft palate who had undergone a one-stage palatal repair. Moderate-to-severe hypernasality was evident in seven (23%) patients. Articulation errors were identified in six (19%) patients; however, it is pertinent to note that oral distortions were apparently not recorded for these patients. The most interesting finding in this investigation was the low correlation (r = .41) obtained between the examiner's assessment and the patient's assessment of their speech. In general, the majority of patients judged their speech to be normal or near normal.

Peterson-Falzone (1995) examined speech outcome in 110 adolescents with cleft palate aged 13 to 19 years. Only 25 (22%) of the adolescents studied demonstrated normal speech. Of the remaining 85 patients, 36 demonstrated standard articulation errors, 6 exhibited audible nasal emission only, and 19 had audible nasal emission in conjunction with other standard articulation errors. Seven patients had hyponasality and standard articulation errors, whereas five patients had compensatory articulation errors alone. The remaining 12 subjects demonstrated a combination of hypernasality, compensatory articulation errors, audible nasal emission, and other articulation problems in some cases. In general, only 61 (55%) of the 110 adolescents demonstrated speech that was considered "acceptable." Peterson-Falzone stated that "with our current technology for visualization of the velopharyngeal system and with the current array of surgical techniques available for both primary and secondary operations on the velopharyngeal mechanism, a failure rate of nearly 50% is unacceptable" (p. 127). She also pointed out, however, many of the patients evaluated at her center had not received consistent team management and so her results are not representative of those that might be associated with "team care."

Finally, Riski (1995) reported more encouraging speech

outcome data for his adolescents with repaired cleft lip and palate. Of the 48 patients studied, 84% demonstrated articulation that was considered normal or acceptable and 71% demonstrated normal resonance. Although mild hypernasality persisted in approximately 8% of the adolescents, a rather large percentage of the subjects (21%) demonstrated hyponasality (most secondary to pharyngoplasty).

The findings of these studies suggest that the articulation performance of individuals with cleft palate improves with age for individual speakers and has improved over time for the population as a whole. Advances in treatment methods during the past 40 years has been credited with much of the improvement observed in patients treated today when compared to younger patients in the same institution. Despite these improvements, an appreciable number of individuals with repaired cleft palate continue to demonstrate articulation and/or resonance problems in adolescence. Although speech production errors related to velopharyngeal dysfunction are evident for some patients, the majority of adolescents with persistent articulation problems demonstrate oral distortion of consonant sounds (primarily sibilant fricatives) related to dental/occlusal status.

Phonological patterns. The speech of children with cleft palate has traditionally been studied by standard articulation analysis. Yet children with cleft palate are at risk for both phonetically and phonologically based speech sound disorders. Phonetic errors in this population occur as a result of structural deviations associated with the cleft (hearing impairment and developmental factors also play a role). Phonological errors may occur in relation to either general expressive language delays or physical constraints imposed by the cleft. According to Chapman (1993), although articulatory errors may initially occur as a result of structural limitations imposed by the palatal cleft, they become integrated into the child's developing phonological system over time. To illustrate this effect, Chapman described a scenario where a young child with a cleft might initially substitute a /g/ for all nonnasal consonants before surgery in an attempt to compensate for velopharyngeal inadequacy. Once surgery is performed, "the errors persist because the child has adopted a rule substituting velar stops for bilabial and alveolar obstruents" (p. 64).

Some young children with velopharyngeal inadequacy have severely restricted consonant inventories that may limit their ability to signal phonological contrasts. According to Stengelhofen (1989), "inability to signal distinctive features leads to reduced phonological contrasts and may be a factor strongly influencing intelligibility" (p. 26).

A consistent finding throughout the literature is the tendency of many children with cleft palate to use the process of backing. This process has been observed in phonologically delayed children but does not occur frequently in the speech of normally developing children (Stoel-Gammon and Dunn, 1985). It has been described by some authors (Russell and Grunwell, 1993) as a "secondary phonological disorder" that originates as a "primary phonetic deviance." Chapman (1993) noted more frequent use of this process in children who had other speech and resonance problems associated with velopharyngeal inadequacy.

In addition to backing, the process of nasal replacement (i.e., the substitution of a nasal consonant for an oral consonant) has also been reported in the speech of children with palatal clefts. Hardin-Jones and Jones (1997) reported that nasal substitutions were produced by 19% of the preschoolers (aged 3 to 5 years) with clefts that they studied. Approximately 15% of the group produced nasal substitutions in combination with backing errors that involved glottal and pharyngeal articulations.

Although the articulatory performance of children with cleft palate has been described in numerous reports detailed throughout this chapter, few investigators have applied distinctive feature analysis and phonological analysis to the speech of children in this population. Chapman (1993) pointed out that the existing reports were limited to descriptions of either a small number of patients (Hodson et al., 1983; Lynch, Fox, and Brookshire, 1983; Powers, Erickson, and Dunn, 1990) or to a single stage of development (Chapman and Hardin, 1992; Estrem and Broen, 1989).

Singh, Hayden, and Toombs (1981) used seven distinctive features to analyze articulation data from 1077 children (18 with cleft palate) receiving speech services in schools. The data analyzed were articulation profiles obtained by speech-language pathologists using different articulation tests. Only substitutions and omissions were evaluated. The children with cleft palate presented a profile different from that of other misarticulating subgroups, performing best on the labiality feature and poorest on the front-back feature.

In a letter concerning problems in the clinical application of phonological theory, Foster, Riley, and Parker (1985) suggested that the studies by Singh, Hayden, and Toomis (1981), Hodson et al. (1983), and Lynch, Fox, and Brookshire (1983) were not compatible with the phonological theory on which their vocabulary and procedure were based because the authors offered no reason to think that the speech disorders of their patients with clefts were psychological or linguistic in nature. Indeed, the analysis described by Lynch, Fox, and Brookshire (1983) more closely reflected traditional articulation analysis than phonological analysis per se.

Only two studies have demonstrated the usefulness of phonological analysis in preschoolers with cleft palate. Powers, Erickson, and Dunn (1990) submitted 1-hour speech samples of four children with repaired clefts (ages 3 years 2 months to 3 years 11 months) to several speech analyses: phonetic inventory, phonological process, and idiosyncratic pattern. A key finding was that the children were similar in phonetic inventory but differed in use of phonological processes. For example, use of fricatives and affricates was restricted in all four children; however, one child used stopping only 8% of the times where it might have occurred and another child used it 48%. This suggests that the children were similar in ability to produce sounds but differed in linguistic use of their phonetic skills. The child thought to have the best language used the fewest processes. The process of backing was used by three of the four subjects and influenced most alveolar and palatal obstruents. Substitution of posterior for anterior place of articulation has been explained as a compensation for velopharyngeal and fistulae leaks. However, three of the subjects in this study were free from audible nasal emission, and all four were thought to be free of "significant problems in velopharyngeal closure." The authors were conservative in interpreting the origin of the children's process usage but noted that an organizational-linguistic phenomenon may have influenced the children's speech.

In a more recent and comprehensive report, Chapman (1993) described the phonological processes of 30 children with repaired cleft palate and 30 noncleft children matched for age and sex (10 each at ages 3, 4, and 5 years). Comparisons were carried out between the groups for overall process use and frequency of occurrence of each phonological process. Significant differences in overall process usage was evident between those 3 and 4 years old in both cleft and noncleft groups. Differences in frequency of occurrence of individual processes were significant only between the 3-year-old children in both cleft and noncleft groups. The following processes occurred more frequently in the responses of the 3-year-old children with clefts: final consonant deletion, syllable reduction, deaffrication, stridency deletion, stopping, cluster simplification, backing, stop replacement, and liquid-glide replacement. Chapman noted, however, that several of these processes (deaffrication, syllable reduction, stop replacement, and liquid-glide replacement) occurred infrequently. She concluded that children with cleft palate use common phonological processes for a protracted time but tend to catch up to their noncleft peers by 5 years of age.

Phonological theory and analysis have contributed little to our understanding and treatment of cleft palate speech to date. Nonetheless, cognitive-linguistic variables probably interact with orofacial variables, including velopharyngeal function, to influence the sound patterns of individual patients. As Russell and Grunwell (1993) concluded, "children with cleft lip and palate can achieve more or less normal phonological systems but the process and pattern of phonological development is affected by the phonetic sequelae of the cleft palate condition" (p. 46). Use of various phonological pattern analysis procedures may help the clinician to recognize and understand patterns that involve multiple phonemes in the speech of patients with clefts. Information gained from such analyses may supplement phonetic information, data about the speech mechanism, and other information from the speech evaluation to help the clinician classify patients and plan treatment that will correct disordered sound patterns in an efficient fashion.

Etiological Factors Contributing to Speech Production Problems

From the review above it is evident that attempts to explain the origins of misarticulation by patients with cleft lip and palate must account for a variety of findings, including delay in the development of articulation skills, nasalization of speech sounds that normally are oral, oral distortions usually of sibilants, and gross substitutions such as glottal stops and pharyngeal fricatives. Palatal clefts influence articulation and the sound system as soon as they start to develop, but children respond to clefts and related conditions in different ways.

Velopharyngeal inadequacy. Velopharyngeal inadequacy is considered to be the major etiological factor influencing the speech production skills of individuals with cleft palate. Certainly errors attributed to this condition, including hypernasality and audible nasal emission, are the most defining speech characteristics of this population. As indicated throughout this chapter, velopharyngeal inadequacy, besides having an obligatory effect on speech production, also appears to influence the strategies that toddlers use when they are learning to talk and older children use when they are attempting to improve their intelligibility. Unfortunately, our casual acceptance of this relationship often leads clinicians to assume a more simplistic association between velopharyngeal inadequacy and speech production than actually exists.

Early attempts to examine the correlation between measures of velopharyngeal function and speech proficiency yielded only moderately high correlations. In a review of previous research, Morris (1968) found that a correlation of 0.50 was a rough average of the correlations that had been reported to date in the literature. These low correlations have been attributed to a number of factors including poor reliability of listener judgments of nasality and simplistic (and in some cases inadequate) measures of velopharyngeal function such lateral cephalometric radiographs (Peterson-Falzone, 1986). As instrumental assessment of velopharyngeal function has improved, so too has the reported correspondence between velopharyngeal closure and judgments of speech (McWilliams et al., 1981).

Another problem that has affected our efforts to examine the correlation between velopharyngeal inadequacy and speech production is the nonlinear relationship that exists between the two variables. Warren (1967) reported that increases in velopharyngeal port size beyond 20 mm^2 were not linearly related to increases in nasal air flow. He and his colleagues (Warren and Devereux, 1966; Warren and Ryon, 1967) have also documented the influence of factors such as respiratory volume, nasal resistance, and oral port constrictions on aerodynamic measurements of velopharyngeal orifice size. More recent findings (Warren, Dalston, and Mayo, 1993) suggest that hypernasality is related to the timing of velopharyngeal port opening and not just the volume of air passing through the nasal cavities.

Much of the research cited above has examined relationships between speech and velopharyngeal closure by analyzing only one pair of variables at a time. Other researchers have performed multivariate analyses to examine these relationships. Early research by Van Demark (1964, 1966) using multiple regression analysis and factor analysis attempted to differentiate articulatory factors attributed to velopharyngeal inadequacy and those that reflected learning or maturation. He found that severity of articulation defectiveness is related primarily to two factors or clusters of variables, one representing velopharyngeal dysfunction and the other maturation-learning. Although both factors were influential in the articulation problems of his subjects, faulty valving emerged as a major source of their errors.

Multivariate statistical analysis was also used by Fletcher (1978) to examine the relationship between articulation and factors related to velopharyngeal function, dentition, malocclusion, fistulae, morphologic features and mobility of the tongue, and syllable repetition time. Once again, velopharyngeal function emerged as an important predictor of articulation proficiency. A coefficient of determination indicated that polysyllable diadochokinesis, palate-pharyngeal contact, velopharyngeal gap, class of cleft, linguapharyngeal aperture, tongue retraction, tongue fronting, vertical interincisor aperture, horizontal interincisor aperture, and velar retraction accounted for 79% of the variance in articulation.

Hardin, Lachenbruch, and Morris (1986) examined the relative contribution of several speech and nonspeech measures to the prediction of speech proficiency for adolescents with cleft palate at age 14 years. The predictor variables, which were measured between 4 and 13 years of age, included articulation test scores, information about manner of production and error type, ratings of articulation defectiveness and nasality, gender, type of primary palatoplasty, age at palatoplasty, and whether the patient had a pharyngeal flap. Gender itself accounted for 40% of the variance in judged speech proficiency—the female subjects had better speech proficiency than the male subjects did. The most efficient subsets of predictors measured at different age levels accounted for 50% to 75% of the variability in the predicted variable. However, except for gender, what constituted an efficient subset of predictors changed from age level to age level. The authors noted that speech proficiency across subjects at age 14 years was restricted in range—a condition that limited the study and may have contributed to the lack of consistency in predictors across age levels.

In summary, the first of the two multivariate studies cited provided information suggesting that articulation errors have their origins both in velopharyngeal function and in learning. The second study suggested that physical and physiological variables in addition to velopharyngeal function also contribute to disordered articulation in cleft palate speakers. These correlational studies are causal in orientation. Theories implicitly or explicitly held by the authors undoubtedly influenced the choice of measures, and that influenced the findings. Each author used multivariate analysis of numerous measures, but the variables studied and the outcomes are quite different. These studies complement each other and help us to understand the complicated interactions that must be taken into account in the clinical management of cleft palate.

Physical characteristics of the vocal tract. Although the primary cause of hypernasality and audible nasal emission is abnormal coupling of the oral and nasal cavities, other physical characteristics of the vocal tract may be influential in minimizing or maximizing the perception of hypernasality (Dalston and Warren, 1986). Some related factors are respiratory effort and the degree of tension in the subglottal, glottal, and supraglottal structures, including the oral and the nasal pharynx. Superimposed on these elements will be the positioning of the tongue, which, riding high posteriorly (McDonald and Baker, 1951), may essentially block oral access of the sound stream. This, in turn, will effectively reduce or almost eliminate the possibility of oral resonance, thus decreasing the relative oral-nasal balance.

Other behaviors will obviously also be involved. Constriction of the oral port by mandibular positioning, limited movement, increased tension, and lip function further serve to restrict or minimize the oral components of speech. Because speakers with cleft palate have a tendency to restrict the size of the oral cavity (Falk and Kopp, 1968) with strategies previously described, hypernasality associated with velopharyngeal inadequacy may be increased. In addition, the size of the velopharyngeal portal during speech will, in relationship to respiratory effort and other tract features, dictate the air and energy loss into the nasal cavities.

Nasal cavities are complex normally and are rendered more so in persons with clefts. Warren, Duany, and Fischer (1969) found higher airway resistance in subjects with clefts even before surgery. Hairfield, Warren, and Seaton (1988) reported that 68% of 85 children and adults with cleft lip and palate were oral, predominantly oral, or mixed oral-nasal breathers, whereas only 32% were nasal or predominantly nasal breathers. The authors attributed this obligatory mouth breathing to such things as a constricted maxilla, large tonsils, a posterior pharyngeal flap, or scarring of the pillars.

It is probable, however, that alterations in the nasal airways are present in fetal specimens as early as 8 to 21 weeks postmenstrual age. Siegel et al. (1987) used computer reconstruction to produce three-dimensional representations of the nasal capsule, nasal septal cartilage, and nasal airway in 20 normal human fetuses and 9 fetuses with clefts. Qualitative assessment revealed that nasal-capsule development in the specimens with clefts appeared to be asymmetrical. The septum was enlarged and distorted and was flanked laterally by reduced nasal airway passages. In those with unilateral clefts, the airway on the cleft side was often enlarged and irregularly shaped. However, the authors found no significant differences in growth rates or size of the nasal capsule between those with and without clefts.

In an effort to explain their earlier findings, Kimes et al. (1988) assessed the relative contributions of the nasal septum and nasal airway to capsule size. They found that the nasal septum in fetal specimens with clefts was enlarged by 45%. The septum was wider, not taller or longer. Mean airway volume, as might be expected, was smaller by 43%. Thus it is clear that velopharyngeal valving and resonance characteristics are likely to be modified by increased nasal resistance.

Such factors as the thickness of the soft palate and the vertical depth of the contact between the velum and the pharyngeal walls may also be factors influencing perceived hypernasality, although the precise nature of these variations remains to be specified. We have seen individuals with hypernasality in the presence of what appeared to be closure accomplished by a thin velum or with a limited contact between the velum and the pharyngeal walls.

Recognition of the influences of the entire vocal tract including oral-nasal coupling on the perception of hypernasality is not new. Schwartz (1979) suggested that ". . . listening to a nasalized vowel involves listening not only to the features produced by the nasal-coupling condition but also to normal variations of quality that are unrelated to nasal coupling" (p. 266). In short, the degree to which hypernasality is perceived by a listener will depend on the characteristics of the entire vocal tract and not only on the size of the functional opening in the velopharyngeal valve (Curtis, 1968).

Oronasal fistulae. As indicated in Chapter 4, palatal fistulae can, depending on their size and location, have a detrimental effect on articulation and resonance. Although few investigators have attempted to correlate size of fistulae with nasalization of speech, clinical accounts of this relationship suggest that, although small fistulae may be nonsymptomatic for speech, large fistulae often result in audible nasal emission and weak pressure consonants with or without hypernasality. Shelton and Blank (1984) conducted aerodynamic assessments for six patients with palatal fistulae in two conditions: with and without palatal obturation. In general, anterior consonants were more affected by fistulae than posterior consonants were. Although the investigators did not measure fistula size, they indicated that patients with large fistulae demonstrated increased nasal airflow and diminished oral pressure when the fistulas were not obturated. Patients with small fistulae demonstrated increased nasal airflow when the fistulae were not obturated; however, oral pressures were essentially unchanged. Shelton and Blank speculated that patients in the latter group may have increased respiratory effort to maintain oral pressures.

Henningsson and her colleagues (Henningsson and Isberg, 1987, 1990; Karling, Larson, and Henningsson, 1993) have devoted considerable effort toward quantifying the impact of a palatal fistula on speech production. In an early report Henningsson and Isberg (1987) used chewing gum to temporarily obturate the fistulae of 10 patients. They reported that a palatal fistula with an area of 4.5 mm^2 resulted in hypernasality, audible nasal emission, and weak pressure consonants. More recently, however, the authors (1990) noted that a fistula of "only a few square millimeters" can have a detrimental effect on speech as well.

The impact of an oronasal fistula on articulation and resonance will also be influenced by its location. A prealveolar fistula does not typically influence resonance but will in rare instances affect articulation. According to Henningsson and Isberg (1990), the upper lip usually prevents loss of air through a fistula in the nasolabial area because of the pressure it naturally exerts on the alveolar ridge. When audible nasal emission occurs as the result of such a fistula, it typically occurs on consonants such as /p/, /b/, /f/, /v/, and /th/ in the presence of a large fistula or when the lip is short or stiff. Fistulae located in the hard or soft palate are those that most often affect speech production. Most palatal fistulae occur at the incisive foramen, and these anterior fistulae typically influence pressure consonants produced with linguapalatal constrictions that are anterior to the fistulae (e.g., /t/, /d/, /s/, /z/, /p/, /b/). A small posterior palatal fistula, on the other hand, tends to influence only /k/ and /g/ (Trost-Cardamone, 1990b).

The work of Henningsson and her group has also demonstrated that the presence of a patent palatal fistula can influence velopharyngeal function. They reported radiographic evidence showing that a palatal fistula can impair velopharyngeal activity in an individual who otherwise demonstrates adequate function, as well as exacerbate existing velopharyngeal inadequacy (Isberg and Henningsson, 1987). Karling, Larson, and Henningsson (1993) examined the relationship between size and site of oronasal fistulae and their influence on speech in three groups of patients: 18 with a fistula affecting speech, 26 with a fistula not affecting speech, and 58 without a fistula. The size of a fistula was measured and a location determined with use of dental impressions. Larger fistulas were found in the affected speech group than the nonaffected speech group. Significant differences in listener judgments of hypernasality, nasal emission, and *n*asal *o*ral *ra*tio *m*eter (NORAM) results were obtained when the fistulae were obturated. The authors interpreted their results as additional evidence that oronasal fistulae can contribute to velopharyngeal dysfunction.

Dental-occlusal status. The relationship between dentition and articulation has long intrigued clinicians working with children having cleft lip and palate. It has been assumed that the numerous dental-occlusal problems evident in these children as well as the changing environment of the oral cavity would place them at risk for oral distortions and other adaptive articulations. Despite the apparent logic of such argument, however, researchers have yet to establish strong causal relationships between any single dental problem and articulation proficiency.

The findings of early studies (Bzoch, 1956; Powers, 1962; Subtelny and Subtelny, 1959) indicated that children with cleft palate who demonstrate varying degrees of articulation proficiency do not differ systematically in specific orofacial relations. These findings were likely influenced by a number of patient factors, including differences in adaptation across speakers and the number of coexisting oral anomalies that may have interacted to influence articulation. McDermott (1962) found that articulation proficiency of /s/ varied according to the number and severity of dental problems. Bishara, Van Demark, and Henderson (1975) examined the relationship between articulation and dentition in 72 individuals with isolated cleft palate who were heterogeneous for velopharyngeal function and articulation proficiency. Although orofacial measurements obtained from lateral cephalograms were significantly correlated with select speech sounds, the correlations were low and "did not demonstrate a uniform relationship for all phonemes in a particular place of articulation" (p. 460). The authors suggested that the combined effects and interaction between several factors may influence articulation.

Several investigators have reported a relationship between maxillary arch width and articulation in children with cleft palate (Counihan, 1956; Foster and Greene, 1960; Starr, 1956). Both Counihan and Starr reported poorer articulation proficiency in children whose maxillary arch was narrower than the mandibular arch. In addition, Foster and Greene found a higher incidence of lateralized sibilant distortions in children with maxillary collapse.

Vallino and Tompson (1993) examined the perceptual characteristics associated with four types of malocclusion (Class II malocclusion, Class II malocclusion with open bite, Class III malocclusion, Class III malocclusion with open bite). Articulation testing was conducted for 33 patients (ages 14 to 39 years) before orthognathic surgery. Of the 33 patients, 29 had articulation errors. The lingua-alveolar sibilants /s/ and /z/ were the most frequently misarticulated sounds, followed by /ʃ/, /ʧ/, /ʤ/, and /ʒ/. Errors on these sounds typically involved combined visual and auditory distortions. Errors involving stop consonants occurred less frequently and, when present, involved visual distortions only. Frontal distortions accounted for the majority of errors on sibilant sounds. The most frequently observed frontal distortion involved placement of the tongue tip "too far distally to the mandibular incisors" with the tongue tip flattened. Distortions created by tongue-tip protrusion between the upper and lower teeth accounted for all the /s/ and /z/ errors produced by patients with Class III malocclusions (+/− open bite). More variability in articulatory posturing was reported in patients with Class II malocclusions (+/− open bite). In contrast to previous reports, Vallino and Tompson did not find distortions of f, v, and th.

In his commentary of the Vallino and Tompson article, Warren (1993) stated:

> In the presence of a malocclusion, the speech system compensates for the structural deficit to maintain pressures at an appropriate level. This would mean compensation using the tongue to close the space present in an anterior open-bite malocclusion. In this way, an acceptable oral constriction can be obtained. Again, the goal is to provide an aerodynamic environment that is compatible with the required turbulence needed for the production of the sound (p. 865).

Despite the inconclusive nature of the findings described above, clinicians who treat children with cleft lip and palate frequently encounter severe oral distortions that appear related to anterior dental deviations and malocclusion. Indeed, these distortions often account for the majority of residual articulation problems seen in adolescents with clefts (Van Demark, Morris, and Vandehaar, 1979). Albery and Grunwell (1993) attributed the palatalization and lateralization of consonants seen in older children with clefts to malocclusion and crossbite. "If the mandible is protruding beyond the maxilla, the tongue may be in an abnormally anterior position during rest. In speech, therefore, there may be a tendency for blade articulations and 'bunching' upwards towards the palate, thus producing the likelihood of palatalisation" (p. 109) Unilateral or bilateral crossbite that occurs secondary to alveolar arch collapse results in a reduction in both intermolar and intercanine width. This in turn may result in an inability to form the anterior seal needed to prevent loss of air laterally for /s/ (Albery and Grunwell, 1993). Dental-occlusal problems frequently seen in this population and their potential impact on articulation are described in Table 7-3. The information provided in this table is intended only to focus the clinician's attention on *possible* relationships that may exist. When one is describing such relationships, it is not possible to fully account for the ability of speakers to adapt to or compensate for dental-occlusal anomalies, nor is it possible to predict the perceptual results when two or more problems interact. The clinician must bear in mind that although many individuals with clefts may demonstrate oral distortions that appear related to their dental-occlusal status, others may demonstrate perceptually adequate speech even in the face of severe dental-occlusal problems.

Tongue posture and mobility. Some authors speculated in early reports that atypical tongue function might be a significant etiological factor underlying some articulation problems in children with cleft palate (see Peterson-Falzone [1986] for a more comprehensive review). Although problems related to tongue coordination and flexibility have not been demonstrated in this population, atypical tongue postures have been reported in some patients. Posterior tongue carriage and abnormal lingual contacts have been

Table 7-3 **Articulation Problems Associated with Dental/Occlusal Anomalies**

Dental/Occlusal Problem	*Potential Effect on Articulatory Posture*	*Potential Perceptual Result*
Protrusive premaxilla	Difficulty approximating lips for bilabials Lack of dental cutting edge	Labiodental production of bilabials and /s/ and /z/ Diffuse sibilant production
Retrusive premaxilla	Difficulty approximating lips for bilabials and labiodentals Linguaalveolar articulation may be difficult to achieve because tongue must retract for placement	Labiodental production of bilabials; inverted /f/ and /v/ Interdental /s/ and /z/
Crossbite		Lateralization of sibilants and fricatives, labiodentals are affected on occasion
Low palatal vault	Restrictive articulatory space	Imprecise articulation of linguaalveolars
Open bite	Difficulty approximating lips in severe cases	Labiodental production of bilabials and interdental articulation of linguoalveolars
Missing teeth	Missing teeth in the buccal region result in redirection of airflow Missing anterior teeth invites tongue protrusion	Lateralization of sibilants, particularly /s/ and /z/ Frontal lisp
Rotated anterior teeth	Linguaverted incisors interfere with tongue placement for tip-alveolar consonants, malposed teeth redirect airflow	Distortion of sibilants and possibly other linguaalveolar consonants
Ectopic teeth	Interferes with tongue placement for lingua alveolar consonants when present in the premaxillary area	Altered tongue placement or oral distortion of linguaalveolar consonants

References: Stengelhofen (1989); Trost-Cardamone (1990a; 1995); Witzel (1995).

documented by a number of investigators (Brooks, Shelton, and Youngstrom, 1965, 1966; Honjow and Isshiki, 1971; Lawrence and Phillips, 1975; Powers, 1962; Trost, 1981) and have been attributed to past or present velopharyngeal inadequacy (see discussion, p. 182). As Peterson-Falzone (1986, p. 282) pointed out, ". . . few if any investigators now view the tongue in cleft palate as being inherently defective in structure or innervation."

Learning. Articulation, like many other capabilities that people acquire, involves development. In this discussion we use the word development to encompass both maturation and learning. The difference between the two has long been controversial in psychology. Maturation is associated with growth of the central nervous system in a satisfactory environment (Kagan, Kearsley, and Zelano, 1978). Learning, on the other hand, is dependent on experience. Although maturation and learning are not always solely responsible for the articulation problems seen in patients with clefts, their influence is frequently evident. The two most obvious articulatory phenomena that invite a learning explanation are phoneme-specific nasal emission and compensatory articulation. In the former case, nasal emission is evident during production of select consonants in the absence of velopharyngeal inadequacy. Even should a physiological component be identified in these patients, their response would be an important contributor to the speech disorder. Compensatory articulation patterns also appear to reflect a strong learning component. Some children with velopharyngeal inadequacy produce these aberrant articulations whereas others do not. Moreover, they persist for some children even after successful surgical management of the mechanism.

Reinforcement has been used to explain some of the articulation errors produced by children with cleft palate. Parents may actually be pleased with the appearance of compensatory articulation behavior in their child's speech and thus knowingly or unknowingly reinforce it. Bzoch (1979) suggested that articulation learning might be negatively influenced by lack of reinforcement of early speech efforts, failure of parents to understand and respond to early speech efforts, deliberate discouragement of speech pending completion of surgery, acceptance of poor speech at least until physical treatment is completed, and anticipation of the child's needs that obviates the need for speech. Each of these variables functions in a reinforcement mode. Morris (1968) noted that communication failure may cause the child with cleft palate to speak less and hence to show less rapid or complete speech development.

Morris (1972) also hypothesized that some persons with velopharyngeal inadequacy use compensatory articulations as a means of avoiding nasal distortions. That is, they use articulatory constrictions inferior to the velopharyngeal port because the resultant productions are considered better perceptual approximations of the target than sounds produced with nasal emission. This type of misarticulation may reflect both speaker preference (albeit at an unconscious level) and past reinforcement. Paynter and Kinard (1979) examined this hypothesis by comparing children's preferences for single words produced with nasal emission to the same words produced with compensatory articulations. Three groups of children (12 noncleft children, 12 cleft palate children with velopharyngeal inadequacy and audible nasal emission, and 12 cleft palate children with velopharyngeal inadequacy and compensatory articulations) were asked to listen to tape-recorded samples of single word pairs (one produced with nasal emission and the other produced with compensatory articulation) and indicate which one sounded better. The noncleft children and the children with cleft palate who did not produce compensatory articulation preferred the test words with compensatory articulation, but the children with cleft palate who produced compensatory articulation preferred the test words produced with audible nasal emission. The authors speculated that children who develop these maladaptive productions may do so because parents and other adults consider their presence in speech production more favorable than nasal emission.

This research was extended by Paynter (1987) and by Bradford and Culton (1987) using the stimulus tape employed by Paynter and Kinard. Children with and without clefts and their parents tended to favor compensatory articulation over audible nasal emission. The finding that children using audible nasal emission and their parents tend to prefer compensatory articulation argues against preference as a variable motivating use of a particular type of articulation error. Paynter noted that the responses provided by both the children and adults in her study were highly variable, and she questioned whether parents would be likely to use reinforcement in a consistent enough manner to influence a child's use of these maladaptive patterns. She interpreted her findings as support for Warren's (1986) hypothesis that compensatory gestures develop as a child attempts to maintain aerodynamic stability in the presence of velopharyngeal inadequacy. Bradford and Culton concluded that, "It may be simplistic to assume that parental preference is the singular, or even the strongest, reinforcing element in determining the use of compensatory articulations by children with cleft palate" (p. 302). They argued that other factors, such as intelligibility of an utterance or early phonological adaptations, might contribute to the development of these aberrant articulations as well. The theories offered by Morris (1972), Bzoch (1979), and Warren (1986) may offer plausible explanations for why compensatory articulation patterns develop in some children, but they do not account for the persistence of these patterns over time nor do they explain why some children develop a number of different compensatory strategies while others never develop them at all. Although these patterns may develop in response to a physiological need for aerodynamic stability and are maintained through parental reinforcement, other factors probably interact over time to influence the development and maintenance of these patterns.

Additional articulatory phenomena appear to reflect learning. For example cinefluorographic and videofluorographic films and tapes have shown speakers using part of the tongue for articulation while, at the same time, using another tongue part to support the velum or a loose obturator. Some patients show palatal surrender (Hagerty, Hess, Mylin, 1968) or what Morris (1968) termed the discouraged /s/, where the patient moves away from velopharyngeal closure during /s/ sounds. Other patients demonstrate better velopharyngeal function during /s/ than on any other sound (Shelton, Brooks, and Youngstrom, 1964). Finally, some persons with clefts maintain closure in nasal contexts (Karnell, Folkins, and Morris, 1985; Shelton and McCauley, 1986), perhaps because the speaker is unable to open and close the velopharyngeal valve at a normal rate. Denasalization of a nasal consonant may be more acceptable than nasalization of nearby sounds.

Generalization is also involved in disordered articulation. In generalization learning, similar stimuli may elicit the same response, and related responses may be associated with a particular stimulus (Mowrer, 1982). Pitzner and Morris (1966), Van Demark, Morris, and Vandehaar (1979), and others have speculated that the misarticulation of high-pressure consonants may generalize to other sounds. Such generalization may account for some articulation errors in cleft palate speakers and may, perhaps, be mediated by shared distinctive features. Placement compensations for velopharyngeal valving dysfunction may also generalize from one speech sound or sound class to others. The speech pathologist working with articulation expects generalization from newly learned behaviors to influence articulation responses not directly taught. Nonetheless, the clinician should be alert for unwanted generalization, which is also known to occur.

Little has been written about the speech maturation variables of individuals with cleft palate. Ewanowski and Saxman (1980) cited evidence that children with clefts start speech sound development slowly and then accelerate this development with the passage of time. They stated that that pattern is the reverse of what is observed in physically normal children.

Phonatory Disorders

As early as the 1950s, clinicians recognized faulty phonation as an important attribute of the speech of individuals with cleft palate (Hess, 1959; McDonald and Baker, 1951; Westlake, 1953). The occurrence of phonatory disorders in individuals with clefts is not well understood because it may vary from one sample to another, depending on such variables as velopharyngeal adequacy and the criteria for determining the presence of a phonatory deviation. It is clear, however, that phonation disorders are more common in this population than in noncleft individuals. Prevalence estimates in early studies ranged from 0.6% to 34% (Brooks and Shelton, 1963; Marks, Barker, and Tardy, 1971; Takagi, McGlone, and Millard, 1965). Deering (1984) also investigated the prevalence of dysphonia in 38 subjects with clefts and found that 50% had aberrant phonation. Of these, 23.7% were described as hoarse, 13.2% as harsh, and 10.5% as breathy. More recently, D'Antonio et al. (1988) reported that 41% of 85 patients with clefts had evidence of laryngeal or phonatory abnormalities.

Although data differ from study to study as do methods, the evidence overwhelmingly supports the conclusion that phonatory disorders are considerably more common in subjects with clefts than in those without clefts.

Hoarseness. Children with cleft palate who demonstrate velopharyngeal inadequacy may well be at increased risk for hoarseness related to vocal hyperfunction. McWilliams, Bluestone, and Musgrave first called attention to this relationship in 1969 when they provided information about 43 children with cleft palate and hoarseness. Thirty-two of the 43 children with chronic hoarseness were successfully laryngoscoped, and 84% had positive vocal fold findings. The most usual pathological condition was bilateral vocal fold nodules, which occurred in 72% of the children. One of the children demonstrated questionable velopharyngeal valving capabilities and was enrolled in a trial period of speech therapy. During the course of therapy, his voice became increasingly hoarse and subsequent laryngoscopy revealed large bilateral vocal fold nodules. The authors speculated that attempts to compensate for inadequate velopharyngeal valving (as was demanded by speech therapy) might be related to the onset of the nodules.

The relationship between faulty valving, hoarseness, and speech therapy was reinforced when it was discovered that 16 of the 22 children with nodules had received speech therapy before the diagnosis of laryngeal pathology. For this reason, the velopharyngeal valving capabilities of all 32 chronically hoarse children were evaluated by lateral videofluoroscopy. Nineteen children fell clearly into the borderline-valving classification. Seven had inconsistent, touch closure and one had touch closure with improper timing. Eleven had wider openings in the hyperextended position, and six failed to achieve closure under any circumstances, although the openings were very narrow. It is of interest to note that the laryngologist did not hear hoarseness in eight children (in addition to the 32 studied). Seven of these underwent laryngoscopy, and all had normal vocal folds. The hoarseness previously heard appeared to have been acute rather than chronic as in the other subjects.

In a companion study, McWilliams, Lavorato, and Bluestone (1973) recalled 27 of the subjects who had participated in the previous study at an average of 4.7 years after their initial assessments. At follow-up, 70% had retained their vocal-fold abnormalities. The eight subjects who demonstrated normal folds at the second study continued to have hoarseness. Subjects who no longer showed vocal-fold pathology but retained hoarseness had an average age of 15 years 8 months, as opposed to an average of 12 years 1 month for those children who retained the vocal-cord abnormalities. This difference was statistically significant and indicated that age probably played a role in the remission of the nodules. Surgical removal of the nodules was usually ineffective unless attention was also given to the faulty velopharyngeal-valving mechanism. When the valve was altered, as it was in seven children, the phonation problem was usually eliminated. No patient failed to show improvement when the valve was made more competent. Vocal-fold pathology also showed improvement after attention to the valve. Nodules either disappeared or were reduced in size.

Greenberg (1982) surveyed 200 speech-language pathologists, of whom 70 responded, about the number of children in their programs with hoarseness. Hoarseness was reported in 5% of 121 hearing-impaired children, 3% of 3244 articulatory cases, 4% of 191 stutterers, and 16% of 38 subjects with cleft palates. It is of interest that the speech-language pathologists referred 42% of children with articulation disorders and 43% of the stutterers for unspecified medical evaluations but referred none of the children with clefts. This failure to recognize the possible meaning of hoarseness in a child with a cleft may result in ill-advised or fruitless therapy.

These findings suggest that children with cleft palate and chronic hoarseness are likely to have vocal fold pathology, and this combination should lead to a suspicion of velopharyngeal valving deficits. Children with clefts and hoarseness who demonstrate evidence of velopharyngeal valving deficiencies should probably not be subjected to the stresses of speech therapy to reduce hypernasality because of the chance that they will compensate laryngeally. Vocal-fold nodules appear to be a danger signal and suggest the need for further evaluation of the valving mechanism and consideration of secondary management.

Intensity and the soft-voice syndrome. The relationship between perceived nasality and vocal intensity has been of interest to clinicians for many years. Excessive nasal resonance results in an increase in the absorption of acoustic energy that in turn leads to a reduction in the intensity of vowels (Curtis, 1968; House and Stevens, 1956). Because of loss of pressure through the velopharyngeal port, some cleft patients have difficulty creating voice of sufficient loudness for conversational purposes. Those who succeed in increasing loudness must use subglottic pressures higher than normal, leading to the perception of increased hypernasality and audible nasal emission.

Anecdotal reports suggest that some patients may use reduced loudness levels as a compensatory strategy to minimize the listener's perception of hypernasality. Bzoch (1979) alluded to this problem in his discussion of "dysphonia characterized by aspirate voice." He found this "weak and aspirate" voice in 323 of 1000 cleft patients and speculated that these voices were developed to compensate for velopharyngeal inadequacy to improve intelligibility.

Additional evidence of altered respiratory demands was supplied by Tronszynska (1972) who found that, on average, people with palatal clefts demonstrate more breath units during speech than do noncleft individuals. They noted that the difference in rates between the two groups becomes increasingly exaggerated with speech therapy. This finding lends support to the notion that an increase in phonatory compensations may occur as a function of speech therapy designed to move speech closer to normal in spite of valving deficits.

D'Antonio et al. (1988) evaluated laryngeal and phonation characteristics in 85 patients aged 3 to 52 years who had evidence of deficient velopharyngeal valving. They assessed subglottic pressures aerodynamically and compared them against normative data for 70 children reported by Lotz and Netsell (1986). Seventy-one percent of the patients with known vocal fold nodules, 58% of those with other laryngeal and phonatory findings, and 25% of those with phonatory symptoms but no pathologic conditions had elevations in subglottic pressures. The authors point out that Lotz et al. (1984) found excessive subglottic pressures for 17 children with vocal nodules and that those authors speculated that increased respiratory effort could be a causal factor in the formation of nodules for some patients.

In summary, many speakers with velopharyngeal inadequacy seem unable to increase loudness. Those who are able often do so at the cost of increasing both nasal emission and the impression of hypernasality. The increase in air flow that results from the increased respiratory effort does not alter intraoral pressure but is simply lost through the ineffective velopharyngeal portal. On the other hand, speakers who produce a breathy voice when asked to increase loudness may sound less hypernasal.

As with other elements that may or may not contribute to the extent to which hypernasality is perceived, the speech pathologist is reminded to experiment carefully to determine whether alterations in loudness seem to make a difference but to exercise restraint in adopting the technique for therapeutic purposes. The laryngeal mechanism is highly vulnerable to stress, and patients with clefts are unusually susceptible when velopharyngeal inadequacy is present.

Pitch. The relationship of perceived nasality to vocal pitch was examined by several investigators in early studies (Hess, 1959; Kelly, 1934; Sherman and Goodwin, 1954). Although authors speculated that changing pitch might reduce the perception of hypernasality, a strong relationship between the two variables was not confirmed.

Curtis (1968) hypothesized that pitch ranges might be reduced by velopharyngeal inadequacy. With the air loss in the vocal system, the greatest subglottic pressure possible with maximum effort would produce less output energy than would be the case if velopharyngeal closure were achieved. Because increases in both subglottic pressure and vocal effort are closely related to increases in intensity and to pitch elevation, it is logical to assume that the speaker with velopharyngeal inadequacy might have a somewhat high voice with limitations in the lower part of the pitch range.

Dickson (1962) lent support to this theory when he reported measurements of fundamental frequencies for vowels produced by male subjects who were either normal speakers, had functional nasality, or had cleft palates. His most nasal speakers tended to have higher fundamental frequencies than did those who were least nasal. Flint (1964) and Rampp and Counihan (1970), on the other hand, reported lower fundamental frequencies for female subjects with clefts, compared with normal subjects, and no difference for male subjects. Tarlow and Saxman (1970) found no differences between normal children and those with clefts between the ages of 7 and 9 years.

Although supportive data have not been forthcoming, some clinicians have reported that a monotonous voice with little pitch variation often accompanies the soft-voice syndrome. Patients with this problem cannot demonstrate pitch variation of more than three or four tones and do not do so even when they attempt to sing.

The best conclusion that can be drawn from these studies is that too little is yet known to permit a working clinical hypothesis about pitch and its relationship to the perception of nasality. Future studies of pitch in speakers with velopharyngeal inadequacy should consider information about perceived hypernasality and the integrity of the velopharyngeal valve. No research to date has specified these variables. Currently we do not recommend either raising or lowering pitch as a therapeutic strategy for obscuring hypernasality because such changes may be injurious to the larynx.

Summary. Although the exact occurrence of phonatory disorders in speakers with clefts is not known, it is clear that they are more prevalent in this group than they are in the general population and that they are manifested in a variety of ways. These include hoarseness, reduction in loudness, monotony, and sometimes extreme systemic tension. Although much remains to be learned about voice production in these patients, data now available suggest alterations in vocal fold vibratory patterns and differences in respiration. These variations are most marked when velopharyngeal inadequacy is also present. The best probable explanation lies in the vocal tract interactions necessary for the regulation of pressures.

LANGUAGE

Little attention has been paid to language development in children with cleft palate. Shames and Rubin (1979) suggested that "the shortcomings of research on language in cleft palate children . . . are directly traceable to the shortcomings of language research in general." They went on to say: "A cleft palate population is homogeneous only with respect to specific structural abnormalities. This population appears to be remarkably heterogeneous with respect to indirect correlates to cleft palate, such as parental attitudes, child rearing practices, medical and hospitalization histories, and speech and language stimulation and reinforcement" (p. 220). In addition, we would add that children with clefts are heterogeneous in the nature of the original deformity, the outcome of treatment, the presence and type of other congenital abnormalities, the degree to which hearing loss is controlled, intelligence, social experience both at and away from home, genetic characteristics, and family constellation. In truth, children with clefts are far more dissimilar than they are similar, and the same factors that combine to make language possible in all children are operative for children with clefts. Thus, if the experience of having a cleft is not in some way detrimental to language development, these children should not be substantially different from their noncleft peers. The early research, which attempted to find out if there were differences, was a reasonable stage in the evolution of language research in children with clefts. Unfortunately, too little effort has been made to move further to understand the variations observed within the context of other aspects of development (McWilliams, 1973).

Vocabulary and Structural Complexity

A limited number of investigations have been conducted to examine language development in children with cleft palate. The findings that are available suggest that these children exhibit a number of linguistic deficits, particularly during the preschool years. Early studies reported that children with clefts demonstrate poorer receptive and expressive vocabulary skills (Morris, 1962; Nation, 1970a, 1970b; Spriestersbach, Darley, and Morris, 1958) than noncleft children. Brennan and Cullinan (1974) compared 14 children with clefts and 14 noncleft children at a mean age of 8 years 10 months and 8 years 11 months, respectively, on tasks involving object identification and naming. Once again, the children with clefts performed less well than did their controls. This study is of special interest because the cleft children, who were older than those in some earlier investigations, appeared to remain at a disadvantage.

Other linguistic deficits, including a shorter mean length of utterance and a reduction in both structural complexity and the variety of words used, have also been reported for children with cleft palate (Horn, 1972; Morris, 1962). Whitcomb, Oschner, and Wayte (1976) explored the language functioning of eight children with clefts and eight normal children between 5 and 6 years of age. The children with clefts, although they had normal hearing and intelligence, were less competent on both the Developmental Sentence Scoring and the Length-Complexity Index (Shriner and Sherman, 1967). Discrepancies between these two small groups were obvious on both instruments but were more marked on the Length-Complexity Index. Again, these preschool children did less well than did their noncleft peers.

More recently, Scherer and D'Antonio (1995) compared the language performance of 30 toddlers with cleft palate (ages 16 to 30 months) with that of 30 age-matched noncleft toddlers on four different measures: the MacArthur Communicative Development Inventory, the Preschool Language Scale, the Rossetti Infant-Toddler Language Scale, and a conversational language sample. The two groups performed comparably on the receptive language subtest of the Preschool Language Scale; however, differences were evident in expressive language performance across the other language measures. The cleft group used fewer total words and fewer different words than the noncleft group. In addition, the cleft group used shorter sentences and less complex sentences than the noncleft group.

Scherer (1995) conducted a longitudinal investigation of early language development in six toddlers (four with cleft lip and palate and two with cleft palate only). The subjects were studied at 20, 24, and 30 months of age. The children with cleft lip and palate achieved higher standard scores on the Bayley Scales of Infant Development and the Preschool Language Scale than the children with cleft palate only. In addition, the cleft lip and palate subjects demonstrated a greater mean length of utterance, frequency of bound morpheme use, number of different words, and frequency of word use than the cleft palate only subjects. Scherer concluded that although children with cleft lip and palate demonstrate "specific deficits in language form," children with cleft palate only showed pervasive delays in receptive and expressive language development. The delays noted in language functioning did not diminish from 20 to 30 months. Although her sample size necessarily limits interpretation of these data, Scherer's study underscores the importance of longitudinal investigation of language functioning in these children.

Some authors have speculated that the linguistic deficits noted in some children with cleft palate may reflect different strategies used by children to enhance speech intelligibility. Faircloth and Faircloth (1971) studied 10 children with cleft palate and concluded that "the child who strives for articulophonetic accuracy" reduces sentence length, word length, and sentence complexity, whereas the child who "relies on language structure for intelligibility" uses a wider variety of linguistic constructions. It seems more likely, however, that bad articulation in association with shorter, less involved sentences would increase intelligibility, whereas subjects able to articulate accurately would not be so constrained. Bland (1974) contributed to the resolution of this issue when she compared preschool subjects who had clefts and intelligible speech with a group of noncleft preschoolers on the Northwest Syntax Screening Tests, a verbal imitation test, and Developmental Sentence Scoring. She found no differences between the two groups.

Pannbacker (1975) shed some light on the study of Faircloth and Faircloth when she compared 20 adults with repaired clefts with 20 normal adults on a number of different language measures. The subjects with clefts were inferior to the normal subjects in mean length of sentence, number of words in the longest response, mean length of the five longest responses, number of different words used, and the intelligibility of speech. However, for the subjects with clefts there were significant correlations between intelligibility and mean length of response, number of words in the longest response, mean number of words in the five longest responses, the number of different words used, and scores on the vocabulary subtest of the Wechsler Adult Intelligence Scale. These findings for adults are in contrast to those of Faircloth and Faircloth (1971) for children and appear to have somewhat greater face validity.

Sociocommunicative Competence

Several authors have described subtle problems in the sociocommunicative skills of children with cleft palate. Long and Dalston (1982) reported that although the 12-month-old infants with clefts that they studied were similar to noncleft infants in expressing communication intentions nonverbally when the total number of communicative attempts was examined, they used intentions that establish social interaction (e.g., pointing, giving) less frequently than their noncleft peers. Shames and Rubin (1979) examined the conversational skills of 75 children with clefts and 75 noncleft children between the ages of 18 and 63 months. They used a standardized interview composed of 135 stimulus episodes to elicit a variety of verbal responses including answering, commenting, and greeting. The children with clefts were 12 to 18 months behind the noncleft children in providing the "expected" response until approximately 45 months of age, when the group with clefts began to resemble their noncleft peers. These findings indicated that children with clefts master some conversational skills at a slower pace than do their peers, but they overcome these lags and are similar to others by age 4 years of age. In spite of this the children with clefts maintained a higher grammatical error rate at all age levels, a result consistent with other studies indicative of slight language differences.

In a more recent investigation, Warr-Leeper et al. (1988) used the Test of Pragmatic Skills (Shulman, 1985) to evaluate the communicative intentions used by 27 preschoolers and school-aged children with clefts. In this study the preschool children with clefts did not differ from their age-matched, noncleft controls. The school-aged children with clefts demonstrated poorer communicative competence than an age-matched comparison group. The authors pointed out that the school-aged cleft group may have received poorer scores because they communicated their responses with shorter sentences, and the test awards longer utterances with higher scores. Differences between the groups may have reflected shorter utterance length rather than difficulty with communicative intentions. Similar findings were obtained by Chapman et al. (1998) for their preschoolers but not for their school-aged subjects. In that study the conversational participation of 10 preschoolers and 10 school-aged children with repaired clefts was compared with that of age-matched noncleft controls. Both groups demonstrated similar conversational skills. Chapman et al. noted that when differences did occur, they were most frequently evident between children in the preschool groups and were related to conversational assertiveness.

The results reported by Warr-Leeper et al. and Chapman et al. were at odds with those reported by Shames and Rubin (1971, 1979) and suggest that, as a group, children with cleft palate do not demonstrate significant sociocommunicative problems. These discrepant findings may be attributed in part to differences in sample size across the studies as well as to differences among subjects in speech proficiency/intelligibility. Chapman and her associates noted that although all their preschoolers with cleft palate "demonstrated normal functioning" on the Test of Pragmatics, a large number revealed a passive conversationalist style. Although this finding could reflect a specific pragmatic deficit, the authors noted that lack of assertiveness in this population could also reflect a reluctance to communicate because of either present or past problems with speech intelligibility and negative listener reactions. Other authors have also described sociocommunicative problems in this population that suggest a reluctance on the part of some children to assert themselves in conversation exchanges. In an early report, Morris (1962) stated that spontaneity of expression decreased with increasing chronological age for his subjects. Although the children improved in usable communicative skills, they grew increasingly unable to respond verbally without inhibition. Chapman and Hardin (1990) speculated that older children with clefts may have acquired the rules that govern sociocommunicative participation but simply limit their participation in conversational exchanges because of previous experience with negative listener reactions. They suggested the use of the model proposed by Fey (1986) as a means of exploring communicative behavior in children with clefts. In this model, conversational assertiveness, described as the ability or willingness to take a conversational turn when there has been no direct solicitation from the conversational partner, and conversational responsiveness, or the child's response when invited to take a turn, are both examined. This system describes children as active conversationalists when they both initiate and respond to the efforts of others, as passive conversationalists when they respond but do not initiate, as inactive communicators when they rarely initiate and are also underresponsive, and as verbal noncommunicators when they initiate but are underresponsive to others. Chapman and Hardin indicated that children with clefts can frequently be described as passive or inactive communicators. Although we know cleft children with and without speech and language problems who fit each of the four categories, we agree that the model is a fascinating one and one that lends itself to research purposes. Of special interest would be relating these conversational styles to various indicators of language and speech deficits and to the many other variables that may help to establish conversational modes. Information from such a study might help to delineate the most reasonable approaches to treatment as well as to clarify the origins of some of the variations we continue to find even though we understand them poorly.

Otitis Media and Language Development

Speech-language pathologists have long been interested in the relationship between otitis media with effusion (OME) and cognitive-linguistic development. Clinicians have speculated that the mild to moderate hearing loss that occurs secondary to OME may be associated with delays in cognitive and language development as well as with delays in later academic performance (Broen et al., 1996). Although early landmark studies (Clark, 1976; Holm and Kunze, 1969; Zinkus, Gottlieb, and Schapiro, 1978) tended to support a relationship between early ear disease and later developmental differences, the studies were faulted on methodological grounds, and disagreement was the rule (Bluestone et al., 1983; Paradise, 1980, 1981; Ventry, 1980). In their review of the literature, Roberts et al. (1991) stated that although investigators have reported differences in receptive language, expressive language, vocabulary diversity, and syntactic complexity, data obtained in other studies have not. They attributed these conflicting findings to methodological constraints (e.g., documentation of OME, timing of data collection) as well as to possible interactions between OME and other risk factors.

More recently, Roberts and Clark-Stein (1994, p. 184) wrote, "The hearing loss associated with OME may place an additional burden on the young child learning to speak who does not have the same ability as older children and adults to use contextual cues or previous experience to decipher a message that often is unclear. Thus, segmenting communication, categorizing speech sounds, and acquiring phonological rules may be difficult for a child with OME." The authors identified three ways in which recurrent otitis media with effusion can influence perception and development during the formative years of speech development. First, fluctuating hearing loss (when present) may result in an inconsistent auditory signal that in turn may lead to inaccurate encoding of information. Second, when disruption to the auditory signal is prolonged or frequent, a child's ability to perceive and discriminate certain speech units (e.g., low energy consonants, morphological markers, inflections) may be impaired. In addition, frequent or prolonged disruption of the auditory signal may lead to attention problems if a child decides to simply "tune out" the signal. Finally, illness that is often associated with middle ear disease may "restrict or alter the child's interactions with people and objects in the environment," resulting in "fewer opportunities to establish a knowledge base from which speech develops."

After an extensive literature review, Roberts and Clark-Stein (1994) concluded that the results of retrospective studies reporting an association between otitis media with effusion and speech processing and speech production were questionable because of methodological problems (e.g., reliance on medical records or parent recall of otitis media with effusion episodes, biased case-control selection). They also argued that although prospective studies have successfully avoided many of the limitations of past research, some methodological problems persist that limit our ability to interpret this association. "First, the findings are inconsistent, some reporting significant findings and others not. Second, when findings are statistically significant, the size of the effect is generally small and of uncertain clinical relevance. Third, the studies did not measure hearing status during OME episodes, even though the hearing loss associated with OME is believed to be the primary factor influencing speech development. Finally, the studies generally did not account for related factors that may have influenced children's speech skills, such as the quality of the child's language environment" (p. 191).

Several investigators have examined the relationship between speech-language development and middle ear disease in children with cleft palate. Although early delays in development have been attributed in part to frequent bouts of otitis media in infancy and early childhood, limited experimental data are available to support such a conclusion.

Axton (1972) evaluated 26 selected children from the Smith and McWilliams studies (1968a, 1968b) between 4 years and 5 years 11 months of age. These subjects, who had not had active ear care from birth, were compared with 31 others of similar age who had had intensive ear care. On the Illinois Test of Psycholinguistic Abilities (ITPA), the mean for the group having aggressive ear care was significantly higher than for the other group. The most significant differences were in manual expression and auditory sequential memory. Verbal expression was also better but remained somewhat below ITPA norms. The children who had not had ear care were also audiologically inferior to those who had been treated from birth. However, because active, continuing ear care depended on the regularity with which parents kept appointments, parental interest may have been a confounding factor. Although this was a small study, it points to a tentative relationship between ear disease and performance on the ITPA.

Hubbard et al. (1985) evaluated 24 closely matched children between 5 and 11 years of age. Management of their palatal clefts had been equivalent, but ear care had differed. One group had had aggressive ear care on an ongoing basis and initial myringotomies at 3 months, whereas the other group had not been consistently followed up and had had myringotomies at a mean age of 30.8 months or, as in two cases, not at all. The children who had had active ear care from birth had significantly better hearing and consonant articulation than did their matched controls. However, the groups did not differ on verbal, performance, or full-scale IQs as determined by the Wechsler Intelligence Scale for Children, Revised, on social maturity measured by the Vineland Social Maturity Scale, on self-esteem indicated by the Coopersmith Self-Esteem Inventory, or on behaviors reported in response to the

Child Behavior Checklist. This study did not support the hypothesis that cognitive, language, and psychosocial development are adversely affected by otitis media.

Bishop and Edmundson (1986) found the same interactions that others have reported but were reluctant to draw the same conclusions. Instead, they speculated that otitis media alone may not be a crucial determinant of language disorder but that it may interact with other risk factors so that it becomes important if the child is already vulnerable because of a hazardous perinatal history. They pointed out that most language research has explored one etiological factor at a time and that we need to design studies specifically to look for interactions among variables. From their own data, they were particularly impressed with family histories of language disorders in first-degree relatives and suggested that it might be fruitful to look for a genetic component in some of these problems.

In a more recent investigation, Broen et al. (1998) compared the early linguistic and cognitive development of 28 children with cleft palate to that of 29 noncleft children during the first 30 months of life. Children in the cleft group scored within the normal range but significantly below the noncleft group on the Mental Scale of the Bayley Scales of Infant Development and select subscales of the Minnesota Child Development Inventory. Significant differences were evident between the groups on the verbal items not the nonverbal items. In addition, the children with cleft palate acquired words more slowly than their noncleft counterparts. Of particular interest in this study was the authors' report that when hearing was added as a covariate in the analysis, differences between the groups on developmental-cognitive measures were not significant. Differences between the groups in rate of word acquisition persisted until velopharyngeal function was added as a covariate in the analysis. These findings underscore the importance of early, aggressive management of middle ear disease and velopharyngeal function.

Despite our conviction that chronic middle ear disease can have a significant negative impact on speech-language development in some young children with cleft palate, we must conclude that the evidence of a one-to-one relationship between otitis media and language deficits does not exist for children with or without clefts. Rather, it is probable that many language disorders are associated with multiple causal factors including genetics, parent-child interactions, variations in neural integrity, intelligence, social competence, social responses to various handicaps, life experience in and out of clinics, and otitis media, among many other things. This interpretation of the literature, on the other hand, in no way denies the importance of providing adequate ear care to children in general and, specifically, to children with clefts, who are at high risk for ear disease, hearing loss, and the complications that occur when otitis media is not treated. It is clinically desirable to minimize possible negative factors, wherever they occur, to maximize a child's developmental potential.

SUMMARY

Children with cleft palate demonstrate a wide range of communication skills. Although a palatal cleft appears to influence babbling in most babies with unrepaired clefts, marked heterogeneity is evident in their speech production performance after palatal repair. At least 25% of these children can be expected to develop normal speech and language without formal interventions. Others will demonstrate sound production errors as a result of velopharyngeal inadequacy, palatal fistulae, dentition, or delays in phonological development.

Our efforts to minimize or circumvent the effects of a cleft on speech and language through early surgical and behavioral intervention have paid off throughout the last several decades. We now see fewer children who demonstrate velopharyngeal inadequacy after the initial palatal repair and fewer children who produce compensatory articulations. Unfortunately, an appreciable number of children with cleft palate do continue to demonstrate significant resonance and articulation problems during the school-age years and into adolescence. The persistence of speech production problems for older patients is particularly alarming in light of (1) recent trends in health care that reject the concept and goals of interdisciplinary management and (2) increasingly limited public school resources that discourage or prevent some practitioners from providing individual, direct therapy services for schoolaged children and, in some cases, from providing any services at all to adolescents.

REFERENCES

Albery E, and Grunwell P: Consonant articulation in different types of cleft lip and palate. In Grunwell P (ed.): *Analysing cleft palate speech.* London: Whurr Publishers, 1993.

Axton S: Hearing loss, otological care, and language retardation in cleft palate children [thesis]. Pittsburgh: University of Pittsburgh, 1972.

Bardach J, Morris HL, Olin W, McDermott-Murray J, Mooney M, and Bardach E: Late results of multidisciplinary management of unilateral cleft lip and palate. *Annals of Plastic Surgery* 12:235-242, 1984.

Bardach J, Morris HL, Olin WH, Gray SD, Jones DL, Kelly KM, Gundlach KKH, Rohrs M, Behlfelt K, and Fricke B: The Iowa-Hamburg Project: late results of multidisciplinary management at the Iowa Cleft Palate Center. In Bardach J, and Morris HL (eds.): *Multidisciplinary management of cleft lip and palate.* Philadelphia: WB Saunders, 1990.

Bardach J, Morris HL, Olin WH, Gray SD, Jones DL, Kelly KM, Shaw WC, and Semb G: Results of multidisciplinary management of bilateral cleft lip and palate at the Iowa Cleft Palate Center. *Plastic Reconstructive Surgery* 89:419-432, 1992.

Bernthal JE, and Weiner FF: A re-examination of the sound omission preliminary considerations. *Journal of Childhood Communication Disorders* 1:132-138, 1976.

Bishara SE, Van Demark DR, and Henderson WG: Relation between speech production and oro-facial structures in individuals with isolated clefts of the palate. *Cleft Palate Journal* 12:452-460, 1975.

Bishop DV, and Edmundson A: Is otitis media a major cause of specific developmental language disorders? *British Journal of Disordered Communication* 21:321-338, 1986.

Bland J: A language comparison of intelligible preschool children with cleft palate and noncleft palate preschool children [thesis]. Chapel Hill: University of North Carolina, 1974.

Bless DM, Ewanowski SJ, and Paul R: A longitudinal analysis of aerodynamic patterns produced by speakers with cleft palates. Proceedings of the annual convention of the American Speech-Language-Hearing Association, San Francisco, 1978.

Bluestone CD, Klein JO, Paradise JL, Eichenwald H, Bess FH, Downs MP, Green M, Berko-Gleason J, Ventry IM, Gray SW, McWilliams BJ, and Gates GA: Workshop on effects of otitis media on the child. *Pediatrics* 71:639-652, 1983.

Bradford PW, and Culton GL: Parents' perceptual preferences between compensatory articulation and nasal escape of air in children with cleft palate. *Cleft Palate Journal* 24:299-303, 1987.

Brennan D, and Cullinan W: Object identification and naming in cleft palate children. *Cleft Palate Journal* 11:188-195, 1974.

Broen PA, Dever MC, Doyle SS, Prouty JM, and Moller KT: Acquisition of linguistic and cognitive skills by children with cleft palate. *Journal of Speech, Language Hearing Research* 41:676-687, 1998.

Broen P, Moller K, Devers M, and Doyle S: Accuracy of speech production of 30 month old children with cleft palate. Proceedings of the 53rd annual meeting of the American Cleft Palate–Craniofacial Association, San Diego, CA, 1996.

Brooks A, and Shelton R: Incidence of voice disorders other than nasality in cleft palate children. *Cleft Palate Bulletin* 13:63-64, 1963.

Brooks AR, Shelton RL, and Youngstrom KA: Compensatory tongue-palate-posterior pharyngeal wall relationships in cleft palate. *Cleft Palate Journal* 30:166-173, 1965.

Brooks AR, Shelton RL, and Youngstrom KA: Tongue-palate contact in persons with palate defects. *Journal of Speech and Hearing Disorders* 31:14-25, 1966.

Byrne MC, Shelton RL, and Diedrich WM: Articulatory skill, physical management, and classification of children with cleft palates. *Journal of Speech and Hearing Disorders* 26:326-333, 1961.

Bzoch KR: An investigation of the speech of pre-school cleft palate children [dissertation]. Chicago: Northwestern University, 1956.

Bzoch KR: Articulatory proficiency and error patterns of preschool cleft palate and normal children. *Cleft Palate Journal* 2:340-349, 1965.

Bzoch KR: Measurement and assessment of categorical aspects of cleft palate speech. In Bzoch KR (ed.): *Communicative disorders related to cleft lip and palate.* Boston: Little, Brown, 1979.

Bzoch KR: Clinical assessment, evaluation, and management of 11 categorical aspects of cleft palate speech disorders. In *Communicative disorders related to cleft lip and palate.* Austin: Pro-Ed, 1997a.

Bzoch KR: Rationale, methods, and techniques of cleft palate speech therapy. In *Communicative disorders related to cleft lip and palate.* Austin: Pro-Ed, 1997b.

Chapman KL: Vocalizations of toddlers with cleft lip and palate. *Cleft Palate–Craniofacial Journal* 28:172-178, 1991.

Chapman KL: Phonologic processes in children with cleft palate. *Cleft Palate–Craniofacial Journal* 30:64-72, 1993.

Chapman KL, and Hardin MA: Communication competence in children with cleft lip and palate. In Bardach J, and Morris HL (eds.): *Multidisciplinary management of cleft lip and palate.* Philadelphia: WB Saunders, 1990.

Chapman KL, and Hardin MA: Phonetic and phonological skills of two-year-olds with cleft palate. *Cleft Palate–Craniofacial Journal* 29:435-443, 1992.

Chapman KL, Graham KT, Gooch J, and Visconti C: Conversational skills of preschool and school-age children with cleft lip and palate. *Cleft Palate–Craniofacial Journal* 35:503-516, 1998.

Clark M: Hearing: a link to IQ? *Newsweek* June 14:46, 1976.

Cohn ER, and McWilliams BJ: Early cleft palate repair and speech outcome [letter]. *Plastic and Reconstructive Surgery* 71:442-443, 1983.

Colton RH, and Cooker HS: Perceived nasality in the speech of the deaf. *Journal of Speech and Hearing Research* 11:553-559, 1968.

Counihan DT: A clinical study of the speech efficiency and structural adequacy of operated adolescent and adult cleft palate persons [dissertation]. Chicago: Northwestern University, 1956.

Counihan DT: Articulation skills of adolescents and adults with cleft palates. *Journal of Speech and Hearing Disorders* 25:181-187, 1960.

Crosby CA: Audience differentiation of recorded samples of cleft and non-cleft palate speech [thesis]. Madison: University of Wisconsin, 1952.

Cullinan WL, and Counihan DT: Ratings of vowel representatives. *Perceptual and Motor Skills* 32:395-401, 1971.

Curtis JF: Acoustics of speech production and nasalization. In Spriestersbach DC, and Sherman D (eds.): *Cleft palate and communication.* New York: Academic Press, 1968.

Dalston RM: Communication skills of children with cleft lip and palate: a status report. In Bardach J, and Morris HL (eds.): *Multidisciplinary management of cleft lip and palate.* Philadelphia: WB Saunders, 1990.

Dalston RM: Timing of cleft palate repair: a speech pathologist's viewpoint. *Problems in Plastic Surgery: Cleft Palate Surgery* 2:30-38, 1992.

Dalston RM, and Warren DW: Comparison of Tonar II, pressure flow, and listener judgments of hypernasality in the assessment of velopharyngeal function. *Cleft Palate Journal* 23:108-115, 1986.

D'Antonio LL: An investigation of speech timing in individuals with cleft palate [dissertation]. San Francisco: University of California, 1982.

D'Antonio LL, Muntz H, Providence M, and Marsh J: Laryngeal/voice findings in patients with velopharyngeal dysfunction. *Laryngoscope* 98:432-438, 1988.

Deering KM: The occurrence of phonatory disorders among cleft palate speakers [thesis]. Akron: University of Akron, 1984.

Dickson DR: An acoustic study of nasality. *Journal of Speech and Hearing Research* 5:103, 1962.

Dorf DS, and Curtin JW: Early cleft palate repair and speech outcome: a ten-year experience. In Bardach J, and Morris HL (eds.): *Multidisciplinary management of cleft lip and palate.* Philadelphia: WB Saunders, 1990.

Estrem T, and Broen PA: Early speech production of children with cleft palate. *Journal of Speech and Hearing Research* 32:12-23, 1989.

Ewanowski SJ, and Saxman JH: Orofacial disorders. In Hixon TJ, Shriberg LD, and Saxman JH (eds.): *Introduction to communication disorders.* Englewood Cliffs (NJ): Prentice-Hall, 1980.

Faircloth S, and Faircloth M: Delayed language and linguistic variations. In Grabb W, Rosenstein S, and Bzoch K (eds.): *Cleft lip and palate.* Boston: Little, Brown, 1971.

Falk ML, and Kopp GA: Tongue position and hypernasality in cleft palate speech. *Cleft Palate Journal* 5:228-237, 1968.

Fey ME: *Language intervention in young children.* San Diego: College-Hill Press, 1986.

Fletcher SG: *Diagnosing speech disorders from cleft palate.* New York: Grune and Stratton, 1978.

Flint R: Fundamental vocal frequency and severity of nasality in cleft palate speakers [thesis]. Norman: University of Oklahoma, 1964.

Foster TD, and Greene MCL: Lateral speech defects and dental irregularities in cleft palate. *British Journal of Plastic Surgery* 12:367-377, 1960.

Foster D, Riley K, and Parker E: Some problems in the clinical application of phonological theory. *Journal of Speech and Hearing Disorders* 50:294-297, 1985.

Gilbert JP, McPeek B, and Mosteller F: Statistics and ethics in surgery and anesthesia. *Science* 198:684, 1977.

Golding-Kushner KJ: Treatment of articulation and resonance disorders associated with cleft palate and VPI. In Shprintzen RJ, and Bardach J (eds.): *Cleft palate speech management: a multidisciplinary approach.* St. Louis: Mosby, 1995.

Gooch JL, Hardin-Jones M, Chapman K, Trost-Cardamone J, and Sussman J: Reliability of listener judgments of compensatory articulations. *Cleft Palate–Craniofacial Journal.* In press.

Greenberg R: The incidence of hoarseness among children enrolled in speech therapy. *Journal of Pennsylvania Speech and Language Hearing Association* 15:20, 1982.

Grunwell P, and Russell J: Vocalisations before and after cleft palate surgery: a pilot study. *British Journal of Disordered Communication* 22:1-17, 1987.

Haapanen ML: Cleft type and speech proficiency. *Folia Phoniatrica Logopedics* 46:57-63, 1994.

Hagerty R, Hess D, and Mylin W: Velar motility, velopharyngeal closure and speech proficiency in cartilage pharyngoplasty: the effect of age at surgery. *Cleft Palate Journal* 5:317-326, 1968.

Hairfield W, Warren DW, and Seaton D: Prevalence of mouth breathing in cleft lip and palate. *Cleft Palate Journal* 25:135-138, 1988.

Hardin MA, Lachenbruch PA, and Morris HL: Contribution of selected variables to the prediction of speech proficiency for adolescents with cleft lip and palate. *Cleft Palate Journal* 23:10-23, 1986.

Hardin-Jones MA, Chapman KL, Schulte J, and Halter KA: Vocal development of 9-month-old babies with cleft palate. Paper presented at the American Speech-Language-Hearing Association annual convention, San Francisco, 1999.

Hardin-Jones MA, and Jones DL: Age of palatoplasty and speech in children with cleft palate. Poster presentation, proceedings of the American Speech-Language-Hearing Association annual convention, Boston, 1997.

Henningsson EG, and Isberg AM: Velopharyngeal movement patterns in patients alternating between oral and glottal articulation: a clinical and cineradiographical study. *Cleft Palate Journal* 23:1-9, 1986.

Henningsson EG, and Isberg AM: Influence of palatal fistula on speech and resonance. *Folia Phoniatrica* 39:183-191, 1987.

Henningsson EG, and Isberg AM: Oronasal fistulas and speech production. In Bardach J, and Morris HL (eds.): *Multidisciplinary management of cleft lip and palate.* Philadelphia: WB Saunders, 1990.

Hess DA: Pitch, intensity and cleft palate voice quality. *Journal of Speech and Hearing Research* 2:113-125, 1959.

Hoch L, Golding-Kushner K, Siegel-Sadowitz V, and Shprintzen RJ: Speech therapy. In McWilliams BJ (ed.): *Current methods of assessing and treating children with cleft palates. Seminars in Speech and Language* 7:313-325, 1986.

Hodson BW, Chin C, Redmond B, and Simpson R: Phonological evaluation and remediation of speech deviations of a child with a repaired cleft palate: a case study. *Journal of Speech and Hearing Disorders* 48:93-98, 1983.

Holm V, and Kunze L: Effect of chronic otitis media on language and speech development. *Pediatrics* 43:833-839, 1969.

Honjow I, and Isshiki N: Pharyngeal stop in cleft palate speech. *Folia Phoniatrica* 23:347-354, 1971.

Horn L: Language development of the cleft palate child. *Journal of South African Speech and Hearing Association* 19:17-29, 1972.

House AS, and Stevens KN: Analog studies of the nasalization of vowels. *Journal of Speech and Hearing Disorders* 21:218-232, 1956.

Hubbard TW, Paradise JL, McWilliams BJ, Elster BA, and Taylor FH: Consequences of unremitting middle-ear disease in early life. *New England Journal of Medicine* 312:1529-1534, 1985.

Hutchinson JM, Robinson KL, and Nerbonne MA: Patterns of nasalance in a sample of normal gerontologic subjects. *Journal of Communication Disorders* 11:469-481, 1978.

Hutters B, and Bronsted K: Strategies in cleft palate speech—with special reference to Danish. *Cleft Palate Journal* 24:126-136, 1987.

Isberg A, and Henningsson G: Influence of palatal fistulas on velopharyngeal movements: a cineradiographic study. *Plastic and Reconstructive Surgery* 79:525-530, 1987.

Jones DL, and Folkins JW: The effect of speaking rate on judgments of disordered speech in children with cleft palate. *Cleft Palate Journal* 22:246-252, 1985.

Jones DL, Folkins JW, and Morris HL: Speech production time and judgments of disordered nasalization in speakers with cleft palate. *Journal of Speech and Hearing Research* 33:458-466, 1990.

Kagan J, Kearsley RB, and Zelazo PR: *Infancy: its place in human development.* Cambridge (MA): Harvard University Press, 1978.

Karling J, Larson O, and Henningsson G: Oronasal fistulas in cleft palate patients and their influence on speech. *Scandinavian Journal of Plastic and Reconstructive Hand Surgery* 27:193-201, 1993.

Karnell MP, and Van Demark DR: Longitudinal speech performance in patients with cleft palate: based on secondary management. *Cleft Palate Journal* 23:278-288, 1986.

Karnell MP, Folkins JW, and Morris HL: Relationships between the perception of nasalization and speech movements in speakers with cleft palate. *Journal of Speech and Hearing Research* 28:63-72, 1985.

Kawano M, Isshiki N, Harita Y, and Tanokuchi F: Laryngeal fricative in cleft palate speech. *Acta Otolaryngologica* 419(Supplement):180-187, 1985.

Kelly JP: Studies in nasality. *Archives of Speech* 1:26-42, 1934.

Kemp-Fincham SI, Kuehn DP, and Trost-Cardamone JE: Speech development and the timing of primary palatoplasty. In Bardach J, and Morris HL (eds.): *Multidisciplinary management of cleft lip and palate.* Philadelphia: WB Saunders, 1990.

Kent RD: Contextual facilitation of correct sound production. *Language, Speech, and Hearing Services in Schools* 13:66-76, 1982.

Kimes K, Siegel M, Mooney M, and Todhunter J: Relative contributions of the nasal septum and airways to total nasal capsule volume in normal and cleft lip and palate fetal specimens. *Cleft Palate Journal* 25:282-287, 1988.

Klinger H: A palatographic and acoustic study of cleft palate speech. *Cleft Palate Bulletin* 6:10-12, 1956.

Kuehn DP, and Trost-Cardamone JE: Speech development and the timing of primary palatoplasty. Proceedings of the annual meeting of the American Cleft Palate Association, Williamsburg, VA, 1988.

Kummer AW, and Neale HW: Changes in articulation and resonance after tongue flap closure of palatal fistulas: case reports. *Cleft Palate Journal* 26:51-55, 1989.

Kummer AW, Curtis C, Wiggs M, Lee L, and Strife JLL: Comparison of velopharyngeal gap size in patients with hypernasality, hypernasality and audible nasal emission, or nasal turbulence (rustle) as the primary speech characteristic. *Cleft Palate Journal* 29:152-156, 1992.

Larson P, and Hamlet S: Coarticulation effects on the nasalization of vowels using nasal/voice amplitude ratio instrumentation. *Cleft Palate Journal* 24:286-290, 1987.

Lass N, and Noll J: A comparative study of rate characteristics in cleft palate and noncleft palate speakers. *Cleft Palate Journal* 7:275-283, 1970.

Lawrence C, and Philips BJ: A telefluoroscopic study of lingual contacts made by persons with palatal defects. *Cleft Palate Journal* 12:85-94, 1975.

Lintz LB, and Sherman D: Phonetic elements and perception of nasality. *Journal of Speech and Hearing Research* 4:381-396, 1961.

Logemann JA: Treatment of articulation disorders in cleft palate children. In Perkins WH (ed.): *Phonologic-articulatory disorders.* New York: Theime-Stratton, 1983.

Lohmander-Agerskov A, Havstam C, Soderpalm E, Elander A, Lilja J, Friede H, and Persson E: Assessment of speech in children after repair of isolated cleft palate. *Scandinavian Journal of Plastic and Reconstructive Hand Surgery* 27:307-310, 1993.

Lohmander-Agerskov A, Soderpalm E, Odont HF, Persson E, and Lilja J: Pre-speech in children with cleft lip and palate or cleft palate only: phonetic analysis related to morphologic and functional factors. *Cleft Palate Journal* 31:271-279, 1994.

Long N, and Dalston RM: Paired gestural and vocal behavior in one-year-old cleft lip and palate children. *Journal of Speech and Hearing Disorders* 47:403-406, 1982.

Lotz W, and Netsell R: Developmental patterns of laryngeal aerodynamics. Proceedings of the midwinter meeting of the Association for Research in Otolaryngology, Clearwater, FL, 1986.

Lotz W, Netsell R, D'Antonio L, et al: Aerodynamic evidence of vocal abuse in children with vocal nodules. Proceedings of the American Speech-Language-Hearing Association Convention, San Francisco, 1984.

Lynch JI, Fox DR, and Brookshire BL: Phonological proficiency of two cleft palate toddlers with school-age follow-up. *Journal of Speech and Hearing Disorders* 48:274-285, 1983.

Marks C, Barker K, and Tardy M: Prevalence of perceived acoustic deviations related to laryngeal function among subjects with palatal anomalies. *Cleft Palate Journal* 8:201-211, 1971.

McDermott RP: A study of /s/ sound production by individuals with cleft palates [dissertation]. Iowa City: University of Iowa, 1962.

McDonald E, and Baker HK: Cleft palate speech: an integration of research and clinical observation. *Journal of Speech and Hearing Disorders* 16:9-20, 1951.

McWilliams BJ: An experimental study of some of the components of intelligibility of the speech of adult cleft palate patients [dissertation]. Pittsburgh: University of Pittsburgh, 1953.

McWilliams BJ: Articulation problems of a group of cleft palate adults. *Journal of Speech and Hearing Research* 1:68-74, 1958.

McWilliams BJ: Cleft palate management in England. *Speech Pathology and Therapy* 3:3-7, 1960.

McWilliams BJ: Language problems. *ASHA Reports* 9:41, 1973.

McWilliams BJ: Cleft palate. In Shames G, and Wiig E (eds.): *Human communication disorders.* Columbus (OH): CE Merrill, 1982.

McWilliams BJ, and Matthews HP: A comparison of intelligence and social maturity in children with unilateral complete clefts and those with isolated cleft palates. *Cleft Palate Journal* 16:363-372, 1979.

McWilliams BJ, and Musgrave RH: Diagnosis of speech problems in patients with cleft palate. *British Journal of Communication Disorders* 6:26–32, 1977.

McWilliams BJ, and Philips BJ: *Audio seminars in speech pathology: velopharyngeal incompetence.* Toronto: BC Decker, 1979; 1989; 1990.

McWilliams BJ, Bluestone CD, and Musgrave RH: Diagnostic implications of vocal cord nodules in children with cleft palate. *Laryngoscope* 79:2072-2080, 1969.

McWilliams BJ, Lavorato AS, and Bluestone CD: Vocal cord abnormalities in children with velopharyngeal valving problems. *Laryngoscope* 83:1745-1753, 1973.

McWilliams BJ, Glaser ER, Philips BJ, Lawrence C, Lavorato AS, Berry QC, and Skolnick ML: A comparative study of four methods of evaluating velopharyngeal adequacy. *Plastic and Reconstructive Surgery* 68:1-9, 1981.

Menyuk P, Liebergott J, and Schultz M: Predicting phonological development. In Lindblom B, and Zetterstrom R (eds.): *Precursors of Early Speech.* New York: Stockton Press, 1986.

Moll KL: Speech characteristics of individuals with cleft lip and palate. In Spriestersbach DC, and Sherman D (eds.): *Cleft palate and communication.* New York: Academic Press, 1968.

Morley ME: *Cleft palate and speech.* 5th ed. Baltimore: Williams & Wilkins, 1962.

Morley ME: *Cleft palate and speech.* 7th ed. Baltimore: Williams & Wilkins, 1970.

Morris HL: Communication skills of children with cleft lip and palate. *Journal of Speech and Hearing Research* 5:79-90, 1962.

Morris HL: Etiological bases for speech problems. In Spriestersbach DC, and Sherman D (eds.): *Cleft palate and communication.* New York: Academic Press, 1968.

Morris HL: Cleft palate. In Weston AJ (ed.): *Communicative disorders: an appraisal.* Springfield (IL): CC Thomas, 1972.

Morris HL, Spriestersbach DC, and Darley FL: An articulation test for assessing competency of velopharyngeal closure. *Journal of Speech and Hearing Research* 4:48-55, 1961.

Morris HL, Bardach J, Ardinger H, Jones D, Kelly KM, Olin WH, and Wheeler J: Multidisciplinary treatment results for patients with isolated cleft palate. *Plastic and Reconstructive Surgery* 92:842-851, 1993.

Mowrer DE: *Methods of modifying speech behaviors.* 2nd ed. Prospect Heights (IL): Waveland, 1982.

Nation J: Determinants of vocabulary development of preschool cleft palate children. *Cleft Palate Journal* 7:645-651, 1970a.

Nation J: Vocabulary comprehension and usage of preschool cleft palate and normal children. *Cleft Palate Journal* 7:639-644, 1970b.

O'Gara MM, and Logemann JA: Phonetic analysis of the speech development of babies with cleft palate. *Cleft Palate Journal* 25:122-134, 1988.

O'Gara MM, Logemann JA, and Rademaker AW: Place features and stop types by babies with cleft palate. Proceedings of the annual meeting of the American Cleft Palate Association, Portland, OR, 1992.

O'Gara MM, Logemann J, and Rademaker AW: Phonetic features by babies with unilateral cleft lip and palate. *Cleft Palate–Craniofacial Journal* 31:446-451, 1994.

Oller DK: Metaphonology and infant vocalizations. In Lindblom B, and Zetterstrom R (eds.): *Precursors of early speech.* Basingstroke, Hampshire: Macmillan, 1976.

Oller DK, and Eilers RE: The role of audition in infant babbling. *Child Development* 59:441-449, 1988.

Olsen DA: A descriptive study of the speech development of a group of infants with cleft palate [dissertation]. Chicago: Northwestern University, 1965.

Pannbacker M: Oral language skills of adult cleft palate speakers. *Cleft Palate Journal* 12:95-106, 1975.

Paradise JL: Otitis media in infants and children. *Pediatrics* 65:917-943, 1980.

Paradise JL: Otitis media during early life: how hazardous to development? A critical review of the evidence. *Pediatrics* 68:869-873, 1981.

Paynter ET: Parental and child preference for speech produced by children with velopharyngeal incompetence. *Cleft Palate–Craniofacial Journal* 24:112-118, 1987.

Paynter ET, and Kinard MW: Perceptual preferences between compensatory articulation and nasal escape of air in children with velopharyngeal incompetence. *Cleft Palate Journal* 16:262-266, 1979.

Peterson-Falzone SJ: Resonance disorders in structural defects. In Lass NJ, McReynolds LV, Northern JL, and Yoder DE (eds.): *Speech, language and hearing.* Volume II: *Pathologies of speech and language.* Philadelphia: WB Saunders, 1982.

Peterson-Falzone SJ: Speech characteristics: updating clinical decisions. *Seminars in Speech and Language* 7:269-295, 1986.

Peterson-Falzone SJ: Compensatory articulations in cleft palate speakers: relative incidence by type. Proceedings of the International Congress on Cleft Palate and Related Craniofacial Anomalies, Jerusalem, Israel, 1989.

Peterson-Falzone SJ: A cross-sectional analysis of speech results following palatal closure. In Bardach J, and Morris HL (eds.): *Multidisciplinary management of cleft lip and palate.* Philadelphia: WB Saunders, 1990.

Peterson-Falzone SJ: Speech outcomes in adolescents with cleft lip and palate. *Cleft Palate–Craniofacial Journal* 32:125-128, 1995.

Philips BJ, and Harrison RJ: Articulation patterns of preschool cleft palate children. *Cleft Palate Journal* 6:245-253, 1969.

Philips BJ, and Kent R: Acoustic-phonetic descriptions of speech production in speakers with cleft palate and other velopharyngeal disorders. In Lass N (ed.): *Speech and language: advances in basic research.* New York: Academic Press, 1984.

Pitzner JC, and Morris HL: Articulation skills and adequacy of breath pressure ratios of children with cleft palate. *Journal of Speech and Hearing Disorders* 31:26-40, 1966.

Powers GR: Cinefluorographic investigation of articulatory movements of selected individuals with cleft palate. *Journal of Speech and Hearing Research* 5:59-62, 1962.

Powers G, Erickson CB, and Dunn C: Speech analyses of four children with repaired cleft palates. *Journal of Speech and Hearing Disorders* 55:542-549, 1990.

Rampp DL, and Counihan DT: Vocal pitch intensity relationships in cleft palate speakers. *Cleft Palate Journal* 3:846-857, 1970.

Renfrew CE: Present day problems in cleft palate speech. Logopeden, June 1960. As cited by Moll KL. Speech characteristics of individuals with cleft lip and palate. In Spriestersbach DC, and Sherman D (eds.): *Cleft palate and communication.* New York: Academic Press, 1968.

Riski JE: Articulation skills and oral-nasal resonance in children with pharyngeal flaps. *Cleft Palate Journal* 16:421-428, 1979.

Riski JE: Speech assessment of adolescents. *Cleft Palate–Craniofacial Journal* 32:109-113, 1995.

Riski JE, and DeLong E: Articulation development in children with cleft lip/palate. *Cleft Palate Journal* 21:57-64, 1984.

Roberts JE, and Clarke-Stein S: Otitis media. In Bernthal JE, and Bankson NW (eds.): *Child phonology: characteristics, assessment, and intervention with special populations.* New York: Theime, 1994.

Roberts JE, Burchinal MR, Davis BP, Collier AM, and Henderson FW: Otitis media in early childhood and later language. *Journal of Speech and Hearing Research* 344:1158-1168, 1991.

Ross BR, and Johnston MC: *Cleft lip and palate.* Baltimore: Williams & Wilkins, 1972.

Russell J, and Grunwell P: Speech development in children with cleft lip and palate. In Grunwell P (ed.): *Analysing cleft palate speech.* London: Whurr, 1993.

Scherer NJ: Longitudinal language development in 20-30 month children with cleft lip/palate. Proceedings of the American Speech-Language-Hearing Association Convention, Orlando, 1995.

Scherer NJ, and D'Antonio LL: Parent questionnaire for screening early language development in children with cleft palate. *Cleft Palate Journal* 32:7-13, 1995.

Schwartz MF: Acoustic measures of nasalization and nasality. In Bzoch KR (ed.): *Communicative disorders related to cleft lip and palate.* 2nd ed. Boston: Little, Brown, 1979.

Shames G, and Rubin H: Psycholinguistic measures of language and speech. In Bzoch K (ed.): *Communicative disorders related to cleft lip and palate.* Boston: Little, Brown, 1971.

Shames G, and Rubin H: Psycholinguistic measures of language and speech. In Bzoch K (ed.): *Communicative disorders related to cleft lip and palate.* 2nd ed. Boston: Little, Brown, 1979.

Shelton RL, and Blank JL: Oronasal fistulas, intraoral air pressure, and nasal air flow during speech. *Cleft Palate Journal* 21:91-99, 1984.

Shelton RL, and McCauley RJ: Use of a hinge-type speech prosthesis. *Cleft Palate Journal* 23:312-317, 1986.

Shelton RL, Brooks AR, and Youngstrom KA: Articulation and patterns of palatopharyngeal closure. *Journal of Speech and Hearing Disorders* 29:390-408, 1964.

Sherman D, and Goodwin E: Pitch level and nasality. *Journal of Speech and Hearing Disorders* 19:423-428, 1954.

Sherman D, Spriestersbach DC, and Noll JD: Glottal stops in the speech of children with cleft palates. *Journal of Speech and Hearing Disorders* 24:37-42, 1959.

Shprintzen R, Lavorato A, Rakoff S, and Skolnick M: Incongruous movements of the velum and lateral pharyngeal walls. *Cleft Palate Journal* 14:148-157, 1977.

Shriberg LD, and Kent RD: *Clinical phonetics.* Boston: Allyn & Bacon, 1995.

Shriner T, and Sherman D: An equation for assessing language development. *Journal of Speech and Hearing Research* 10:41-48, 1967.

Shulman BB: *Test of pragmatic skills.* Tucson (AZ): Communication Skill Builders, 1985.

Siegel M, Mooney M, Kimes K, and Todhunter J: Analysis of the size variability of the human normal and cleft palate fetal nasal capsule by means of 3-dimensional computer reconstruction of histologic preparations. *Cleft Palate Journal* 24:190-199, 1987.

Singh S, Hayden ME, and Toombs MS: The role of distinctive features in articulation errors. *Journal of Speech and Hearing Disorders* 46:174-183, 1981.

Smith, and McWilliams: Psycholinguistic considerations in the management of children with cleft palate. *Journal of Speech and Hearing Disorders* 33:26-32, 1968a.

Smith, and McWilliams: Psycholinguistic abilities of children with clefts. *Cleft Palate Journal* 5:238-249, 1968b.

Spriestersbach DC, Darley FL, and Morris HL: Language skills in children with cleft palate. *Journal of Speech and Hearing Research* 1:279-285, 1958.

Spriestersbach DC, Darley FL, and Rouse V: Articulation of a group of children with cleft lips and palates. *Journal of Speech and Hearing Disorders* 21:436-445, 1956.

Spriestersbach DC, Moll KL, and Morris HL: Subject classification and articulation of speakers with cleft palates. *Journal of Speech and Hearing Research* 4:362-373, 1961.

Starr C: A study of some of the characteristics of the speech and speech mechanism of a group of cleft palate children [dissertation]. Chicago: Northwestern University, 1956.

Stengelhofen J: The nature and causes of communication problems in cleft palate. In Stengelhofen J (ed.): *Cleft palate: the nature and remediation of communication problems.* Edinburgh: Churchill-Livingstone, 1989.

Stoel-Gammon C: Prelinguistic development: measurement and predictions. In Ferguson CA, Menn L, and Stoel-Gammon C (eds.): *Phonological development: models research, implications.* Timonium (MD): York Press, 1992.

Stoel-Gammon C: Measuring phonology in babble and speech. *Clinics in Communication Disorders* 4:1-11, 1994.

Stoel-Gammon C, and Cooper JA: Patterns of early lexical and phonological development. *Journal of Child Language* 11:247-271, 1984.

Stoel-Gammon C, and Dunn C: *Normal and disordered phonology in children.* Baltimore: University Park Press, 1985.

Subtelny J, and Subtelny JD: Intelligibility and associated physiological factors of cleft palate speakers. *Journal of Speech and Hearing Research* 2:353-360, 1959.

Takagi Y, McGlone R, and Millard R: A survey of the speech disorders of individuals with clefts. *Cleft Palate Journal* 2:28-31, 1965.

Tarlow A, and Saxman JA: Comparative study of the speaking fundamental frequency characteristics in children with cleft palate. *Cleft Palate Journal* 7:696-705, 1970.

Tronczynska J: Electrorhinopneumography as an objective method of assessment of velopharyngeal insufficiency in cleft palate patients. *Folia Phoniatrica* 24:371-380, 1972.

Trost JE: Articulatory additions to the classical descriptions of the speech of persons with cleft palate. *Cleft Palate Journal* 18:193-203, 1981.

Trost-Cardamone JE: Differential diagnosis of velopharyngeal disorders. In *Communicative disorders: an audio-journal for continuing education.* New York: Grune and Stratton, 1987.

Trost-Cardamone JE: Speech: anatomy, physiology, and pathology. In Kernahan DA, and Rosenstein SW (eds.): *Cleft lip and palate: a system of management.* Baltimore: Williams & Wilkins, 1990a.

Trost-Cardamone JE: The development of speech: assessing cleft palate misarticulations. In Kernahan DA, and Rosenstein SW (eds.): *Cleft lip and palate: a system of management.* Baltimore: Williams & Wilkins, 1990b.

Trost-Cardamone JE: Diagnosis and management of speakers with craniofacial anomalies. Short course presented at the American Speech-Language-Hearing Association Convention, Orlando, FL, 1995.

Trost-Cardamone JE: Diagnosis of specific cleft palate speech error patterns for planning therapy or physical management needs. In Bzoch KR (ed.): *Communicative disorders related to cleft lip and palate.* Austin: Pro-Ed, 1997a.

Trost-Cardamone JE: Speech compensatory misarticulations. Proceedings of the American Cleft Palate–Craniofacial Association preconference symposium, New Orleans, 1997b.

Vallino LD, and Tompson B: Perceptual characteristics of consonant errors associated with malocclusion. *Journal of Oral and Maxillofacial Surgery* 51:850-856, 1993.

Van Demark DR: Misarticulations and listener judgments of the speech of individuals with cleft palates. *Cleft Palate Journal* 1:232-245, 1964.

Van Demark DR: A factor analysis of the speech of children with cleft palate. *Cleft Palate Journal* 3:159-170, 1966.

Van Demark DR: Consistency of articulation of subjects with cleft palate. *Cleft Palate Journal* 6:254-262, 1969.

Van Demark DR, and Hardin MA: Speech therapy for the child with cleft lip and palate. In Bardach J, and Morris HL (eds.): *Multidisciplinary management of cleft lip and palate.* Philadelphia: WB Saunders, 1990.

Van Demark DR, and Morris HL: Stability of velopharyngeal competency. *Cleft Palate Journal* 20:18-22, 1983.

Van Demark DR, and Van Demark AH: Misarticulations of cleft palate children achieving velopharyngeal closure and children with functional speech problems. *Cleft Palate Journal* 4:31-37, 1967.

Van Demark DR, Morris HL, and Vandehaar C: Patterns of articulation abilities in speakers with cleft palate. *Cleft Palate Journal* 16:230-239, 1979.

Van Demark DR, Hardin MA, O'Gara MM, Logemann J, and Chapman KL: Identification of children with and without cleft palate from tape-recorded samples of early vocalizations and speech. *Cleft Palate–Craniofacial Journal* 30:557-563, 1993.

Ventry IM: Effects of conductive hearing loss: fact or fiction. *Journal of Speech and Hearing Disorders* 45:143-156, 1980.

Vihman M, and Greenlee M: Individual differences in phonological development: ages one and three years. *Journal of Speech and Hearing Research* 30:503-521, 1987.

Vihman MM, Macken MA, Miller R, Simmons H, and Miller J: From babbling to speech: A re-assessment of the continuity issue. *Language* 61:397-445, 1985.

Warr-Leeper G, Crone L, Carruthers A, and Leeper H: A comparison of the performance of preschool children with cleft lip and/or palate on the test of pragmatic skills. Proceedings of the annual meeting of the American Cleft Palate–Craniofacial Association, Williamsburg, VA, 1988.

Warren DW: Nasal emission of air and velopharyngeal function. *Cleft Palate Journal* 4:148-155, 1967.

Warren DW: Compensatory speech behaviors in individuals with cleft palate: a regulation/control phenomenon? *Cleft Palate Journal* 23:251-260, 1986.

Warren DW: Discussion: perceptual characteristics of consonant errors associated with malocclusion. *Journal of Oral and Maxillofacial Surgery* 51:856, 1993.

Warren DW, and Devereux JL: An analog study of cleft palate speech. *Cleft Palate Journal* 3:103-114, 1966.

Warren DW, and Ryon WE: Oral port constriction, nasal resistance, and respiratory aspects of cleft palate speech: an analog study. *Cleft Palate Journal* 4:38-46, 1967.

Warren DW, Dalston RM, and Mayo R: Hypernasality in the presence of "adequate" velopharyngeal closure. *Cleft Palate–Craniofacial Journal* 30:150-154, 1993.

Warren DW, Duany LF, and Fischer ND: Nasal pathway resistance in normal and cleft lip and palate subjects. *Cleft Palate Journal* 6:134-140, 1969.

Webb M, Starr CD, and Moller K: Effects of extended speaking on resonance of patients with cleft palate. *Cleft Palate–Craniofacial Journal* 29:22-26, 1992.

Westlake H: Understanding the cleft palate child. *Quarterly Journal of Speech* 38:165-172, 1953.

Whitcomb L, Ochsner G, and Wayte R: A comparison of expressive language skills of cleft palate and non-cleft palate children: a preliminary investigation. *Journal of Oklahoma Speech and Hearing Association* 3:25, 1976.

Witzel MA: Communicative impairment associated with clefting. In Shprintzen RJ, and Bardach J (eds.): *Cleft palate speech management.* St. Louis: Mosby, 1995.

Wood KS: Terminology and nomenclature. In Travis LE (ed.): *Handbook of speech pathology and audiology.* New York: Appleton-Century-Crofts, 1971.

Yamashita Y, and Michi K: Misarticulations caused by abnormal lingual-palatal contact in patients with cleft palate with adequate velopharyngeal function. *Cleft Palate Journal* 28:360-368, 1991.

Zinkus PW, Gottlieb M, and Schapiro M: Developmental and psychoeducational sequelae of chronic otitis media. *American Journal of Diseases of Children* 132:1100-1104, 1978.

Chapter 8

Noncleft Velopharyngeal Problems

Speech-language pathologists are sometimes confronted with children or adults whose speech is characterized by nasal air loss, hypernasal resonance, or other perceptual stigmata of an inadequately functioning velopharyngeal system but whose history does not indicate cleft palate. There are many structural and neurologic conditions that may lead to such speech problems and some behavioral or learning bases as well. The first and perhaps most difficult lesson to learn about this topic is that the multiple causes of inadequate velopharyngeal closure[1] in the absence of overt or submucous clefts may occur in combinations of two or more in any given individual.

LEARNING TO THINK IN COMBINATIONS

In Chapter 1, you learned about submucous clefts of the palate (Fig. 8-1) and how they vary in terms of what the clinician can see and what the effects may or may not be on speech. Historically, undetected or incompletely diagnosed submucous defects have obviously composed a large percentage of supposedly "noncleft" cases of velopharyngeal inadequacy.[2] However, much of the literature even today assumes that inadequate closure in a given patient can have only one etiology. Several highly detailed classification systems for causes of inadequate closure were devised in the 1950s, 1960s, and 1970s (Calnan, 1957b, 1959, 1961a, 1976; Minami et al., 1975; Pitt and Ingram, 1975a; Pruzansky et al., 1977; Randall, Bakes, and Kennedy, 1960), but each system essentially ignored the possibility of a combination of causes. In 1983 Cotton and Nuwayhid offered a rather simplified system for classifying causes of "velopharyngeal insufficiency" but their system did recognize the possibility of combinations of etiologies in a single patient. In the 1980s and 1990s the imaging techniques described in Chapter 10 became increasingly routine diagnostic tools, and as a result we learned much more about the multiple etiologies of what had often been termed in the past "cleft palate speech without cleft palate."

Each time you see a patient with inadequate velopharyngeal closure in the absence of a history of known cleft palate or submucous cleft palate, you will need to consider the possibility of one *or more* of the following problems:

1. A previously undiagnosed "occult" submucous cleft as described in Chapter 1, with a muscular deficiency on the upper surface of the velum (Fig. 8-2).
2. Palatopharyngeal disproportion (that is, a mismatch between the length of the velum and the depth of the pharynx), with or without stigmata of a submucous cleft. The possible contributing factors to palatopharyngeal disproportion include a short hard palate, a short soft palate, and abnormal pharyngeal depth (Figs. 8-3 and 8-4). In addition to these congenital problems, some cases are "iatrogenic," often attributable to incautious adenoidectomy or tonsillectomy that creates an excessively deep pharynx. (If the bony and soft tissue structures of the velopharyngeal system are normal in size and position, an adenoidectomy or tonsillectomy should not have a permanent deleterious effect on speech, although there may be transitory effects.) Of course, ablative surgery on any part of the palate or pharynx carried out to remove malignant or nonmalignant growths can also result in inadequate velopharyngeal closure.
3. Mechanical obstruction to complete velopharyngeal closure
   a. Tonsils
   b. Irregularly shaped adenoid pad
   c. Irregularities of the faucial pillars

[1]In the literature on cleft palate and on inadequate velopharyngeal closure the student will find that the terms velopharyngeal "inadequacy," "incompetency," and "insufficiency" are typically used interchangeably. Trost (1981) suggested segregating use of these terms as follows: "incompetency" for deficiencies of movement, "insufficiency" for deficiencies of tissue, and "inadequacy" for cases of mixed or undiagnosed etiology. Folkins (1988) pointed out that we cannot always separate speakers on the basis of neuromuscular versus structural deficits. In this book "velopharyngeal inadequacy" is used as a generic or umbrella term.

[2]As pointed out in Chapter 1, diagnosis of velopharyngeal abnormalities is much different from what it was even a decade ago. Chapter 10 describes current instrumental approaches to diagnosis.

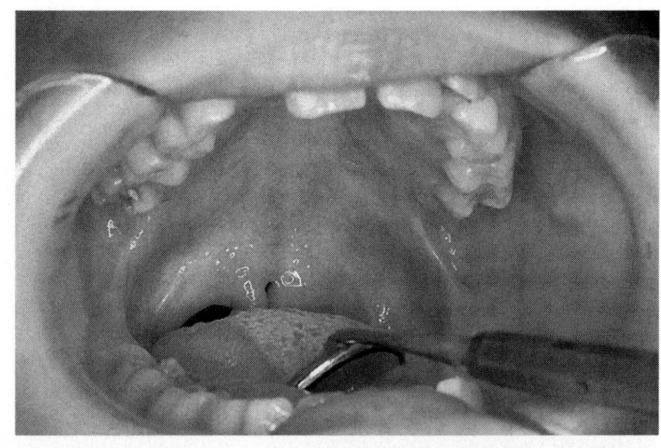

Figure 8-1 Patient with the classic triad of intra-orally visible stigmata of a submucous cleft of the secondary palate: bifid uvula, zona pellucida of the soft palate (extending into the hard palate), and a notch in the posterior border of the hard palate (digitally palpable but not always easily visible).

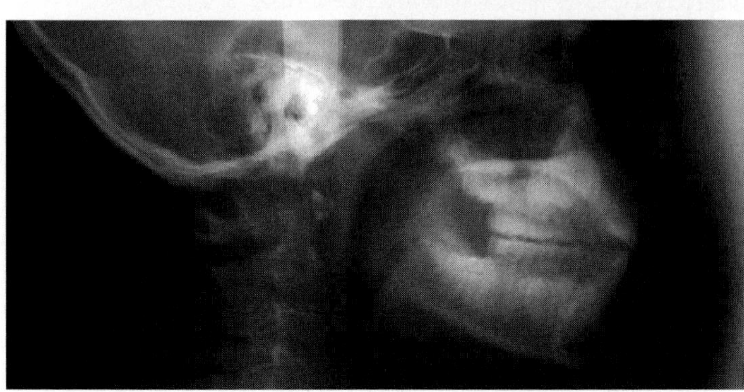

Figure 8-2 The velum in this individual is thin, suggesting a lack of normal muscle bulk. There is also a very large pharyngeal space, with no adenoid pad.

4. Deficient movement of the velum or pharyngeal components of velopharyngeal closure occurring
   a. In apparent isolation
   b. In association with neuromotor impairment of other parts of the speech mechanism (dysarthria, apraxia)
5. Mislearning (phoneme-specific nasal emission)

In this chapter we will discuss each of these topics but with the caveat that considering any of these factors as de facto discrete, mutually exclusive entities will lead to diagnostic and therapeutic errors.[3]

ARCHITECTURAL LESSONS ABOUT THE VELOPHARYNGEAL SYSTEM

Bony Architecture

When a baby is born with a cleft of the secondary palate, the obvious anatomical abnormalities are accompanied by other rather subtle differences in the bony architecture of the nasopharynx and contiguous structures. These same anatomical differences may be found in individuals who have more obscure palatal problems. Several decades ago, investigators found the lateral dimensions of the pharynx to be wider in individuals with clefts (Kirkham as quoted by Peyton, 1931; Moss, 1956; Psaume, 1950; Ricketts, 1954; Subtelny, 1955; Wardill, 1928). In fact, Moss (1956) stated, "... cleft palate should be considered to be but one of a continuous series of cephalic malformations," meaning that clinicians must be aware of the likelihood of abnormal structures or dimensions in other areas of the craniofacial complex. Fletcher (1960) made a similar point, describing anatomical differences in the velopharyngeal system as being part of a "regional growth disturbance."

Of particular concern are abnormalities of the cervical spine that occur in patients with clefts, which may cause abnormal depth of the pharynx (Osborne, 1968; Ross and Lindsay, 1965).[4] In a landmark study in 1968 Osborne (Osborne, 1968; Osborne, Pruzansky, and Koepp-Baker, 1971) found a high prevalence of cervical anomalies in individuals with submucous cleft palate and with noncleft velopharyngeal inadequacy, once again demonstrating that individuals with overt clefts and those with more subtle abnormalities of the velopharyngeal system should be viewed as being on the same continuum. Fig. 8-4 illustrates cervical anomalies in noncleft patients and the effect on the position of the posterior pharyngeal wall. If the posterior processes of two or more cervical vertebrae are fused, or if one or more vertebrae are displaced posteriorly, the effect is to pull the posterior wall back, creating an abnormally deep pharyngeal space. Anomalies of the cervical spine often

[3]For an extensive review of the literature up to 1984 on the topic of velopharyngeal inadequacy in the absence of cleft palate, see Peterson-Falzone (1985).

[4]The sample in the Ross and Lindsay study (1965), however, was biased toward cervical anomalies because more than one half of the cases had a diagnosis of Klippel-Feil syndrome, for which cervical anomalies are a key or pathognomonic feature.

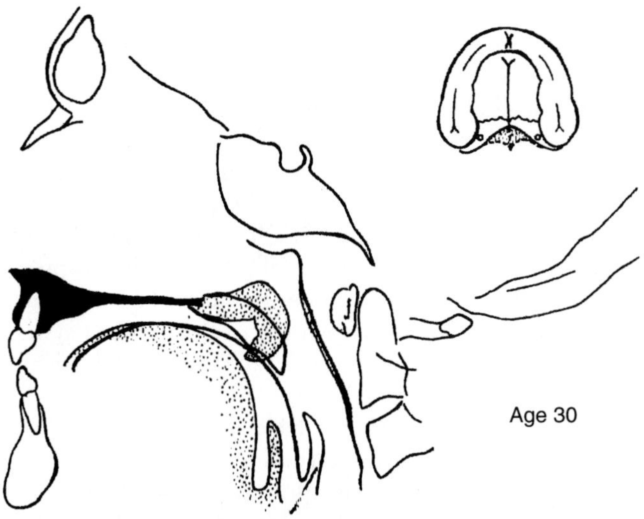

Figure 8-3 Tracing from an x-ray film taken during production of a sustained fricative by a patient with a submucous cleft (see upper diagram showing the bony notch in the hard palate). This patient had good muscular bulk and length of the velum, but the defect in the hard palate meant that the attachment of the velum was displaced anteriorly, preventing velopharyngeal closure.

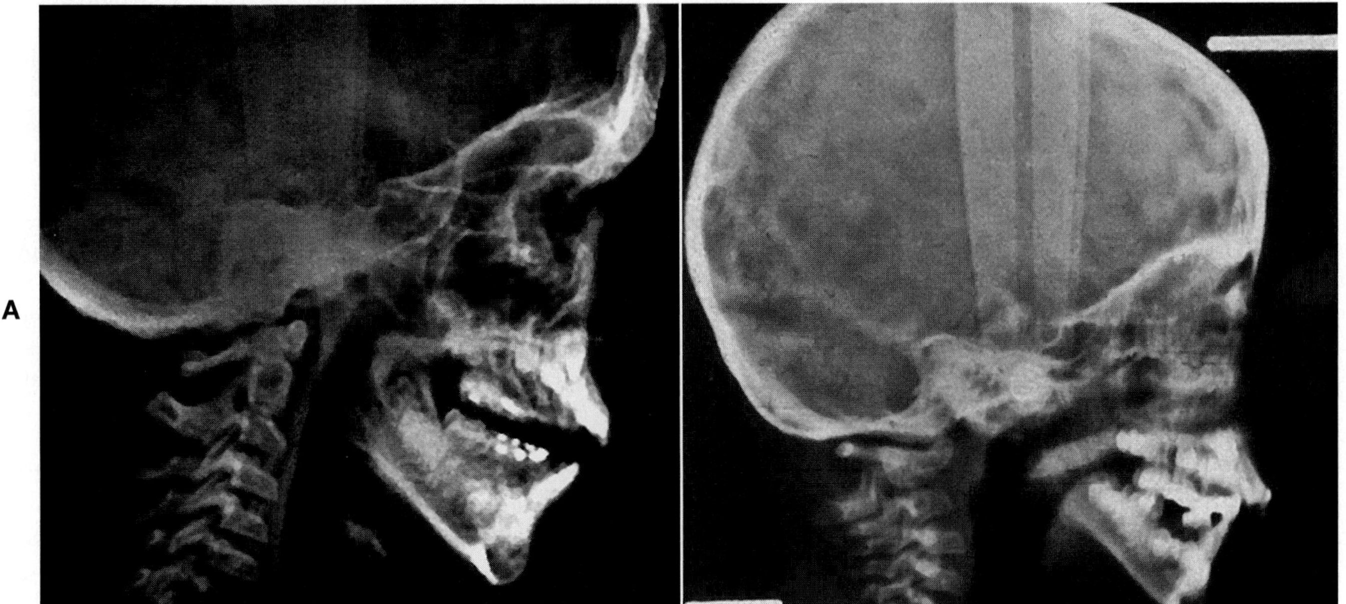

Figure 8-4 Both these patients exhibit excessive pharyngeal depth attributable to malformations of the cervical spine. **A,** Fusion of the posterior processes of the second and third cervical vertebrae. **B,** Severe posterior displacement of the second vertebra, in addition to other malformations. Note also that this patient has a velum that seems to lift throughout its length, rather than showing a normal velar eminence or "knee" action.

result in decreased range of motion of the neck,[5] and some include displacement of part of the atlas (first cervical vertebra) up into the foramen magnum, a condition that can be life threatening if the head is extended, as in surgery on the palate.

Another cause of an abnormally deep pharynx is a rather flattened cranial base angle (Fig. 8-5), which also has the effect of moving the posterior pharyngeal wall backward.

In theory, a foreshortened hard palate could cause inadequate velopharyngeal closure because the velar musculature would be anteriorly displaced (Crikelair et al., 1964). However, a short hard palate has not been described as an independent or "stand-alone" cause of inadequate closure but as part of the anatomical abnormalities in either frank or occult submucous clefts (Kaplan, 1975; Kelly, 1910; Ricketts, 1954).

Some persons with clefts and some without clefts undergo surgical advancement of the midface to bring the maxilla and mandible into better alignment, improving occlusion and facial appearance. This involves a change in both bony and soft tissue architecture of the velopharyngeal system because surgical repositioning of the maxilla will automatically take the soft palate with it. To date, however,

[5]Be on the alert for signs of limited neck motion, such as decreased ability to turn the head from side to side, as you examine your patient.

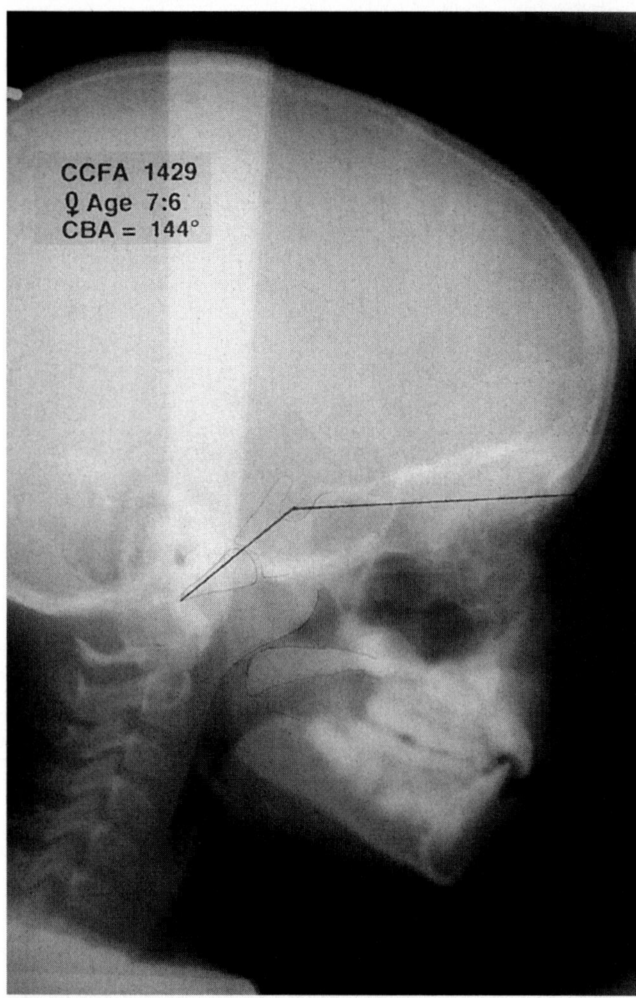

Figure 8-5 A flattened cranial base angle, leading to posterior displacement of the posterior pharyngeal wall (the cranial base angle should usually be around 120 degrees, although it is normal for there to be a few degrees of change in angulation as the child grows).

there has been no report of onset of velopharyngeal inadequacy after maxillary advancement in speakers without clefts or other abnormalities of the velopharyngeal system. The topic of maxillary advancement is discussed in Chapter 4.

Soft Tissue Architecture

Soft palate. Obviously the length, thickness, and muscular integrity of the soft palate are principal concerns when velopharyngeal closure is inadequate. Although congenital anatomic abnormalities of the velum have most often been described as part of the spectrum of findings in frank or occult submucous clefts, there is a dilemma in that very few of the patients described as having a "congenital short palate" in the older literature (Kelly 1910; Winters, 1966, 1975), and in some current literature as well (Spauwen, 1988), underwent the types of diagnostic procedures currently used for detection of occult abnormalities.[6] Kaplan (1975) reported that 75% of his 240 cases of velopharyngeal inadequacy had a short soft palate, but all of these proved to have either classic or occult submucous clefts. For a description of how the abnormal muscular insertions or deficiencies of muscular bulk in submucous clefts affect closure, see Chapter 3.

Tonsils and adenoids.[7,8] The tonsils and adenoids are part of the reticulo-endothelial system and thus play a part in the production of immunoglobulins. However, they constitute a relatively small portion of the immune system and can fulfill their protective role only so long as the tissues themselves are not diseased.

The tonsils and adenoids have different embryologic origins and different cytologic features (Pruzansky, 1975). They do not follow the same growth cycles, which means that the size of one is not predictive of the size of the other. Both can have effects on velopharyngeal function but in quite different ways.

The adenoid pad is generally visible in radiographic views of the nasopharynx by the time a child is 6 weeks old. The pad increases in size in the childhood years, reaches a peak size, and then begins to recede or involute until, by the adult years, it has usually disappeared altogether. However, clinical investigators have been unable to identify a single age or definite age span during which the adenoids can be expected to reach maximum size. Subtelny and Koepp-Baker (1956) reported the age for maximum adenoid size to be as early as 9 to 10 years and as late as 14 to 15 years. Handelman and Pruzansky (1967) found large adenoids to be most frequent in children between 4 and 6 years old, and less frequent in older groups. Pruzansky's (1975) radiographic data on 291 normal children showed considerable variation in adenoid size in all age groups from 4 to 16 years.[9] In 1983, Linder-Aronson and Leighton derived longitudinal data on 53 normal children and found that adenoid size peaked at 5 years, then decreased, but showed another slight regrowth at age 11 years.

While the adenoid pad is increasing in size, the nasopharynx itself is growing. The major increase in size is

[6]Winters (1966) credited Passavant (1865) with being the first to "discover" that the palate could be congenitally short without the presence of a submucous or overt cleft.

[7]There are actually two sets of tonsils. The tonsils that are discussed here are termed the "faucial tonsils" and normally reside between the anterior and posterior faucial pillars. There are also "lingual tonsils," clusters of lymphoid tissue on the lower portion of the dorsum of the tongue. To make matters more confusing, the adenoids are sometimes referred to as the "pharyngeal tonsils."

[8]There is really just one adenoid pad, and some authors therefore object to using the plural noun "adenoids." However, the plural form "adenoids" is the one most often found in the literature.

[9]All these studies were cross-sectional and did not include longitudinal radiographic data on children as they grew.

vertical because of the descent of the hard palate away from the cranial base (Handelman and Osborne, 1976; Subtelny and Koepp-Baker, 1956). This is the result of the natural pattern of growth of the face, which is downward and forward. Usually the growth of the adenoids and the growth of the nasopharyngeal space maintain a balance, but sometimes adenoidal growth outpaces that of the nasopharynx, resulting in impaired nasal breathing (Fig. 8-6) (Handelman and Osborne, 1976; Linder-Aronson, 1970; Weimert, 1987). The immediate concerns in such cases include abnormal sleep, reduced exercise tolerance, reduced appetite, daytime sleepiness, and, if symptoms are prolonged, possible deleterious effects on the heart, termed "cor pulmonale." In terms of speech, the only effect is denasality.[10]

For speech-language pathologists, there are four important points to remember about adenoids: (1) In the young child, "velopharyngeal closure" is actually "velum-adenoid closure" Fig. 8-7. (2) The adenoids are not visible on your intraoral examination of the child, because they are up *behind* the velum. (Similarly, velopharyngeal closure cannot be seen on the oral examination because the closure takes place on the upper or nasal side of the velum, out of your line of view.) (3) The adenoids may be literally either "coming or going" in the child you see, meaning that they may get larger or smaller over the next few months or years. (4) The adenoids may be critical for closure, particularly in individuals with abnormalities of velopharyngeal structure or function.

The literature is replete with warnings against performing adenoidectomies in children with overt or submucous clefts (Calnan, 1953, 1954, 1956, 1957a, 1957b, 1959, 1961a, 1961b, 1971a, 1971b, 1976; Chaco and Yules, 1969; Cotton and Nuwayhid, 1983; Croft, Shprintzen, and Ruben, 1981; Gereau and Shprintzen, 1988; Seid, 1990; Subtelny and Koepp-Baker, 1956; Witzel et al., 1986).[11] Paradise (1983) also pointed out the potential deleterious effects of removing the adenoids in individuals with neurologically impaired palatal function or "the unusually capacious pharynx." For the child with any of these conditions, the natural involution of adenoids also carries the risk of onset of velopharyngeal inadequacy (Goode and Ross, 1972; Mason and Warren, 1980; Massengill and Quinn, 1974; Morris et al., 1990; Shapiro, 1980).[12,13] Mason and Warren (1980) reported that the initial cue to the gradual onset of velopharyngeal inadequacy was found in longitudinal aerodynamic (pressure-flow) data, in some cases as much as a year or more before speech became symptomatic.

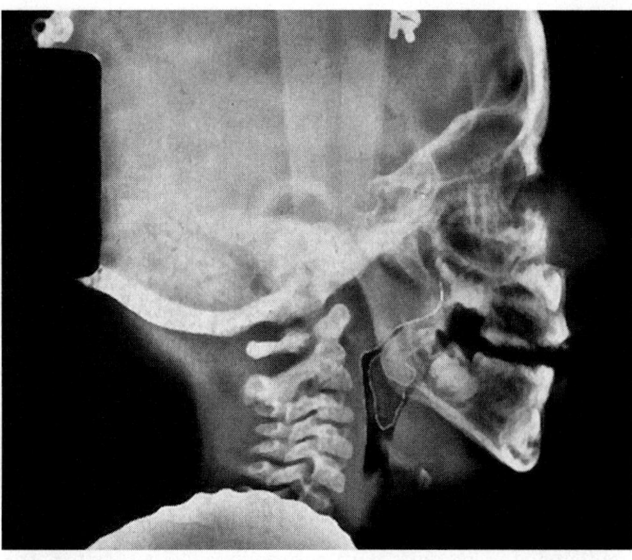

Figure 8-6 A youngster with an extremely large adenoid pad (outlined in white, above the velum), and fairly large tonsils (outlined in white, below the velum).

When inadequate velopharyngeal closure becomes evident after performance of an adenoidectomy, the speech-language pathologist may be one of the first people (after the surgeon) approached by the patient or parents with the questions, "How long is this going to last? What can we do to make it go away?" The first response from clinicians is a concern that an anatomic or neurogenic abnormality of the velopharyngeal mechanism may have gone undetected before the surgical removal of the adenoids. In 1981 Croft, Shprintzen, and Ruben reported that surgical removal of the adenoids was the major "cause" of velopharyngeal

[10]There is an extensive body of literature about the possible effects of nasal obstruction on orofacial structures, with some unresolved controversy about the exact nature of the cause-effect relationship. This topic will not be covered here, but a supplemental list of readings is appended to the references for this chapter. For the clinician, it is important to remember that some abnormal findings on an oral examination *may* be due to impaired nasal breathing, the most frequently cited examples being a narrowed or constricted maxillary arch, hypertrophy of soft tissue in the palatal vault, and malocclusion.

[11]For a more extensive list of references on this point, see Peterson-Falzone, 1985.

[12]The articles by Mason and Warren (1980) and by Morris et al. (1990) were on patients with clefts. Each of the cases reported by Goode and Ross (1972), Massengill and Quinn (1974), and Shapiro (1980) appears to have had palatopharyngeal disproportion, unmasked by natural involution of the adenoids.

[13]In their article on the functional role of the adenoids in speech, Finkelstein et al. (1996) made a misleading and undocumented statement (p. 67): "It is probable that patients with palatal anomalies as a group show a greater frequency of residual adenoidal tissue in young adult life," citing as a source an article in which this topic was not even discussed. Finkelstein et al. went on to hypothesize that adenoid tissue is retained in patients with palatal anomalies due to "recurrent upper airway infections in childhood" and "reduced mechanical force of the velum against the adenoidal pad." There are no data, either in their own article or in the literature to date, to support their statements.

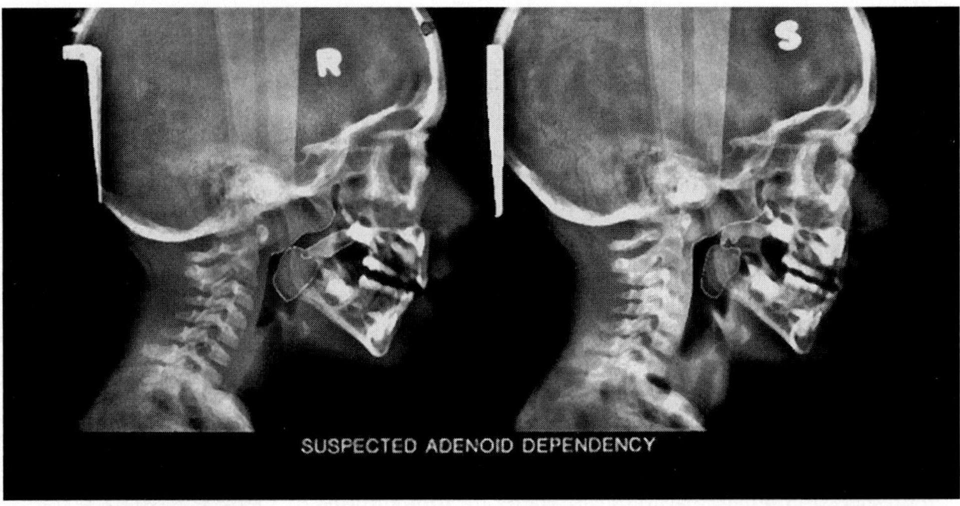

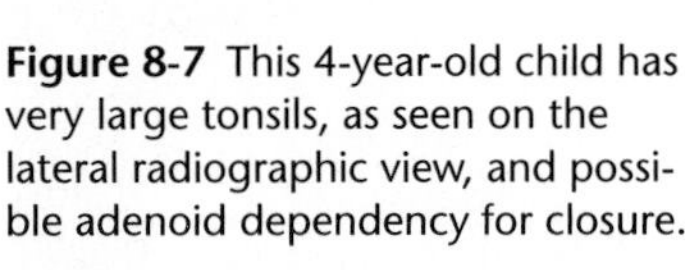
Figure 8-7 This 4-year-old child has very large tonsils, as seen on the lateral radiographic view, and possible adenoid dependency for closure.

inadequacy in patients with submucous clefts. That is, the adenoid pad had masked the underlying velopharyngeal problem. Overall, in their 120 cases of postadenoidectomy velopharyngeal inadequacy, 29% were found to have submucous clefts. In the report of Witzel et al. (1986), 27% of 137 patients referred after adenoidectomy had submucous clefts. In at least one case in the latter report, the adenoidectomy had been undertaken to "cure" pre-existing hypernasal speech. Although the number of articles in the medical literature on apparently unexpected cases of postadenoidectomy velopharyngeal inadequacy has dropped in the past decade, they have not disappeared. In reality, the preoperative assessment of any child scheduled for an adenoidectomy rarely meets even the minimal criteria proposed by Croft, Shprintzen, and Ruben (1981): visual inspection and digital palpation of the hard and soft palate, and lateral cephalometric films, including one taken "in phonation."[14]

Estimates of how long temporary velopharyngeal inadequacy may be evident after adenoidectomy have ranged in the literature from days or hours (Morris, 1975) to a day or two (Morris, Krueger, and Bumsted, 1982) to 2 to 3 weeks (Calnan, 1954), to 4 to 6 weeks (Greene, 1957). Witzel et al. (1986) stated that, in their experience, spontaneous improvement in speech may occur for up to 1 year after adenoidectomy. The first step is to ascertain whether there are any previously undetected structural or neurologic problems, but the timing of such studies depends on two factors: the potential cost-benefit ratio (e.g., is the radiation exposure worth the information) and the comfort or discomfort of the parents in simply waiting out the problem for a while versus undertaking diagnostic studies. If diagnostic studies such as videofluoroscopy or nasopharyngoscopy show a small or inconsistent velopharyngeal defect, speech therapy, especially with some form of biofeedback, would be preferable to further physical intervention (surgery or prosthesis). However, if the defect is larger, or consistent, or if the small gap persists despite behavioral therapy, consideration should be given to further physical management.[15]

Another potential influence of adenoids on velopharyngeal closure came to light in a recent report by Ren, Isberg, and Henningsson (1995) on velopharyngeal inadequacy in speech in 16 children between 4 and 9 years old. For some of those children, the reported cause was irregular contour of the adenoid pad after partial adenoidectomy, making it impossible for the velum to achieve full closure around the pad. For others the cause was enlarged tonsils intruding between the velum and posterior pharyngeal wall.

The tonsils as a potential obstruction to velopharyngeal closure first came to our attention about a decade ago (MacKenzie-Stepner et al., 1987; Shprintzen, Sher, and Croft, 1987). In the aggregate of 22 cases described in these two reports, tonsillectomy alone eliminated velopharyngeal inadequacy because the upper poles of the tonsils had simply been interposed between the velum and the posterior pharyngeal wall, preventing complete closure. In three cases, speech therapy reportedly eliminated some residual velopharyngeal inadequacy in speech, and in one additional case a temporary speech bulb[16] was used (Shprintzen, Sher, and Croft, 1987). Kummer, Billmire, and Myer (1993) reported one case in which enlarged tonsils inhibited velopharyngeal closure and speech was characterized by intermittent bursts of nasal emission and hypernasality, hyponasality, and cul-de-sac resonance; acoustic studies confirmed mixed nasality. Other reports also mentioned "muffled" resonance as a possible consequence of enlarged tonsils (Finkelstein, Nachmani,

[14]The velum elevates on production of a sustained vowel, but a better index of closure or the potential for closure may be obtained by taking the static film during sustained production of a voiced or voiceless fricative. In the latter case, of course, phonation is not actually taking place.

[15]Although these remarks about management are based on the stated assumption of no underlying structural or neurologic abnormalities, in reality they also apply even in the presence of such abnormalities *if* the velopharyngeal deficit in speech is found to be small or inconsistent. In other words, therapy alone may eradicate the problem.

[16]See Chapter 13 for a description of various types of prosthetic devices, including speech bulbs.

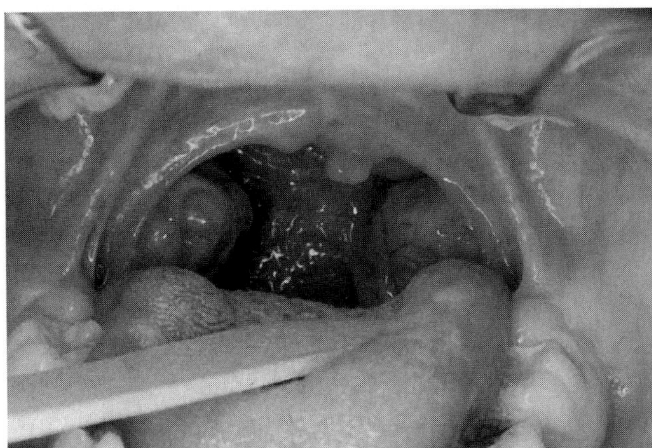

Figure 8-8 Moderately enlarged tonsils. This youngster also has a repaired palatal cleft, which is why the uvula is small and displaced a little to one side.

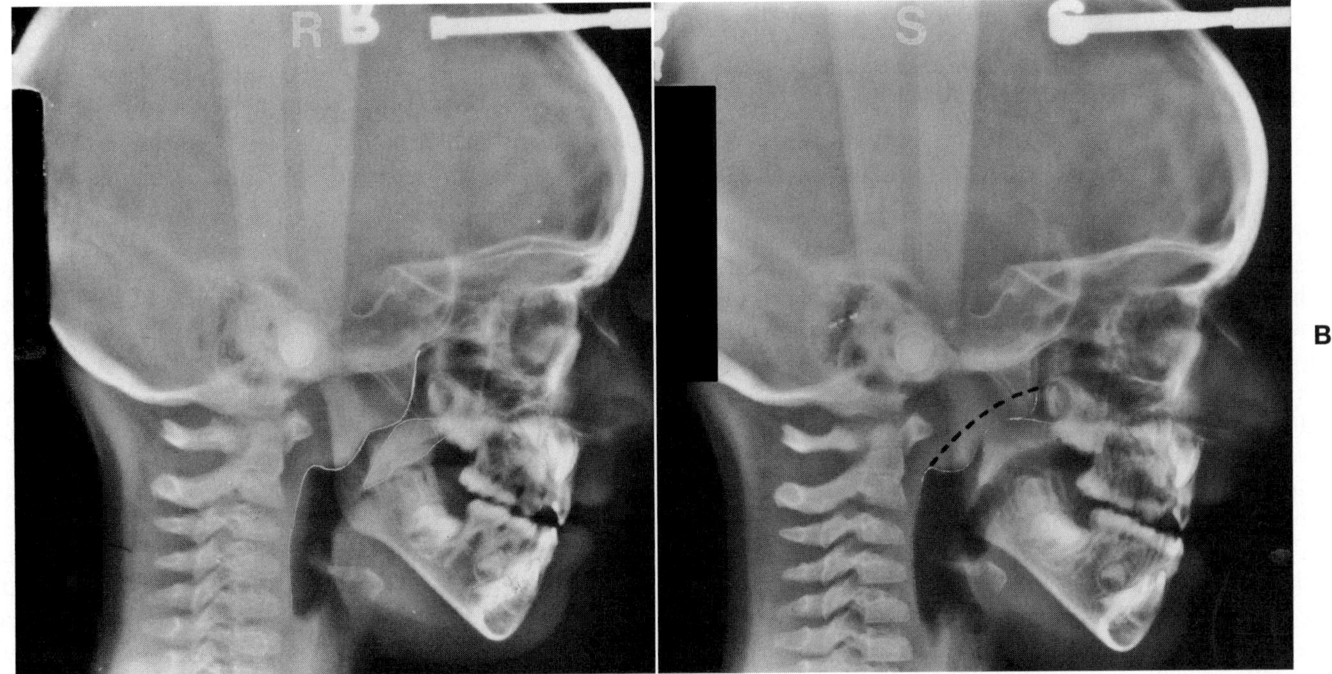

Figure 8-9 **A** and **B,** Large adenoid pad in a 5-year-old child who was evaluated because his otolaryngologist was concerned that removing the adenoid pad might lead to velopharyngeal inadequacy for speech. The film taken during sustained production of a fricative *(right)* shows the velum lifted into the adenoid pad; *dashed line,* theoretical configuration of the nasopharynx at the midsagittal plane if the adenoid tissue was "subtracted."

and Ophir, 1994; Morris, 1975; Shprintzen, Sher, and Croft, 1987). Fig. 8-8 shows moderately enlarged tonsils as seen on the intraoral view (more severely enlarged tonsils may meet in the midline), and Fig. 8-9 demonstrates tonsillar hypertrophy as seen radiographically in a 5-year-old child.

In a speaker exhibiting perceptual evidence of inadequate velopharyngeal closure and in whom tonsils are present, accurate delineation of the role the tonsils may be playing in the problem requires nasopharyngoscopy or multiview videofluoroscopy. In the absence of such studies, a surgeon may erroneously decide to place a pharyngeal flap as an aid to closure (see Chapter 13). There are two dangers in such a decision: tonsillectomy alone may eliminate the problem[17] and a pharyngeal flap residing between two large tonsils could very well precipitate significant airway problems.

Pharyngeal musculature. In the chapter on velopharyngeal anatomy and physiology, you learned that complete

[17]Some of the older literature spoke of a potential danger to velopharyngeal closure if tonsils were removed, particularly in children with cleft palate. However, the reports of "posttonsillectomy" problems in closure generally described postoperative scarring of the velum and/or faucial pillars causing restriction in velopharyngeal movement. See Peterson-Falzone (1985) for a review.

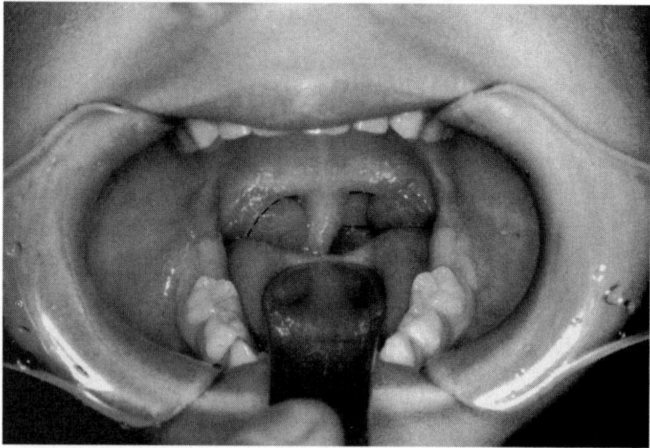

Figure 8-10 Anteriorly positioned uvula in a child who also has a very large tonsil on his right and a slightly smaller one on his left. The two top *dashed lines* indicate the position of the anterior pillars. The *lower dashed line* indicates the posterior faucial pillar on the left side (obscured from view on the right by the large tonsil), which is behind the uvula. It is normal for the tonsils to be positioned between the anterior and posterior pillars. This child had normal speech.

closure in many noncleft speakers as well as speakers with repaired cleft palates is dependent on the action of the pharyngeal musculature in addition to (or sometimes instead of) full elevation of the velum. In some multi-anomaly conditions, the pharyngeal musculature may be abnormal in structure and/or function (see Chapter 2). However, even in patients without clefts and without multi-anomaly conditions, you may occasionally see a variation in pharyngeal anatomy that could be a mechanical obstruction to closure. Some very interesting case reports of anatomical abnormalities of the faucial pillars began to appear in the French and English literature at least 100 years ago (Peterson-Falzone, 1985). As you would expect, descriptions of speech in these reports, if any description was given at all, were casual. In 1978 Warren, Bevin, and Winslow described "posterior pillar webbing" (that is, the posterior pillars were joined behind the uvula) as a cause of inadequate velopharyngeal closure in two speakers and described a third speaker with "palatopharyngeus displacement." However, some speakers in whom the uvula appears to be positioned in front of the posterior faucial pillars (Fig. 8-10) may actually have normal speech (Peterson-Falzone, 1985). In fact, we do not know how many normal speakers have such anatomical findings.

NEUROLOGICAL IMPAIRMENT OF VELOPHARYNGEAL FUNCTION

Both congenital and acquired neurological conditions may impair velopharyngeal function. The literature on this topic, as well as the literature on neurological impairment of speech in general, is difficult to follow and collate because of the variety of approaches used to categorize or label cases. To make matters worse, more than one name may be applied to a certain disease or set of symptoms. To some extent, the latter problem is an inevitable consequence of the growth of medical expertise.

"Isolated" Neurological Impairment of the Velopharyngeal System

Impairment of movement of the velum alone or together with the pharyngeal musculature, with normal control of the remainder of the oral musculature, has been described by many clinicians (Ardran and Kemp, 1975; Ashley et al., 1961; Blackfield et al., 1962; Calnan 1957b, 1959, 1961a, 1976; Crikelair et al., 1964; Davison, Razzell, and Watson, 1990; Hoopes et al., 1970a, 1970b; Jackson, McGlynn, and Huskie, 1980; Jafek et al., 1979; Johns, 1985; Kelly, 1910; Keogh, 1956; Lawshe et al., 1971; Mazaheri, Millard, and Erickson, 1964; Minami, Kaplan, and Wu, 1975; Owsley et al., 1967; Pitt and Ingram, 1975a, 1975b; Pollack, Shprintzen, and Zimmerman-Manchester, 1979; Shprintzen et al., 1977; Stueber and Wilhelmsen, 1984; Sturim and Jacob, 1972; Worster-Drought, 1956, 1968). Some of the patients in these reports had congenital conditions,[18] and others had acquired diseases or trauma. In 1956 Worster-Drought wrote, "The most frequent example of congenital suprabulbar paresis[19] affecting a single peripheral organ, I believe to be that of paralysis or weakness of the soft palate; this may be accompanied by an increased jaw jerk, but by no other manifestations of the disorder. Paresis of the soft palate may also co-exist with only a minor degree of weakness of the tongue or of the orbicularis oris. . . . I have come to regard an isolated congenital palsy of the soft palate as a manifestation of a mild form of congenital suprabulbar paresis" (pp. 454-455).

Several reports in the last two decades have described *temporary* unilateral or bilateral palatal paresis as an apparent result of various types of infections assumed to be affecting one or more of the cranial nerves IX, X, XI, or XII (Auberge et al., 1979; Crovetto et al., 1988; Dunn, 1983; Edin et al., 1976; Nussey, 1977; Roberton and Mellor, 1982; Sullivan and Carlson, 1976).[20] Most of the affected individuals in these reports were male. Typically, the case histories are of sudden onset of dysphagia, nasal regurgitation, and some perceptual indication of velopharyngeal inadequacy in speech, with some patients also exhibiting a hoarse voice quality. Time from onset of the first symptoms to complete remission has been reported to be 1 to 6 weeks. Complete recovery was documented in the majority of cases, the exception being nine cases reported by Auberge et al. (1979). For speech-language pathologists, the lesson to be learned from these case descriptions is that you *might* encounter a child in whom velopharyngeal inadequacy in speech is part of a transitory medical condition.

---

[18]One congenital condition in which there is often unilateral or bilateral decreased movement of the velopharyngeal system is hemifacial microsomia, discussed in Chapter 2.

[19]A synonym for "cerebral palsy" in some of the older literature.

[20]Interestingly, one case of a 28-year-old with transitory involvement of cranial nerves IX, X, and XII occurred following performance of cerebral angiography (Lapresle, Lasjunias, and Thevenier, 1980).

Descriptions of speech in the reports of "palatal myoclonus" or "nystagmus" are typically vague or absent. For a list of references on this topic, see Peterson-Falzone (1985). Interestingly, Duffy (1995) stated that the only type of dysarthria that may result in abnormalities of movement at only one level of speech production is hyperkinetic dysarthria (an involuntary movement disorder), one clinical characteristic of which may be "palatal myoclonus."[21]

Impairment of Velopharyngeal Function in the Dysarthrias

Duffy's 1995 text on motor speech disorders contained extensive information on seven forms of dysarthria: flaccid, spastic, ataxic, hypokinetic, hyperkinetic, unilateral upper motor neuron, and mixed. In his table of etiologic bases for the dysarthrias (pp. 348-349), he listed 23 degenerative diseases, four demyelinating diseases, three muscle diseases (muscular dystrophy, myopathy, and myotonic dystrophy), and two neuromuscular diseases, together with several dozen conditions classified as vascular, traumatic, neoplastic, toxic or metabolic, infectious, inflammatory, anatomic malformation, undetermined etiology, and "other." As detailed as Duffy's table was, it is important to recognize that many of the conditions listed as etiologies are themselves varied in type and severity. For example, there are many forms of muscular dystrophy, at least one of which—oculopharyngeal muscular dystrophy—does not become evident until the fifth or sixth decade of life.

The following is a synopsis of Duffy's (1995) information specific to velopharyngeal function in each of the dysarthrias, based on the categorization systems of Darley, Aronson, and Brown (1969a, 1969b, 1975) and Duffy's own clinical observations in Mayo Clinic patients:

1. Flaccid dysarthria: velopharyngeal inadequacy dependent on site of damage in the final common pathway. Hypernasality, imprecise consonants, nasal emission, short consonants. In unilateral involvement, the velum pulls toward the nonparalyzed side on phonation.
2. Spastic dysarthria: Hypernasality, pressure consonants more severely involved than in other dysarthrias; gag possibly hyperactive, but velar movement may be minimal or slow on phonation.
3. Ataxic dysarthria: Abnormal resonance rare. Infrequent reports of hyponasality, presumably reflecting timing problems between velar and articulatory gestures. Oral examination often normal.
4. Hypokinetic dysarthria: Increased nasal airflow on intended non-nasal consonants; slow velopharyngeal movements in speech.
5. Hyperkinetic dysarthria: Possible palatopharyngeal myoclonus, possibly no effect on speech.
6. Unilateral upper motor neuron dysarthria: "hypernasality" in 11% of Mayo cases. Duffy (1995) attributes motor innervation of the velum only to cranial nerve X (the vagus nerve), but most anatomists currently attribute the motor innervation of the velar musculature to the pharyngeal plexus, receiving fibers from cranial nerves IX (glossopharyngeal) and X (vagus). In addition, cranial nerves VII and XI play a role in velar elevation (Nishio et al., 1976a, 1976b; Zemlin, 1998).
7. Mixed dysarthria: According to Duffy (1995), mixed dysarthrias account for more that 34% of the dysarthric patients seen at the Mayo Clinic, the most common mixture being flaccid and spastic. Clearly, speech symptoms, including velopharyngeal inadequacy, depend on the particular combinations of dysarthria in the individual patient.

When you encounter a patient with velopharyngeal inadequacy of unknown but probable neurogenic origin, you may want to search for information either by specific medical diagnosis or by details of the symptoms in your own patient. Box 8-1 provides a list of medical conditions in which velopharyngeal inadequacy has been documented, although this can only be current up to the date of publication and grows so rapidly that the clinician is advised to conduct an on-line research of the literature rather than rely solely on archival data.

Impairment of Velopharyngeal Function in Apraxia

If apraxia of speech is conceptualized as a problem in the neuromotor programing of articulation, it is reasonable that the programing for the velopharyngeal system (which accomplishes the task of nasal-versus-nonnasal contrasts) could be affected as well as the programming for other articulators. As of this writing, "developmental apraxia of speech" in children is a highly controversial diagnosis, although that controversy will not be covered here. In adults with traumatic brain damage, apraxia of speech is a much better understood phenomenon. There are a few reports of inappropriate nasalization of speech in children with apraxia (Bowman, Parsons, and Morris, 1984; Dabul, 1971; Davison, Razzell, and Watson, 1990; Hall, Hardy, and LaVelle, 1990; Weiss, Gordon, and Lillywhite, 1987; Yoss and Darley, 1974). One report on an adult patient with apraxia (Itoh, Sasanuma, and Ushijima, 1977) described abnormal movements patterns of the velum as well as other articulators, but did not describe perceptual evidence of inadequate velopharyngeal closure. It is of interest that major reviews of the clinical findings in adult apraxia (Duffy, 1995; Rosenbek, 1985) do not mention problems in control of the velopharyngeal mechanism.

For the clinician, the possibility nevertheless remains that one part of the symptomatology in apraxia of speech may be inadequate velopharyngeal closure. In fact, the symptoms may include both "hyponasality" (not enough normal nasal resonance on nasal consonants and vocalic

[21]For the student or new clinician, a complete review of the speech symptoms in the various types of dysarthria as presented by Duffy (1995) or other comprehensive texts on neurologic disorders of speech is a necessary part of professional preparation, but it is not provided here.

Box 8-1 A Sampling of the Categories or Diagnostic Labels Under Which Neuromotor Deficits of Velopharyngeal Function May Be Found in the Literature*

BY TYPE OF DYSARTHRIA (AFTER DUFFY, 1995)

Ataxic (Darley et al., 1969a, 1969b, 1975; Duffy, 1995)
Flaccid (Darley et al., 1969a, 1969b, 1975; Duffy, 1995; Rosenbek and LaPointe, 1985; Wertz, 1985)
Hyperkinetic (Darley et al., 1969a, 1969b, 1975; Rosenbek and LaPointe, 1985)
Hypokinetic (Darley et al., 1969a, 1969b, 1975; Duffy, 1995)
Spastic (Canter, 1967; Darley et al., 1969a, 1969b, 1975; Duffy, 1995; Schweiger, Netsell, and Sommerfeld, 1970; Wertz, 1985)
Mixed (Darley et al., 1969a, 1969b, 1975; Duffy, 1995; Rosenbek and LaPointe, 1985; Wertz, 1985)
Unilateral upper motor neuron (Duffy, 1995)

BY SITE OF DAMAGE

Cerebellar (Darley et al., 1969a, 1969b, 1975)
Chiari malformation type I (Gerard et al., 1992; Pollack, Shprintzen, and Zimmerman-Manchester, 1979)
Malignant brainstem tumor (Lefaivre et al., 1997)
Extrapyramidal (Canter, 1967; Darley et al., 1969a, 1969b, 1975; Randall, Bakes, and Kennedy, 1960; Rosenbek and LaPointe, 1985)
Lower motor neuron (Canter, 1967; Darley et al., 1969a, 1969b, 1975; Davison, Razzell, and Watson, 1990; Rosenbek and LaPointe, 1985; Wertz, 1985)
Upper motor neuron (Darley et al., 1969a, 1969b, 1975; Davison, Razzell, and Watson, 1990; Randall, Bakes, and Kennedy, 1960; Wertz, 1985; Worster-Drought, 1956, 1968)
Pyramidal (Canter, 1967)

BY DISEASE (NOMENCLATURE AS USED IN CITED SOURCES)

Amyotrophic lateral sclerosis (Darley et al., 1969a, 1969b, 1975; Hirose, Kiritani, and Sawashima, 1982; Minami et al., 1975; Randall, Bakes, and Kennedy, 1960; Rosenbek and LaPointe, 1985; Wertz, 1985)
Bulbar palsy (Darley et al., 1969a, 1969b, 1975; Honjow, Isshiki, and Kitajima, 1969; Rosenbek and LaPointe, 1985; Pitt and Ingram, 1975a)
Bulbar poliomyelitis (Blackfield et al., 1962; McWilliams and Musgrave, 1965; Minami et al., 1975; Pitt and Ingram, 1975a; Worster-Drought, 1968)
Chorea (Hoopes et al., 1970a, 1970b; Rosenbek and LaPointe, 1985)
Congenital suprabulbar paresis (Worster-Drought, 1956, 1968)
Dystonia (Hoopes et al., 1970a, 1970b)
Gilles de la Tourette syndrome (Rosenbek and LaPointe, 1985)
Multifocal eosinophilic granuloma (Cohn et al., 1982)
Multiple sclerosis (Rosenbek and LaPointe, 1985)
Muscular dystrophy (McCoy and Zahorski, 1972; Minami et al., 1975; Mullendore and Stoudt, 1961; Randall, Bakes, and Kennedy, 1960; Rosenbek and LaPointe, 1985)
Myasthenia gravis (Canter, 1967; Hagstrom et al., 1979; Honjow, Isshiki, and Kitajima, 1969; Minami et al., 1975; Wolski, 1967)
Myotonic dystrophy (Cadieux et al., 1984; Hillarp et al., 1994; Leach, 1962; Pitt and Ingram, 1975a; Pollack, Shprintzen, and Zimmerman-Manchester, 1979; Salomonson, Kawamoto, and Wilson, 1988; Weinberg et al., 1968)
Neurofibromatosis (Hoopes et al., 1970a, 1970b; Minami et al., 1975; Pollack and Shprintzen, 1981)
Parkinson's disease (Darley 1969a, 1969b, 1975; Duffy, 1995)
Pseudobulbar palsy (Darley 1969a, 1969b, 1975; Hirose, Kiritani, and Sawashima, 1982; Hoopes et al., 1970a, 1970b; Minami et al., 1975; Pitt and Ingram 1975a, 1975b; Pollack, Shprintzen, and Zimmerman-Manchester, 1979; Randall, Bakes, and Kennedy, 1960)
Suprabulbar palsy (Davison, Razzell, and Watson, 1990)
Syringomyelia (Randall, Bakes, and Kennedy, 1960)
Wilson's disease (Rosenbek and LaPointe, 1985)

BY SOME OTHER NAMED SYNDROMES

Fetal anticonvulsant syndrome (Pearl, Dickens, and Latham, 1984)
Moebius syndrome (Davison, Razzell, and Watson, 1990; Henderson, 1939; Languth, 1972; Meyerson and Foushee, 1978; Pitt and Ingram, 1975a, 1975b; Rubin, 1976)
Oculodentodigital syndrome (Pollack, Shprintzen, and Zimmerman-Manchester, 1979)
Sedlackova syndrome or velocardiofacial syndrome (multiple sources, see Chapter 2)

BY LESS SPECIFIC DIAGNOSES

Antenatal infection (Pollack et al., 1979)
Arrested hydrocephalus (Davison, Razzell, and Watson, 1990)
Cerebral palsy (Blackfield et al., 1962; Davison, Razzell, and Watson, 1990; Hardy et al., 1961, 1969; Hegarty, 1960; Heller et al., 1974; Jackson, McGlynn, and Huskie, 1980; Kent and Netsell, 1978; McWilliams and Musgrave, 1965; Netsell, 1969; Owsley et al., 1967; Pitt and Ingram, 1975a; Randall, Bakes, and Kennedy, 1960; Worster-Drought, 1968)
Generalized hypotonia (Davison, Razzell, and Watson, 1990)
Hypoxia (Pollack et al., 1979)
Myopathy (Pollack et al., 1979)
Stroke or "CVA" (Pollack et al., 1979; Wertz, 1985; Yorkston, Beukelman, and Honsinger, 1989)
Trauma (Pollack et al., 1979; Wertz, 1985; Yorkston, Beukelman, and Honsinger, 1989)

*Because authors approach the topic of neuromotor problems in speech from different perspectives, many of these listings are duplicated or overlapping.The student or clinician is encouraged to conduct an on-line search for current information under any selected disease, syndrome, site-of-lesion, etc.

segments) and hypernasality or nasal emission on pressure consonants. As you would expect, treatment of such mixed symptoms is not simple (Hall, Hardy, and LaVelle, 1990).

Impairment of Velopharyngeal Function in Other Conditions

There are some reports in the literature of individuals with various types and degrees of developmental disability and also of individuals with severe hearing loss who manifested inappropriate nasalization of speech (Daly and Johnson, 1974; Heller et al., 1974; Hoopes et al., 1970a, 1970b; McWilliams and Musgrave, 1965). The report of Heller et al. (1974) included individuals with "mental retardation" (n = 4), "emotional disturbance" (n = 6), "neurologic impairment" (n = 15), and "mixed handicap" (n = 17). The 15 patients with velopharyngeal problems of neurological origin were described as having neurological impairment ranging from minimal brain dysfunction (a popular term in the 1970s) to severe cerebral palsy.

Clearly, as our ability to diagnose more subtle problems in velopharyngeal anatomy and function increases, the diagnosis of cases reported in earlier literature becomes increasingly suspect. The article of Heller et al. (1974) may be an example of a clinical report that might have been much different if today's diagnostic armamentaria had been available. Certainly the report of Pruzansky et al. (1977) was restricted by just such limitations. However, the possibility of *nonstructural* impairments or dysfunctions of the velopharyngeal system should always be borne in mind, even in patients with clefts.

Some speakers in the overly large and often amorphous categories of developmental disabilities, as well as those with significant hearing loss, may have genetic or chromosomal abnormalities causing craniofacial disorders in which abnormal velopharyngeal function is a part of the expected symptomatology. For individuals with hearing impairment, a hearing loss of sufficient degree that could easily impair the ability to monitor the nasal-nonnasal contrast in speech would be expected. However, in any summary describing speech problems in individuals with hearing loss, consider the possibility of a coexisting problem such as a structural craniofacial abnormality.

TWO SPECIAL TYPES OF VELOPHARYNGEAL INADEQUACY OF HETEROGENEOUS OR UNKNOWN ETIOLOGY

It is important for you to know that *neither* of the next two topics actually constitutes a diagnostic category because the etiologies of these problems are typically mixed or unknown.

Stress Velopharyngeal Incompetency in Wind Instrument Players

In 1970 Weber and Chase described an oboe player who had nasal air loss after 10 minutes of continuous play. The authors labeled this phenomenon as "stress velopharyngeal incompetence." Nasal air loss did not occur in this musician's speech, and no structural abnormality of the velopharyngeal mechanism was detected on oral examination, oral endoscopy, or cineradiographic examination. Palatal length was reported as 30 mm and pharyngeal depth 31 mm, suggesting a possibility of a marginal mechanism (Subtelny, 1957), although the authors did not comment on this point. There have been several subsequent reports of wind instrument players who had incomplete velopharyngeal closure after a period of play (Argamaso and Shprintzen, 1983; Conley, Beecher, and Marks, 1995; Dibbell, Ewanowski, and Carter, 1979; Gordon, Astrachan, and Yanagisawa, 1994; Massengill and Quinn, 1974; Peterson-Falzone, 1985). The physical findings in these cases varied, and the documentation of each patient did not always include nasopharyngoscopy. The case of Massengill and Quinn was ascribed to adenoid involution, but such involution is normal. This is the only case in which there was also some perceptual evidence of velopharyngeal inadequacy in speech. One of the two cases reported by Dibbell, Ewanowski, and Carter (1979) had an obvious submucous cleft, whereas the other had a reportedly normal palate but the uvula herniated into the nasopharynx under the stress of wind instrument playing. The case reported by Peterson-Falzone (1985) had an occult submucous defect; the case reported Argamaso and Shprintzen was one of posttonsillectomy scarring. In the two latest reports (Conley, Beecher, and Marks, 1995; Gordon, Astrachan, and Yanagisawa, 1994) there was no sign of an occult cleft on endoscopy but there was a small velopharyngeal gap on playing. The musicians seen by Massengill and Quinn (1974) and by Conley, Beecher, and Marks (1994) were amateur musicians, and the treatment approach was use of palatal exercise. Each of the other reported cases was of a professional musician or someone in training for such a career, playing for long periods of time,[22] and in each case surgical management was carried out (Argamaso and Shprintzen, 1983; Dibbell, Ewanowski, and Carter, 1979; Gordon, Astrachan, and Yanagisawa, 1994; Peterson-Falzone, 1985; Weber and Chase, 1970).

Phoneme-Specific Nasal Emission

There are speakers in whom the velopharyngeal port is capable of complete closure in speech, even at the relatively rapid rate required in normal conversational speech, but in whom the mechanism does not close on specific pressure consonants. These speakers show adequate closure of the mechanism on other pressure consonants and no hypernasal resonance. In 1972 Lawson et al., writing about effects of adenoidectomy on children with potential velopharyngeal problems, observed "For some patients, the nasal emission appeared only on specific phonemes or combinations." Sporadic references to this phenomenon have appeared in

[22]See Dibbell, Ewanowski, and Carter (1979) for a table listing the intraoral pressure requirements for the playing of wind instruments.

the literature since at least 1937 (Beebe, 1946; Berry and Eisenson, 1942, 1956; Edwards and Shriberg, 1983; Hall and Tomblin, 1975; Powers, 1971; Van Dantzig, 1940; Van Riper, 1972; West and Ansberry, 1968; West, Ansberry, and Carr, 1957; West, Kennedy, and Carr, 1937, 1947). Peterson (1975) described nasal emission as a component of the misarticulation of sibilants and affricates both in children who had been treated for cleft palate and in children with no history of palatal structural problems. The lateral radiographs taken on these children during production of sustained sibilants showed the tongue to be retracted and elevated. In 1981 Trost described the "posterior nasal fricative" and commented that this articulation had "a notable occurrence in non-cleft velopharyngeal disorders, including the neurogenic problems of the dysarthrias and phoneme-specific velopharyngeal inadequacy." She used the latter term ". . . to define the occurrence of nasal air emission and audible posterior frication on certain pressure consonants only." Since the Trost article (1981), this phenomenon has become commonly labeled in the literature as "phoneme-specific nasal emission" or sometimes "phoneme-specific velopharyngeal inadequacy."

In some speakers who exhibit this behavior, the nasal emission simply accompanies oral placement of a pressure consonant, whereas in others either nasal emission or a posterior nasal fricative as described by Trost (1981) completely replaces the oral placement. In the latter case a child may actually be observed to try to produce /s/ (or whatever his own "vulnerable" consonant[s] may be) with the lips closed, completely prohibiting oral direction of the air stream. Peterson-Falzone and Graham (1990) documented various patterns of phoneme-specific use of nasal emission or nasal frication in 32 children, 13 of whom had histories of repaired clefts or other structural abnormalities of the velopharyngeal mechanism and 19 of whom had normal oral mechanisms. As in previous reports (Peterson, 1975; Trost, 1981), the phonemes that were most often vulnerable were the sibilants alone or the sibilants plus affricates. Radiographic and endoscopic imaging confirmed the perceptual impression that the velopharyngeal system consistently closed on all other pressure consonants. Some of these children had substantial delays in phonological development, but others did not.

The pattern of phoneme-specific nasal emission and the variety of patients in whom this phenomenon has been observed certainly indicates that the etiology is heterogeneous. In patients with repaired clefts or other structural abnormalities of the velopharyngeal system, it seems reasonable that this articulatory behavior represents a vestige from a time when the velopharyngeal system could not effectively close for any pressure consonants. Many of these children, although not all, have a history of early ear disease and hearing loss (Peterson-Falzone and Graham, 1990). Either a previous history of true physiological velopharyngeal inadequacy or hearing loss could easily be a basis for "mislearning" of how to produce a normal sibilant or affricate or other fricatives. We do not yet know what may explain its occurrence in children without such histories. Fortunately, this particular speech behavior is typically responsive to appropriate speech therapy (Hall and Tomblin, 1975; Peterson-Falzone and Graham, 1990). Even more important, such behaviors are not changed through palatal surgery because they are learned patterns.[23]

[23]Similarly, the compensatory articulations often heard in speakers with repaired clefts cannot be "repaired" with further palatal surgery but require speech therapy for acquisition of oral placements to replace the glottal and pharyngeal placements.

REFERENCES

Ardran GM, and Kemp FH: Radiology in the study of neurological diseases affecting the pharynx and larynx. *Proceedings of the Royal Society of Medicine* 18:641-644, 1975.

Argamaso RV, and Shprintzen RJ: Fanfare for a pharyngeal flap. Videotape presentation before the American Cleft Palate Association, Denver, 1983.

Ashley FL, Sloan RF, Hahn E, Hanafee W, and Miethke J: Cinefluorographic study of palatal incompetency cases during deglutition and phonation. *Plastic and Reconstructive Surgery* 28:347-364, 1961.

Auberge C, Ponsot G, Gayraud P, Bouygues D, and Arthuis M: Les hemiparalysies velopalatines isolees et adquises chez l'enfant. *Archives Francaises de Pediatre* 3:283-286, 1979.

Beebe HH: Sigmatismus nasalis. *Journal of Speech Disorders* 11:35-37, 1946.

Berry MF, and Eisenson J: *The defective in speech.* New York: Appleton-Century-Crofts, 1942.

Berry MF, and Eisenson J: *Speech disorders, principles, and practices of therapy.* New York: Appleton-Century-Crofts, 1956.

Blackfield HM, Miller ER, Owsley JQ, and Lawson LI: Cinefluorographic evaluation of patients with velopharyngeal dysfunction in the absence of overt cleft palate. *Plastic and Reconstructive Surgery* 30:441-451, 1962.

Bowman SN, Parsons CL, and Morris DA: Inconsistency of phonological errors in developmental verbal dyspraxic children as a factor of linguistic task and performance load. *Australian Journal of Human Communication Disorders* 12:109-119, 1984.

Cadieux RJ, Kales A, McGlynn TJ, Jackson D, Manders EK, and Simmonds MA: Sleep apnea precipitated by pharyngeal surgery in a patient with myotonic dystrophy. *Archives of Otolaryngology* 110:611-613, 1984.

Calnan JS: Movements of the soft palate. *British Journal of Plastic Surgery* 5:286-296, 1953.

Calnan JS: Submucous cleft palate. *British Journal of Plastic Surgery* 7:264-282, 1954.

Calnan JS: Diagnosis, prognosis, and treatment of "palato-pharyngeal incompetence," with special reference to radiographic investigations. *British Journal of Plastic Surgery* 8:265-282, 1956.

Calnan JS: Modern views on Passavant's ridge. *British Journal of Plastic Surgery* 10:89-113, 1957a.

Calnan JS: The investigation of nasality (nasal escape) in speech. *Speech* 21:59-74, 1957b.

Calnan JS: The surgical treatment of nasal speech disorders. *Annals of the Royal College of Surgeons of England* 25:119-141, 1959.

Calnan JS: Palatopharyngeal incompetence in speech. In Pruzansky S (ed.): *Congenital anomalies of the face and associated structures.* Springfield (IL): CC Thomas, 1961a.

Calnan JS: The mobility of the soft palate: a radiological and statistical study. *British Journal of Plastic Surgery* 14:33-38, 1961b.

Calnan JS: Congenital large pharynx: a new syndrome with a report of 41 personal cases. *British Journal of Plastic Surgery* 24: 263-271, 1971a.

Calnan JS: Permanent nasal escape in speech after adenoidectomy. *British Journal of Plastic Surgery* 24:197-204, 1971b.

Calnan JS: Surgery for speech. In Calnan JS (ed.): *Recent advances in plastic surgery, I.* Edinburgh: Churchill Livingstone, 1976, pp. 39-57.

Canter C: Neuromotor pathologies of speech. *American Journal of Physical Medicine* 46:659-666, 1967.

Chaco J, and Yules R: Velopharyngeal incompetence post tonsillo-adenoidectomy. *Acta Oto-Laryngologica* 68:276-278, 1969.

Cohn ER, Garver KL, Metz HC, McWilliams BJ, Skolnick ML, and Garrett WS: Velopharyngeal incompetence in a patient with multifocal eosinophilic granuloma (Hand-Schuller-Christian disease). *Journal of Speech and Hearing Disorders* 47:320-323, 1982.

Conley SF, Beecher RB, and Marks S: Stress velopharyngeal incompetence in an adolescent trumpet player. *Annals of Otology, Rhinology, and Laryngology* 104:715-717, 1995.

Cotton R, and Nuwayhid N: Velopharyngeal insufficiency. In Bluestone C, and Stool S (eds.): *Pediatric otolaryngology.* Volume 2. Philadelphia: WB Saunders, 1983, pp. 1521-1542.

Crikelair GF, Kastein S, Fowler EP, and Cosman B: Velar dysfunction in the absence of cleft palate. *New York State Journal of Medicine* January 15:263-269, 1964.

Croft CB, Shprintzen RJ, and Ruben RJ: Hypernasal speech following adenotonsillectomy. *Otolaryngology–Head and Neck Surgery* 89:179-188, 1981.

Crovetto MA, Aguirre JM, Municio A, Perez-Rojo A, and Saint-Gerons S: Idiopathic paralysis of the palate in childhood. *British Journal of Oral and Maxillofacial Surgery* 26:241-243, 1988.

Dabul BL: Lingual incoordination-language delay. *California Journal of Communication Disorders* 2:30-33, 1971.

Daly DA, and Johnson HP: Instrumental modification of hypernasal voice quality in retarded children: case reports. *Journal of Speech and Hearing Disorders* 39:500-507, 1974.

Darley FL, Aronson AE, and Brown J: Clusters of deviant diagnostic patterns of dysarthria. *Journal of Speech and Hearing Research* 12:462-496, 1969a.

Darley FL, Aronson AE, and Brown J: Differential diagnostic patterns of dysarthria. *Journal of Speech and Hearing Research* 12:246-269, 1969b.

Darley FL, Aronson AE, and Brown J: *Motor speech disorders.* Philadelphia: WB Saunders, 1975.

Davison PM, Razzell RE, and Watson ACH: The role of pharyngoplasty in congenital neurogenic speech disorders. *British Journal of Plastic Surgery* 43:187-196, 1990.

Dibbell DG, Ewanowski S, and Carter WL: Successful correction of velopharyngeal stress incompetence in musicians playing wind instruments. *Plastic and Reconstructive Surgery* 64:662-664, 1979.

Duffy JR: *Motor speech disorders: substrates, differential diagnosis, and management.* St. Louis: Mosby, 1995.

Dunn DH: Glossopharyngeal neuropathy. *Southern Medical Journal* 76:542, 1983.

Edin M, Sveger T, Tegner H, and Tjernstrom O: Isolated temporary pharyngeal paralysis in childhood. *Lancet* 1:1047-1048, 1976.

Edwards ML, and Shriberg LD: *Phonology: applications in communication disorders.* San Diego (CA): College-Hill Press, 1983.

Finkelstein Y, Nachmani A, and Ophir D: The functional role of the tonsils in speech. *Archives of Otolaryngology, Head and Neck Surgery* 120:846-851, 1994.

Finkelstein Y, Berger G, Nachmani A, and Ophir D: The functional role of the adenoids in speech. *International Journal of Pediatric Otorhinolaryngology* 34:61-74, 1996.

Fletcher SG: Hypernasal voice as an indication of regional growth and developmental disturbance. *Logos* 3:3-12, 1960.

Folkins J: Velopharyngeal nomenclature: incompetence, inadequacy, insufficiency, and dysfunction. *Cleft Palate Journal* 25:413-416, 1988.

Gerard CL, Dugas M, Narcy P, and Hertz-Pannier J: Chiari malformation type I in a child with velopharyngeal insufficiency. *Developmental Medicine and Child Neurology* 34:174-176, 1992.

Gereau SA, and Shprintzen RJ: The role of adenoids in the development of normal speech following palate repair. *Laryngoscope* 98:299-303, 1988.

Goode RI, and Ross J: Velopharyngeal insufficiency after adenoidectomy. *Archives of Otolaryngology* 96:223-226, 1972.

Gordon NA, Astrachan D, and Yanagisawa E: Videoendoscopic diagnosis and correction of velopharyngeal stress incompetence in a bassoonist. *Annals of Otology, Rhinology, and Laryngology* 103:595-600, 1994.

Greene MCL: Speech of children before and after removal of tonsils and adenoids. *Journal of Speech and Hearing Disorders* 22:361-370, 1957.

Hagstrom W, Parsons R, Landa S, and Robson M: Familial velopharyngeal incompetence caused by myasthenia gravis. *Annals of Plastic Surgery* 3:555-557, 1979.

Hall PK, and Tomblin JB: Case study: therapy procedures and remediation of a nasal lisp. *Language, Speech, and Hearing Services in Schools* 6:29-32, 1975.

Hall PK, Hardy JC, and LaVelle WE: A child with signs of developmental apraxia of speech with whom a palatal lift prosthesis was used to manage palatal dysfunction. *Journal of Speech and Hearing Disorders* 55:454-460, 1990.

Handelman CS, and Osborne GS: Growth of the nasopharynx and adenoid development from one to eighteen years. *Angle Orthodontist* 46:243-259, 1976.

Handelman CS, and Pruzansky S: The size of the adenoids in normal and C.P.I. children. Proceedings of the International Association of Dental Research, Washington (DC), 1967.

Hardy JC, Rembolt R, Spriestersbach DC, and Jayapathy B: Surgical management of palatal paresis and speech problems in cerebral palsy: a preliminary report. *Journal of Speech and Hearing Disorders* 26:320-325, 1961.

Hardy JC, Netsell R, Schweiger J, and Morris HL: Management of velopharyngeal dysfunction in cerebral palsy. *Journal of Speech and Hearing Disorders* 34:123-127, 1969.

Hegarty IE: Case study of velar and facial paralysis. *Journal of Speech and Hearing Disorders* 25:409-411, 1960.

Heller JC, Gens GW, Moe DG, and Lewin ML: Velopharyngeal insufficiency in patients with neurologic, emotional and mental disorders. *Journal of Speech and Hearing Disorders* 39:350-359, 1974.

Henderson J: The congenital facial diplegia syndrome: clinical features, pathology and etiology. *Brain* 62:381-403, 1939.

Hillarp B, Ekberg O, Jacobsson S, Nylander G, and Aberg M: Myotonic dystrophy revealed in videoradiography of deglutition and speech in adult patients with velopharyngeal insufficiency: presentation of four cases. *Cleft Palate–Craniofacial Journal* 31:125-133, 1994.

Hirose H, Kiritani S, and Sawashima M: Patterns of dysarthric movement in patients with amyotrophic lateral sclerosis and pseudobulbar palsy. *Folia Phoniatrica* 34:106-112, 1982.

Honjow I, Isshiki N, and Kitajima K: Congenital and acquired hypernasalities. *Folia Phoniatrica* 21:266-276, 1969.

Hoopes JE, Dellon AL, Fabrikant JI, Edgerton MT, and Soliman AH: Cineradiographic definition of the functional anatomy and pathophysiology of the velopharynx. *Cleft Palate Journal* 7:443-453, 1970a.

Hoopes JE, Dellon AL, Fabrikant JI, and Soliman AH: Idiopathic hypernasality: cineradiographic evaluation and etiologic considerations. *Journal of Speech and Hearing Disorders* 35:44-50, 1970b.

Itoh M, Sasanuma S, and Ushijima T: Velar movements during speech in a patient with apraxia of speech. *Annual Bulletin of the Research Institute of Logopedics and Phoniatry, University of Tokyo* 11:67-75, 1977.

Jackson IT, McGlynn MJ, and Huskie CF: Velopharyngeal incompetence in the absence of cleft palate: results of treatment in 20 cases. *Plastic and Reconstructive Surgery* 66:211-213, 1980.

Jafek BW, Balkany TJ, Wong ML, and Bryant K: Surgical management of the hypodynamic palate. *Archives of Otolaryngology* 105:347-350, 1979.

Johns DF: Surgical and prosthetic management of neurogenic velopharyngeal incompetency in dysarthria. In Johns DF (ed.): *Clinical management of neurogenic communicative disorders.* 2nd ed. Boston: Little, Brown, 1985, pp. 153-177.

Kaplan EN: The occult submucous cleft palate. *Cleft Palate Journal* 12:356-368, 1975.

Kelly AB: Congenital insufficiency of the palate. *Journal of Laryngology, Rhinology, and Otology* 25:281-358, 1910.

Kent RD, and Netsell R: Articulatory abnormalities in athetoid cerebral palsy. *Journal of Speech and Hearing Disorders* 43:353-373, 1978.

Keogh C: Paralysis of the pharynx. *Journal of Laryngology and Otology* 70:344-351, 1956.

Kummer AW, Billmire DA, and Myer CM III: Hypertrophic tonsils: the effect on resonance and velopharyngeal closure. *Plastic and Reconstructive Surgery* 91:608-611, 1993.

Languth P: Speech with palatal dysfunction. *Proceedings of the Royal Society of Medicine* 65:413-416, 1972.

Lapresle J, Lasjunias P, and Thevenier D: Attentitetransitoire des IX, X et XII ainsi que du VII gauches au decours d'une angiographie. *Revue Neurologique* (Paris) 11:787-791, 1980.

Lawshe BS, Hardy JC, Schweiger JW, and Van Allen MW: Management of a patient with velopharyngeal incompetency of undetermined origin. *Journal of Speech and Hearing Disorders* 36:547-551, 1971.

Lawson LI, Chierici G, Castro A, Harvold EP, Miller E, and Owsley JQ: Effects of adenoidectomy on the speech of children with potential velopharyngeal dysfunction. *Journal of Speech and Hearing Disorders* 37:390-402, 1972.

Leach W: Generalized muscular diseases presenting as pharyngeal dysphagia. *Journal of Laryngology and Otology* 76:237-240, 1962.

Lefaivre J-F, Cohen SR, Riski JE, and Burstein FD: Velopharyngeal incompetence as the presenting symptom of malignant brainstem tumor. *Cleft Palate–Craniofacial Journal* 34:154-158, 1997.

Linder-Aronson S: Adenoids—their effect on mode of breathing and nasal airflow and their relationship to characteristics of the facial skeleton and the dentition. *Acta Otolaryngologica Supplement* 265, 1970.

Linder-Aronson S, and Leighton BC: A longitudinal study of the development of the posterior nasopharyngeal wall between 3 and 16 years of age. *European Journal of Orthodontics* 5:47-58, 1983.

MacKenzie-Stepner K, Witzel MA, Stringer DA, and Laskin R: Velopharyngeal insufficiency due to hypertrophic tonsils: a report of two cases. *International Journal of Pediatric Otorhinolaryngology* 14:57-63, 1987.

Mason RM, and Warren DW: Adenoid involution and developing hypernasality in cleft palate. *Journal of Speech and Hearing Disorders* 45:469-480, 1980.

Massengill R, and Quinn G: Adenoidal hypertrophy, velopharyngeal incompetence, and sucking exercises: a two year follow-up case report. *Cleft Palate Journal* 11:196-199, 1974.

Mazaheri M, Millard RT, and Erickson DM: Cineradiographic comparison of normal to noncleft subjects with velopharyngeal inadequacy. *Cleft Palate Journal* 1:199-209, 1964.

McCoy F, and Zahorski C: A new approach to the elusive dynamic pharyngeal flap. *Plastic and Reconstructive Surgery* 49:160-164, 1972.

McWilliams BJ, and Musgrave R: Differential diagnosis and management of hypernasal voices in children. *Transactions of the American Academic of Ophthalmology and Otolaryngology* March-April:322-331, 1965.

Meyerson MD, and Foushee D: Speech, language and hearing in Moebius syndrome: a study of 22 patients. *Developmental Medicine and Child Neurology* 20:357-365, 1978.

Minami RT, Kaplan EN, Wu G, and Jobe RP: Velopharyngeal incompetence without overt cleft palate. *Plastic and Reconstructive Surgery* 55:573-587, 1975.

Morris HL: The speech pathologist looks at the tonsils and the adenoids. *Annals of Otology, Rhinology, and Laryngology* 84(Supplement 19):63-66, 1975.

Morris HL, Krueger L, and Bumsted R: Indications of congenital palatal incompetence before diagnosis. *Annals of Otology, Rhinology, and Laryngology* 91:115-118, 1982.

Morris HL, Miller Wroblewski SK, Brown CK, and Van Demark DR: Velar-pharyngeal status in cleft patients with expected adenoidal involution. *Annals of Otology, Rhinology, and Laryngology* 99:432-437, 1990.

Moss M: Malformations of the skull base associated with cleft palate deformity. *Plastic and Reconstructive Surgery* 17:226-234, 1956.

Mullendore J, and Stoudt R: Speech patterns of muscular dystrophic individuals. *Journal of Speech and Hearing Disorders* 26:252-257, 1961.

Netsell R: Evaluation of velopharyngeal function in dysarthria. *Journal of Speech and Hearing Disorders* 34:113-122, 1969.

Nishio J, Matsuya T, Ibuki K, and Miyazaki T: Roles of the facial, glossopharyngeal and vagus nerves in velopharyngeal movement. *Cleft Palate Journal* 13:201-214, 1976a.

Nishio J, Matsuya T, Machida J, and Miyazaki T: The motor nerve supply of the velopharyngeal muscles. *Cleft Palate Journal* 13:20-30, 1976b.

Nussey AM: Paralysis of palate in a child. *British Medical Journal* 2:165-166, 1977.

Osborne GS: The prevalence of anomalies of the upper cervical vertebrae in patients with cranio-facial malformations and their effect on osseous nasopharyngeal depth [dissertation]. Carbondale: Southern Illinois University, 1968.

Osborne GS, Pruzansky S, and Koepp-Baker H: Upper cervical spine anomalies and osseous nasopharyngeal depth. *Journal of Speech and Hearing Research* 14:14-22, 1971.

Owsley JQ, Chierici G, Miller ER, Lawson LI, and Blackfield HM: Cephalometric evaluation of palatal dysfunction in patients without cleft palate. *Plastic and Reconstructive Surgery* 39:562-568, 1967.

Paradise JL: Tonsillectomy and adenoidectomy. In Bluestone C, and Stool S (eds.): *Pediatric otorhinolaryngology.* Volume 2. Philadelphia: WB Saunders, 1983, pp. 992-1006.

Passavant G: Ueber die Beseitigung der naselnden Sprache bei angeborenen Spalten des harten und Weichen Gaumens. *Archiv fuer Klinisch Chirurgie* 6:333-349, 1865.

Pearl KN, Dickens S, and Latham P: Functional palatal incompetence in the fetal anticonvulsant syndrome. *Archives of Disease in Childhood* 59:989-990, 1984.

Peterson SJ: Nasal emission as a component of the misarticulation of sibilants and affricates. *Journal of Speech and Hearing Disorders* 40:106-114, 1975.

Peterson-Falzone SJ: Velopharyngeal inadequacy in the absence of overt cleft palate. *Journal of Craniofacial Genetics and Developmental Biology Supplement* 1:97-124, 1985.

Peterson-Falzone SJ, and Graham MS: Phoneme-specific nasal emission in children with and without physical anomalies of the velopharyngeal mechanism. *Journal of Speech and Hearing Disorders* 55:132-139, 1990.

Peyton W: The dimensions and growth of the palate in the normal infant and in the infant with gross maldevelopment of the upper lip and palate. *Archives of Surgery* 22:704-737, 1931.

Pitt M, and Ingram TTS: The radiology of speech disorders in childhood. I: Disorders and their study. *Radiography* 41:53-59, 1975a.

Pitt M, and Ingram TTS: The radiology of speech disorders in childhood. II: Radiology in the diagnosis of speech disorders. *Radiography* 41:90-104, 1975b.

Pollack MA, and Shprintzen RJ: Velopharyngeal insufficiency in neurofibromatosis. *International Journal of Pediatric Otorhinolaryngology* 3:257-262, 1981.

Pollack MA, Shprintzen RJ, and Zimmerman-Manchester KL: Velopharyngeal insufficiency: the neurological perspective: a report of 32 cases. *Developmental Medicine and Child Neurology* 21:194-201, 1979.

Powers MH: Functional disorders of articulation—symptomatology and etiology. In Travis LE (ed.): *Handbook of speech pathology.* New York: Appleton-Century-Crofts, 1971, pp. 837-876.

Pruzansky S: Roentgencephalometric studies of tonsils and adenoids in normal and pathologic states. *Annals of Otology, Rhinology, and Laryngology* 84(Supplement 19):55-62, 1975.

Pruzansky S, Peterson-Falzone SJ, Laffer J, and Parris P: Hypernasality I the absence of overt cleft: commentary on nomenclature, diagnosis, classification, and research design. Proceedings of the 3rd International Congress on Cleft Palate and Related Craniofacial Anomalies, Toronto, 1977.

Psaume J: Contribution a l'etude du squelette du bec de lievre et de la division palatine non-operes [dissertation]. Paris, 1950.

Randall P, Bakes F, and Kennedy C: Cleft palate-type speech in the absence of cleft palate. *Plastic and Reconstructive Surgery* 25:484-495, 1960.

Ren Y-F, Isberg A, and Henningsson G: Velopharyngeal incompetence and persistent hypernasality in children without palatal defect. *Cleft Palate–Craniofacial Journal* 32:476-482, 1995.

Ricketts RM: The cranial base and soft structures in cleft palate speech and breathing. *Plastic and Reconstructive Surgery* 14:47-61, 1954.

Roberton DM, and Mellor DH: Asymmetrical palatal paresis in childhood: a transient mononeuropathy? *Developmental Medicine and Child Neurology* 24:842-846, 1982.

Rosenbek JC: Treating apraxia of speech. In Johns DF (ed.): *Clinical management of neurogenic communicative disorders.* 2nd ed. Boston: Little, Brown, 1985, pp. 267-312.

Rosenbek JC, and LaPointe LL: The dysarthrias: description, diagnosis, and treatment. In Johns D (ed.): *Clinical management of neurogenic communicative disorders.* 2nd ed. Boston: Little, Brown, 1985, pp. 95-152.

Ross RB, and Lindsay W: The cervical vertebrae as a factor in the etiology of cleft palate. *Cleft Palate Journal* 2:273-281, 1965.

Rubin L: The Moebius syndrome: bilateral facial diplegia. *Clinics in Plastic Surgery* 3:625-636, 1976.

Salomonson J, Kawamoto H, and Wilson L: Velopharyngeal incompetence as the presenting symptom of myotonic dystrophy. *Cleft Palate Journal* 25:296-300, 1988.

Schweiger J, Netsell R, and Sommerfeld R: Prosthetic management and speech improvement in individuals with dysarthria of the palate. *Journal of the American Dental Association* 80:1348-1353, 1970.

Seid AB: Velopharyngeal insufficiency versus adenoidectomy for obstructive apnea: a quandary. *Cleft Palate Journal* 27:200-202, 1990.

Shapiro RS: Velopharyngeal insufficiency starting at puberty without adenoidectomy. *International Journal of Pediatric Otorhinolaryngology* 2:255-260, 1980.

Shprintzen RJ, Sher AE, and Croft CB: Hypernasal speech caused by tonsillar hypertrophy. *International Journal of Pediatric Otorhinolaryngology* 14:45-56, 1987.

Shprintzen RJ, Rakoff SJ, Skolnick ML, and Lavorato AS: Incongruous movements of the velum and lateral pharyngeal walls. *Cleft Palate Journal* 14:148-157, 1977.

Spauwen PHM: Het congenitaal te korte verhemelte. *Nederlands Tijdschrift voor Geneeskundf* 132:965-967, 1988.

Stueber K, and Wilhelmsen HR: Use of the pharyngeal flap in the treatment of congenital velopharyngeal incompetence. *Plastic and Reconstructive Surgery* 73:219-222, 1984.

Sturim HS, and Jacob CT: Teflon pharyngoplasty. *Plastic and Reconstructive Surgery* 49:180-185, 1972.

Subtelny JD: Width of the nasopharynx and related anatomic structures in normal and unoperated cleft palate children. *American Journal of Orthodontia* 41:889-909, 1955.

Subtelny JD: A cephalometric study of the growth of the soft palate. *Plastic and Reconstructive Surgery* 19:49-62, 1957.

Subtelny JD, and Koepp-Baker H: The significance of adenoid tissue in velopharyngeal function. *Plastic and Reconstructive Surgery* 71:235-250, 1956.

Sullivan JL, and Carlson CB: Isolated temporary pharyngeal paralysis in childhood [letter]. *Lancet* 2:863, 1976.

Trost JE: Articulatory additions to the classical description of the speech of persons with cleft palate. *Cleft Palate Journal* 18:193-203, 1981.

Van Dantzig G: The nomenclature of certain forms of sigmatism. *Journal of Speech Disorders* 5:209-210, 1940.

Van Riper CR: *Speech correction: principles and methods.* 5th ed. Englewood Cliffs (NJ): Prentice-Hall, 1972.

Wardill W: Cleft palate. *British Journal of Surgery* 16:127-148, 1928.

Warren DW, Bevin A, and Winslow R: Posterior pillar webbing and palatopharyngeus displacement: possible causes of congenital incompetence. *Cleft Palate Journal* 15:68-72, 1978.

Weber J, and Chase RA: Stress velopharyngeal incompetence in an oboe player. *Cleft Palate Journal* 7:858-861, 1970.

Weimert TA: Evaluation of the upper airway in children. *Ear, Nose, and Throat Journal* 66:196-200, 1987.

Weinberg B, Bosma JF, Shanks JC, and DeMyer W: Myotonic dystrophy initially manifested by speech disability. *Journal of Speech and Hearing Disorders* 33:51-59, 1968.

Weiss CE, Gordon ME, and Lillywhite HS: *Clinical management of articulatory and phonologic disorders.* Baltimore: Williams & Wilkins, 1987.

Wertz RT: Neuropathologies of speech and language: an introduction to patient management. In Johns D (ed.), *Clinical management of neurogenic communicative disorders.* 2nd ed. Boston: Little, Brown, 1985, pp. 1-96.

West R, and Ansberry M: *The rehabilitation of speech.* New York: Harper & Row, 1968.

West R, Ansberry M, and Carr A: *The rehabilitation of speech.* New York: Harper & Row, 1957.

West R, Kennedy L, and Carr A: *The rehabilitation of speech.* New York: Harper & Row, 1937.

West R, Kennedy L, and Carr A: *The rehabilitation of speech.* New York: Harper & Row, 1947.

Wharton P, and Mowrer DE: Prevalence of cleft uvula among school children in kindergarten through grade five. *Cleft Palate–Craniofacial Journal* 29:10-12, 1992.

Winters H: Some historical remarks on congenital short palate. *British Journal of Plastic Surgery* 19:308-312, 1966.

Winters H: *Congenital short palate* [monograph]. Lochem: Kerkard, 1975.

Witzel MA, Rich RH, Margar-Bacal F, and Cox C: Velopharyngeal insufficiency after adenoidectomy: an 8-year review. *International Journal of Pediatric Otorhinolaryngology* 11:15-20, 1986.

Wolski W: Hypernasality as the presenting symptom of myasthenia gravis. *Journal of Speech and Hearing Disorders* 32:36-38, 1967.

Worster-Drought C: Congenital suprabulbar paresis. *Journal of Laryngology and Otology* 70:453-463, 1956.

Worster-Drought C: Speech disorders in children. *Developmental Medicine and Child Neurology* 10:427-440, 1968.

Yorkston KM, Beukelman DR, and Honsinger MJ: Perceived articulatory adequacy and velopharyngeal function in dysarthric speakers. *Archives of Physical Medicine and Rehabilitation* 70:313-317, 1989.

Yoss KA, and Darley FL: Developmental apraxia of speech in children with defective articulation. *Journal of Speech and Hearing Research* 17:399-416, 1974.

Zemlin WR: *Speech and hearing science: anatomy and physiology.* 4th ed. Needham Heights, MA: Allyn & Bacon, 1998.

SUPPLEMENTARY READING LIST

Cheng M-C, Enlow DH, Papsidero M, Broadbent HH Jr, Oyen O, and Sabat M: Developmental effects of impaired breathing in the face of the growing child. *The Angle Orthodontist* 58:309-320, 1988.

Coccaro PJ, and Coccaro PJ Jr: Dental development and the pharyngeal lymphoid tissue. *Otolaryngologic Clinics of North America* 20:241-257, 1987.

Harvold EP, Chierici G, and Vargervik K: Experiments on the development of dental malocclusions. *American Journal of Orthodontics* 61:39-44, 1972.

Linder-Aronson S: Dimensions of the face and palate in nose breathers habitual mouth breathers. *Odontologisk Revy* 14:187-200, 1963.

Linder-Aronson S: Respiratory function in relation to facial morphology and the dentition. *British Journal of Orthodontics* 6:59-71, 1979.

Linder-Aronson S, and Backstrom A: A comparison between mouth and nose breathers with respect to occlusion and facial dimensions. *Odontologisk Revy* 11:343-376, 1960.

McNamara J (ed.): *Naso-respiratory function and craniofacial growth.* Monograph 9, Craniofacial Growth Series, Center for Human Growth and Development. Ann Arbor: University of Michigan, 1979.

McNamara J: Influence of respiratory pattern on craniofacial growth. *Angle Orthodontist* 51:269-300, 1981.

O'Ryan F, Gallagher D, LeBanc J, and Epker B: The relation between nasorespiratory function and dentofacial morphology: a review. *American Journal of Orthodontics* 83:403-410, 1982.

Quick CA, and Gundlach KKH: Adenoid facies. *Laryngoscope* 88:327-333, 1978.

Warren DW, Duany I, and Fischer N: Nasal pathway resistance in normal and cleft lip and palate subjects. *Cleft Palate Journal* 6:134-140, 1969.

Chapter 9

Assessment of Speech-Language Problems

Differential diagnosis of articulation and resonance problems in children with cleft palate requires a thorough understanding of oropharyngeal anatomy and physiology. Although many of the tests and procedures used to assess performance in these children can be used to examine any child's speech production patterns, the nature of the disorders in this population must be carefully examined because a myriad of factors can contribute to the error patterns. It is often assumed that the primary goal in assessment of children with palatal clefts is identifying and treating the speech production problems associated with velopharyngeal inadequacy. This is undoubtedly true for many children; however, factors such as dental occlusion, palatal fistulae, and learning will also play a role in the assessment. The inexperienced clinician may hear audible nasal emission and assume that velopharyngeal inadequacy exists. The experienced clinician knows that certain patterns of audible nasal emission may be more indicative of a palatal fistula or may reflect a learned behavior. The more knowledgeable a clinician is about clefts and their associated problems, the more successful he or she is likely to be in accurately diagnosing the problem.

Children with cleft lip and palate provide a unique opportunity to explore the interaction between anatomical and physiological deficits and speech learning. The impact of a palatal cleft can vary dramatically across individuals even when the severity of the cleft and surgical management regimens are similar. A palatal cleft that might have negligible impact on speech production for one child can have a profound impact for another because of the way the cleft interacts with other oropharyngeal structures and because of differences between the children with regard to learning style. Velopharyngeal inadequacy will lead some children, but not all, to adopt compensatory articulations. Poor dental and occlusal status that results in oral distortion of sibilant consonants will lead some children, but not all, to adaptive articulations. The adaptations and compensations that these children produce offer insight into the flexibility of the speech production mechanism.

As you proceed through this chapter, remember that the evaluation of a patient with cleft lip and palate is an interdisciplinary effort, and findings contributed by all team members will be used in planning comprehensive services for the patient. The speech pathologist must be informed about the dental and surgical management that has been performed as well as services that are being planned. The type and timing of such management often influences the treatment recommendations that we make.

HISTORY

Regardless of whether you serve on an interdisciplinary team or are an independent practitioner and despite the age of the child you are scheduled to see, a comprehensive clinical history should always be obtained. Because children with cleft palate receive continuing interdisciplinary care throughout childhood and adolescence, the history obtained during the initial interview will provide only a glimpse of an ever-changing story that will unfold with time. Our goal during this interview is to obtain as much pertinent information as possible about the child, the cleft, and any related medical and surgical intervention that has taken place. We are also interested in obtaining some insight into the parents' perspective of the cleft condition and their responses to it. Speech-language pathologists who serve on an interdisciplinary team typically have a child's medical and surgical history available to them when they see that child for an initial consultation. This information may not be readily available to clinicians in the field who are called on to evaluate or treat these patients but should always be obtained to ensure continuity of care. In addition to the basic history that would be obtained for any noncleft patient, the following information should be obtained.

Surgical History

It is important to remember that professionals who serve on craniofacial–cleft palate teams are individuals with different educational backgrounds and clinical experiences. As you know from your own experience, educational and clinical experiences lead us to develop biases that have an impact on both the type and timing of treatment that we deliver. It should come as no surprise then that different cleft palate teams advocate different management regimens. What is standard practice for one team may not be recommended at all by another. And what is deemed an appropriate surgical regimen for the typical child seen by a team may be inappropriate for a particular child for a number of reasons. Therefore you should make no assumptions regarding the surgical management that a particular child has or will receive. The types of surgeries that are planned for a child and the estimated timing of those surgeries should be identified. In most cases in the United States, the exact procedure used to close the palatal cleft will be of less interest to the practicing speech pathologist than when the surgery is to be performed, unless a two-stage closure is performed. When the soft palate is scheduled for early repair and the intent is to delay closure of the hard palate, the clinician should determine whether the hard palate will be obturated in the interim and obtain an estimate of the child's age at time of hard palate repair. This information should be considered when counseling parents regarding the impact of the cleft on early speech-language development.

Medical History

An inventory of other health problems that the child may have (or may have had) should be obtained. Although many of the children you will see will have isolated cleft palate, others will have multiple congenital anomalies with a host of accompanying medical problems. Medical problems that appear totally unrelated to the cleft in infancy can become an important part of the diagnostic puzzle in later years.

The frequency of middle ear infections as well as information pertaining to their management should be ascertained. The child's early feeding history should also be documented as carefully as possible. Although the majority of babies with cleft palate can be successfully fed with minor modifications to the feeding process (e.g., changes in positioning, use of special bottles or nipples), some babies have significant long-term feeding problems that may or may not be attributed to the cleft condition. Parents (and professionals) frequently assume that the child's feeding difficulties are directly related to the cleft, when in fact they may be due to a compromised airway or neurological condition.

Speech-Language Therapy

Information regarding speech-language therapy that the child has received should always be obtained. Specifically, we are interested in how long the child has been enrolled in therapy, how many times a week the child is being seen, whether the child is being seen for individual or group therapy, and what goals have been addressed in therapy. It has been our experience that although most parents can provide information about duration, frequency, and type (individual or group) of therapy, they are frequently uncertain of the specific goals being addressed. Because parents may not always be as informed about their child's therapy as we would like, it is a good idea to have them bring a copy of the child's treatment plan for you to examine. You will not only be able to monitor the child's progress in therapy but will also be able to determine whether the services being provided are appropriate for the child's needs. The importance of receiving written documentation of a child's intervention was underscored in the following case study.

S. D. was a noncleft child with suspected velopharyngeal inadequacy who was seen by one of the authors for an initial evaluation through a craniofacial clinic. She was 5 years old at the time of the assessment and demonstrated severe hypernasality and poor consonant development (consonant production was limited to glottals, nasals, and glides). Her mother reported that S. D. had been enrolled in therapy for 2 years through the local school system but was unable to provide specific information about therapy goals. A letter was written to her therapist summarizing the clinical findings, providing treatment recommendations, and recommending individual, intensive therapy. On follow-up examination 6 months later, S. D. demonstrated essentially no improvement in speech production. A quick phone call to the child's preschool teacher revealed that S. D. was receiving "therapy" one time a week along with the rest of her classroom—a therapist spent 30 minutes reading a story to the class every Thursday. Not only was the focus of this therapy inappropriate for S. D.'s needs, the frequency of therapy was inadequate as well. S. D.'s story is not unusual in the current economic climate.

As D'Antonio and Scherer (1994) have pointed out, public law may have mandated special services for children with special health care needs, but there is no guarantee that those services, when available, will be appropriate or adequate.

Parent Perspective of Impact of Cleft on Speech

Parents with clefts and those who have relatives with clefts may make assumptions about their child's management or treatment outcome that is based on their own previous experience. When a history of clefting is present (and even when it is not!), it is a good idea to spend time discussing a parent's experiences and identify any preconceived notions that he or she has regarding treatment of the cleft and its impact on speech. There have been many advances in management during the past several decades that have led to better speech results. Parents should understand that the presence of an isolated cleft lip and palate does not sentence a child to life-long speech problems. There is every reason to believe that these children will achieve normal or near-normal speech and this message must be conveyed to parents.

What information has the parent been given by health care providers and others about the disorder of cleft lip and palate? Booklets that talk about the infant's inability to achieve velopharyngeal closure for adequate production of pressure consonants before surgical repair of the palate are often misleading to parents who interpret that information to mean that their baby will not talk before palatal surgery. Parents may (and often do) assume that there is little to be gained by stimulating their child's vocalizations before surgical repair of the palate. Identifying any preconceived notions that parents may have about the relationship between clefting and speech is often helpful in determining what their educational needs are.

ASSESSING EARLY COMMUNICATIVE BEHAVIORS

If you serve on an interdisciplinary cleft palate team, chances are you will see an infant with a cleft for an initial consultation before surgical repair of the palate.[1] Parents invariably ask about the impact that the cleft will have on their child's speech after surgery and will frequently ask you to predict whether the child is likely to need secondary surgical management for velopharyngeal inadequacy. Although we are unable to identify those infants before surgery who will go on to demonstrate velopharyngeal inadequacy after surgery, we can assess the baby's receptive and expressive language development early on to obtain an estimate of the child's level of developmental functioning and identify those babies who appear at risk for speech-language delays. Parents (and other professionals as well) often focus on the potential long-term impact of a cleft on speech (velopharyngeal inadequacy) and neglect the impact that a cleft may have on early language development. Lack of concern regarding early development is readily apparent in the surprise that some parents express when they learn that their child is scheduled to receive a communication screening before surgical repair of the cleft. ". . . but she can't talk yet!" It is important that we counsel parents about early communicative behaviors and emphasize that receptive language develops and communicative intents emerge long before the first word appears. Most babies will demonstrate comprehension of some words at 9 months of age. By the time they produce their first word (typically at 13 months for most babies), a receptive vocabulary of approximately 50 words may be evident (Stoel-Gammon, 1992).

The speech-language pathologist who serves on a cleft palate–craniofacial team rarely has the time to conduct comprehensive language assessments for either toddlers or older children. Informal observations of language functioning are typically made during the team visit, with referral for a more comprehensive work-up when indicated. For children functioning at a developmental level of 8 to 18 months, we are particularly interested in determining whether intentional communication exists. Observation of normally developing babies of this age interacting with their parents should reveal the following communicative functions: request for objects, requests for actions, rejections/protest, pointing, and commenting. The gestural form of these intentions is considered evidence of a normal 8- to 12-month-old performance; a gesture used along with a wordlike vocalization (or a vocalization used alone) is indicative of a 12- to 18-month communicative performance, and more frequent use of words or word combinations is suggestive of an 18- to 24-month level performance (Paul, 1995). More advanced intentions, including requests for information, answering, and acknowledgment, emerge at about 18 to 24 months of age in normally developing toddlers.

The assessment of comprehension skills in toddlers during the emerging language stage typically focuses on whether a child can comprehend single words and, if so, on whether he or she can process words within a sentence and comprehend semantic relations (Paul, 1995). Paul summarized a series of comprehension activities previously described by Miller and Paul (1995) that can easily be incorporated into an informal assessment. She recommended interviewing parents by phone before an assessment to obtain some information about the child's comprehension skills and asking the parents to bring objects whose names are known to the child. Comprehension of these single words is then examined without the support of nonlinguistic cues by placing six to eight objects in front of the child during the assessment and asking the child to "Give me the _____." In a similar fashion, the clinician can determine the child's understanding of body parts and people by asking the child "Where's _____?" After correct identification of a series of nouns, comprehension of verbs can be examined by giving the child an object and asking him or her to "kiss/pat/throw it" (parents should provide the action words they think the child knows). Once the child successfully identifies several nouns and several verbs without the use of nonlinguistic cues (12- to 18-month level), his or her ability to understand two-word instructions (e.g., action-object semantic relation) can be examined. Unexpected word combinations (e.g., kiss the ball, hug the shoe) should be used to avoid the child's natural tendency to perform common actions when he or she hears an object's name. Comprehension of two-term relations is typically seen at 18 to 24 months, with comprehension of three-term relations (e.g., agent-action-object) expected at the 24- to 36-month level.

Depending on the time available to you for assessment, information regarding early language development may be obtained with any one (or more) of a number of instruments on the market such as the Preschool Language Scale (Zimmerman, Steiner, and Pond, 1992) and the Rosetti Infant-Toddler Language Scale (Rosetti, 1990). When time is limited (and even when it is not!), parent questionnaires are often useful in screening early language development. One such tool that has been normed and

---

[1] It is not uncommon for speech-language pathologists to see an infant and his or her parents as early as the first week of life, when feeding concerns arise. In fact, in some hospitals the speech-language pathologist may be one of the cleft palate team representatives who counsels the family immediately after the birth of a child with a cleft. We have seen infants who were less than 12 hours old.

validated is the MacArthur Communicative Development Inventory (Fenson, Dale, and Reznick, 1993). The inventory is composed of two forms that assess parental judgment of language development between 8 and 30 months of age. The Words and Gestures Form assesses comprehension and production of vocabulary as well as use of communicative gestures between 8 and 16 months. The Words and Sentences Form examines expressive vocabulary and grammatical use between 16 and 30 months. The usefulness of the MacArthur Communicative Development Inventory in screening language development in toddlers with cleft palate was reported by Scherer and D'Antonio (1995).

In addition to obtaining an estimate of overall receptive and expressive language functioning, it is important to examine or inquire about the baby's babbling behavior. Measurement of vocal development during the prelinguistic period of development is generally based on independent analysis of a child's productions. As indicated in Chapter 7, different measures that have been used to examine prelinguistic vocal development have been associated with later phonological and linguistic development. Such measures include amount of vocalization before 6 months, age at onset of canonical babbling, frequency of consonantal babble, frequency of canonical syllables, and diversity of consonant production. Since babies with cleft palate are known to vocalize less frequently, show delays in onset of babbling, and produce fewer true consonants than their noncleft peers, it is imperative that the speech pathologist examine early vocalizations to identify those babies who appear at risk for later delays in expressive language or phonological development. Particular attention should be directed toward examining the baby's consonant/vowel inventory, syllable shapes, and the presence of any maladaptive articulations. When examining the prelinguistic utterances of babies with cleft palate, the clinician should be alert for the presence or absence of supraglottal consonants. The total lack of supraglottal consonants is abnormal, even during the prelinguistic stage of development (Stoel-Gammon and Stone, 1991), and should serve as a signal that the baby's speech sound development is not progressing satisfactorily. We agree with Devers, Broen, and Moller (1997) who wrote, "Infants whose speech-like vocalizations are composed primarily of nasal phones, even before the emergence of their first words, may be candidates for early behavioral intervention to determine the extent to which those children are capable of achieving and maintaining velopharyngeal closure and to prevent compensatory articulation patterns from developing."

Once the child begins producing meaningful speech, phonological measures can be obtained from either independent analyses of the child's production or relational analyses that compare the child's production with that of the adult target. Stoel-Gammon pointed out, "whereas the absolute number of phones in an inventory might be a convenient and valid means of comparing children with normal development, it is important to consider both size and make-up of the inventories in comparisons involving children with delayed speech and language" (1994, p. 5). Consonant inventory, syllable shape, and presence of maladaptive articulations should be described. In addition, the consistency of the child's productions can be examined by first listing all different productions of the same words and then calculating a measure of variability: ratio of number of different words produced/ number of phonetic forms. Lexical selectivity can also be examined for toddlers in the first 50-word stage of development by documenting the adult targets that the child attempted to produce and determining whether the child is selecting or avoiding production of certain sounds or syllable shapes. Finally, another phonological measure that has been used by clinicians to identify children who are experiencing significant delays is the Percentage of Consonant Correct (PCC) score. The PCC score is calculated by dividing the number of consonants in the child's productions that are correctly produced by the total number of consonants produced and then multiplying by 100. The resultant percentage is frequently used as a general measure of phonological development. Although phonological process analysis (discussed later in this chapter, p. 225) is appropriate for older children, it is not appropriate when the speech of children in the first 50-word stage of phonological development is analyzed because children appear to learn words as whole units during this time.

Once information regarding the toddler's phonological and linguistic development have been obtained, the clinician can estimate the child's overall level of functioning to determine whether intervention is indicated. Although standardized language tests frequently provide normative data regarding general receptive and expressive language functioning, fewer data are available to characterize the typical phonological performance of toddlers less than 3 years old. This is due, at least in part, to the substantial variability evident among children in early phonological development. Some general guidelines for interpreting early phonetic inventories and phonological development can be discerned from the work of Stoel-Gammon and others (1985, 1987, 1991). Children with a productive vocabulary of less than 50 words should be producing supraglottal consonants that reflect both an oral-nasal and a labial-lingual distinction; that is, the child should be producing at least one oral and one nasal consonant and at least one labial and one lingual consonant. Two-year-old children should be producing nasal consonants, voiced and voiceless stop consonants, glides, and one to two fricatives (Table 9-1). The clinician should be alert for toddlers with cleft palate functioning in the first 50-word phonology stage (as well those who are demonstrating more advanced expressive language) who produce only glottals, nasals, and vowels. These children should be considered for early intervention services to facilitate babbling and imitation.

Table 9-1 **General Profile of Linguistic and Phonological Performance of Normally Developing Toddlers**

Characteristic	*First 50-Word Phonology*	*24 Month Olds*
Expressive vocabulary		250-350 words
Consonant inventory		9-10 word-initial phones 5-6 word-final phones
Sound classes		
Word initial	Anterior stops and nasals	Nasals, glides, stops, fricatives
Word final	1-2 glides	Nasals, glides, stops (mostly), fricatives
Syllable shapes	V, CV	CV, CVC, CVCV, CVCVC

References: Stoel-Gammon, 1987, 1998; and Stoel-Gammon and Stone, 1991.

ASSESSING SPEECH PRODUCTION PROBLEMS

A primary concern for the speech-language pathologist who is called on to assess a child with repaired cleft palate is whether the child demonstrates misarticulations that are related to the cleft. As indicated in Chapter 7, children with cleft palate are not only susceptible to the same developmental speech sound errors that are observed in their noncleft peers, they are also at risk for misarticulations associated with both dental/occlusal anomalies and velopharyngeal inadequacy. Identifying and sorting out the nature of the errors present will be a primary goal of the assessment. This goal, however, may not always be accomplished in a single session. The age of a child and the type of errors produced will limit the scope of any assessment. For example, although excessive nasalization of speech is frequently observed in toddlers and young children with repaired cleft palate, speech sound development is often too immature and the child is too young to permit a comprehensive assessment of velopharyngeal function. These children are typically referred for speech therapy to establish appropriate articulation placement and, although articulation and resonance will be reassessed periodically, comprehensive assessment of velopharyngeal function is generally deferred until the child is four years of age or older. The primary reason for waiting is the ability of the child to cooperate for instrumental assessment.

Protocol for Assessment

The protocol for assessment of speech production problems in children with cleft palate will vary somewhat depending on the age of the child and the goals of the clinician. In a typical speech screening, the clinician generally looks for the presence or absence of speech production problems. Diagnostic testing is then conducted to more closely examine the patterns and nature of the problem. For individuals with cleft palate, screening assessment is frequently conducted to identify the presence of hypernasality or misarticulations suggestive of velopharyngeal dysfunction. Once these are identified, diagnostic evaluation is then initiated to carefully examine patterns of errors and obtain objective information about velopharyngeal function. Philips (1986, p. 299) stated, " When conducting a diagnostic evaluation, the speech pathologist's objectives shift to defining the nature and severity of the speech-language problems, determining contributing etiologies, making certain of the adequacy of language development, and recommending management options . . . use of instrumentation may be necessary." Instrumental assessment of velopharyngeal function is discussed in Chapter 10 and will not be further described here. We will simply underscore our conviction that a comprehensive assessment of velopharyngeal function involves both a perceptual speech evaluation and an instrumental assessment.

A typical protocol for the speech pathology assessment is provided in Table 9-2; it includes a variety of sampling procedures. A sample of the child's conversational speech is typically obtained to determine the impact of any articulation and resonance problems on general speech intelligibility. Connected speech also provides information about the consistency of the child's errors and the influence of context (Trost-Cardamone and Bernthal, 1993). Articulation testing is performed to identify the child's phonetic inventory as well as to identify patterns of errors that the child may be producing. A series of syllable and sentence repetition tasks designed to examine patterns of nasalization is also included. These assessment tasks are further described below. In addition, different clinical tools that can be used to augment the perceptual evaluation will be described. A good-quality tape recorder is always a good investment. Whenever possible, an individual's performance on each of the tasks described below should be audiorecorded for documentation and future reference.

Conversational Speech Sample

The analysis of a conversational sample is essential to a thorough understanding of the articulatory behavior of individuals with clefts. Although the procedures listed above (and described below) are helpful in identifying patterns of errors that the child produces, the interaction of these errors and their full impact on speech intelligibility can only be assessed when the child engages in spontaneous conversation. In addition, although much of the information obtained from single-word articulation testing will correspond highly with that perceived in a child's conversational speech, the effect of context and the consistency of errors can only be fully appreciated when a conversational speech sample is obtained. There are many reasons for

Table 9-2 **Sample Protocol for Assessment of Resonance and Articulation**

Task	*Rationale for Inclusion*
Articulation testing	Facilitates pattern analyses and comparison to developmental norms
Repeated productions of high-pressure consonants + vowel	Helpful in examining patterns of nasal emission
Repetition of words containing oral consonants adjacent to nasal consonants	Assists in examining effect of rapidly alternating velopharyngeal movements
Production of sentences containing only oral consonants	Patterns of nasal emission can be more easily examined
Production of sentences containing nasal consonants	Facilitates identification of assimilative nasality and hyponasality
Production of sentences containing no high-pressure consonants or nasal consonants	Facilitates identification of hypernasality by eliminating consonants that can be accompanied by audible nasal emission or hyponasality
Conversational speech	Most representative sample of performance; can examine (1) general speech intelligibility, (2) influence of context on production of sounds, and (3) consistency of sound production errors
Stimulability testing	Identify sounds that are readily modified with auditory and visual cues; identify strategies that facilitate correct production of target sounds

variations in articulatory performance between test and conversational conditions. In some cases the careful articulation of single words or of cued sentences is not possible under the demands of connected discourse. In other cases, improved articulation is possible in conversational contexts but has not become automatic. Finally, engaging a child in spontaneous conversation also provides the examiner an opportunity to examine sociocommunicative performance and to identify nonverbal behaviors (such as nasal grimace) that may negatively influence the listener.

Intelligibility has been described as the "complex product of language formulation, phonological organization, and motor execution" (Kent, Miolo, and Bioedel, 1994, p. 82). Any measurement of intelligibility is thus vulnerable to a number of influences from the spoken material, environmental factors that influence the clarity of the message, characteristics of the speaker, and listener biases such as familiarity with the speaker. Consequently, most speakers probably have a "range of intelligibility potentials" (Kent, Miolo, and Bioedel, 1994) that cannot be adequately measured with any single score. With that in mind, the clinician must identify those procedures that are most applicable to their immediate purposes. Kent, Miolo, and Bioedel summarized 19 different procedures that have been used to assess intelligibility and noted that although some were developed for immediate clinical use, others were developed for research or specific populations. They categorized the procedures into five major categories including procedures that focus on (1) phonetic contrast analysis, (2) phonological process analysis, (3) word identification (excluding phonetic and phonological analysis), (4) the derivation of phonetic index values from continuous speech, and (5) rating scales. The authors concluded from their review that rating scales and simple clinical measurements (such as the PCC index previously described by Shriberg and Kwiatkowski [1982b]) are probably sufficient when assessing the intelligibility of children who are intelligible enough to engage in conversation with an unfamiliar listener. They noted, however, that these procedures may be inappropriate for use with children who have severe phonological disorders or limited expressive language and advised the use of closed-set testing. In this latter type of testing, the speaker is recorded while reading or repeating a series of words. A listener is then asked to identify the words, and an intelligibility score is derived from the percentage of words that are correctly identified.

Measurement of intelligibility was once the most commonly used procedure for assessing the effects of palatal surgery for children with cleft palate. Intelligibility was estimated in some reports by recording speakers as they produced a list of syllables, words, or sentences. The recordings were then played to listeners who were asked to write down what they heard. The resultant number or percentage of correct responses was used as an index of intelligibility (Prins and Bloomer, 1968; Subtelny and Subtelny, 1959; Subtelny, Koepp-Baker, and Subtelny, 1961). Subtelny, Van Hattum, and Myers (1972) noted that these write-down techniques are so time consuming that the technique is more appropriate to research than to clinical application. They recommended the use of rating scales when judging articulation, intelligibility, nasal emission, and other characteristics of speech in patients with cleft palate. Other speech pathologists have also used rating scales to assess speech intelligibility in this population (Wells, 1971).

Ultimately, judgments of speech intelligibility made from conversational speech samples will have a large influence on treatment decisions for children with cleft palate. Rating scales that allow you to characterize overall speech intelligibility are often helpful when conveying your findings to other professionals. Subtelny, Van Hattum, and Myers (1972) presented rating scales for use in measuring articulation, intelligibility, nasal emission, and other characteristics of speech as studied in patients with cleft palate. They described their scales as reliable and recommended that they be applied to conversational speech samples. A modification of their intelligibility scale is as follows: (1) normal for age and sex, (2) mild difficulty in understanding, repetition not required, (3) moderate difficulty, repetition required infrequently, (4) marked difficulty, repetition required frequently, and (5) unintelligible even with repetition. Paul (1995) reported guidelines for estimating intelligibility that were based on previous work by Shriberg and Kwiatkowski (1982a). Intelligibility is considered good if the child correctly produces approximately 85% or more of consonants in a short conversational sample. Mild-to-moderate unintelligibility is the subjective rating assigned when 65% to 84% of consonants are correct, and speech is judged as moderately to severely unintelligible when only 50% to 64% of consonants are correctly produced. When a child produces less than 50% of consonants in the conversational sample, speech is judged as severely unintelligible.

Articulation Testing

Articulation testing is one of the most expedient ways of obtaining information about a child's phonetic inventory. The target word is always known (which is particularly useful with children who demonstrate speech that is highly unintelligible) and the clinician can control the inventory of sounds that the child will attempt to produce (Bernthal and Bankson, 1993). Many articulation tests are available for use with all types of patients, including those with cleft palate. The specific test used with any patient depends on the information to be obtained and the age of the child. Although we are particularly interested in the interaction between speech sound development and any oropharyngeal problems that may be present as a result of a cleft, the test or test battery that you use to examine a child's speech production patterns should also permit developmental comparisons with published norms.

The Templin-Darley Tests of Articulation (1969) include a 50-item screening test that is used to identify speakers who are in need of more thorough testing as well as a 176-item diagnostic test for more detailed assessment of articulation. Although frequently cited in many early published reports of articulation in cleft palate children, this test appears to be less frequently used today—probably in part because it is more lengthy than other tests on the market, with some stimulus items that are relatively difficult for preschoolers to produce. A commonly used articulation test for both cleft and noncleft children today is the Goldman-Fristoe Test of Articulation (1986). It samples consonant sounds under several stimulus conditions, one of which is story retelling. Short stories, accompanied by pictures, are read to the child, who is asked to retell the stories with the aid of the pictures. The result is a sample of connected speech that contains consonants of interest. The test also examines consonants in words elicited by naming pictures and in syllables and sentences repeated after the examiner. The majority of test stimuli on the Goldman-Fristoe test are appropriate for children as young as 2 to 3 years old, although several of the items are clearly inappropriate for the very young child (e.g., gun, matches). This test is particularly attractive to clinicians who serve on cleft palate teams and have restricted amounts of time to spend with each patient. Strengths of the Templin-Darley and the Goldman-Fristoe tests include the attractiveness of the stimulus items and the normative data available for both tests. The Fisher-Logemann Test of Articulation Competence (1971) also has pictorial stimuli that are attractive and appropriate for children as young as 2 to 3 years old; however, normative data are not available. This test is distinguished by a system of pattern analysis that uses place of articulation, manner of articulation, and voicing features.

Special articulation tests for patients with cleft palate. The Iowa Pressure Articulation Test (IPAT), which is included in the Templin-Darley Tests of Articulation, is often included in descriptions of articulation assessments for children with cleft palate (Trost-Cardamone and Bernthal, 1993). It is composed of 43 fricative, plosive, and affricative sounds identified by Morris, Spriestersbach, and Darley (1961) and by others as likely to be misarticulated by persons with poor velopharyngeal function. That is, the test emphasizes sounds that are produced with high intraoral air pressure and it is used to identify people with velopharyngeal dysfunction. Paynter (1984) published norms for Spanish-speaking Mexican-American children imitating words in English from the Templin-Darley Screening Test of Articulation and from the IPAT.

Van Demark and Swickard (1980) noted that the IPAT contains many consonants that are not developed by 3 and 4 years of age. They concluded that there was a need for a pressure articulation test suitable for use with 3- and 4-year-old children and suggested a test that emphasized /p/ and /b/ sounds. Those sounds are acquired early, and previous work by Van Demark (1979) had indicated that these sounds are useful in discriminating between young children who eventually required secondary palatal surgery and those who did not. The authors developed a set of words and corresponding pictures that were recognized, named, and correctly articulated by most of the noncleft children who were studied. As is true of the IPAT, this test is directed toward identification of velopharyngeal inadequacy. The person who passes the test may, nonetheless, have nasal emission during production of more demanding speech sounds, such as sibilants. Thus, this test can undoubtedly identify children with gross valving problems but may fail to auditorily isolate those with marginal velopharyngeal inadequacy. Obviously, the clinician can informally assess the production of many words containing /p/ and /b/.

Bzoch (1979) constructed the Bzoch Error Patterns Diagnostic Articulation Test for use with patients with cleft palate. The scoring system distinguishes among five articulation error types: nasal emission, distortion, simple substitution, gross substitution, and omission. These errors are considered to fall on a severity continuum in the order presented above with omission representing the most severe type of misarticulation. The test samples fricatives, affricates, and plosives, the sound classes that children with cleft palates are most likely to misarticulate. Bzoch recommended that the clinician administering this test observe both the visual and auditory aspects of the patient's speech.

The articulation tests described above have all been developed with one common characteristic: they include words loaded with pressure consonants. These particular tests are useful to the clinician who is attempting to examine patterns of nasalization. However, the results of these tests should be interpreted cautiously. An individual can fail any one of these tests because of misarticulations related to factors other than velopharyngeal inadequacy. Children who perform poorly on these tests because of velopharyngeal inadequacy are likely to produce unique error types that involve nasal emission and weak pressure consonants. Thus, observations of error type are even more important than test score for differentiating between the disordered articulation associated with past or present velopharyngeal dysfunction and that associated with other origins and patterns.

A major limitation of single-word articulation tests is that they typically elicit only one production of a sound in different word positions. Because variability in sound production is common during phonological development, it may be inaccurate to assume that a child's production of a sound during a single stimulus item is representative of his typical production. To more accurately assess a child's speech sound inventory, whole word transcription should be performed to increase the number of sounds sampled during articulation testing.

Patterns of Cleft Palate Misarticulations

Scoring articulation responses as correct or incorrect provides only a gross description of speech and offers little help in diagnosing problems associated with velopharyngeal inadequacy. Comparing the number of correct responses a child produces with normative data provides information about the severity of misarticulation and may contribute to decision making; however, such a score does not provide clues about the types of therapy or other interventions that are likely to be beneficial to the patient (Turton, 1973), nor does it offer prognostic information. Information descriptive of the type and severity of misarticulation is used to decide whether a problem exists and, if so, whether it requires speech therapy or some other kind of management.

The clinician scoring articulation responses must first decide whether a particular response was correct or incorrect. If the response was incorrect, the nature of the error should be determined or estimated and transcribed. The speech pathologist may also supplement response classification and transcription with descriptions of how the speech mechanism is used in the production of sounds. Examples of possible observations include incomplete bilabial closure, tongue tip deflected into spaces created by missing or misplaced teeth or maxillary collapse, placement of the tongue within or outside the maxillary arch and in or out of contact with lateral teeth for coronal sounds, unusual adjustments of the mandible, or posterior tongue placement for anterior consonants. In short, the articulation errors of subjects with cleft palate should be detailed as thoroughly and as reliably as possible. When the speech of individuals with cleft palate is transcribed, diacritics should be used to indicate the occurrence of audible nasal emission and weak pressure consonants. Some of the symbols and diacritics that are commonly used are provided in Table 9-3.

Nasal emission. During transcription of articulation test responses, it is important that the clinician make note of patterns of nasal emission that may be evident in the child's speech. As pointed out by Trost-Cardamone (1990), the pattern of nasal emission observed during production of pressure consonants appears highly correlated with its source. She identified four distinct sources of nasal emission that are associated with different patterns of nasal emission, including (1) the velopharyngeal port, (2) an anterior fistula, (3) a posterior fistula, and (4) sound-specific nasal

Table 9-3 **Diacritics**

Description	*Diacritic*
Nasalized	C̃
Nasal emission	C͋
Denasalized	C^{+}
Palatalized	C,
Dentalized	C̪
Lateralized	C̭
Fronted	$C_{<}$
Backed	$C_{>}$
Inverted	C˞

Reference: Shriberg and Kent, 1995.

emission (Table 9-4). Although velopharyngeal inadequacy tends to be associated with nasal emission on most if not all pressure consonants, the latter three sources are associated with nasal emission on only select groups of consonants. It is essential that the suspected source(s) of nasal emission be identified during the perceptual evaluation when possible to circumvent inappropriate assessment and management recommendations. For example, sound-specific nasal emission typically occurs only during production of one or more of the sibilant fricative (s, z, ʃ) or affricate (ʧ, ʤ) consonants. Although often confused with disorders of velopharyngeal inadequacy, phoneme-specific nasal emission is an articulatory disorder that can easily be identified through perceptual evaluation alone; it is appropriately managed with speech therapy.

Occasionally, a child will demonstrate perceptual evidence of both velopharyngeal inadequacy and phoneme-specific nasal emission. In such cases, hypernasality is perceived and audible nasal emission is evident on obstruent consonants. In addition to this nasalization of speech, posterior nasal frication is also present during production of selected fricative consonants. Although surgery can eliminate the perceptual consequences of velopharyngeal inadequacy, the posterior nasal frication will persist as a learned behavior until eliminated through speech therapy. In cases where nasalization of speech is relatively mild, it is sometimes appropriate to refer the child for therapy before surgical management is considered. The severity of nasalization may not warrant surgery once the severe nasal snorts have been eliminated with therapy.

Determining the source of nasal emission when a palatal fistula is present may be more problematic for the clinician.

Table 9-4 Articulatory Evidence of Nasal Emission: Four Distinct Sources

Sources of Nasal Emission	*Consonants Distorted*
Velopharyngeal port	All high pressure consonants: /p/, /b/, /t/, /d/, /k/, /g/, /θ/, /ð/, /f/, /v/, /s/, /z/, /ʃ/, /ʒ/, /ʧ/, /ʤ/
Fistula	
Anterior	Anterior pressure consonants: /t/, /d/, /s/, /z/, /p/, /b/ ± /f/, /v/, /θ/, /ð/
Posterior	Posterior pressure consonants: /k/, /g/
Phone-specific nasal emission	Sibilant fricatives, affricates: /s/, /z/, /ʃ/ ± /ʧ/, /ʤ/

From Trost-Cardamone JE: The development of speech: assessing cleft palate misarticulations. In Kernahan DE, and Rosenstein SW (eds.): *Cleft lip and palate: a system of management.* Baltimore: Williams & Wilkins, 1990.

When nasal emission occurs only on anterior pressure consonants (e.g., p, b, t, d, s, z), the clinician should be alert for an anterior palatal fistula. A posterior palatal fistula is usually responsible when nasal emission is restricted to /k/ and /g/. Although some patients will have patterns of nasal emission that are readily attributed to a fistula, others will demonstrate patterns that may not be easily interpreted without temporary obturation of the fistula. For example, some children demonstrate nasal emission related to both velopharyngeal inadequacy and a palatal fistula. The relative contribution of each is best examined by first obturating the fistula and then observing any changes in the perceptual signal. Isberg and Henningsson (1987) and others (Karling, Larson, and Henningsson, 1993; Lohmander-Agerskov et al., 1996; Tachimura et al. 1997) have demonstrated that obturating a fistula results in improved velopharyngeal valving for some patients. Different materials have been used for temporarily obturating a fistula, including chewing gum, stoma adhesive, and dental wax. When any of these materials are used, it is recommended that a dentist or physician be present to extract the material from the fistula should it migrate after application.

The clinician should be aware that a fistula that is asymptomatic during one examination may not remain so over time. Henningsson and Isberg (1990) reported that an asymptomatic fistula can become symptomatic after pharyngeal flap surgery. They attributed this change to the increase in intraoral pressure that results after surgery.

Although the patterns of nasal emission described above are often readily identified when appropriate test stimuli are used, it is not uncommon for audible nasal emissions to be perceived on an inconsistent basis and thus complicate interpretation of the data. When inconsistent audible nasal emission is perceived, explanations for the inconsistency should be sought. Such a finding may reflect actual inconsistent behavior or simply reflect our inability to identify the patterns described above in conversational speech. It is also possible in some cases that nasal emission is consistently present but simply inaudible at times. The speech-language pathologist should attempt to identify inaudible nasal emission during the syllable and sentence repetition tasks by placing a mirror under the child's nares and documenting the presence or absence of condensation (fogging) during each pressure consonant. A useful alternative to the mirror during such an examination is a dental reflector. Unlike cold mirrors that retain moisture and must be continually wiped, condensation on dental reflectors clears rapidly and spontaneously. One such device, known as the Detail Reflector,[2] is a magnifying plastic mirror that can also be inserted in the mouth to reflect the palate and teeth. Speech pathologists have long used such devices to supplement the ear when nasal emission is suspected. Although clinically useful, a mirror

[2]The Detail Reflector is sold by the Floxite Company, Inc., 1 Lethbridge Plaza, Mahwah, NJ 07430.

examination is imprecise and provides only gross information about nasal air escape. It does not quantify air pressure or air flow, and it is sometimes difficult to differentiate between abnormal air leakage and normal nasal exhalation.

Other devices with similar purposes and similar limitations are the listening tube (Blakeley, 1972, 2000) and plastic "scopes" that resemble water manometers. The listening tube is a catheter with a nasal olive in each end, one for the patient's nose and one for the examiner's ear. The scopes consist of glass or plastic tubing containing a float or piston that is displaced by nasal emission of air. These devices supplement the clinician's ear in the evaluation of velopharyngeal function. However, as Glaser and Shprintzen (1979) noted, these devices do not provide information about the size of the orifice responsible for the nasal emission or the utterance segment associated with nasal air leakage.

Compensatory articulation patterns. Compensatory articulation patterns should also be carefully evaluated during the speech assessment. The presence of these atypical errors will not only influence general speech intelligibility, but velopharyngeal function as well. Henningsson and Isberg (1986) provided radiographic evidence to indicate that patients demonstrate poorer velopharyngeal function during glottal stop productions than during oral stop productions. The limited velopharyngeal activity that occurs during glottal and pharyngeal productions prevents adequate assessment of the *functional potential* of the mechanism. If glottal stops and pharyngeal articulations are frequently observed during the perceptual evaluation, direct assessment of velopharyngeal function should be deferred until these atypical patterns of articulation are eliminated (or substantially reduced) through speech therapy.

A cautionary statement seems appropriate here. It is tempting to assume that if you are knowledgeable about compensatory articulation errors, you can reliably identify and transcribe them. Knowledge of these atypical errors will certainly facilitate transcription of them. However, there is no adequate substitute for good transcription experience. If you have never heard these patterns of articulation or have limited experience transcribing these errors, you should seek out these experiences either through continuing education workshops or through the use of teaching audiotapes and videotapes (McWilliams and Philips, 1990; Trost-Cardamone, 1987).

Analyzing Patterns of Articulation

Once the articulation test has been administered and scored, the responses must be analyzed to determine the child's phonetic inventory and identify any patterns of errors that may be influencing entire classes of sounds. Three procedures are used: (1) place-manner-voice analysis, (2) distinctive feature analysis, and (3) phonological process analysis. The latter two procedures are generally considered extensions of the place-manner-voice analysis (Bernthal and Bankson, 1993) and all three procedures are interpreted similarly so far as therapy planning is concerned. If several sounds that are misarticulated share place or manner of articulation or distinctive features or are influenced by the same phonological processes, therapy may be organized so that treatment that favorably influences one or two sounds will also influence related sounds. In patients with cleft palate and related disorders, the possibility of structural or physiological constraints must be considered.

Stoel-Gammon and Dunn (1985) wrote that analysis of a child's speech should provide information about (1) consonant inventory, (2) positional and sequential constraints on the production of those sounds, (3) contrastive units present in the child's speech, and (4) comparison of the child's sound system with the adult system. The child's speech is first studied as an independent system and then as it relates to the adult system. These authors determine the phonetic inventory, identify syllable and word shapes that the child uses, and then record positional and sequential constraints operating in the child's speech. The relational analysis includes identification of phonological processes used, including those of a presumably idiosyncratic (provisionally unique) nature. Phonemic contrasts and variability in production are also considered. The texts by Bernthal and Bankson (1988) and Paul (1995) provide a catalog of many published articulatory and phonological analysis materials.

In a traditional sound-by-sound analysis, the focus is on individual speech sounds that require treatment. Error sounds identified on the articulation test are listed by word position, and factors such as consistency of error, stimulability, and age appropriateness of the error are considered when arriving at treatment recommendations. This approach to analysis is considered most appropriate for children who demonstrate a limited number of errors that are phonetic in nature. Since errors are considered motor production problems, subsequent therapy typically focuses on discrimination training, articulatory placement, and motor practice (Bernthal and Bankson, 1988).

In contrast to the traditional analysis, pattern analyses typically focus on the relationship among error sounds in the phonological system. The place-manner-voice analysis is used to classify substitution errors according to the place, manner, and voicing characteristics of each target production (Bernthal and Bankson, 1993). Once a child's errors have been subjected to such an analysis, patterns of errors can be readily identified for remediation. The Fisher-Logemann Tests of Articulation (1971) have a built-in place-manner-voice analysis.

Another type of pattern analysis is the distinctive feature analysis. This analysis provides a means of organizing misarticulated sounds according to shared and unshared features. This information may be taken into account in selecting sounds for training in the hope of encouraging generalization of gains with therapy along feature lines. Bernthal and Bankson (1993) pointed out that distinctive feature analysis may not be appropriate when analyzing speech sound errors because the binary nature of these features may not appropriately characterize the variety of errors seen in the speech of children with phonological disorders. Sound deletions and distortions are ignored in this type of analysis—a factor that certainly limits its application in young children with cleft palate.

Phonological process analysis is commonly used to identify patterns of misarticulation, arrive at a prognosis, and organize therapy to influence the articulation of two or more sounds that share one or more common characteristics. Different authors have used different lists of phonological processes in analyzing disordered articulation. Ingram (1976) used three process categories: syllable structure, assimilation, and substitution. These process constructs are used to explain articulatory behaviors such as deletion of consonants from syllables and clusters, alteration of a sound to resemble a neighboring sound, and replacement of sounds in one phonetic category with sounds from another category. For example, a child may replace fricatives with stops. Use of processes drops out with maturation, and authors have published information relating process usage and age (Grunwell, 1985; Preisser, Hodson, and Paden, 1988; Vihman and Greenlee, 1987). Guidelines for determining when to perform a phonological analysis were suggested by Paul (1995) and are shown in Table 9-5.

Several phonological analysis kits have been published (Compton and Hutton, 1978; Grunwell, 1985; Hodson, 1980; Ingram, 1981; Khan and Lewis, 1986; Shriberg and Kwiatkowski, 1980; Weiner, 1979). These materials differ in the processes studied, in the procedures for obtaining speech samples, in the techniques for analysis, and perhaps most importantly, in their theoretical bases. The Khan-Lewis kit was developed on a psychometric base and may be interpreted as a test. Dinnsen (1984) wrote that an adequate phonological analysis cannot be performed in a mechanical fashion but rather that the clinician should have the capability of adapting the analysis to the child. He noted that many of the analytical procedures that have been published compare the child's pattern with that of the ambient language. He would relate the child's spoken utterances to the child's underlying representations, which may or may not be the same as those used in the child's community. Procedures for generative phonological analysis such as that recommended by Dinnsen (1984) are described by Elbert and Gierut (1986).

McReynolds and Elbert (1981) recommended that we not consider a phonological process to be operative unless we have observed several appropriate contexts in which it occurred. They also listed qualitative criteria that might be applied in identifying the operation of processes:

1. That speech sounds influenced by processes in certain contexts be correctly articulated in contexts where those processes are not operative.
2. That the correctly articulated speech sound serve to establish contrast between minimal pairs.
3. That the sound not be articulated correctly in contexts where the process is expected to be operative.

When phonological process analysis is applied in the evaluation of patients with cleft palate, the speech pathologist must consider whether the analysis used captures pattern information important to decision making and whether that information is a valuable addition to that obtained from articulation testing. We view phonological process analysis in descriptive terms. Inferring causation from this type of analysis alone is unwarranted. We agree with Trost-Cardamone and Bernthal (1993, p. 324) who wrote, ". . . often process-based approaches yield little useful data on organic- structural or physiological disorders. For compensatory articulation in particular, and organic disorders in general, we recommend a place-manner-voicing analysis."

Clinical Judgments of Resonance

Perceptual assessment of oral-nasal resonance balance involves at least two clinical judgments. First, the type of resonance demonstrated by the child must be identified. That is, resonance should be described as normal, hypernasal, hyponasal, mixed, or cul-de-sac. If resonance is

Table 9-5 **Guideline for Deciding To Do Phonological Analysis of Continuous Speech**

DO a Phonological Analysis If:	*DO NOT Do Phonological Analysis If:*
There are many substitutions and deletions on an articulation test.	Almost all errors on an articulation test are distortions.
Errors on an articulation test are inconsistent.	Errors on an articulation test are consistent. Sounds are almost always produced with the same errors, regardless of position or context.
Errors are made on classes of sounds, such as fricatives or velars, on an articulation test.	Errors are made on individual sounds and do not generalize across the class of the sound on an articulation test.
Conversational speech intelligibility is moderately poor to poor.	Conversational speech intelligibility is fair to good.

From Paul R: *Language disorders from infancy through adolescence.* St. Louis: Mosby, 1995.

judged to be abnormal, then the severity of the disorder should be identified. Obviously, the easiest and most reliable way of rating a resonance disorder, including hypernasality, is to make a decision that the problem is either present or absent. Bzoch (1979) felt that this is the only reliable decision that can be made in most cases. However, that decision by itself is not useful clinically because it does not discriminate between the nasality that is environmental or idiosyncratic and the nasality that is associated with velopharyngeal dysfunction. The next decision that must be made, then, is whether the speech, in spite of its nasal elements, falls within a normal distribution or whether its characteristics suggest that it is pathological. To overcome that problem, many writers have recommended the use of scales designed to provide information about the degree of perceived hypernasality. Needless to say, the more choices listeners have, the harder it is to develop reliability. However, many studies carried out in the past have used rating scales reliably.

Rating scales. Sherman (1954) and Morris, Shelton, and McWilliams (1973) have discussed "equal-appearing-interval" scales, usually containing five, seven, or nine points. On such scales the uppermost point is indicative of the most severe form of hypernasality. Box 9-1 provides examples of several different rating scales that may be used. Our preference is to rate hypernasality separately and then to indicate the presence or absence of other possible features. Hyponasality, if present, can be rated on a three-point scale, whereas cul-de-sac resonance and combined hyponasality-hypernasality can be evaluated as present or absent. Any person with the latter combination will already have been rated on the two resonance characteristics, and the severity of the cul-de-sac attribute will be reflected in the ratings of hyponasality. It is important to understand that cul-de-sac resonance reflects hyponasality or denasality. It is helpful to test the two nostrils separately because the goal is to determine as much as possible about the characteristics of the nasal resonating system.

In our view, a rating scale is a useful device provided reliability is consistently monitored and provided speech is heard in a variety of contexts ranging from a sentence containing neither high-pressure consonants nor nasals (e.g., Willie lay low) through one loaded with sibilants (e.g., Suzy sees the sky). Sentence repetition tasks are often used by clinicians to examine resonance characteristics and patterns of nasal emission during clinical assessments—particularly when time is limited as it so often is during cleft palate clinics. Such tasks permit you to control the phonetic composition of a speech sample and thus facilitate identification of error patterns. It is not difficult for the trained speech-language pathologist to perceive hypernasal-

Box 9-1 Methods of Rating Resonance

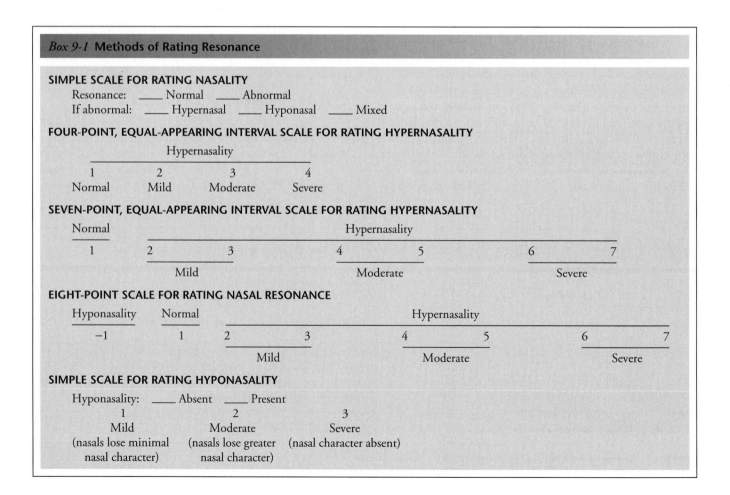

SIMPLE SCALE FOR RATING NASALITY

Resonance: ____ Normal ____ Abnormal

If abnormal: ____ Hypernasal ____ Hyponasal ____ Mixed

FOUR-POINT, EQUAL-APPEARING INTERVAL SCALE FOR RATING HYPERNASALITY

Hypernasality			
1	2	3	4
Normal	Mild	Moderate	Severe

SEVEN-POINT, EQUAL-APPEARING INTERVAL SCALE FOR RATING HYPERNASALITY

Normal	Hypernasality					
1	2	3	4	5	6	7
	Mild		Moderate		Severe	

EIGHT-POINT SCALE FOR RATING NASAL RESONANCE

Hyponasality	Normal	Hypernasality					
−1	1	2	3	4	5	6	7
		Mild		Moderate		Severe	

SIMPLE SCALE FOR RATING HYPONASALITY

Hyponasality: ____ Absent ____ Present

1	2	3
Mild	Moderate	Severe
(nasals lose minimal nasal character)	(nasals lose greater nasal character)	(nasal character absent)

ity and audible nasal emission; however, special sampling contexts are often helpful in identifying patterns of distortion (Trost-Cardamone, 1990). Most clinicians include at least three general types of sentences in their sentence repetition task: (1) sentences containing only oral consonants, (2) sentences loaded with nasal consonants, and (3) sentences containing no pressure consonants or nasal consonants. The use of sentences composed only of oral consonants can aid in identifying patterns of nasal emission as well as in examining the general influence of velopharyngeal inadequacy on speech production (see Table 9-2). Sentences loaded with nasal consonants are helpful in identifying assimilative nasality or hyponasality. Finally, sentences that are devoid of pressure consonants and nasal consonants provide a good context for the identification of hypernasality. Sentences that have been reported by other investigators are shown in Table 9-6. Note that there is nothing sacred about these particular combinations of words and that other writers suggest other tasks, such as counting from 60 to 100. Concentrate on vowels in these short speech samples and then listen in the same way to conversational speech. Try to discern the influence of consonant context. To begin with, you may wish to experiment with a four-point scale for rating hypernasality, as shown in Box 9-1. From there, you can move into the expanded scales also shown to provide for more variations in the speech patterns you are rating. Always carry out ratings so that reliability is provided for. McWilliams and Philips (1979, 1990) developed a series of training audiotapes that may be used to help listeners learn to make reliable judgments about hypernasality as well as about other speech attributes discussed throughout this book.

Cul-de-sac test. Bzoch (1979) used an old approach to assessing resonance, which he referred to as the cul-de-sac test. More recently, the test has been referred to as the hypernasality test and the hyponasality test (Bzoch, 1997). Simply stated, the tests involve the alternate compressing and releasing of the nares during speech and listening for a shift in resonance when the nares are occluded. The short test used by Bzoch involved having patients repeat a series of 10 words beginning with /b/. Each word is produced first with the nares unoccluded and then with the nares pinched. If hypernasality is present when the nares are unoccluded, a shift to cul-de-sac resonance will be heard. Patients may also (or alternatively) be asked to sustain various vowels while their nostrils are alternately compressed and released. The test is invalidated if hyponasality is present with or without hypernasality or if cul-de-sac resonance is already a characteristic of the speech being tested.

In our clinical experience, we use the cul-de-sac test but do not always find it useful, especially for small children, who sometimes demonstrate a shift although they do not sound hypernasal in conversational speech and have no unusual behaviors that would tend to invalidate the test. In addition, some children are deeply embarrassed by the procedure. For these reasons, we view the test as one that is sometimes useful but cannot always be relied on to provide valid data.

Stimulability

Stimulability testing is typically conducted to determine whether an individual can produce an articulatory gesture that was not previously identified in his or her phonetic repertoire when provided with strong auditory and visual stimulation. When an individual correctly articulates a

Table 9-6 **Sentence Repetition Protocols**

	Sentences		
Target Sound	*Sell, Harding, and Grunwell (1994)*	*Kummer and Lee (1996)*	*McWilliams and Philips (1979)*
/p/	Paul likes apple pie.	Popeye plays baseball.	Put the baby in the buggy.
/b/	Ben is a baby boy.		
/t/	Tim told Pete, "Put a hat on."	Take Teddy to town.	
/d/	Daddy mended the door.		
/k/	Katy's baking a cake.	Give Kate the cake.	Kindly give Kate the cake.
/g/	Gary's got a bag of Lego.		Go get the wagon for the girl.
/f/	The phone fell off the shelf.	Fred has five fish.	
/v/	Vicky's very clever.		
/s/	I saw Sam sitting on a bus.	Sissy sees the sun in the sky.	Sissy sees the sun in the sky.
/z/	The zebra lives at the zoo.		
/ʃ/	The fish shop was shut.	The ship goes in shallow waters.	
/ʧ/	Charlie's watching a football match.		
/ʤ/	John jumped off a bridge.	John told a joke to Jim.	Jim and Charlie chew gum.
/m/	Mum came home early.		Mama made lemon jam.
/n/	I saw a robin in a nest singing a song.		

sound in imitation of an examiner who directs the patient's attention to information regarding place and manner of articulation, then it is inferred that the patient is capable of improving his or her articulation with therapy (and perhaps without it). The concept of this "stimulability" as a predictor was first suggested by Milisen (1954) and Snow and Milisen (1954a, 1954b) and was further developed by Carter and Buck (1958). The latter authors developed a predictive articulation test with cutoff scores for use in making articulation predictions. Persons who met the authors' subject selection criteria and whose scores exceeded the cutoff score tended to develop normal articulation without therapy. Unfortunately, from the viewpoint of predicting change in individuals, so did most persons who had lower predictor scores. This same problem exists with other predictive articulation tests that have been published. Weiss, Lillywhite, and Gordon (1980) cited evidence that persons who perform well on stimulability measures may not progress rapidly in therapy. However, poor performance on stimulability measures tends to be associated with poor speech improvement.

Many authors have advocated the treatment of stimulable sounds as opposed to nonstimulable sounds (Winitz, 1975; see discussion by Bernthal and Bankson, 1993). Data reported by Powell, Elbert, and Dinnesen (1991), however, suggest that treatment of nonstimulable sounds may be a more productive strategy. They found that treatment of sounds that were not stimulable resulted in change in both the targets and untreated, stimulable sounds. Treatment of stimulable sounds, on the other hand, did not prompt changes in either untreated stimulable sounds or nonstimulable sounds.

The Miami Imitative Ability Test (Harrison, 1969; Jacobs et al., 1970) was developed for use in a research project intended to evaluate the speech of preschool children with cleft palate. The test samples the subject's ability to imitate lingual and labial placement when producing 24 consonants in CV syllables. Children were instructed to watch and listen as the examiner presented each test syllable three times. After the three presentations, the examiner said, "Now you do it." Each response was scored for placement and acceptability to the examiner's ear.

Harrison (1969) administered both a word articulation test and the Miami Imitative Ability Test to a control group and to 24 preschool cleft palate children who later received stimulation therapy for 12 months. The word articulation test was readministered to each group after the 12 months. Harrison found that the children made greater articulation gains over the course of the study on those sounds on which they were initially stimulable. This was true for both the treated and the untreated subjects. However, the treated subjects made greater articulation gains than did the untreated subjects. Data in the report do not indicate whether sounds in different manner or place categories differed in stimulability. If the sounds on which the subjects were stimulable and on which they improved were a subset of the total set of consonants studied, that information might influence the interpretation of the study. It would be interesting to know how highly Harrison's syllable imitation scores correlated with the difference between his pretreatment and posttreatment word articulation scores. We have no basis from this or other studies to predict articulation change in individual cleft palate children with or without therapy.

Although stimulability testing does not provide a basis for predicting articulation change in individual children, stimulability data do contribute to our understanding of a child's articulatory status and capability. Use of stimulability techniques to sample production of target sounds in isolation, syllables, words, and other units can help the clinician select units for use in therapy. Success at stimulability tasks suggests that the child has the phonetic capability to produce sounds of interest. The clinician must always recognize, however, that failure to use stimulable sounds in spontaneous speech could reflect either phonetic-physiological or phonological variables or both. Children with cleft palate sometimes succeed in imitating sounds that they are physically unable to maintain in more complex contexts, especially in running speech. For example, a child with a repaired cleft lip and palate may be stimulable for /s/ in isolation or CV syllables but be unable to adequately produce the sound in connected speech despite months of therapy because of dental or occlusal hazards. Further, it may be possible at times for a child with borderline velopharyngeal inadequacy to generate enough oral pressure to adequately produce a stop consonant during simple syllable repetition tasks. When that consonant is produced in connected speech, however, it may be more difficult to impound the oral pressure needed to achieve an acceptable production because the physiological demands of the task have increased.

Oral-Peripheral Examination

An oral-peripheral examination should always be performed in individuals with cleft palate. The information derived from such an examination is invaluable to the speech pathologist attempting to integrate all the information obtained in an assessment and to identify the etiological factors responsible for them. Before identifying the observations that should be made in such an examination, it seems appropriate to first address several issues that should be considered when such an assessment is performed. The first issue is related to when an oral-peripheral examination should be performed. Some clinicians feel it is important to examine a patient's oral cavity before the speech assessment to identify factors that likely will influence the speech they will hear. Other clinicians prefer to listen to the child's speech first, make their clinical judgments and then examine the patient's oral cavity. Because children with cleft palate often have multiple oral anomalies that may or may not be influencing speech, it is probably best, certainly for the inexperienced clinician, to perform the oral-peripheral examination after articulation testing has been performed and clinical judgments of articulation defectiveness, resonance, and general intelligibility have been made. In this way, you will not be biased by structural anomalies that may look significant but are actually having little-to-no effect on the patient's speech. All too often clinicians identify oral anomalies and assume a causal relationship exists between that problem and the speech production errors that are present.

The second issue that should be considered is that of the clinician's experience. Speech pathologists are frequently called on to make qualitative judgments about a child's oral anatomy and physiology. Although the presence or absence of oral anomalies is readily evident in many cases, it is far more difficult to characterize the severity/extent of the problem. How large do the tonsils have to be before their size is considered to be a significant finding? How high does a palatal vault have to be before it is considered "high"? How do we differentiate a palate that is moderately mobile from one that is markedly mobile? The answers to these questions cannot be found in any textbook. They come from experience. To adequately describe the oral anatomy and physiology that you will see in children with cleft palate (as well as other children) and to develop your own mental template for what "normal" is, it is essential that you become familiar with "normal" mouths. Only when you have examined the mouths of many normally developing children will you have an appreciation of the variability that characterizes a "normal" mouth and be able to identify and describe abnormalities when you encounter them. We know of no substitute for experience here.

Children with cleft palate are accustomed to professionals asking them to open their mouth. For some children, this means that oral examinations have become routine and are easily accomplished. Other children may be fearful of the procedure and be reluctant to cooperate. It is always wise to assume that your first look in a child's mouth may be your last look during this particular session. Do not ask a child to open the mouth and then scan your checklist for observations to make. Know the observations you want to make before soliciting the child's cooperation. Clinicians who take a systematic approach to oral examinations are more likely to obtain a child's cooperation and complete the examination quickly. Checklists and rating scales are available to ensure systematic study of the speech mechanism (Bateman and Mason, 1984; Dworkin and Cullata, 1980; Spriestersbach, Morris and Darley, 1978; St. Louis and Ruscello, 1987). These tools will guide the examiner in the observation of lips, dentition, maxillary arch width, occlusion, tongue, faucial pillars, tonsils, hard palate, soft palate, uvula, and pharyngeal walls. An exhaustive account of the observations typically made in an oral-peripheral examination will not be provided here. Instead, our discussion will be limited to those observations that are of special significance to individuals with cleft palate.

Face. It is often valuable to observe a patient at rest before initiating an oral-peripheral examination. Observation of a child playing can provide important information about habitual mouth posture as well as the ability to achieve different oral gestures. The coexistence of several minor or major anomalies of the head and neck may suggest the possibility of a multiple anomaly syndrome. Other external characteristics may provide some indication of what to expect during the oral examination. Facial asymmetries should alert the clinician to the possibility of oral and pharyngeal asymmetries. In addition, the presence of drooling or poor muscle tone may signal the presence of an oral-motor problem.

Lips. The repaired cleft lip rarely influences speech production. Nonetheless, the presence of an abnormally short upper lip should be noted, as should any discrepancy in upper-lower lip approximation related to maxillary retrusion. As indicated in Chapter 7, individuals with an extremely short upper lip may produce bilabial consonants as labiodentals. Severe Class III malocclusions may prevent bilabial contact and lead to inverted labiodentals as well as tongue tip-labial production of tongue tip-alveolar consonants.

Dentition. Special attention should be given to the child's dental/occlusal status. The type of occlusion as well as any anterior dental anomalies that could potentially influence the production of consonant sounds, particularly sibilant fricatives, should be recorded. These observations might include problems such as crossbite, anterior open bite, closed bite, and the presence of ectopic teeth in the palatal vault. Remember that although severe Class II and Class III malocclusions can lead to adaptive articulatory gestures that may introduce auditory or visual distortions of speech, malposed or rotated anterior teeth alone can have a significant impact on the precision of articulation for some children.

Treatment planning for children with dental/occlusal anomalies must account for changes in the condition that will naturally occur with growth and development. According to Moller (1994, p.18), "there is a marked decrease in anterior open bite from ages 7 to 9 and from 10-12." Therapy for children who have mild oral distortions that are presumed related to an anterior open bite might be deferred in anticipation of some closure that will occur with additional growth.

What are the long-term plans for orthognathic surgery or orthodontia for this child? The plan of treatment developed by the dental specialists on the cleft palate team will have a direct impact on the timing of speech therapy for some patients. When oral distortions are unresponsive to direct articulation therapy, it may be more cost-effective to delay therapy until orthodontic management is well under way or complete.

The presence of dental appliances such as obturators, expanders, and braces should also be noted. Children are always growing, so a dental appliance that fits one day may be too small the next time you see the child. Appliances that do not fit well and those that take up too much vertical space in the palatal vault can interfere with the precision of consonant production.

Tongue. Children with nonsyndromic cleft lip and palate do not typically have anatomical or physiological problems involving the tongue. However, speech-language pathologists who serve on cleft palate–craniofacial teams are called on periodically to make judgments about the contribution of a child's tongue size to articulation problems. Those judgments can be difficult ones to make for some children because many factors (e.g., poor neuromuscular control, airway obstruction) can lead a child to favor an anterior tongue posture at rest and during speech. Any clinical judgment of tongue size must be made in relation to the size of space that is available to house the tongue. The fact that a child always has his tongue between his teeth at rest and during speech should not be viewed as evidence that the tongue is too large or as justification to recommend surgical reduction. To identify possible airway obstruction problems, Moller (1994) recommended that the patient be instructed to place his tongue postdentally within the oral cavity, occlude the teeth, and breathe nasally for a period of approximately 10 seconds. He went on to recommend that observations of the tongue be made during linguoalveolar sounds to determine whether the tongue tip or blade is typically used for these sounds. Moller noted that both tongue blade–alveolar productions and tongue tip–incisal edge of teeth productions can result in acceptable speech.

Patients with syndromes such as Beckwith-Wiedemann syndrome often have obvious macroglossia. They typically cannot position their tongue within the postdental oral space and the resultant anterior tongue position influences appearance as well as the accuracy of lingual consonants. Dental anomalies such as labioverted anterior teeth and open bite may also occur (Moller, 1994). Surgical reduction of the tongue is often indicated these cases.

Other problems that might be observed in children with syndromes include lobules (oral-facial-digital syndrome), tumors (neurofibromatosis), and tongue deviation in response to deficient cranial nerve innervation (hemifacial microsomia) (Witzel, 1994).

Hard palate. The contour and width of the hard palate should be assessed. A high palatal vault rarely influences speech production; however, the "narrowed maxillary arch which accompanies it provides insufficient space for the tongue to carry out articulatory movements" (Stenglehofen, 1990, p. 32). An extremely low palatal vault can also influence articulation, particularly when an anterior open bite is present. Both of the aforementioned conditions invite interdental tongue carriage—particularly for linguoalveolar consonants. The presence of ectopic teeth may contribute to anterior tongue carriage as well.

The palate should be carefully examined for oronasal fistulae. When malposed teeth and narrowed maxillary arches impede your view, a dental reflector mirror can be used to closely examine the anterior palate. Henningsson and Isberg (1990) have reported that a "slit-like" fistula in the hard palate may be difficult to visualize because the surrounding mucosa may occlude it until intraoral pressure is great enough to open it. Remember that a fistula that appears patent on the oral surface of the palate is not necessarily patent on the nasal side. Many small palatal fistulae that are observed in children with repaired cleft palate have minimal to no impact on either speech or loss of liquids or food through the nose. Therefore, identification of a fistula should not lead to a recommendation for palatal surgery/obturation unless your findings demonstrate that the fistula is having a significant effect on a specific behavior (this will be discussed in more detail below).

Faucial pillars or tonsils. When tonsils are present, note their size. Although it is rare for tonsils to have an impact on speech production, occasionally they may become so hypertrophied that they restrict velar movement. (Note: The adenoid pad is located in the nasopharynx and is typically not visible on intraoral examination. Only on rare occasions will the inferior border of a hypertrophied adenoid pad be visible.)

Soft palate. The soft palate should initially be examined at rest. If the palate is obstructed from view by the tongue, visualization can frequently be accomplished by having the child take short, rapid breaths (i.e., pant). When present, a bifid uvula is likely to be the first observation made. Although the presence of a bifid uvula does not always indicate the presence of a submucous cleft, the clinician should examine the palate for other overt signs of a submucous cleft, including bluish translucency of the palate at midline (zona pellucida) and bony notching of the posterior border of the hard palate. The latter observation should be made by palpating the palate at the juncture of the hard and soft palate. Finally, the symmetry and length of the palate should be examined at rest.

Palatal movement should be examined as the patient phonates /a/. If a tongue blade is needed to ensure visualization of the palate, care should be taken not to depress the tongue with too much force. Peterson-Falzone (1994, p. 345) cautioned, "In the child with a repaired cleft the muscular link between the tongue and the velum—the palatoglossus muscle—may be tighter than normal and pushing down on the tongue dorsum may interfere with upward movement of the velum, thus giving false information about velar movement." The speech pathologist can make limited observations of the rate, extent, and direction of movement of the velum and portions of the pharyngeal walls during sustained phonation or gag. However, the information derived from observation has little value in predicting velopharyngeal closure during connected speech except in cases of severe inadequacy caused by very short, scarred immobile palates. The speech pathologist must be aware that velopharyngeal inadequacy may have anatomical or physiological origins that are not evident on intraoral inspection. Factors such as enlarged tonsils and pharyngeal webbing can mechanically interfere with velar movement. Other factors that may influence velopharyngeal valving include ". . . a deficieny of muscle mass on the nasal surface of the velum, abnormal direction of pull of the velar musculature, and inadequate movement of pharyngeal musculature towards closure" (Peterson-Falzone, 1994, p. 345). Finally, it is pertinent to reiterate that velopharyngeal closure cannot be viewed on direct intraoral examination. The site of closure is hidden from view by the velum. Although observations regarding velar movement can be made, velopharyngeal function cannot be assessed from this type of examination, no matter who performs it.

Pharyngeal walls. Any movement of the pharyngeal walls that is observed during sustained /a/ should be noted. Occasionally, a Passavant's ridge may be apparent on the posterior pharyngeal wall. Obviously, such movement is not contributing to velopharyngeal closure when it is occurring below the level of the velum.

VOICE ASSESSMENT

The majority of individuals with cleft palate who are referred for a speech-language assessment typically demonstrate problems associated with articulation and/or resonance, if they have clinical problems at all. When voice disorders are encountered in this population (or in patients with velopharyngeal inadequacy from other causes), they generally include hoarseness and soft-voice syndrome. As Philips (1986) pointed out, these problems likely "have their origin in excessive respiratory effort and laryngeal tension, which may be used as the speaker attempts to reduce nasal airflow or compensate for the damping effects of nasal airflow" (p. 305).

A screening assessment for voice disorders can easily be incorporated into any speech-language assessment protocol. Wilson (1987) recommended that a child be asked to (1) count from 1 to 10, (2) read orally for 1 minute, (3) produce continuous speech for 1 minute, and (4) prolong five different vowels for 5 seconds each. Vocal characteristics (including laryngeal tone, pitch, and loudness) are evaluated and then rated on a five-point rating scale. If perceptual signs of a voice problem are identified, additional assessment is indicated. Although the protocol for assessment will vary depending on a number of factors (including the age of the patient, the nature of the problem, and the instrumental tools available) a comprehensive assessment of voice disorders typically includes a perceptual assessment of vocal characteristics, acoustic or aerodynamic assessment, and direct examination of the laryngeal structures and their function. A comprehensive discussion of voice disorders and their management is beyond the scope of this book. For a detailed account of voice examinations, the reader is referred to Boone and McFarlane (1994) and Colton and Casper (1996).

When a voice problem is present, a careful history should be taken to discover whether the symptom is of recent origin, is chronic or acute, or is associated with an allergy, upper respiratory infection, or unusual vocal abuse. People who have had voice problems for a long time may not realize it, and their families, accustomed to hearing their speech, may not recognize that there is anything unusual. For this reason, it is necessary to be alert for such statements as, "This is the way I always talk," or "I don't notice anything different about my voice," or "My voice sounds all right to me." These comments may suggest that the phonation is not different from what the patient views as "normal." If the voice disorder appears to be chronic, a behavioral history is important to determine whether there are environmental factors or patterns of vocal abuse that might account for laryngeal hypofunction or hyperfunction. Frequent screaming, excessively loud talking, frequent coughing or throat clearing, imitating motor noises, and making animal sounds are activities common among children who develop various types of hyperfunctional phonatory disorders. Although we have no systematic information about these vocal abuses in children with clefts, it is our clinical impression that we fail more often than not to find evidence of such vocal misuse. Nevertheless, the information must be sought and acted on in those cases where it is appropriate. Special attention should be paid to the child with hypernasality and hoarseness. Speech therapy with the goal of reducing hypernasality may contribute to either hypofunctional or hyperfunctional disorders in some children.

A second area that should be explored is personality and interpersonal relationships. Phonatory problems with origins in hyperfunction often occur in tense people who are loud and somewhat aggressive. Although such behaviors are no more prevalent in children with clefts than their noncleft peers, the possibility of their existence outside the clinic should be investigated. The socially reticent, somewhat withdrawn individual may also develop voice problems, which reflect confusion about the need to communicate and the desire to remain quiet.

The third step in the voice evaluation is to determine the nature of the deviation. We are interested in the appropriateness of vocal pitch, pitch range, loudness, and voice quality. Several authors have reported simple systems for scoring these dimensions of voice (Boone and McFarlane, 1994; Wilson, 1987). These systems provide the clinician with the information required to decide whether the voice is or is not defective and, if defective, what the severity of the problem is. Aronson (1980) considered the sustaining of /a/ to be the single most revealing voice test available. He recommended assessing quality, pitch, loudness, and steadiness with vowel prolongation.

In addition to judging the adequacy of a patient's vocal behaviors during speech, excessive throat clearing, frequent phonation breaks, and any unusual vocal behaviors such as inhalatory/expiratory stridor, vocal tics, and grunts should be noted. The presence of stridor in infants may signal the presence of laryngomalacia. Stridor typically occurs secondary to airway obstruction related to problems such as laryngeal webs, obstructive lesions, abductor vocal fold paralysis, or ankylosis of the cricoarytenoid joints (Colton and Casper, 1996). Vocal tics and other unexpected vocal behaviors (e.g., barks, growls) may be symptomatic of a neurological disorder.

Acoustic studies, aerodynamic studies, and physiological studies are routinely used at major voice centers today to examine different vocal parameters. Some of the instrumentation used to study the acoustic and aerodynamic characteristics of phonation will be described later in this text (see Chapter 10). For additional information regarding instrumental assessment, refer to Boone and McFarlane (1994) and Colton and Casper (1996).

Some authors (Boone and McFarlane, 1994; Colton and Casper, 1996) have described the use of simple, noninstrumental screening measures to obtain gross information about an individual's respiratory function and laryngeal control. *Maximum phonation time* is obtained by instructing the patient take a deep breath and sustain an /a/ for as long as possible. The longest duration over three trials is typically designated as the maximum phonation time. Colton and Casper (1996) reported normative data for this measure, noting that both age and sex influence an individual's ability to sustain phonation. The *s/z ratio* described by Boone and McFarlane (1988) can also be used as a screening tool in a voice assessment to obtain gross information about laryngeal efficiency. In this procedure the patient is instructed to take a deep breath and sustain /s/ and then /z/ for as long as possible. The procedure is typically replicated several times, then the s/z ratio is calculated. Presumably, when a vocal cord pathologic condition is present, the patient may show a differential between the two, with /z/ being shorter. Eckel and Boone (1981) reported that 95% of the adults with laryngeal pathologic conditions that they examined had s/z ratios greater than 1.4. Ratios obtained by subjects without these laryngeal conditions approximated 1.0. The validity of this measure with children has been questioned by several authors (Hufnagle and Hufnagle, 1988; Rastatter and Hyman, 1982) who reported s/z ratios of 1.0 in their children with vocal nodules. Colton and Casper stated that, although the measures of maximum phonation time and s/z ratio may be used as screening tools or in conjunction with other tests, the information derived from these tests should be interpreted cautiously (particularly with children).

The fourth step in the evaluation is to determine whether the voice can be modified. For hyperfunctional voice deviations, it is often beneficial to have the patient produce reflexive sounds (e.g., cough, laugh, clearing the throat, and production of "uh-huh") to determine whether the quality of voice changes during nonspeech tasks. Production of such sounds may provide a glimpse of the patient's normal voice because the unwanted behaviors that led to the phonatory problem will not likely be present during these nonspeech behaviors (Colton and Casper, 1996). Other "facilitating approaches" that are useful in diagnostic therapy to reduce excessive muscular tension and promote easy onset of phonation include lowering the back of the tongue, chant talk, chewing with phonation, and coupling phonation with a yawn-sigh (Boone and McFarlane, 1994; Colton and Casper, 1996).

Finally, we recommend that an audiological evaluation be included as part of all voice examinations. Hearing losses, usually conductive, occur more frequently in children with clefts than in those without. Conductive losses, when great enough, can be associated with a reduction in loudness as well as with variations in loudness, whereas sensorineural losses may be accompanied by an increase in loudness. If hearing loss is found, the patient will, of course, be referred to an otologist before any other recommendations are made.

Laryngeal Examination

If hoarseness or any other condition that may accompany vocal cord pathology is present, the patient should be examined by an otolaryngologist to obtain definitive information about the condition of the vocal cords. When hoarseness and a cleft occur together, chances are that the diagnosis will be bilateral vocal cord nodules or some preliminary condition such as edema or inflammation. Unless the nodules are unusually large, surgery is not likely to be recommended (Aronson, 1980; Boone, 1977; Boone and McFarlane, 1988; Colton and Casper, 1996). Rather, the preferred treatment will undoubtedly be to eliminate the vocal hyperfunction usually associated with nodules.

LANGUAGE

All children born with clefts or other craniofacial malformations should be routinely followed up for language development just as they are for hearing, dental problems, facial growth, special pediatric needs, and psychosocial well-being. They are prone to the same developmental problems that may occur in any child, but special factors create added risks that should not be ignored. The speech-language pathologist working with individual children has no foundation on which to assume that language will be either normal or aberrant, although, as we saw earlier, language deficits over a wide range occur more frequently in children with clefts than in noncleft children. For this reason, surveillance is always indicated, with routine testing as a regular part of clinical care and special testing in response to need. A comprehensive diagnostic evaluation of language typically includes assessment of form, content, and use of language within the modalities of both comprehension and production. According to Paul (1995), a comprehensive assessment should also include investigation of "collateral" areas such as hearing, speech-motor functioning, social functioning, and nonverbal cognition.

Psychosocial/Environmental Factors

The child's social environment should be examined through conversations with parents as well as through observations of parent-child interactions when possible to obtain information about the child's language needs. Such an assessment may be useful in identifying factors that may contribute to a language deficit. Differential treatment in the family, poor parent-child relationships, child management problems, overprotection, parental anxiety, general health of the child and the family, socioeconomic factors, the parents' marital stability and happiness, the kind of verbal interaction in the family and with the child—any one of these factors alone or in combination with one another can play a role in influencing language development. Although the quality of parent-child interaction is always of interest in such an assessment and may provide useful information about the parent's communicative style, Paul (1995) cautioned against assuming that differences observed in interaction styles are responsible for the language deficits noted. "Except in cases of extreme abuse or neglect, parents are almost never the primary source of their child's communication difficulty" (p. 35). According to Paul, there are five goals that should be addressed in an assessment of social functioning. First, information regarding the child's use of communication skills should be obtained and the influence of communication problems on the development of daily living skills should be examined. Useful information about social functioning and daily living skills can be obtained with instruments such as the *Vineland Adaptive Behavior Scales* (Sparrow, Balla, and Cicchetti, 1984). Second, the emotional and behavioral status of a child should be examined. If problems in adjustment are suspected, then referral to a psychologist may be indicated. The final three goals include exploring the family's perceptions of the child's needs, identifying the support available to the parents from friends and professionals, and obtaining information about language and cultural differences in the home that may have an impact on the child's communication.

Developmental Evaluation

In our zeal to recognize and treat language impairments, we sometimes forget that language in all its forms is a part of the total fabric of human development. If a child's language is not maturing as we would wish, all aspects of development should be assessed. It may be that language is out of keeping with the rest of development or that it is consistent with other developmental characteristics. A 2-year-old child doing well in almost every way except language would be a candidate for language management. A 2-year-old child showing, in addition, deficits in motor, cognitive, and interpersonal skills might more reasonably be considered for placement in a program designed to stimulate general development including language.

A word of caution is necessary here. Speech-language pathologists should be developmental specialists who understand normal development and recognize variations when they occur. Not all young children reach the same developmental milestones at precisely the same ages. Thus, a child who is using little expressive language at 18 months may or may not require intervention. This is especially true if the child has had life experiences that may reasonably explain the delay. For example, surgery at 12 and 18 months may be incompatible with the onset of speech in some children but not in others. A child who understands appropriately for chronological age but does not talk is different from one who neither talks nor understands. The same may be said for slow acquisition of early motor behaviors. The pieces of the puzzle must fit together in a reasonable way, or the clinician is pursuing the wrong course. Only careful study will provide the evidence needed to decide.

Few speech-language pathologists are well qualified to administer psychological tests, and some seem not to recognize the importance of these in reaching even tentative conclusions about the nature of language disorders. We think that it is a mistake to attempt language therapy without evaluation of the patient by a competent psychologist experienced in testing young children, especially those with clefts, craniofacial abnormalities, and disordered speech. Even when such information is not available, the speech-language pathologist can screen nonverbal cognition through the use of informal instruments such as the *Cognitive Behavior Scales* or the *Uzgiris-Hunt Scales of Infant Development* or through play assessments such as the *Communication and Symbolic Behavior Scales* (Paul, 1995).

Language Evaluation

Children with clefts are at an increased risk for language problems because of a host of interacting factors such as negative social-emotional status and hearing impairment. This is especially true if they have isolated palatal clefts (as opposed to cleft lip and palate) or associated malformations, including syndromes. All children with clefts or other craniofacial malformations should be carefully followed up from birth, with developmental and language screenings performed routinely and in-depth testing recommended if there is any doubt about the level of functioning. Language assessment of children with clefts is not fundamentally different from that of any other child except that the examiner needs to be especially alert for low levels of expressivity used by these children, quite apart from their language capabilities, and to the inhibitions that may mediate between the child and the examiner.

A comprehensive assessment of language functioning is typically performed using a combination of standardized tests, developmental scales, criterion-referenced procedures, and behavioral observations. A number of standardized language tests investigate both receptive and expressive language either for screening or for diagnostic purposes. There is dissatisfaction with many of the testing tools now available because, in addition to their other problems, they are often too simplistic to address in any detail the complex issues involved in language disorders. However, they do offer systematic approaches and can be useful in helping the clinician delineate general problems that can then be explored in greater depth. Huang, Hopkins, and Nippold

(1997) surveyed 216 speech-language pathologists and found that the most commonly used language tests for preschoolers included the *Peabody Picture Vocabulary Test-Revised,* the *Expressive One Word Picture Vocabulary Test,* the *Preschool Language Scale-3,* the *Sequenced Inventory of Communication,* and the *Test of Language Development Primary.* The former two tests were also frequently used with the elementary school-aged child, as was *The Word Test- Revised* and the *Test of Language Development 2-Intermediate.* An inventory of tests commonly used to assess language can be found in Paul (1995).

As indicated earlier in this chapter, speech-language pathologists who serve on cleft palate–craniofacial teams often face time constraints that do not permit a comprehensive assessment of language functioning during the team assessment. In such cases, information obtained through parent report and informal observation is frequently used to screen patients for language impairments during routine clinic visits and to make decisions about referral for additional assessment. Inventories that make use of parent report and informal observations (e.g., *MacArthur Communicative Development Inventory)* were described earlier in this chapter. Informal assessment of language in children should include observation of syntax-morphology, semantics, and pragmatics.

Receptive language. The goal of receptive language testing is to discover how complicated verbal expression can become before the child ceases to understand it and what, if any, particular forms cause breakdown in performance. Receptive language can be examined by both formal and informal assessment procedures. Miller and Paul (1995) and Paul (1995) provide an excellent catalog of many standardized language tests that are used to examine receptive language functioning. In addition to standardized tests, many authors also recommend the use of nonstandard measures to obtain more specific information about a child's linguistic functioning. Weiss, Tomblin, and Robin (1994) identified three basic tasks that are used to assess receptive language functioning. The first, *recognition/identification tasks,* require the child to listen to a language stimulus and then identify the object or event that was described in the stimulus. In an *acting out task,* the child is provided with objects and asked to manipulate them in some way (e.g., kiss the ball). The third type of task described was a *judgment task,* where the child is asked to listen to a statement produced by the examiner and then judge how acceptable it is.

The outcome of both formal and informal receptive-language testing is closely related to the child's ability and desire to cooperate, to his or her comfort in the testing situation, to the sophistication of the examiner, and to his or her rapport with the child. The speech pathologist who undertakes testing of this sort on an informal basis must be knowledgeable about the levels of difficulty and abstraction of the requests made to the child and must recognize the structural elements involved.

Expressive language. Children fail to acquire and develop the complex use of expressive language at the expected ages for a variety of reasons. One child may have extensive problems encompassing both receptive and expressive language, whereas another will have relatively minor deficits involving only verbal communication. Although neither talks, their clinical pictures differ markedly and so should their treatment.

Expressive language is typically examined through analysis of a spontaneous language sample. A sample of at least 50 spontaneous utterances are transcribed and then analyzed to obtain information about syntax and morphology as well as other components of language. In addition to measures of sentence complexity that might be obtained with analyses such as the Developmental Sentence Scoring (Lee, 1974), measures of sentence length can also be obtained. Mean length of response or mean length of utterance is an important area for investigation because children with clefts appear to have their most significant problems in the amount of verbal output they use. On average, most of the children will be mildly deficient, but some will have significant problems in this regard. Analysis of language samples may be time consuming to carry out, but they do provide what is probably the best information that can be gathered about language usage. When necessary, clinicians who audiorecord their sessions can simply identify the morphemes and syntactic patterns heard without transcribing the entire sample. Paul (1995) noted that, although some morphemes might be missed in such an analysis, this method is more practical for use in clinical settings. In her discussion of language assessment in children with cleft palate, Philips (1986) cautioned that "Pervasive glottal stops, pharyngeal plosives and fricatives, and nasal-airflow substitutions can make morphological markers, and specific words used, difficult, if not impossible to discern" (p. 306).

Narratives are a popular strategy used for examining a child's productive language. A narrative sample can be elicited by asking the child to describe a personal narrative, retell a story, describe a movie, or narrate a picture book. Expressive language can also be examined using tasks such as confrontation naming, imitation, and the Cloze technique (Weiss et al., 1994). These tasks are used in formal language tests and can be used informally as well to probe for certain language constructs. Confrontation naming tasks, such as that used in *The Expressive One-Word Vocabulary Test,* involve presenting a child with a picture or object then asking him or her to name it. Imitation tasks require the child to repeat exactly what the examiner says either immediately after the examiner (direct imitation) or after some delay (delayed imitation). The Cloze technique elicits language by having the child fill in a missing element from a sentence spoken by the examiner (e.g., A bicycle is fast, but a plane is _____). Finally, role playing and games (e.g., I spy) can be used to elicit particular linguistic forms. Paul (1995) pointed out elicited imitations can result in errors that a child would not normally produce in spontaneous speech. She recommended that this technique be used as a "last resort."

The sociocommunicative skills of children with cleft palate should always be considered in any language assessment. In our efforts to identify and treat the salient aspects of *cleft palate speech* (e.g., hypernasality, audible nasal emission, compensatory articulation patterns), we often neglect to examine their impact on the child as a communicator. We may be concerned that the presence of severe nasalization in conjunction with a severe phonological delay is compromising the child's speech intelligibility, thus resulting in frequent communication failure. We may develop strategies to further examine and treat the patterns of errors. Unfortunately, once those errors are eradicated, we frequently assume that the job is done. Chapman and Hardin (1990), reviewing the research literature describing sociocommunicative functioning in children and adolescents with clefts, speculated that these individuals may differ from their noncleft peers in the dimension of conversational participation. They recommended the use of a model described by Fey (1986) that evaluates two components of language: conversational assertiveness and conversational responsiveness. Fey defined conversational assertiveness as the "ability or willingness (or both) to take a conversational turn when none has been solicited by a partner" (p. 69). Conversational responsiveness refers to the child's response to a conversational turn that was previously initiated by a communication partner. According to Fey, four different patterns of conversational participation can be described using this model: (1) *active conversationalists* (initiates conversation and responsive to conversation initiated by others), (2) *passive conversationalists* (responsive to conversation initiated by others but does not routinely initiate conversation), (3) *inactive conversationalists* (rarely initiates conversation and not highly responsive to conversations initiated by others), and (4) *verbal noncommunicators* (initiates conversations but not highly responsive to partner's needs).

Chapman and Hardin (1990) observed that as a child matures ". . . negative peer reactions and negative self-perceptions about facial appearance and communication effectiveness may lead a child to withdraw from the verbal limelight and avoid verbal interactions when possible" (p. 725). Models of sociocommunicative effectiveness like the one proposed by Fey can assist the clinician in differentiating children with cleft palate who avoid or limit conversational exchanges as a result of poor speech intelligibility problems (or perceptions of self as a poor communicator) from those who do not understand the rules of communication as well as those who are reluctant to talk as a result of personality style.

Other protocols developed for assessing pragmatic skills in children are described elsewhere (Creaghead, 1984; Paul, 1995; Shipley and McAfee, 1992). The pragmatic behaviors sampled across protocols may differ; however, Shipley and McAfee (1992) point out that, regardless of the specific protocol used, pragmatic skills should be examined across a variety of situations because they can be situationally and environmentally specific. They identified 15 pragmatic behaviors and provided suggestions for eliciting the behaviors in a semistructured setting. The behaviors included response to greetings, describing events, taking turns, making requests, following commands, making eye contact, repeating, attending to tasks, maintaining the topic, role playing, sequencing actions, defining words, categorizing, understanding object functions, and initiating activity or dialogue.

Hearing

Hearing evaluations are always important for all children, especially for those who have a language delay. They are essential for children with clefts because, as we have already seen, they all begin life with ear disease and remain at increased risk for conductive hearing losses in the preschool years and even later. Any sign of even a mild hearing loss should be cause for referral to an otolaryngologist for examination and treatment as indicated. No loss is too minimal to be ignored because it may mean that hearing sensitivity is fluctuating, a condition difficult for any child to deal with. Although the evidence is far from clear that these conductive losses are implicated in a major way in language deficits in children with clefts, we do know that such sensory variations do nothing to enhance language development and that, left untreated, they may grow progressively worse. The need for careful audiological assessment, including tympanometry, cannot be overemphasized.

RELIABILITY AND VALIDITY ISSUES

The single most important assessment tool that the speech-language pathologist will use in clinical practice is the ear. Perceptual judgments are used each time an articulation test is scored, speech intelligibility is estimated, rate and volume are described, and voice and resonance are scaled. Moll (1964) made a strong case for the desirability and necessity of making listener judgments the basis of all assessments of speech, including resonance deviations. He suggested that listener judgments provide the only measures that are direct and logically valid, given the basic perceptual nature of speech, and that any instrumental approach to measuring hypernasality, if it is to be useful, must provide reliable data that are closely related to listener judgments. We are in agreement with this position but recognize with others (Bradford, Brooks, and Shelton, 1964; Wells, 1971) that listeners do not always agree on the presence, absence, or amount of nasality in normal speech. The same statement applies to the assessment of other resonance and articulatory disorders found in speakers with cleft palate.

Although listener judgments intuitively appear to be the most valid indicator of a communication problem, they are subject to numerous threats to reliability. Indeed, both speaker and listener variables have the potential to influence speech ratings. Kent (1996) wrote, "Clinical applications of auditory judgments are predicated on the assumptions that listeners (a) have a common understanding of perceptual labels such as *hoarse, nasal, rough, monoloud, excess and equal stress, or stuttering;* (b) use essentially the same verbal descriptors and associated scale values to assess a given sample of speech or voice; (c) can isolate for judgment one perceptual dimension from several co-occurring dimensions; (d) have a uniform reliability in judging the various dimensions that give a complete clinical portrait of speech or voice disorders; and (e) can make perceptual judgments for which the interjudge differences are smaller than the differences needed for clinical classification or to discern changes in clinical status" (p. 7).

Articulation Testing

Reliability in articulation testing is an important concern of speech pathologists. Articulation tests are usually administered in a clinic by one examiner whose judgments may or may not be consistent from one session to the next or with those assigned by other clinicians. Clinicians can improve the reliability of articulation testing by recognizing several problems such as anchoring and sequencing effects (Young, 1970). *Anchors* are the standards against which responses are to be judged. In psychophysical scaling test responses may be compared with a recorded standard. Clinically, the standard is likely to be in the examiner's head, that is, remembered from previous experience. The clinician should strive to maintain a consistent standard or at least to be aware of a shift in the standard against which a patient's articulation is evaluated. *Sequencing* is the interacting influence of neighboring sounds. As an example, if the /s/ sound in a test word follows a very well articulated /s/ in a previous word, the second /s/ might be scored as incorrect, whereas the same response might be scored as correct if it occurred after a poorly articulated /s/. We think that the effects of anchoring and sequencing can be tempered by the instructions examiners give themselves. For example, they may arbitrarily decide to score marginal or questionable responses as incorrect. This instruction would be expected to reduce the occurrence of sequencing effects, but it would do so at the cost of sensitivity to marginal articulation that might well be acceptable. Again, the clinician may instruct himself or herself to categorize a response as correct or incorrect and then, if possible, to specify additional information: correct but slightly dentalized; incorrect because of lateral emission, or correct in place of articulation but accompanied by audible nasal emission.

Sometimes comparison of articulation judgments by two speech pathologists will show that examiner disagreement was of a semantic rather than a perceptual nature. The two examiners may agree, for example, that the /s/ sounds are slightly dentalized but are free from tongue protrusion. However, one examiner chose to accept those responses as correct, whereas the other classified them as incorrect. Another factor that may influence reliability is repeatedly listening to the same stimulus. It has been demonstrated that some individuals evaluating repeated productions of a particular consonant classify some as correct and some as incorrect when, unknown to them, they are listening to dubbings of a single utterance (Ruscello et al., 1980; Shelton, Johnson, and Arndt, 1974). When informed of the deception, some listeners express the conviction that the articulation of the target sound differed in correctness from one time to another. Our ears can play tricks on us in different ways. Diedrich and Bangert (1980) found that clinicians who have provided training to misarticulating children are more likely to hear improvement in the articulation of those children than are other clinicians who are equally qualified but who do not know the children.

Determining examiner reliability for research purposes is done in a variety of ways. One involves computation of correlation coefficients on the basis of total test scores. If total articulation scores obtained through testing done by two examiners are similar, the resulting correlation will be high, and reliability will appear to be adequate. However, total score agreement can mask disagreements on particular test sounds. Consequently, agreement between observers is often expressed as a percentage of agreement based on an item-by-item analysis. Again, item agreement tends to be lower when the examiners must determine the exact nature of the error than it is when the judgment is only whether the sound is correct or incorrect. Studies with cleft subjects have indicated that the identification of the type of error is considerably less reliable than is scoring the response as correct or incorrect (Bzoch, 1979; Philips and Bzoch, 1969). Moreover, articulation judgments made from tapes are less likely to be reliable than are live judgments (Stephens and Daniloff, 1977). A distinction has been drawn between agreement among observers on all test items (speech sounds) under consideration and observer agreement regarding responses that occur infrequently. For example, agreement may be high on clearly correct or grossly distorted responses but marginal on marginal responses (Byrne, Shelton, and Diedrich, 1961). McReynolds and Kearns (1983) and Kearns and Simmons (1988) recommend that observer agreement be identified for the infrequently occurring responses and that the agreement be tested to determine whether it exceeds that which would be expected on the basis of chance.

Clinicians may improve interobserver reliability by analyzing live speech samples that are also recorded for repeated study. The recording is used as a referent, and disagreements are discussed and, when possible, resolved.

Rating Scales

The reliability of speech ratings assigned to patients with clefts has also been studied. Moller and Starr (1984) compared speech ratings obtained under three listening conditions: face-to-face with the patient, observing by a mirror and sound system, and listening to tape recordings.

The study was motivated by evidence that data obtained by individual observers sometimes lack reliability. Speech samples from 100 consecutive patients (age range 2 to 42 years) were rated on eight-point scales for intelligibility, resonance distortion, articulation deviation, voice deviation, and overall speech acceptability. Multiple listeners, including graduate students and speech pathologists, participated. Each underwent listening training. For each measure data obtained from students correlated highly with that obtained from speech pathologists (for articulation, $r = 0.92$). The speech sample included 2 or more minutes of conversation, a standard paragraph, selected sentences, counting to 10, and sustained /i/ and /a/ vowels. The authors found no statistically significant difference among the three listening conditions for any measure except voice. They questioned whether a single rating can successfully represent voice quality, which is multidimensional. Speech ratings made by panels of observers trained for the task constitute good data for use in study of patients with cleft palate. There is the difficulty, however, in reliable distinction between oral and nasal distortion from tape-recorded samples.

Reliability in using scales of these types rests with the rater(s). Many studies have, through training listeners, reported acceptable levels of agreement among listeners (McWilliams, 1954; McWilliams and Philips, 1979). However, rating reliably remains a difficult task and one that has been approached in several different ways. Scales are most reliable when groups of listeners participate and the central tendencies of the pooled ratings are used as the final ratings. This is so because of the wide variations found among raters assessing the same speech sample. This system is not an appropriate clinical tool because it is far too cumbersome, expensive, and time consuming. A more effective technique that has been successfully used in clinics has speech pathologists first test their reliability against group ratings by listening to and independently rating speech samples previously rated by a group of listeners. They then discuss their ratings, attempting to decide what elements in the speech pattern led them to respond as they did, and gradually they reach agreement on the nature of the speech that is to be associated with a particular point on the scale. Then, if the individual clinicians doing the ratings also agree with each other and frequently re-establish their agreement, they may have confidence in their ratings. All these steps are necessary to ensure that the ratings are reliable. Anyone working with patients who have velopharyngeal incompetence should routinely collect data on interjudge agreement and establish clinical protocols to ensure that this important aspect is not neglected.

The validity of rating scales is also a matter of concern. The evidence is somewhat ambiguous (Ramig, 1982; Sinko and Hedrick, 1982), but speech ratings may be influenced by facial appearance or vice versa and ratings of nasality may be influenced by the presence of misarticulations (Hess, 1971; Sherman, 1970). Listeners have difficulty separating hypernasality from the other speech characteristics associated with velopharyngeal incompetence. The more "other" symptoms, the higher the ratings of nasality (McWilliams, 1954). Thus it seems that raters, in reality, rate their global perceptions and are not able to rate the single element of nasality. This always means that ratings, even those on which listeners agree, may be invalid.

Sherman (1954) theorized that ratings of nasality might be more valid and more reliable if the contaminating cues were eliminated by playing audiotapes backward and having judges rate nasality under that condition. Black (1973) showed, however, that backward play of speech alters some characteristics of the signal to a greater extent than it does others. Of interest in the assessment of hypernasality is the finding that vowels are changed more than are such consonants as /k/, /z/, /r/, /s/, and /f/. All but the /r/ are elements of extreme importance when velopharyngeal competence is a factor. In addition, frication was identifiable on backward play. These findings suggested that the backward play of speech samples may be questionable in the rating of hypernasality, and this was the conclusion of Fletcher (1976) as well.

There is modest evidence that speech rated from tape recordings may, in some cases, lead to somewhat different conclusions from those achieved from live ratings (McWilliams and Philips, 1979). Thus, if taped samples are to be used for rating hypernasality, it is wise to have data from live ratings as well. If the two do not agree, additional evaluations are in order because questions of validity arise.

The problem of rating hypernasality as a single entity persists. Bzoch (1979), as noted earlier, stated that hypernasality can be reliably rated only under conditions of clear phonation and normal articulation. We agree that those conditions make the task easier, but the clinical reality is that hypernasality is one of several characteristics associated with velopharyngeal incompetence and we have to continue our efforts to make valid and reliable judgments concerning it. Bzoch also recognized this need.

MAKING TREATMENT RECOMMENDATIONS

Once information about speech and language have been gathered, the patterns of articulation and resonance analyzed, and the prognosis considered, a plan of treatment must be developed. The clinician will use knowledge of the speech mechanism, of the child's articulatory pattern, and of speech development to decide whether disordered articulation is likely to improve spontaneously, whether articulation and/or resonance improvement appears to be contingent on medical or dental treatments, or whether therapy appears to be warranted. Other decisions, such as need for language intervention, must also be made.

Treatment planning for children with clefts who demonstrate conventional (developmental) speech-language problems is fairly straightforward and does not really differ from that initiated for children without clefts. Management decisions for children who demonstrate articulation and resonance problems associated with poor dental/occlusal status or velopharyngeal dysfunction is more complex.

The Problem of Dentition

If the results of articulation testing, stimulability testing, and oral peripheral examination suggest that the child's dentition is influencing the precision of articulation of sibilant consonants, the clinician must decide whether to attempt articulation therapy before orthodontics is completed. If the clinician waits for that completion, the patient will probably have entered puberty and may have passed through the "sensitive period" during which speech learning is relatively easy. On the other hand, the behavioral modification of articulatory errors related to structural deviations is often difficult or impossible, and speech may improve spontaneously with successful orthodontic correction or midface advancement so that therapy will not be required. The potential for change is always a factor in making recommendations either for or against speech therapy.

Most speech-language pathologists will enroll a child with dental/occlusal problems in a trial therapy to assess the child's potential for change. The actual improvement noted, however, should drive future decisions to retain the child in therapy or to defer treatment. We should not keep a child in therapy simply because he or she has a problem.

Velopharyngeal Inadequacy: Surgery, Therapy, or Both?

Velopharyngeal dysfunction manifests itself in different ways in different children. Some children have severe nasalization of speech and are immediately referred for instrumental assessment of velopharyngeal function. The referral is made with the assumption that once the problem has been confirmed and studied, surgical (or prosthetic) management will be the obvious treatment of choice. Unfortunately, management decisions are not easily made for all patients with velopharyngeal valving problems. Some children may demonstrate evidence of velopharyngeal dysfunction but may not be candidates for anything other than speech-language therapy at the time of their initial referral. These children are discussed in the section below. Other children may demonstrate mild hypernasality, inconsistent audible nasal emission, and weak pressure consonants—although the nasalization is readily perceived during conversational exchanges with the child, it is not severe enough to compromise general intelligibility and so management decisions are deferred and the child's resonance is simply monitored over time. For some children with severe speech sound deficits, improvement in articulation alone may decrease the *perception* of nasality to the point that surgical management is not warranted. The point here is that the presence of hypernasality and audible nasal emission does not necessarily mean that a child should be referred for surgical management. The severity of the problem, its influence on speech intelligibility, and the child's and parents' reaction to the problem should all be considered when making treatment recommendations.

Referral for Objective Assessment of Velopharyngeal Function

The decision to refer for an objective assessment of velopharyngeal function is an easy one to make for many patients that we see. When a speaker with good articulation demonstrates nasalization of speech that is severe enough to distract a listener and when that speaker is mature enough to cooperate for an objective assessment of velopharyngeal function, then the referral is easily made. Unfortunately, not all patients who demonstrate perceptual evidence of velopharyngeal inadequacy are appropriate candidates for instrumental assessment. A number of factors can interfere with our ability to evaluate the functional potential of the velopharyngeal mechanism in some patients.

Age or maturity. Toddlers and young children with hypernasality and audible nasal emission are frequently referred to cleft palate teams by speech-language pathologists for physical management of velopharyngeal inadequacy. It is assumed that because a problem exists it should be treated without delay. Frequently, however, the child is too young to cooperate for an objective assessment of velopharyngeal function. Is it best to proceed with a recommendation for surgical management in the hopes that the surgeon will be able to eliminate the problem without documenting the nature of the problem? Or should we defer decisions regarding surgical management until the child is a little older and more likely to cooperate for instrumental assessment? We believe in such cases that it is not always in a child's best interests to proceed with a recommendation for physical management. Even when the results of the perceptual examination lead you to believe without hesitation that velopharyngeal inadequacy exists, a better speech result may be obtained if treatment is deferred until the speech-language pathologist and surgeon are able to view the velopharyngeal mechanism. Procedures such as nasoendoscopy and videofluoroscopy are performed not only to verify that a problem exists but also to obtain information about the child's anatomy and physiology. Identifying those structures that move well and those that offer limited to no movement potential often determines the type of pharyngoplasty that should be performed to provide the best possible speech result.

Severe phonological delay. Children with extremely poor consonant development who demonstrate severe nasalization of speech are often referred by professionals who presume that the child will be a good candidate for surgical management. Parents and professionals alike may be disappointed when informed by the speech-language pathologist on the cleft palate team that the child's speech is not developed enough to permit an assessment of velopharyngeal function. It is not uncommon for speech-language pathologists who have made the referral to argue that therapy is simply not working and infer that progress is being compromised by velopharyngeal inadequacy. Other professionals may argue that speech intelligibility will be enhanced by eliminating velopharyngeal inadequacy, whereas others adopt the "it can't hurt" philosophy. Unfortunately, it is not possible to adequately assess velopharyngeal function in children who are making no attempt toward production of pressure consonants. As an example, consider the young child with repaired cleft palate whose consonant inventory is limited to nasals, glides, and glottal productions. These children may be referred for velopharyngeal function studies because speech sounds "nasal," yet the nature of their errors (particularly the nasal and glottal substitutions of oral consonants) obligates them to sound nasal. Speech therapy should be recommended for these children with a goal of establishing appropriate articulatory placements. Only when the child is attempting to produce pressure consonants can velopharyngeal function be adequately assessed.

Children with severe apraxia and those with severe oral motor deficits may also have excessive nasalization of speech, but surgical management may not always be an appropriate recommendation. It is important to carefully consider the impact of velopharyngeal inadequacy on the child's global speech intelligibility problem and the extent to which it is simply a manifestation of a larger oral motor problem. Surgical management of velopharyngeal inadequacy is unlikely to have a large impact on a child's intelligibility when the speech sound inventory is composed largely of vowels or when a generalized oral motor deficit is present. All too often, however, children are referred for surgical management because therapy is either "going nowhere" or progress is slow. Neither concern is adequate justification to refer a child for surgery. Surgery should never be recommended unless results of the perceptual or objective evaluation suggest that it is likely to improve a child's speech. As D'Antonio (1992) wrote, "It is incumbent on the speech pathologist to interpret the available evaluation data and determine whether management of any form will improve speech intelligibility, speech quality, or quality of life" (p. 101).

Glottal and pharyngeal articulations. The presence of glottal and pharyngeal articulations should be documented during the perceptual evaluation and their influence on velopharyngeal function carefully considered before referral for an objective assessment. Radiographic evidence previously reported by Henningsson and Isberg (1986) indicated that patients demonstrate poorer velopharyngeal function during glottal stop articulations than during production of oral stops. The limited movement that occurs during these productions makes it virtually impossible to determine the functional potential of the velopharyngeal mechanism when these compensatory articulations are frequently produced. Therefore, direct assessment of velopharyngeal function should be deferred until these patterns of articulation have either been eliminated or substantially reduced in speech therapy—at least for those children who substitute these productions for most oral consonants. In cases where children substitute glottal or pharyngeal productions for only one or two consonants, it is possible to obtain valid information about velopharyngeal function by simply using a speech sample that contains oral stops and fricatives that the child is capable of producing.

Palatal fistula. Isberg and Henningsson (1987) provided radiographic evidence to suggest that patients with palatal fistulae demonstrate better velopharyngeal movements when the fistula is covered than when it is left unobturated. Because the "velopharyngeal surrender" that takes place in the presence of a fistula can complicate interpretation of nasoendoscopic and/or videofluoroscopic findings, the fistula should be temporarily obturated during the assessment to determine the contribution of each.

SUMMARY

Assessment of speech-language problems in individuals with cleft palate begins in infancy and, for some, will extend through adolescence and beyond. The protocol for assessment of children who demonstrate normal speech-language development and those who produce developmental errors will not differ from that used for any noncleft child learning language. Children with cleft palate who produce errors related to poor dental/occlusal status, palatal fistula, and/or velopharyngeal inadequacy typically present a more complex diagnostic puzzle that requires interdisciplinary teamwork to solve. The significance of errors produced by these children may change over time as factors such as maturation, physical growth, and physical management converge to alter the mechanism that the child has to work with. The challenge for clinicians working with this population will be in sorting out the relative contribution of each etiological factor to the errors produced by each child. The more you know about clefting and its impact on speech production, oropharyngeal anatomy and physiology, and the basic regimens used in dental and surgical management, the greater your contribution will likely be to the diagnostic process.

REFERENCES

Aronson AE: *Clinical voice disorders.* New York: Thieme-Stratton, 1980.

Bateman HE, and Mason RM: *Applied anatomy and physiology of the speech and hearing mechanism.* Springfield (IL): CC Thomas, 1984.

Bernthal JE, and Bankson NW: *Articulation and phonological disorders.* 2nd ed. Englewood Cliffs (NJ): Prentice Hall, 1988.

Bernthal JE, and Bankson NW: *Articulation and phonological disorders.* 3rd ed. Englewood Cliffs (NJ): Prentice Hall, 1993.

Black JW: The phonemic content of backward-reproduced speech. *Journal of Speech and Hearing Research* 16:165-174, 1973.

Blakely RW: *The practice of speech pathology: a clinical diary.* Springfield (IL): CC Thomas, 1972.

Blakely RW: *Palate dysfunction and speech disorders: evaluation and treatment planning program for children and adults.* Austin (TX): Pro-Ed, 2000.

Boone DR: *The voice and voice therapy.* Englewood Cliffs (NJ): Prentice-Hall, 1977.

Boone DR, and McFarlane S: *The voice and voice therapy.* Englewood Cliffs (NJ): Prentice-Hall, 1994.

Bradford LF, Brooks AR, and Shelton RL: Clinical judgment of hypernasality in cleft palate children. *Cleft Palate Journal* 1:329-335, 1964.

Byrne MC, Shelton RL, and Diedrich WM: Articulatory skill, physical management, and classification of children with cleft palates. *Journal of Speech and Hearing Disorders* 26:326-333, 1961.

Bzoch KR: Measurement and assessment of categorical aspects of cleft palate speech. In Bzoch KR (ed.): *Communicative disorders related to cleft lip and palate.* 2nd ed. Boston: Little, Brown, 1979.

Bzoch KR: Clinical assessment, evaluation, and management of 11 categorical aspects of cleft palate speech disorders. In Bzoch KR (ed.): *Communicative disorders related to cleft lip and palate.* Austin: Pro-Ed, 1997.

Carter ET, and Buck M: Prognostic testing for functional articulation disorders among children in the first grade. *Journal of Speech and Hearing Disorders* 23:124-133, 1958.

Chapman KL, and Hardin MA: Communicative competence in children with cleft lip and palate. In Bardach J, and Morris HL (eds.): *Multidisciplinary management of cleft lip and palate.* Philadelphia: WB Saunders, 1990.

Colton R, and Casper J: *Understanding voice problems: a physiological perspective for diagnosis and treatment.* Baltimore: Williams & Wilkins, 1996.

Compton AJ, and Hutton JS: *Compton-Hutton phonological assessment.* San Francisco: Carousel House, 1978.

Creaghead, N: Strategies for evaluating and targeting pragmatic behaviors in young children. *Seminars in Speech and Language* 5:241-252, 1984.

D'Antonio LL: Evaluation and management of velopharyngeal dysfunction. In Lehman JA (ed.): *Cleft Palate Surgery. Problems in Plastic and Reconstructive Surgery* 2:86-111, 1992.

D'Antonio LL, and Scherer NJ: The evaluation of speech disorders associated with clefting. In Shprintzen RJ, and Bardach J (eds.): *Cleft palate speech management: a multidisciplinary approach.* St. Louis: Mosby, 1994.

Devers M, Broen P, and Moller K: Prelinguistic vocalizations of children requiring secondary management for velopharyngeal inadequacy. Poster presentation, proceedings of the 54th annual meeting of the American Cleft Palate–Craniofacial Association, New Orleans, 1997.

Diedrich WM, and Bangert J: *Articulation learning.* Houston: College-Hill, 1980.

Dinnsen DA: Methods and empirical issues in analyzing functional misarticulation. In Elbert M, Dinnsen D, and Weismer G (eds.): *Phonological theory and the misarticulating child.* ASHA Monographs No. 22, 1984.

Dworkin JP, and Culatta RA: *Dworkin-Culatta oral mechanism examination.* Nicholasville (KY): Edgewood Press, 1980.

Eckel FC, and Boone DR: The s/z ratio as an indicator of laryngeal pathology. *Journal of Speech and Hearing Disorders* 46:147-149, 1981.

Elbert M, and Gierut JA: *Handbook of clinical phonology: approaches to assessments and treatment.* San Diego: College-Hill, 1986.

Fenson L, Dale PS, Reznick S, Thal D, Bates E, Hartung J, Pethick S, and Reilly J: *The MacArthur Communicative Development Inventories.* San Diego: Singular Publishing Group, 1993.

Fey M: *Language intervention in young children.* San Diego: College-Hill, 1986.

Fisher MB, and Logemann JA: *The Fisher-Logemann test of articulation competence.* New York: Houghton Mifflin, 1971.

Fletcher SG: "Nasalance" vs. listener judgments of nasality. *Cleft Palate Journal* 13:31-44, 1976.

Glaser ER, and Shprintzen RJ: A review of See-Scape: instrument and manual. *Cleft Palate Journal* 16:213, 1979.

Goldman R, and Fristoe M: *Goldman-Fristoe articulation test.* Circle Pines: American Guidance Services, 1986.

Grunwell P: *Phonological assessment of child speech (PACS).* San Diego: College-Hill, 1985.

Harrison RJ: A demonstration project of speech training for the preschool cleft palate child. Final report, Project No. 6-1101, Grant No. OEG-2-6-061101-1553. US Office of Education, Bureau of the Handicapped, HEW, 1969.

Henningsson GE, and Isberg AM: Velopharyngeal movement patterns in patients alternating between oral and glottal articulation: a clinical and cine radiological study. *Cleft Palate Journal* 23:1-9, 1986.

Henningsson GE, and Isberg AM: Influence of palatal fistulae on speech and resonance. *Folia Phoniatrica* 39:183-191, 1987.

Henningsson GE, and Isberg AM: Oronasal fistulas and speech production. In Bardach J, and Morris HL (eds.): *Multidisciplinary management of cleft lip and palate.* Philadelphia: WB Saunders, 1990.

Hess DA: Effects of certain variables on speech of cleft palate persons. *Cleft Palate Journal* 8:387-398, 1971.

Hodson BW: *The assessment of phonological processes.* Danville: Interstate Press, 1980.

Huang R, Hopkins J, and Nippold MA: Satisfaction with standardized language testing: a survey of speech-language pathologists. *Language, Speech, and Hearing Services in Schools* 28:12-23, 1997.

Hufnagle J, and Hufnagel K: S/Z ratio in dysphonic children with and without vocal cord nodules. *Language, Speech, and Hearing Services in Schools* 19:418-422, 1988.

Ingram D: *Phonological disability in children.* New York: Elsevier, 1976.

Ingram D: *Procedures for the phonological analysis of children's language.* Baltimore: University Park Press, 1981.

Isberg A, and Henningsson G: Influence of open versus covered fistulas on velopharyngeal movements: a cineradiographic study. *Plastic and Reconstructive Surgery* 79:525-530, 1987.

Jacobs RJ, Philips BJ, and Harrison RJ: A stimulability test for cleft-palate children. *Journal of Speech and Hearing Disorders* 35:354-360, 1970.

Karling J, Larson O, and Henningsson G: Oronasal fistulas in cleft palate patients and their influence on speech. *Scandinavian Journal of Plastic and Reconstructive Hand Surgery* 27: 193- 201, 1993.

Kearns KP, and Simmons NN: Interobserver reliability and perceptual ratings: more than meets the ear. *Journal of Speech and Hearing Research* 31:131-136, 1988.

Kent RD: Hearing and believing: some limits to the auditory-perceptual assessment of speech and voice disorders. *American Journal of Speech-Language Pathology* 5:7-23, 1996.

Kent RD, Miolo G, and Bioedel S: The intelligibility of children's speech: a review of evaluation procedures. *American Journal of Speech-Language Pathology* 3:81-95, 1994.

Khan ML, and Lewis NP: *Khan-Lewis phonological analysis.* Circle Pines: American Guidance Service, 1986.

Kummer A, and Lee L: Evaluation and treatment of resonance disorders. *Language, Speech, and Hearing Services in Schools* 27:271-281, 1996.

Lee L: *Developmental sentence analysis.* Evanston (IL): Northwestern University Press, 1974.

Lohmander-Agerskov A, Dotevall H, Lith A, and Soderpalm E: Speech and velopharyngeal function in children with an open residual cleft in the hard palate, and the influence of temporary covering. *Cleft Palate–Craniofacial Journal* 33:324-332, 1996.

McReynolds LV, and Elbert M: Criteria for phonological process analysis. *Journal of Speech and Hearing Disorders* 46:197-204, 1981.

McReynolds LV, and Kearns KP: *Single-subject experimental designs in communicative disorders.* Austin: Pro-Ed, 1983.

McWilliams BJ: Some factors in the intelligibility of cleft palate speech. *Journal of Speech and Hearing Disorders* 19:524-527, 1954.

McWilliams BJ, and Philips BJ: Velopharyngeal incompetence. Audio Seminars in Speech Pathology. Philadelphia: WB Saunders, 1979.

McWilliams BJ, and Philips BJ: Velopharyngeal incompetence. Audio Seminars in Speech Pathology. Toronto: BC Decker, 1990.

Milisen R: A rationale for articulation disorders. *Journal of Speech and Hearing Disorders Supplement* 4:5-17, 1954.

Miller J, and Paul R: *The clinical assessment of language comprehension.* Baltimore: Paul H Brookes, 1995.

Moll KL: "Objective" measures of nasality. *Cleft Palate Journal* 1:371-374, 1964.

Moller KT: Dental-occlusal and other oral conditions and speech. In Bernthal JE, and Bankson NW (eds.): *Child phonology: characteristics, assessment, and intervention with special populations.* New York: Thieme Medical Publishers, 1994.

Moller KT, and Starr CD: The effects of listening conditions on speech ratings obtained in a clinical setting. *Cleft Palate Journal* 21:65-69, 1984.

Morris HL, Shelton RL, and McWilliams B: Assessment of speech. In Speech, language, and psychosocial aspects of cleft lip and cleft palate: the state of the art. *ASHA Reports,* No. 9, 1973.

Morris HL, Spriestersbach DC, and Darley FL: An articulation test for assessing competency of velopharyngeal closure. *Journal of Speech and Hearing Research* 4:48-55, 1961.

Paul R: *Language disorders from infancy through adolescence.* St. Louis: Mosby, 1995.

Paynter ET: Articulation skills of Spanish-speaking Mexican-American children: normative data. *Cleft Palate Journal* 21:313-316, 1984.

Peterson-Falzone S: Cleft palate. In Tomblin JB, Morris HL, and Spriestersbach DC (eds.): *Diagnosis in speech-language pathology.* San Diego: Singular, 1994.

Philips BJ: Speech assessment. In McWilliams BJ (ed.): *Seminars in Speech and Language* 7:297-326, 1986.

Philips BJ, and Bzoch KR: Reliability of judgments of articulation of cleft palate speakers. *Cleft Palate Journal* 6:24-34, 1969.

Powell TW, Elbert M, and Dinnesen DA: Stimulability as a factor in the phonologic generalization of misarticulating preschool children. *Journal of Speech and Hearing Research* 34:1318-1328, 1991.

Preisser DA, Hodson BW, and Paden EP: Developmental phonology: 18-29 months. *Journal of Speech and Hearing Disorders* 53:125-130, 1988.

Prins D, and Bloomer HH: Consonant intelligibility: a procedure for evaluating speech in oral cleft subjects. *Journal of Speech and Hearing Research* 11:128-137, 1968.

Ramig LA: Effects of examiner expectancy on speech ratings of individuals with cleft lip and/or palate. *Cleft Palate Journal* 19:270-274, 1982.

Rastatter MP, and Hyman M: Maximum phoneme duration of /s/ and /z/ by children with vocal nodules. *Language, Speech, and Hearing Services in Schools* 13:197-199, 1982.

Rosetti L: *The Rosetti Infant-Toddler Language Scale: a measure of communication and interaction.* East Moline (IL): LinguiSystems, 1990.

Ruscello DM, Lass JJ, Bosch W, and Jones C: The verbal transformation effect as studied in judgments of misarticulations. Proceedings of the annual convention of the American Speech-Language-Hearing Association, Detroit, 1980.

Scherer NJ, and D'Antonio LL: Parent questionnaire for screening early language development in children with cleft palate. *Cleft Palate–Craniofacial Journal* 32:7-13, 1995.

Sell D, Harding A, and Grunwell P: A screening assessment of cleft palate speech (Great Ormond Street Speech Assessment). *European Journal of Disorders of Communication* 29:1-15, 1994.

Shelton RL, Johnson A, and Arndt WB: Variability in judgments of articulation when observer listens repeatedly to the same phone. *Perceptual and Motor Skills* 39:327-332, 1974.

Sherman D: The merits of backward playing of connected speech in the scaling of voice quality disorders. *Journal of Speech and Hearing Disorders* 19:312-321, 1954.

Sherman D: Usefulness of the mean in psychological scaling of cleft palate speech. *Cleft Palate Journal* 7:622-629, 1970.

Shipley KG, and McAfee JG: *Assessment in speech-language pathology: a resource manual.* San Diego: Singular Publishing Group, 1992.

Shriberg LD, and Kent RD: *Clinical phonetics.* Boston: Allyn & Bacon, 1995.

Shriberg LD, and Kwiatkowski J: *Natural process analysis (NPA): a procedure for phonological analysis of continuous speech samples.* New York: Wiley, 1980.

Shriberg LD, and Kwiatkowski J: Phonological disorders. II: A conceptual framework for management. *Journal of Speech and Hearing Disorders* 47:242-256, 1982a.

Shriberg LD, and Kwiatkowski J: Phonological disorders. III: A procedure for assessing severity of involvement. *Journal of Speech and Hearing Disorders* 47:256-270, 1982b.

Sinko GR, and Hedrick DL: The interrelationships between ratings of speech and facial acceptability in persons with cleft palate. *Journal of Speech and Hearing Research* 25:402-407, 1982.

Snow K, and Milisen R: Spontaneous improvement in articulation as related to differential responses to oral and picture articulation tests. *Journal of Speech and Hearing Disorders Supplement* 4:45-49, 1954a.

Snow K, and Milisen R: The influence of oral versus pictorial presentation upon articulation testing results. *Journal of Speech and Hearing Disorders Supplement* 4:29-36, 1954b.

Sparrow S, Balla D, and Cicchetti D: *Vineland Adaptive Behavior Scales.* Circle Pines (MN): American Guidance Service, 1984.

Spriestersbach DC, Morris HL, and Darley FL: Speech mechanism examination. In Darley FL, and Spriestersbach DC (eds.): *Diagnostic methods in speech pathology.* New York: Harper & Row, 1978.

St. Louis KO, and Ruscello DM: *Oral speech mechanism screening examination,* revised. Austin: Pro-Ed, 1987.

Stenglehofen J: *Working with cleft palate.* Bichester: Winslow Press, 1990.

Stephens MI, and Daniloff R: A methodological study of factors affecting the judgment of misarticulated /s/. *Journal of Communication Disorders* 10:207-220, 1977.

Stoel-Gammon C: Phonetic inventories, 15-24 months: a longitudinal study. *Journal of Speech and Hearing Research* 28:505-512, 1985.

Stoel-Gammon C: Phonological skills of 2-year-olds. *Language, Speech, and Hearing Services in Schools* 18:323-329, 1987.

Stoel-Gammon C: Prelinguistic vocal development: measurement and predictions. In Ferguson C, Menn L, and Stoel-Gammon C (eds.): *Phonological development: models, research, implications.* Timonium (MD): York Press, 1992.

Stoel-Gammon C: Measuring phonology in babble and speech. *Clinics in Communication Disorders* 4:1-11, 1994.

Stoel-Gammon C: Sounds and words in early language acquisition: The relationship between lexical and phonological development. In Paul R (ed.): *Exploring the speech-language connection.* Baltimore: Paul H. Brookes Pub, 1998.

Stoel-Gammon C, and Dunn C: *Normal and disordered phonology in children.* Baltimore: University Park Press, 1985.

Stoel-Gammon C, and Stone JR: Assessing phonology in young children. *Clinics in Communication Disorders* 1:25-39, 1991.

Subtelny J, and Subtelny JD: Intelligibility and associated physiological factors of cleft palate speakers. *Journal of Speech and Hearing Research* 2:353-360, 1959.

Subtelny J, Koepp-Baker H, and Subtelny JD: Palatal function and cleft palate speech. *Journal of Speech and Hearing Disorders* 26:213-224, 1961.

Subtelny JD, Van Hattum RJ, and Myers BA: Ratings and measures of cleft palate speech. *Cleft Palate Journal* 9:18-27, 1972.

Tachimura T, Hara H, Koh H, and Wada T: Effect of temporary closure of oronasal fistula on levator veli palatini muscle activity. *Cleft Palate–Craniofacial Journal* 34:505-511, 1997.

Templin MC, and Darley FL: *The Templin-Darley tests of articulation.* 2nd ed. Iowa City: Bureau of Educational Research and Service, University of Iowa, 1969.

Trost-Cardamone JE: *Cleft palate misarticulations: a teaching tape.* Videotape produced by the Instructional Media Center, California State University, Northridge, 1987.

Trost-Cardamone JE: The development of speech: assessing cleft palate misarticulations. In Kernahan DE, and Rosenstein SW (eds.): *Cleft lip and palate: a system of management.* Baltimore: Williams & Wilkins, 1990.

Trost-Cardamone JE, and Bernthal JE: Articulation assessment procedures and treatment decisions. In Moller KT, and Starr CD (eds.): *Cleft palate: interdisciplinary issues and treatment.* Austin: Pro-Ed, 1993.

Turton LJ: Diagnostic implications of articulation testing. In Wolfe WD, and Goulding DJ (eds.): *Articulation and learning: new dimensions in research, diagnostics, and therapy.* Springfield (IL): CC Thomas, 1973.

Van Demark DR: Predictability of velopharyngeal competency. *Cleft Palate Journal* 16:429-435, 1979.

Van Demark DR, and Swickard SL: A pre-school articulation test to assess velopharyngeal competency: normative data. *Cleft Palate Journal* 17:175-179, 1980.

Vihman MM, and Greenlee M: Individual differences in phonological development: ages one and three years. *Journal of Speech and Hearing Research* 30:503-521, 1987.

Weiner FF: *Phonological process analysis.* Baltimore: University Park Press, 1979.

Weiss A, Tomblin JB, and Robin DA: Language disorders. In Tomblin JB, Morris HL, and Spriestersbach DC (eds.): *Diagnosis in speech-language pathology.* San Diego: Singular Publishing, 1994.

Weiss CE, Lillywhite HS, and Gordon ME: *Clinical management of articulation disorders.* St. Louis: Mosby, 1980.

Wells CC: *Cleft palate and its associated disorders.* New York: McGraw-Hill, 1971.

Wilson DK: *Voice problems of children.* Baltimore: Williams & Wilkins, 1972, 1979, 1987.

Winitz H: *From syllable to conversation.* Baltimore: University Park Press, 1975.

Witzel MA: Communicative impairment associated with clefting. In Shprintzen RJ, and Bardach J (eds.): *Cleft palate speech management: a multidisciplinary approach.* St. Louis: Mosby, 1994.

Young MA: Anchoring and sequence effects for the category scaling of stuttering severity. *Journal of Speech and Hearing Research* 13:360-368, 1970.

Zimmerman I, Steiner V, and Pond R: *Preschool language scale-3.* San Antonio: Psychological Corporation, 1992.

Chapter 10

Instrumentation for Assessing the Velopharyngeal Mechanism

No instrument can surpass the trained human ear for assessing velopharyngeal insufficiency and associated speech disorders. That being said, the use of instruments is essential in the evaluation and documentation of velopharyngeal function. Many advancements in speech pathology have been based on insights derived from use of new instrumentation. The instruments described below have proven clinical and research value for assessing velopharyngeal valving. Emphasis is placed on radiography, endoscopy, acoustic analyses, and aerodynamics. Other measures that are historically significant or that demonstrate potential for the future are also briefly discussed. A historical perspective may be found in a review by Hirschberg (1986).

RADIOGRAPHY

Radiography permits the imaging of internal body parts. The roentgen ray (x-ray) is projected through the body directly to photographic film or to a fluoroscopic screen (Fig. 10-1). The fluoroscopic screen converts invisible photons to visible light, which may be photographed or videorecorded. There are a number of radiographic methods from which the researcher or clinician may choose. Each has its strengths and limitations. Scheier reported radiographic studies of speech in 1909, and over the years radiography has contributed much to our understanding of the function of the speech mechanism, especially the velopharyngeal valve. Radiographic techniques have evolved considerably and continue to be used frequently in research as well as in diagnosis and treatment planning.

Regardless of whether still or motion radiographic techniques are selected, ionizing radiation is used. The radiation dosage differs from one technique to another, and although radiation is always potentially hazardous, technological advances have reduced the risks to clinically acceptable levels. To further reduce radiation hazard, exposure time is kept to the minimum required to obtain needed information, lead shielding is used, the roentgen ray beam is filtered and coned down to the target area, and image intensifiers are used. Isberg et al. (1989) stated that use of a head fixation device permits the radiologist to cone the field of exposure, thus protecting the eyes and thyroid gland while permitting study of the velopharyngeal mechanism. They described speech study sequences as requiring 5 seconds for coning the field, 3 seconds for setting of the automatic exposure control, and 40 seconds for recording speech. This was repeated for additional views. They found that videofluoroscopy (fluoroscopic images obtained with a video camera and recorded on videotape) required only one tenth the radiation of cinefluorography (fluorographic images obtained with a moving picture camera and recorded on photographic film). For this reason and others, cinefluorography is no longer used for evaluation of the velopharyngeal mechanism.

Lead shields should be worn by the patient, the radiologist, and the participating speech pathologist during the examination. Staff exposure must be monitored closely by radiation experts, and equipment must be checked for safe function. The use of radiographic procedures in research is closely monitored by institutional internal review committees concerned with the rights and well-being of patients, research subjects, and staff.

CINEFLUOROSCOPY AND VIDEOFLUOROSCOPY

The use of cinefluoroscopy in the study of speech of patients with cleft palate was introduced at the Lancaster Cleft Palate Clinic in the 1950s. Since then video recording technology has effectively replaced motion picture recording for essentially all clinical and research applications having to do with assessing speech. Use of videofluoroscopy in the study of patients with clefts was first reported by McWilliams and Girdany (1964). Video recording has the advantage of instant playback with synchronized sound, avoiding the delays required to process and develop cinefluorographic film. Fig. 10-2 shows a person in position for midsagittal videofluorography and the equipment used. At the time of this writing, digital video recording is

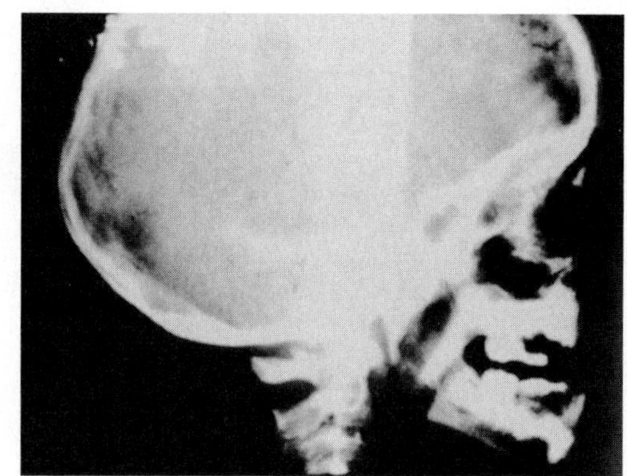

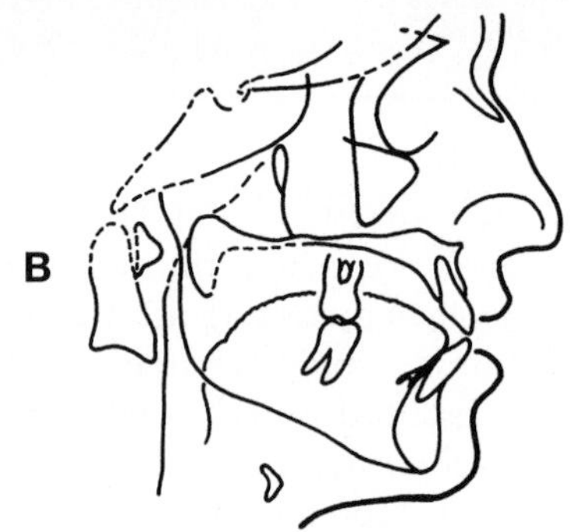

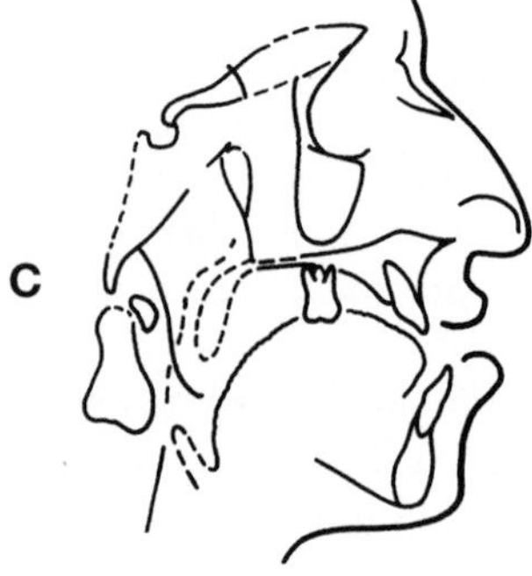

Figure 10-1 A, Cephalometric radiography. **B,** Tracing of a cephalometric film taken during normal /s/ production. **C,** Tracing of a cephalometric film taken during production of /s/ associated with velopharyngeal opening and tongue protrusion. *(From McWilliams BJ: Cleft palate. In Shames GH, and Wiig EH (eds.):* Human communication disorders. *Columbus: CE Merrill, 1982.)*

replacing analog video recording, making storage, enhancement, retrieval, and processing of images more efficient and ultimately less costly.

When motion techniques for speech study first became available, only midsagittal and occasionally frontal studies were done. The midsagittal view provides information about movement of the velum and posterior pharyngeal wall and about height and length of the velum and velar relationships to the adenoids and posterior pharyngeal wall. It does not provide information about the velum lateral to midline nor does it enable assessment of movement of the lateral pharyngeal walls. Frontal views provide information about movement of the lateral

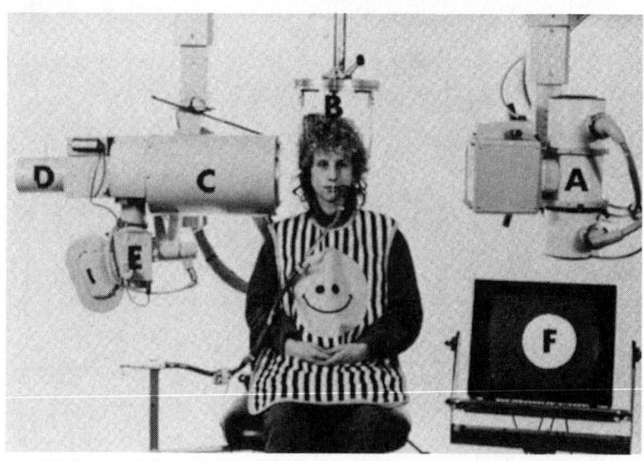

Figure 10-2 Radiographic equipment. **A,** X-ray tube. **B,** Cephalostat. **C,** Image intensifier. **D,** Vidicon camera. **E,** Cinecamera. **F,** TV monitor. *(From Isberg A, Julin P, Kraepelien T, and Henrickson CO: Absorbed doses and energy imparted from radiographic examination of velopharyngeal function during speech.* Cleft Palate Journal *26:106, 1989.)*

pharyngeal walls but do not show clearly their relationship to the velum. The two views supplement each other but may leave unanswered the question of whether a velopharyngeal opening during speech exists, and if so where it is in the horizontal plane. A gap that appears in the midsagittal view may actually be filled by the lateral pharyngeal walls. A gap that appears in the frontal view may actually be filled by the velum. It is important to obtain a view that permits simultaneous recording of velar and lateral wall movement.

Toward this end, Skolnick (1970) introduced what he described as multiview videofluoroscopy, a technique that adds a base view to the traditional lateral and frontal projections. When considered together, this series of three views provides a more complete picture of the velopharyngeal valve. For base-view videofluoroscopy, the patient is placed in a sphinx-like position, with the neck extended as shown in Fig. 10-3. In this way, the x-ray beam can be directed upward, from under the chin through the velopharyngeal portal. Fig. 10-4 shows the radiographic positioning required for all three views. These views are usually obtained sequentially.

Skolnick et al. (1975) wrote that the multiview system allows the clinician to estimate the location of the base view plane within the vocal tract by considering information from all three views. The frontal view shows the vertical location of maximum pharyngeal wall movement; the midsagittal view shows the soft palate and the posterior pharyngeal wall relative to each other; and the base view shows all of these except vertical location. What is observed on the base view must be consistent with what is seen on the other views. For example, the study is improperly done if the midsagittal view shows closure, but the base view shows a large midline opening or vice versa. It is possible, however, to see a small central opening on base view or a unilateral

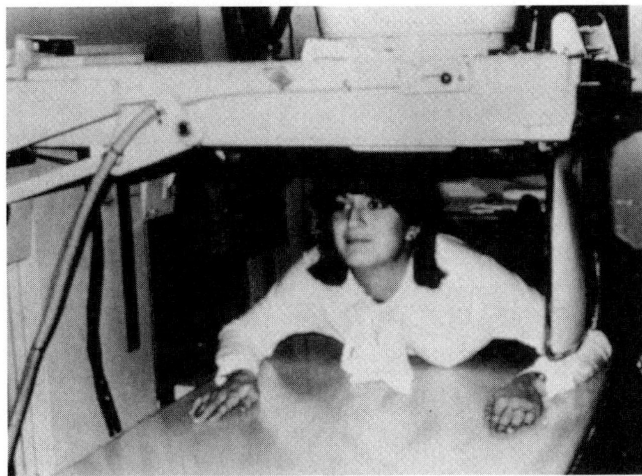

Figure 10-3 Sphinx-like position used in taking base views of the velopharyngeal valve. *(From McWilliams BJ: Communication problems associated with cleft palate. In Van Hattum RJ (ed.):* Communication disorders. *New York: Macmillan, 1980.)*

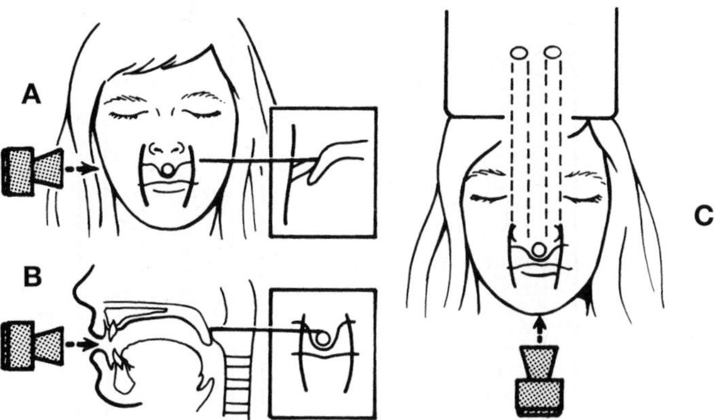

Figure 10-4 Radiographic positioning of a patient for **(A)** lateral, **(B)** frontal, and **(C)** base views of velopharyngeal portal. *(From Skolnick ML, and McCall GN: Velopharyngeal competence and incompetence following pharyngeal flap surgery: videofluoroscopic study in multiple projections.* Cleft Palate Journal *9:1, 1972.)*

opening that could not be seen on midsagittal projection. The three views complement each other when they are interpreted together.

Kuehn and Dolan (1975) and Schwartz (1975) questioned the accuracy of the base view due to ". . . the difficulty in specifying the exact inferior-superior level of mesial LPW [lateral pharyngeal wall] movement" (p. 201). Skolnick (1982), however, reiterated his position that the vertical location of the sphincter visualized in base view can be satisfactorily estimated by comparing the cross-sectional dimensions with those measured from frontal and midsagittal views. He noted that, in base views, bulges into the vocal tract that occur at two different levels will appear to be located at the same level (Fig. 10-5). However, reference to midsagittal and frontal views will protect against erroneous interpretations.

Other views of the velopharyngeal valve have been devised and recommended for clinical use as supplements or alternatives to the base view. Zwitman, Gyepes, and Sample (1973, p. 474) studied a submentovertical projection in which the upright patient is turned to face the image amplifier. ". . . he is asked to step forward and to tilt his head back until it rests against the upright x-ray table." The patient is then standing with the neck extended and the face directed to the ceiling. This view is similar to Waters' view described by Stringer and Witzel (1986, 1989) and Witzel and Stringer (1990) (Fig. 10-6) who reported that the Waters projection permits visualization of the lateral walls in a fashion equal or superior to that associated with the frontal view. The authors further noted that head extension may unmask marginal velopharyngeal disfunction.

Stringer and Witzel (1986, 1989) and Witzel and Stringer (1990) also described Towne's view (Fig. 10-6), in which the radiographic beam is perpendicular to the velopharyngeal sphincter, thus resembling the base view. In Towne's view, the patient may sit upright or lie supine on the x-ray table with the head, neck, and shoulders flexed forward. In the supine position, the patient's head and shoulders are supported by a wedge. This permits recording of the velopharyngeal sphincter on a quasitransverse plane. However, the authors noted that in Towne's view the main radiographic beam is not directed to the thyroid gland and that the eyes can be protected by careful coning of the beam. We frequently obtain Towne's view by having the patient sit upright with the head rotated forward and downward as if reading a book. With some radiographic systems, it is possible to obtain Towne's views by adjusting equipment to the patient rather than the reverse. In this approach the patient can be studied in an upright posture, thus avoiding the narrowing of the velopharyngeal port that may be associated with cervical flexion (Fig. 10-7). Stringer and Witzel (1989) reported Towne's view provided information comparable to that provided by videoendoscopy. This seems reasonable given the similarities in the plane of view obtained by both approaches.

Rotation of the videofluorographic camera around the patient provides a means of relating structures and movements observed in one plane of view to structures and movements observed in another (Massengill et al., 1966). A similar effect can be achieved by rotating the patient as he or she is positioned relative to a standard cineradiographic unit (Skolnick, 1982). A simple version of this approach involves having the subject positioned for a midsagittal view gradually rotate the head over the shoulder to approximate a frontal view. Tomography, described by Kuehn and Dolan (1975) for evaluation of lateral pharyngeal wall movement, also involves a rotating view around the patient.

CT and MRI scans (Honjo, 1984; McGowan et al., 1992; Yamawaki, Nishimura, and Suzuki, 1996) have been applied to velopharyngeal research and may soon become sufficiently evolved and affordable to be applied to routine

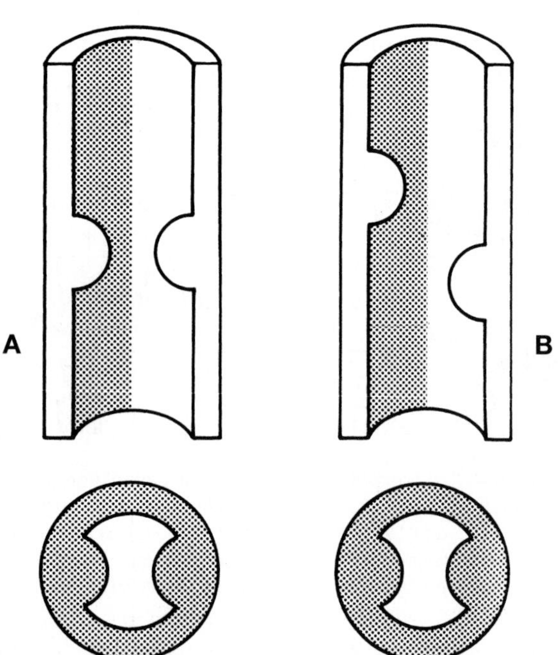

Figure 10-5 A, Ridges intruding into a tube at the same level. B, Comparable ridges intruding at two different levels. The relationships in A and B would be indistinguishable in base view.

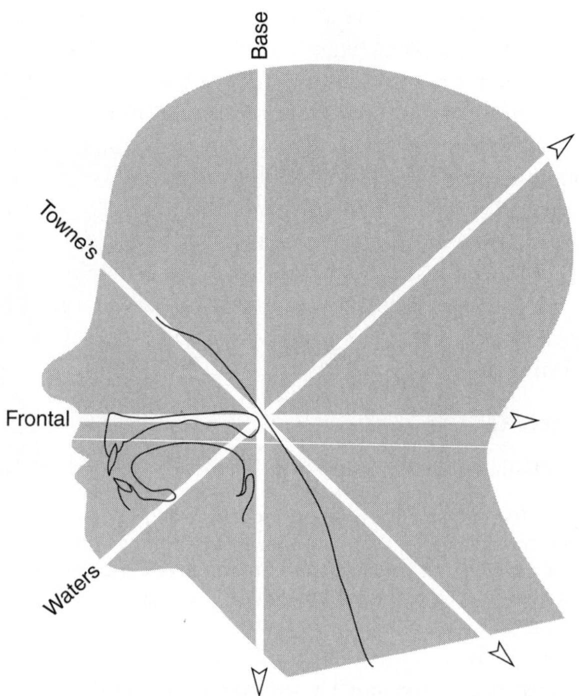

Figure 10-6 Schematic drawing of the direction of the x-ray beam through the velopharyngeal valve for the base, Towne's, frontal, and Water's views. *(From Witzel MA, and Stringer DA: Speech and language diagnosis and treatment. In Bardach J, and Morris HL:* Multidisciplinary management of cleft lip and palate. *Philadelphia: WB Saunders, 1990, p. 766.)*

clinical evaluation of the velopharyngeal mechanism. Improvements are needed in the ability of these approaches to capture velopharyngeal movements with adequate temporal resolution. An image-capture rate of 60/s is needed before MRI or CT scans can equal the temporal resolution of standard videofluoroscopic recordings.

Head Positioners

When calibrated measurements of velopharyngeal or other speech articulator movements are to be obtained from fluoroscopic images, an important aspect of the procedure is the use of a headholder. Early lateral view cineradiographic studies routinely used some type of cephalostat. Use of such standard cephalometric procedures can provide data that speak a common language to all who use them, and measurements derived in one situation are comparable to those generated in another.

Although the use of head stabilization techniques remains important for measurement purposes, it is certainly not universally used when dynamic speech is evaluated in children as part of routine clinical assessments. Recording quality may vary across institutions because there is no assurance that equipment and procedures are consistent from one institution to another. No universally accepted standards exist for measurement of speech movements, although there tend to be similarities across studies that obtained such measurements. For clinical purposes, the rigid standards needed when measurements are desired usually give way to priorities such as patient compliance, clarity of view, and time limitations.

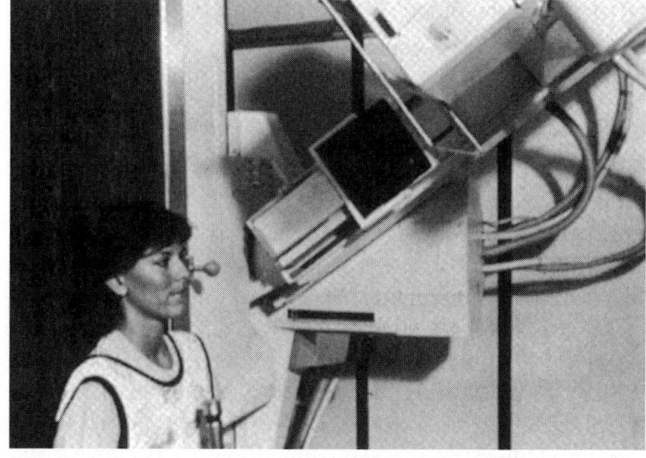

Figure 10-7 Patient in the upright position for Towne's view with overtable x-ray equipment. *(From Stringer DA, and Witzel MA: Comparison of multi-view videofluoroscopy and nasopharyngoscopy in the assessment of velopharyngeal insufficiency.* Cleft Palate Journal *26:91, 1989.)*

Contrast Materials

Fluorographic studies of speech usually employ methods designed to outline or enhance the view of soft tissues that otherwise may be difficult to see on fluorographic images. For some research applications, radiopaque markers have been glued to the tongue, velum, and pharyngeal walls so that they will show up clearly on the radiograph, whereas the soft tissue alone would not. Application of a liquid radiopaque material (e.g., barium sulfate) that clearly outlines the structures of interest is commonly used for clinical purposes. Liquid contrast material must be applied carefully because application of excessive amounts may obscure rather than clarify the surfaces of interest.

Fastening an external marker of known size, such as a metal ball bearing, at the subject's midline is a technique that has been used often, particularly in research. This marker enables calibration of the displayed image to life size, provided the orientation of the subject, marker, and recording apparatus remain constant.

Measurement Techniques

For many research and some clinical purposes, image-by-image measurement has been necessary (Moll, 1964). Historically, such analysis has been productive in studies of speech of both healthy subjects and those with pathological conditions. Image-by-image tracings and measurement of different structures combined with use of a sound track to identify acoustical phenomena allows identification of movement relationships among different speech organs and specification of the timing relationships among structures and contexts.

Although early cineradiographic frame-by-frame measurement required a stop-frame projector and a tracing device, similar measurements from video fields may now be obtained from standard analog or digital video recording media. Moll (1960) demonstrated that measurements made from projected images or from tracings of the image are usually highly reliable. Mean discrepancies between repeated measurements were small. He measured the distance between the velum and the posterior pharyngeal wall, the distance from tongue to alveolus, the size of the incisal opening, and the extent of contact between the velum and the posterior pharyngeal wall. The extent-of-contact measurement was less reliable than the others.

Scientific approaches to clinical ratings of videofluorographic images have long been advocated. McWilliams-Neely and Bradley (1964) prepared psychophysical rating scales to establish standard procedures for the analysis of videofluorographic images. Variables to be rated included approximation or contact between the velum and the posterior pharyngeal wall, thickness of the soft palate, length of the soft palate, extent of vertical contact between velum and posterior pharyngeal wall, location of velopharyngeal closure relative to the anteriormost projection of the tubercle of the first cervical vertebra, and location of closure relative to the hard palate. Timing factors were later added. Ratings made by two observers of 16 subjects were analyzed in terms of the percentages of agreement between the two ratings and in terms of Pearson correlations between the pairs of ratings. Most of the correlations were in the 0.70s and 0.80s, and the percentages of agreement ranged from 38% to 81% with a mean of 65%. Only five of 288 paired observations differed by more than one scale value. The authors noted that rating scales provide consistency in reporting and that the ratings take much less time to perform than other methods do. They stressed that those doing the ratings must be trained for the task. Such training would be facilitated by demonstration tapes serving as standards against which to compare ratings made by clinicians in training.

McWilliams and Bradley (1965) illustrated the rating scale for velopharyngeal closure and used it later in a study that compared connected speech, blowing with the nares open, and blowing with the nares closed. Fig. 10-8 shows the ratings used. Reliability coefficients for repeated ratings of three performances by 37 cleft palate patients ranged from 0.84 to 0.96, indicating that high levels of agreement can be developed with use of this system. Their procedure was later adapted for use in evaluating still radiographs by Van Demark, Kuehn, and Tharp (1975). Lewis and Pashayan (1980) illustrated a scale for use in rating medial movement of the lateral pharyngeal walls in frontal motion radiographic views (Fig. 10-9).

Skolnick et al. (1975) and later Croft et al. (1981) described patterns of velopharyngeal valving based on the relative contribution of the velum and pharyngeal walls to velopharyngeal closure. The "coronal pattern" was described as consisting primarily of velar movement with relatively little lateral or posterior wall movement. The "circular pattern" consists of velar and lateral wall movements of approximately equal magnitude, with little or no posterior wall movement. "Circular with Passavant's ridge" was the pattern description when Passavant's ridge occurred along with the circular closure pattern. The "sagittal pattern" was described as consisting primarily of lateral wall displacement, with the lateral walls touching at the midline of the velopharyngeal port during maximum movement. These patterns are graphically presented in Fig. 10-10.

Golding-Kushner et al. (1990) reported the results of an international working group convened to establish recommended standards for reporting videofluorographic and videoendoscopic data. Their system was based on relative ratings or measurements. Displacement of structures was considered relative to the position of the structure at rest and the maximum position to which the structure could be expected to move. For example, velar movement was considered as a ratio ranging from 0 (velum in its rest position) to 100% (velum in maximum contact with the posterior pharyngeal wall) (Fig. 10-11). Similar ratios were proposed that would characterize movements of the lateral and posterior pharyngeal walls and the size of the velopharyngeal port (Figs. 10-12 to 10-14). The system is attractive because it has both research and clinical utility. For research applications, when precise measurement of physiologic movements is critical, measures can be obtained from the video screen or from digitized images by use of digital video processing techniques. For clinical purposes, when time constraints dictate the need for quick estimates rather than precise measurements, the system can accommodate clinical judgments that, if necessary, may subsequently be validated using more objective measurements.

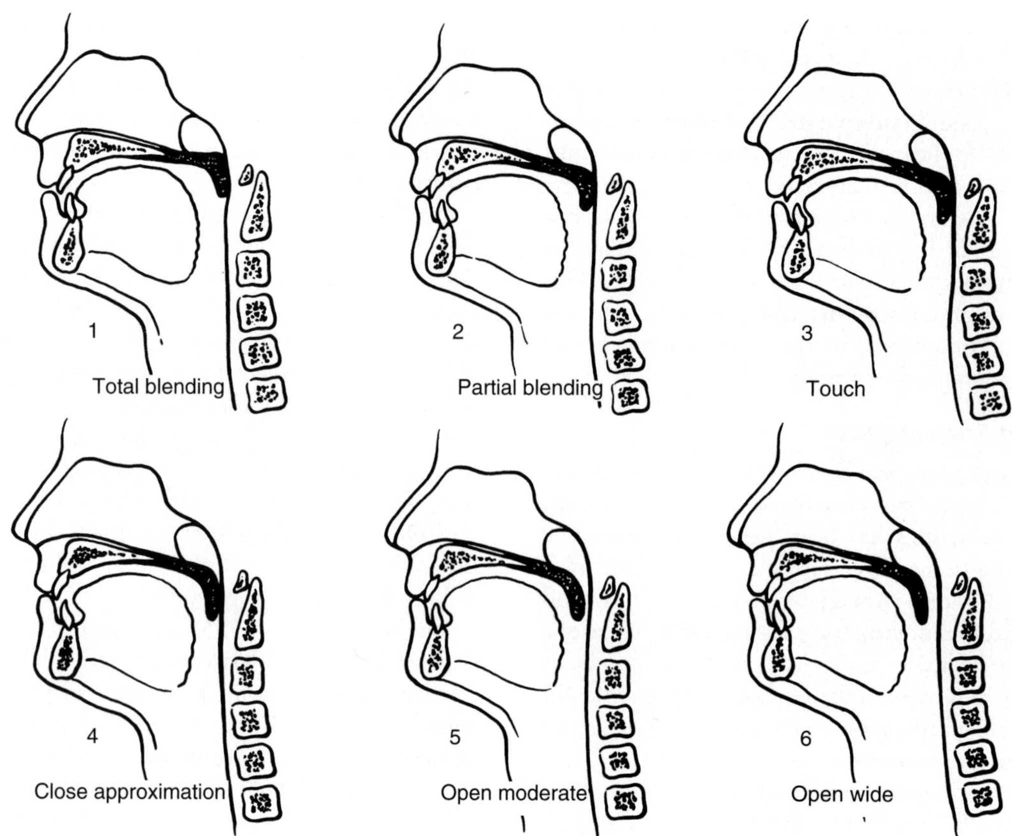

Figure 10-8 Six different relationships between the soft palate and the posterior pharyngeal wall. *(From McWilliams BJ, and Bradley DP: Ratings of velopharyngeal closure during blowing and speech.* Cleft Palate Journal *2:46, 1965.)*

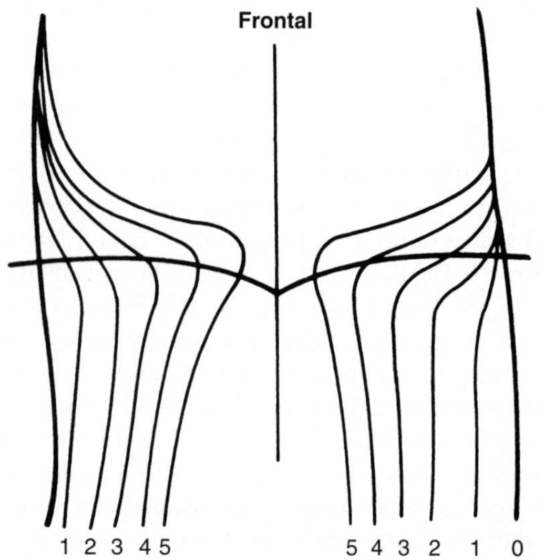

Figure 10-9 Diagrammatic scheme for the grading of lateral pharyngeal wall motion as seen on frontal view. *(From Lewis MB, and Pashayan HM: The effects of pharyngeal flap surgery on lateral pharyngeal wall motion: a video radiographic evaluation.* Cleft Palate Journal *17:302, 1980.)*

Image Resolution

Standard video frame rates of 30 frames per second actually yield 60 separate images per second. This is due to the interlacing of successive separate video images that occurs during real-time video display. Each video frame consists of two interlaced video fields, each of which is separated in time by 1/60th of a second (16.7 ms) and each of which consists of illumination of every other horizontal line of resolution. That is, if a video frame is made up of 500 horizontal lines of video resolution, each of the two fields that make up the frame consists of 250 illuminated lines. The first field would be made up of lines 1, 3, 5, 7, 9, . . . 499, and the second would be made up of lines 2, 4, 6, 8, 10, . . . 500.

When movements are measured from recorded video images, the images are presented individually, as fields, rather than frames, by today's standard four-head videocassette recorders. Although this temporal resolution is probably adequate for most studies of velar movement, Bjork (1961b) found that velum moves as much as 3 mm between cineradiographic frames at 50 frames per second (20 ms interframe interval). Studies requiring more precise recordings of movement must use faster frame rates. For many research purposes, particularly when movements of

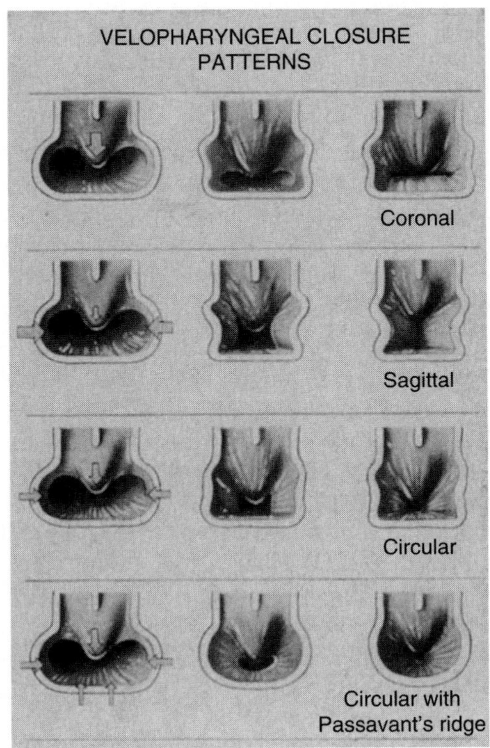

Figure 10-10 Artist's representation of the four types of velopharyngeal valving patterns. *(From Siegel-Sadewitz VI, Shprintzen RJ: Nasopharyngoscopy of the normal velopharyngeal sphincter; an experiment of biofeedback.* Cleft Plate Journal *19:196, 1982.)*

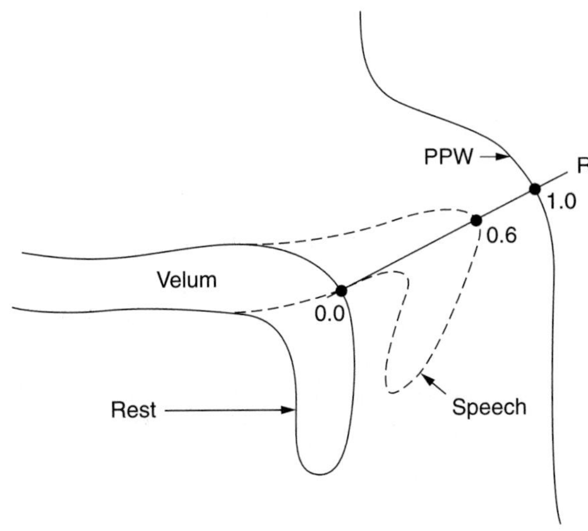

Figure 10-11 Lateral view videofluoroscopy: velar displacement along trajectory of movement (referant line *R*) resulting in a rating of 0.6 toward the posterior wall. *(Redrawn from Golding-Kushner KJ, et al.: Standardization for the reporting of nasopharyngoscopy and multiview videofluoroscopy: a report from an international working group.* Cleft Palate Journal *27:344, 1990.)*

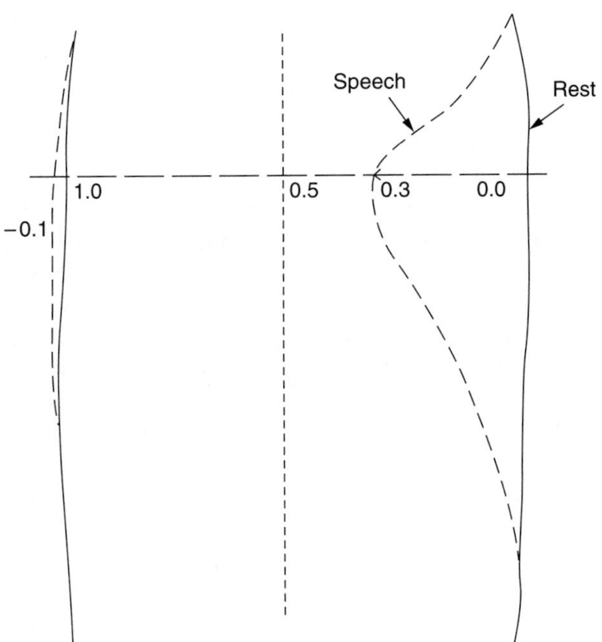

Figure 10-12 Frontal view videofluoroscopy: lateral pharyngeal wall displacement as assessed along the point of maximal medial excursion toward the opposite lateral wall (which as a value of 1.0). In this case the left lateral wall moves 0.3 toward the right wall at rest, and the right wall moves passively outward resulting in a score of −0.1. *(Redrawn from Golding-Kushner KJ, et al.: Standardization for the reporting of nasopharyngoscopy and multiview videofluoroscopy: a report from an international working group.* Cleft Palate Journal *27:343, 1990.)*

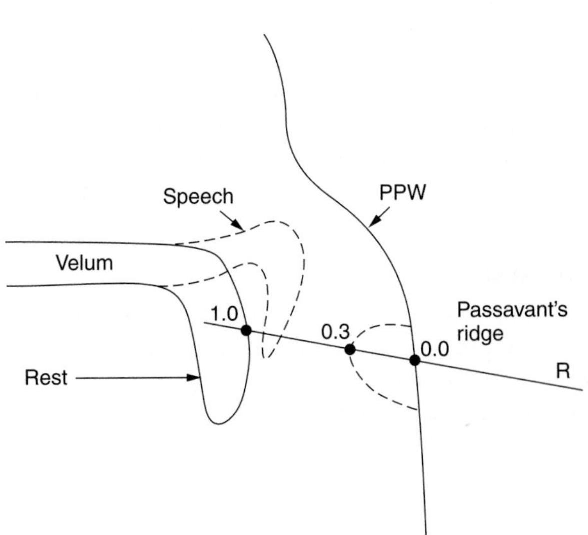

Figure 10-13 Lateral view videofluoroscopy: Passavant's ridge displacement along its trajectory of movement (referant line *R*) toward the resting velum (1.0) resulting in a rating of 0.3. *(Redrawn from Golding-Kushner KJ, et al.: Standardization for the reporting of nasopharyngoscopy and multiview videofluoroscopy: a report from an international working group.* Cleft Palate Journal *27:344, 1990.)*

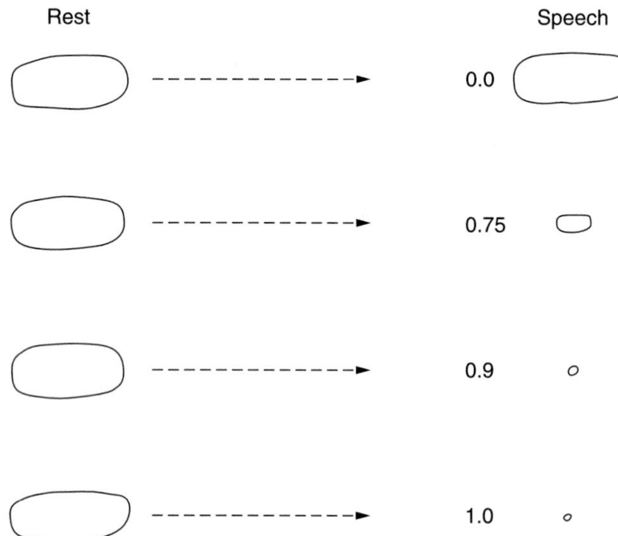

Figure 10-14 Nasopharyngoscopy or en face videofluoroscopy: velopharyngeal gap size as estimated compared with the size of the velopharyngeal valve at rest. The gap may be estimated or calculated by computer programs that compute surface areas. *(Redrawn from Golding-Kushner KJ, et al.: Standardization for the reporting of nasopharyngoscopy and multiview videofluoroscopy: a report from an international working group.* Cleft Palate Journal *27:341, 1990.)*

the tongue or vocal folds are of interest, frame advancement rates up to 5000 cine frames-per-second have been used. High-speed video recording devices are currently available that exceed these rates and will likely become clinically accessible as technology advances further. Currently, however, for clinical purposes and many research purposes, 60 video fields-per-second provides adequate temporal resolution where velopharyngeal movements are of interest. Sharper image resolution is also on the horizon as higher resolution display and digital video recording technology advances.

ENDOSCOPY

Endoscopes are optical instruments consisting of viewing lens, fiberoptic insertion tube, and an eyepiece that can be attached to a camera (Fig. 10-15). They require a high-intensity light source. Both end-viewing and side-viewing rigid and flexible endoscopes have been used. Endoscopes can be passed through body openings and pathways to reach internal organs, including the velopharyngeal area, that cannot otherwise be directly visualized. These instruments have wide application in medicine and are especially useful in viewing the velopharyngeal valve, pharynx, and larynx (Bell-Berti and Hirose, 1975; Croft et al., 1981; Karnell, 1994; Karnell and Morris, 1985; Osberg and Witzel, 1981; Pigott, 1969; Pigott and Makepeace, 1982; Shelton et al., 1978; Shprintzen, McCall, and Skolnick, 1980; Taub, 1966; Zwitman, 1982; Zwitman, Sonderman, and Word, 1974). Ideally, endoscopic examination of the velopharyngeal port provides a view similar to the base or Towne's view obtained in motion fluorographic studies. The endoscope permits observation of the velum and pharyngeal walls as they move in relationship to one another for speech and swallowing. The examiner may visualize, photograph, or record structures in the field of view.

Application of endoscopy for evaluation of the velopharyngeal mechanism for speech was introduced by Taub in 1966. He described a rigid endoscope, which he called the "panendoscope," to study the velopharyngeal mechanism and larynx. This scope, too large for passage through the nasal cavities, was introduced through the mouth to the oropharynx for a view of the velopharyngeal mechanism from below. The panendoscope included an incandescent light bulb at the side of the lens, a feature that created troublesome heat and a potential electrical hazard in the patient's mouth. This instrument, although it was cumbersome and interfered with speech production, represented a breakthrough in assessment of velopharyngeal function (Willis and Stutz, 1972) (Fig. 10-16).

Later rigid endoscopes used fiberoptic bundles to transmit light from a remote source to target structures (Fig. 10-17). These evolved from pediatric urethroscopes, and they have excellent optics and fields of view (Pigott, 1969). With the fiberoptic feature, no heat associated with illumination was introduced into the patient's mouth. Moreover, the diameter of these rigid scopes was considerably smaller than the panendoscope. They could be inserted orally (Beery, Armany, and Katenberg, 1985; Zwitman, 1982) or transnasally (Pigott, 1969; Pigott, Bensen, and White, 1969), although transnasal insertion required additional care and control.

Various problems arise when oral endoscopy is used for the study of velopharyngeal valving. Placement of the scope in the mouth restricts speech to bilabial stops and fricatives combined with low vowels. Gagging is a problem for some patients, and even when it is not, time is needed to teach the patient to accept the scope and to assume a position that permits viewing of the velopharyngeal port. These problems combined with the advent of small-diameter flexible endoscopes led to the prevalent use of nasal endoscopy in the United States today. Use of rigid nasal endoscopy continues to be advocated by some, particularly in the United Kingdom (Gilbert and Pigott, 1982). Karnell and Morris (1985) reported data yielding complementary data from oral and nasal endoscopic examinations performed on the same individual.

Nasal endoscopy performed with flexible fiberoptic endoscopes provides a good view of the nasal surface of the velopharyngeal structures during speech (Croft et al., 1981; Finkelstein et al., 1995; Henningsson and Isberg, 1991; Karnell, 1994; Ramamurthy et al., 1997; Siegel-Sadewitz and Shprintzen, 1982; Witt et al., 1995; Yamaoka et al., 1983) (Fig. 10-18). A description of

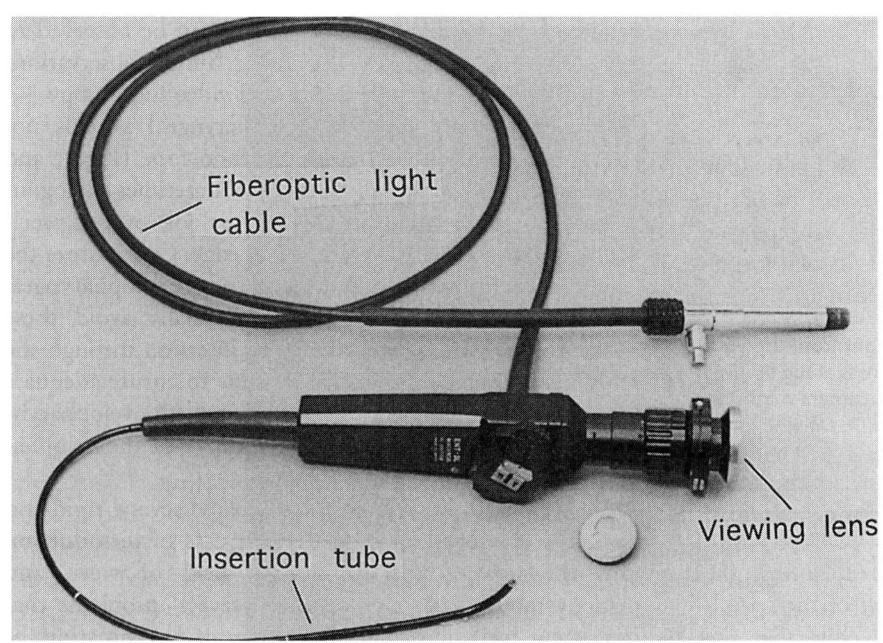

Figure 10-15 Common components of all endoscopes include a viewing lens, insertion tube, and the fiberoptic light cable. *(From* Videoendoscopy From Velopharynx to Larynx, 1st edition, *by Karnell © 1995. Reprinted with permission of Delmar, a division of Thomson Learning. Fax 800-730-2215.)*

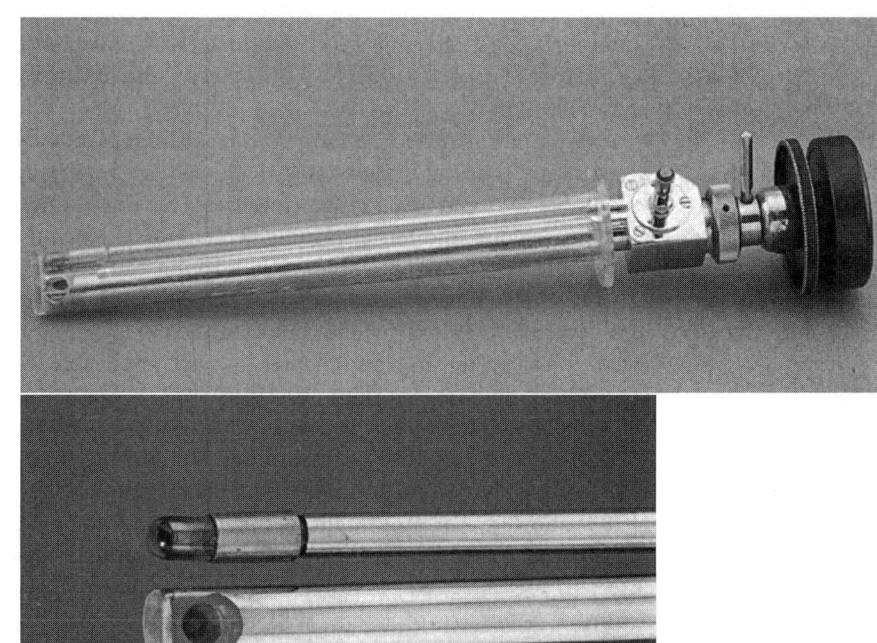

Figure 10-16 The Taub oral panendoscope. The insertion tube was encased in a heat shield to protect the patient from the heat generated by the incandescent bulb **(A).** A closeup of the insertion tube without the heat shield is shown **(B).** *(From* Videoendoscopy From Velopharynx to Larynx, 1st edition, *by Karnell © 1995. Reprinted with permission of Delmar, a division of Thomson Learning. Fax 800-730-2215.)*

videoendoscopic equipment (scope, light source, camera, videorecorder, and television monitor) and procedures for its use including patient preparation is found in Karnell (1994). The development of solid-state, light-sensitive camera technology (Wilson, 1988; Yanagisawa, Godley, and Muta, 1987) and high-resolution videorecorders have further contributed to the utility of nasal videoendoscopy when applied to the evaluation of velopharyngeal insufficiency.

Use of nasal endoscopy in children requires special considerations and procedures. D'Antonio et al. (1986) described techniques for use of videonasendoscopy with

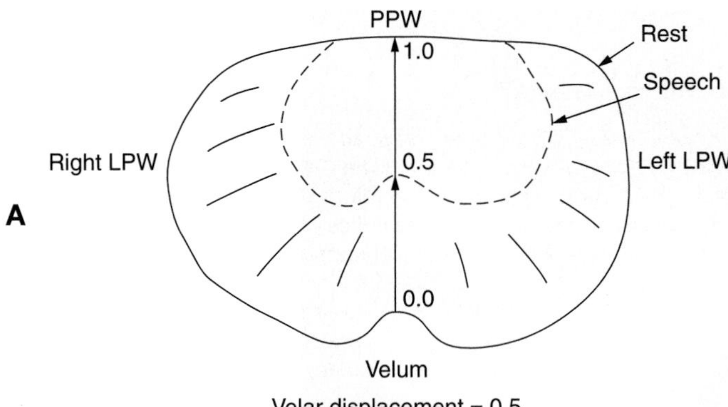

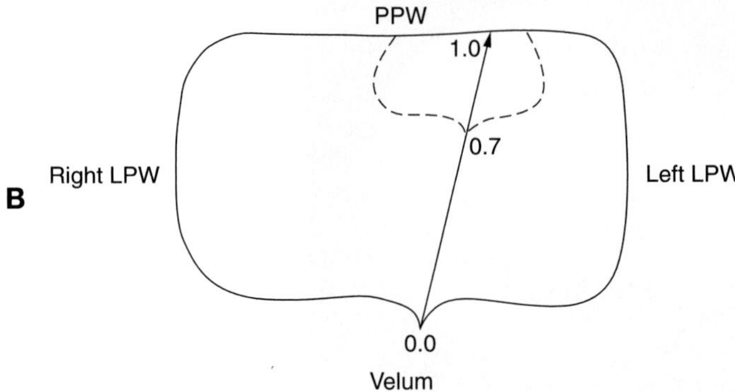

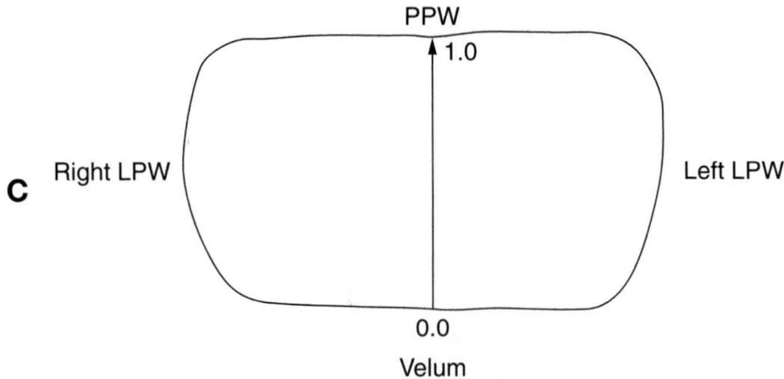

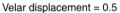

Figure 10-19 A, Nasopharyngoscopy or en face videofluoroscopy (e.g., base or Towne view) demonstrating degree of velar movement as rated by the standardized system. Velopharyngeal valve with normal palate and musculus uvula. The velum (0.0) moves half the distance to the posterior pharyngeal wall (*PPW,* 1.0), which is scored as 0.5. **B,** In submucous cleft palate or repaired cleft palate, where a notch is apparent on the superior surface of the velum, the midline of this notch represents 0.0. The trajectory of the velum is asymmetric and the degree of motion (0.7) is measured along this asymmetric trajectory. **C,** When the superior surface of the vellum is flat, the anatomic midline represents 0.0. Movement to PPW represents a value of 1.1. *(From Golding-Kushner KJ, et al.: Standardization for the reporting of nasopharyngoscopy and multiview videofluoroscopy: a report from an international working group.* Cleft Palate Journal *27:339, 1990.)*

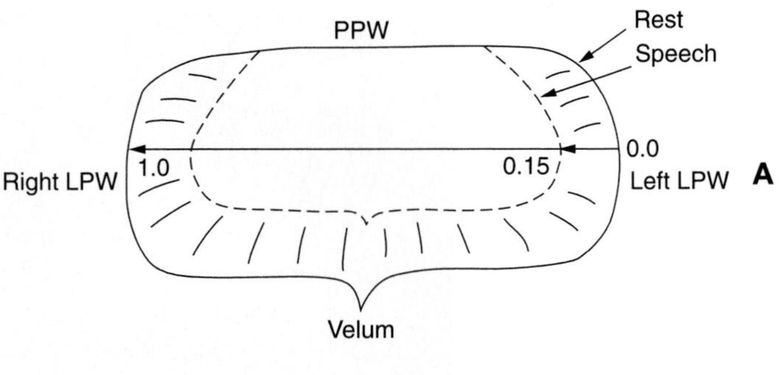

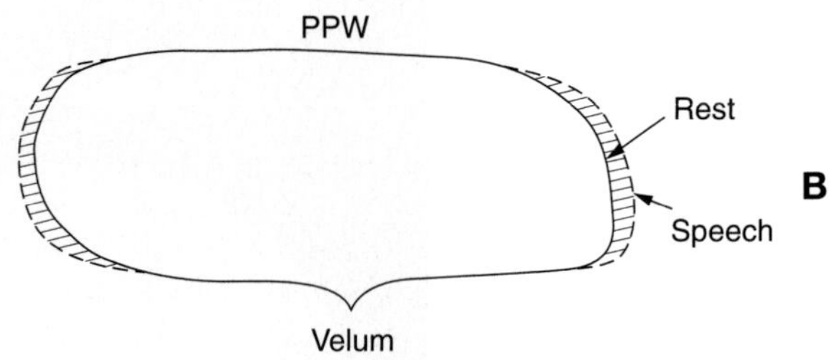

Figure 10-20 A, Nasopharyngoscopy or en face videofluoroscopy: degree of lateral pharyngeal wall *(LPW)* displacement. The opposite lateral wall represents 1.0. The left lateral wall moves 0.15 (distance ration) toward the right lateral pharyngeal wall. **B,** The lateral walls move outward, resulting in a rating of –0.1. *(From Golding-Kushner KJ, et al.: Standardization for the reporting of nasopharyngoscopy and multiview videofluoroscopy: a report from an international working group.* Cleft Palate Journal *27:340, 1990.)*

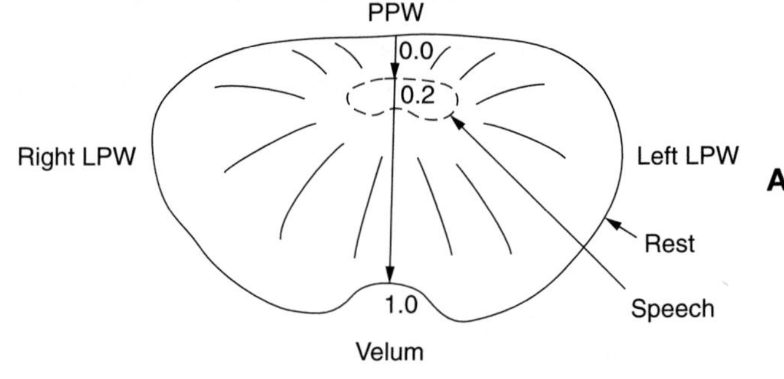

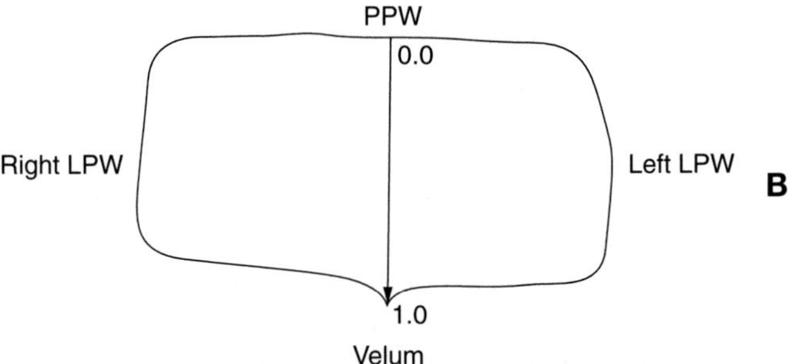

Figure 10-21 A, Nasopharyngoscopy or en face videofluoroscopy: degree of posterior pharyngeal wall displacement. In the case of a structurally normal palate, the posterior pharyngeal wall represents 0.0 and the midline of musculus uvulae is 1.0. In this case the posterior wall moves 0.2 of the distance toward the velum at rest. **B,** In the case of a notched soft palate, the midline of the notch represents 1.0. *LPW,* Lateral pharyngeal wall. *(From Golding-Kushner KJ, et al.: Standardization for the reporting of nasopharyngoscopy and multiview videofluoroscopy: a report from an international working group.* Cleft Palate Journal *27:340, 1990.)*

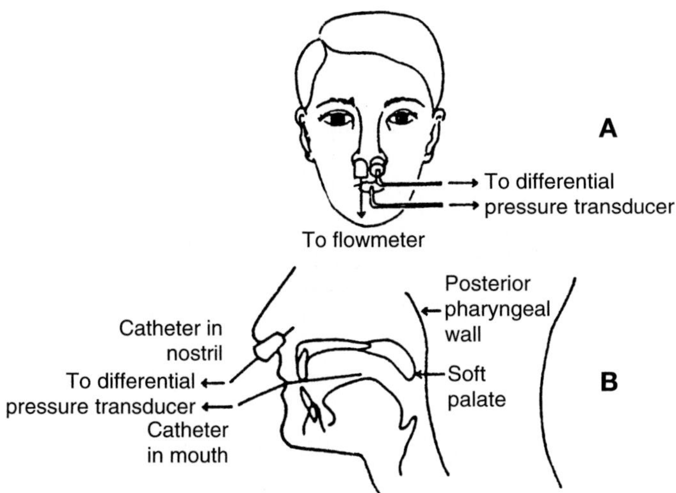

Figure 10-22 Catheters are placed above and below the orifice to measure the differential pressure. The catheter placed in the left nostril is secured by a cork, which plugs the nostril and creates a stagnant air column above the orifice **(A)**. The second catheter is placed in the mouth **(B)**. Both catheters are connected to a differential pressure transducer. The pneumotachygraph is connected to the right nostril and collects orifice airflow through the nose. *(From Warren DW: Aerodynamics of speech production. In Lass NJ [ed.]:* Contemporary issues in experimental phonetics. *New York: Academic Press, 1976.)*

Speech-language pathologists use various endoscopic procedures to describe structure and function of the larynx, pharynx, and velopharynx to assist in development of treatment planning and, where appropriate, behavioral therapy. Nasal videoendoscopy should be performed with primary consideration for patient health and safety. For this reason, we feel nasal endoscopy should only be performed in facilities where full medical support is readily available.

AERODYNAMICS

Aerodynamics is a branch of mechanics that deals with the motion of air and other gases and with the effects of that motion on bodies in the air (Flexner, 1987). In this section we review instrumentation and procedures for the aerodynamic evaluation of velopharyngeal physiology, including the estimation of the narrowest cross-sectional areas of the velopharyngeal port and of the nasal pathway. Data collected for those measures may also be used to quantify the resistance of each passage to airflow. Attention is given to precautions that should be observed in using aerodynamic equipment. Estimation of velopharyngeal area and other applications of aerodynamics in the study of velopharyngeal function is commonly discussed with reference to the expression "pressure-flow technique."

Measurement of the Area of Velopharyngeal Opening at Its Narrowest Cross Section

The area of an orifice can be determined by measuring the fluid flow through and fluid pressure drop across that orifice. The narrowest constriction of the velopharyngeal port during production of a pressure consonant /p/ may be determined by measuring the nasal airflow through one nasal passage and the difference in air pressure between pressure-sensing tubes placed in the mouth and in the second nasal passage. The data can also be used to calculate the resistance of the velopharyngeal pathway (Warren, 1984, 1989; Warren and Du Bois, 1964).

Dalston and Warren (1986, p. 110) summarized their use of aeromechanical instrumentation for estimation of velopharyngeal area:

> Briefly, the adequacy of the velopharyngeal port was assessed by simultaneously measuring the airflow through it and the pressure drop across it. Nasal airflow (V_n) was recorded by means of a heated pneumotachograph connected to plastic tubing of sufficient size to fit snugly in the subject's more patent nostril. The pressure drop across the velopharyngeal orifice (AP) was obtained by placing one catheter within the mouth and a second catheter in the subject's other nostril. The nasal catheter was secured by a cork stopper that occluded the nostril, thereby creating a stagnant air column.

Their placement of pressure and flow sensing tubing and use of transducers, pneumotachograph, and computer are shown in Figs. 10-22 and 10-23.

The area of the velopharyngeal opening is obtained by multiplying the differential air pressure by 980, which converts to dynes, and entering that value and nasal airflow in the following equation provided by Warren and DuBois (1964):

$$A = \frac{\dot{V}_n}{k\sqrt{\dfrac{2\,(P_1 - P_3)}{D}}}$$

where

A is area in cm^2

$\dot{V}_n$ is nasal air flow in liters per second

P_1 and P_3 are oral and nasal air pressures in dynes

D is density of air (0.001 g/cm^3)

k is a correction factor (0.65)

The correction factor of 0.65 was obtained by Warren and DuBois through use of a model of the vocal tract with known velopharyngeal orifices. Their model—and others—and the correction factor have been studied by many investigators (Guyette and Carpenter, 1988; Lubker, 1969; Selley et al., 1987; Smith and Weinberg, 1980, 1982; Smith, Maddox, and Kostinski, 1985; Yates, McWilliams, and Vallino, 1990). Zajac and Yates (1991) reported findings that indicated that the error of aerodynamic estimates of velopharyngeal orifice area measurements was 7% when the accurate correction factor was known,

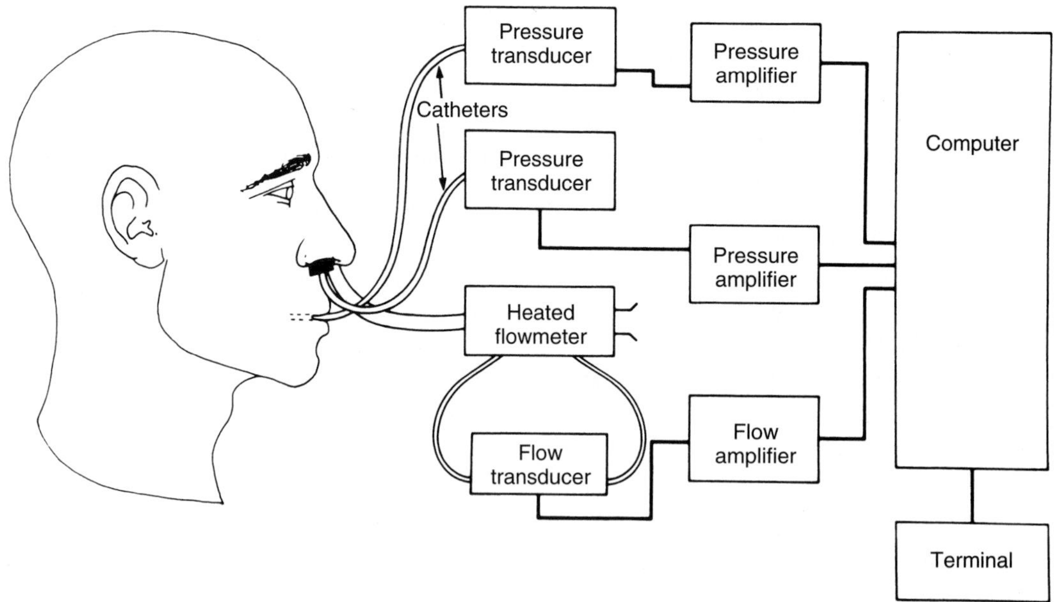

Figure 10-23 Equipment used to record intraoral pressures. *(From Dalston RM, Warren DW, Morr KE, and Smith LR: Intraoral pressure and its relationship to velopharyngeal inadequacy.* Cleft Palate Journal *25:212, 1988.)*

suggesting that errors in excess of this amount may be expected when an accurate correction factor was unknown. Normative pressure, flow, and estimated velopharyngeal area data for selected oral and nasal speech segments were reported by Andreassen, Smith, and Guyette (1991) and appear in Tables 10-1 through 10-3.

The resistance of the passage between two pressure-sensing tubes is calculated by dividing oral-nasal differential air pressure by nasal airflow. The resistance is expressed in centimeters of water per liter per second:

$$R = \frac{\Delta P}{\dot{V}_n}$$

where

R is resistance expressed in centimeters of water per liter per second

ΔP is oral-nasal differential air pressure

$\dot{V}_n$ is nasal airflow in liters per second

Although this formula is used to measure laminar flows, which we do not have in velopharyngeal assessment, it provides adequate estimates of resistance if the measurement is always obtained at a given rate of nasal air flow. Commonly, resistance is measured at 0.25 or 0.5 L/s/cm H_2O. If one of the pressure-sensing tubes used to measure oral-nasal differential air pressure is placed at the nares, the resistance measured reflects the influence of the velopharyngeal port and the nasal pathways combined. Isshiki, Honjow, and Morimoto (1968) wrote that any resistance calculated is the sum of the resistances present, including those of the velopharyngeal port, the nasal pathways, and the pneumotachometer itself. Hixon, Bless, and Netsell (1976) discussed the matter of differentiating between velopharyngeal and nasal pathway resistance to nasal air flow. We assume that during /p/ the resistance measured primarily reflects the influence of the velopharyngeal port and that during nasal breathing the anterior nasal passages have the greatest influence on the resistance measure.

Patients with cleft palate or craniofacial anomalies frequently have some degree of upper air way obstruction that may have implications for breathing as well as speech. Smith and Guyette (1993) described a technique for differentiating nasal airway resistance into anterior nasal and velopharyngeal components. They used their approach to measure nasal passage and velopharyngeal resistance before and after pharyngeal flap surgery in two subjects with clefts. Results from one of the two subjects, shown in Table 10-4, shows a dramatic increase in velopharyngeal resistance before and after surgery while nasal cavity resistance remained essentially unchanged. Henrich et al. (1995) examined subjects' responses to sudden changes (within 10 ms) in airway size. They found that subjects appeared to recognize the change before the airway became self-limiting or obstructed. They interpreted their findings as evidence that breathing behaviors follow the rules of a physiologic regulating system. Warren et al. (1976), in a similar report, stated that subjects appeared to sense breathing difficulty when nasal airway resistance reached approximately 5 cm/L/s. Patients were found to begin to change from nasal breathing to oral breathing when resistance values were measured between 3.5 and 4.5 cm/L/s.

Pressure-flow assessment of velopharyngeal function requires pressure transducers, a pneumotachograph, a recorder, and calibration equipment. An example of a com-

Table 10-1 **Peak Oral-Nasal Pressures (cm H_2O) for Oral Consonants**

Sex/Utterance Type	*Group Mean*	*SD*	*Range of Subject Means*	*Range of Individual Productions*
Men				
/pi/	6.68	1.31	4.79-9.49	4.31-10.39
/fi/	6.25	1.93	4.03-10.03	2.85-12.09
/pa/	6.44	1.52	4.32-9.64	2.93-11.40
/p/ in "hamper"	6.03	1.19	4.41-8.29	4.00-10.55
Women				
/pi/	6.50	1.11	5.17-9.09	4.62-9.93
/fi/	5.51	1.15	4.34-8.14	3.23-8.93
/pa/	6.07	1.10	4.66-8.55	4.00-9.24
/p/ in "hamper"	5.69	1.64	3.41-8.83	3.00-9.70

From Andreassen ML, Smith BE, and Guyette TW: Pressure flow measurements for selected oral and nasal sound segments produced by normal adults. *Cleft Palate Journal* 28:398-406, 1991.

Table 10-2 **Nasal Airflow Rates (ml/s) at Peak Pressures for Oral Consonants**

Sex/Utterance Type	*Group Mean*	*SD*	*Range of Subject Means*	*Range of Individual Productions*
Men				
/pi/	3.96	4.31	0.00-13.09	0.00-26.95
/fi/	4.19	4.64	0.38-15.40	0.00-50.05
/pa/	17.82	29.98	2.69-101.64	0.00-150.15
/p/ in "hamper"	30.03	16.52	2.57-51.33	0.00-57.75
Women				
/pi/	2.04	1.52	0.00-5.00	0.00-7.70
/fi/	1.62	1.88	0.00-6.16	0.00-7.70
/pa/	6.66	8.22	0.00-28.49	0.00-42.35
/p/ in "hamper"	12.19	10.91	0.00-37.22	0.00-42.35

From Andreassen ML, Smith BE, and Guyette TW: Pressure flow measurements for selected oral and nasal sound segments produced by normal adults. *Cleft Palate Journal* 28:398-406, 1991.

Table 10-3 **Velopharyngeal Orifice Areas (mm^2) at Peak Pressures for Consonants**

Sex/Utterance Type	*Group Mean*	*SD*	*Range of Subject Means*	*Range of Individual Productions*
Men				
/pi/	0.15	0.15	0.00-0.46	0.00-1.06
/fi/	0.19	0.20	0.03-0.61	0.00-1.96
/pa/	0.78	1.31	0.10-4.46	0.00-6.49
/p/ in "hamper"	1.40	0.95	0.29-3.04	0.19-4.80
Women				
/pi/	0.09	0.07	0.00-0.22	0.00-0.39
/fi/	0.11	0.14	0.00-0.40	0.00-0.47
/pa/	0.29	0.34	0.00-1.19	0.00-1.68
/p/ in "hamper"	0.63	0.41	0.00-1.34	0.00-1.80

From Andreassen ML, Smith BE, and Guyette TW: Pressure flow measurements for selected oral and nasal sound segments produced by normal adults. *Cleft Palate Journal* 28:398-406, 1991.

Table 10-4 **Preoperative and Postoperative Resistance Data (cm H_2O/L/s) for Patient 2**

	Preoperative	*8 Weeks Postoperative*	*7 Months Postoperative*
Right nasal cavity	2.11	1.71	4.84
Left nasal cavity	2.34	2.39	1.86
Total nasal cavities (% contribution)	1.11 (100%)	1.00 (10%)	1.34 (20%)
Velopharynx (% contribution)	0.00 (0%)	9.17 (90%)	5.33 (80%)
Total nasal airway (100%)	1.11 (100%)	10.17 (100%)	6.67 (100%)

From Smith BE, and Guyette TW: Component approach for partitioning nasal airway resistance: pharyngeal flap case studies. *Cleft Palate Journal* 30:78-81, 1993.

puter printout of pressure-flow data and their computer analysis from Warren's laboratory is shown in Fig. 10-24.

Warren (1989) and colleagues at the University of North Carolina used pressure-flow instrumentation to measure velopharyngeal opening during /p/ in various contexts. Production of /mp/ as in hamper requires the velopharyngeal mechanism to open and close quickly. Performance during that word is contrasted with performance in less-demanding nonnasal contexts such as "papa." Individuals who are able to achieve closure during /p/ in "papa," but who fail to achieve closure during "hamper," are believed to have difficulty with timing of velopharyngeal closure. Zajac and Mayo (1996) interpreted timing data obtained with this approach as evidence that aerodynamic parameters are more constrained in the temporal domain than in the amplitude domain in normal speakers. Leeper, Tissington, and Munhall (1998) provided some normative data about duration aspects of pressure-flow measures obtained during production of the word "hamper." Although there was a trend for temporal measures to decrease as age increased, durational values were similar to those previously reported for normal speaking adults. Low variability was reported across age groups of children tested.

Velopharyngeal area is measured during /p/ because during that sound the air in the oral and nasal passages is theoretically stagnant or still. Also, the pressure detected at the mouth presumably is the same as the pressure just below the velopharyngeal port. The pressure detected at one naris is the same as that just above the velopharyngeal port. Thus the pressure drop recorded is across the velopharyngeal port. Warren (1989, p. 244) wrote that application of the equation is most appropriate when measurements are made at the flow peak when the rate of change of flow is zero. However, because the oral air pressure and the nasal airflow peaks during /p/ approximately coincide when the velopharyngeal port is not closed and because the oral air pressure waveform is more stable than the air flow waveform at that moment, the area estimate is commonly described as being made at the moment of peak oral air pressure or oral-nasal differential air pressure.

For sounds other than /p/, the pressure drop might be across a constriction other than the one formed by the velopharyngeal valve. The production of /b/ is not used because of the reduction in air pressure associated with voicing. During /p/ produced with a velopharyngeal opening, change in respiratory effort influences oral and nasal pressures equally.

Vowel effects on pressure-flow measurements have been reported by Smith and Guyette (1996) who described 8 of 51 patients who demonstrated inadequate velopharyngeal closure during production of /pi/ syllables but who achieved adequate velopharyngeal closure during /pa/ syllables. They suggested the downward pull on the palate by the palatoglossus muscle may have influenced velopharyngeal closure in these individuals.

Velopharyngeal Closure Categories and Variables that May Confound Aerodynamic Measurement

Warren and colleagues used pressure-flow assessment to categorize patients with clefts into three categories of velopharyngeal competence: adequate, borderline, and inadequate or incompetent (Warren, 1979). Dalston and Warren (1986, p. 113) indicated that their terms adequate, borderline, and inadequate pertain to ". . . velopharyngeal function in terms of the respiratory requirements of speech. The pressure-flow technique does not evaluate speech performance. . . . When velopharyngeal closure is less than total, [its influence on speech] depends upon the anatomic configuration of the oral and nasal cavities as well as the extent to which other speech structures adapt to the incompetency" (p. 113). They went on to indicate that oral closure may shunt acoustic energy into the nasal passages and that timing of speech events contributes to the quality of speech in individuals within a given closure category.

Selley et al. (1987), using CT scans in construction of a "fully anatomical" model of the vocal tract, confirmed that resistance associated with tongue posture and the nasal pathways influences nasal air flow when the velopharyngeal opening is kept constant. The model was constructed so that oral port size and tongue posture as well as velopharyngeal opening could be varied. Data obtained with the model indicated that nasal air flow was similar with velopharyngeal openings of 55 and 16 mm^2, respectively, if the larger opening were associated

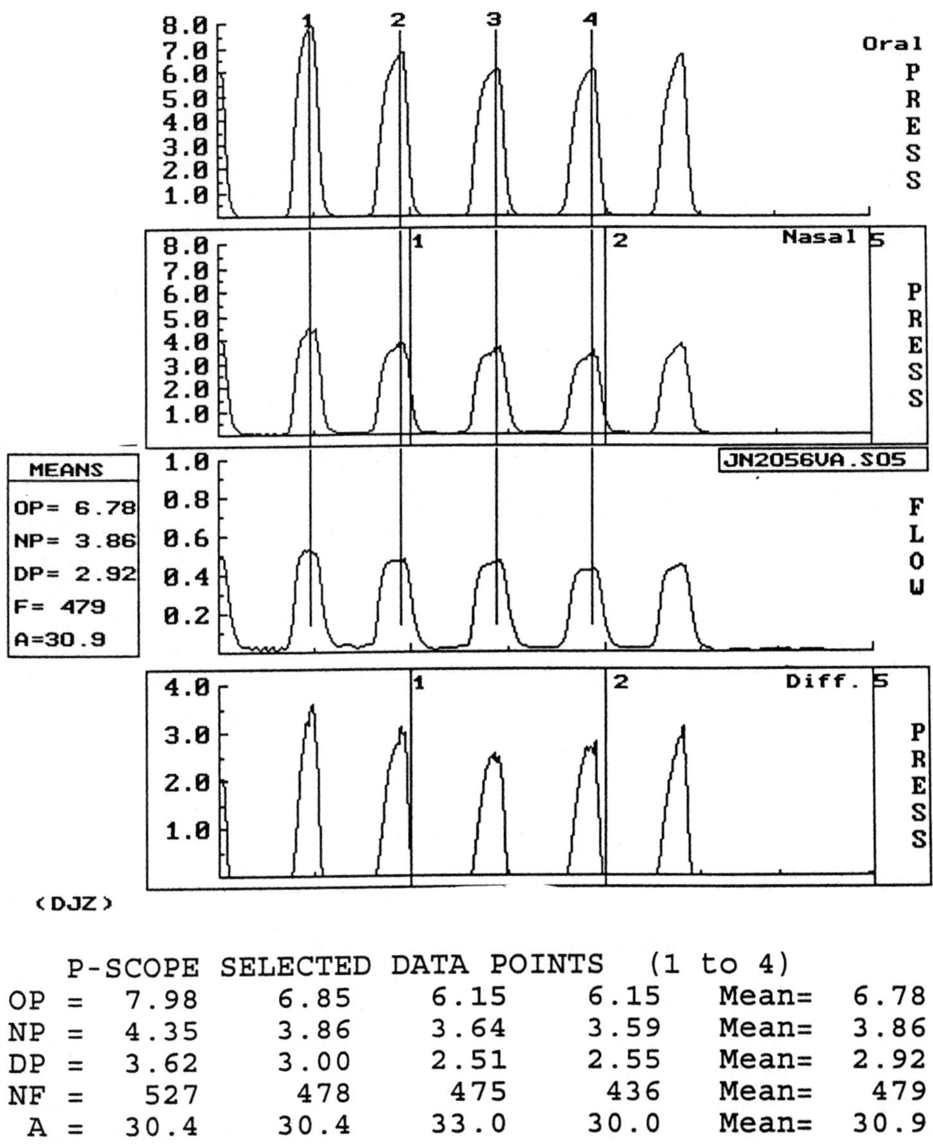

P-SCOPE SELECTED DATA POINTS (1 to 4)

OP =	7.98	6.85	6.15	6.15	Mean= 6.78
NP =	4.35	3.86	3.64	3.59	Mean= 3.86
DP =	3.62	3.00	2.51	2.55	Mean= 2.92
NF =	527	478	475	436	Mean= 479
A =	30.4	30.4	33.0	30.0	Mean= 30.9

Figure 10-24 A pressure-flow recording obtained during six productions of /pa/ by an adult speaker with repaired cleft palate. Graphs are (top to bottom): oral air pressure (OP), nasal air pressure (NP), nasal airflow (NF), and differential oral-nasal air pressure (DP). Pressures are measured in centimeters of water (cm H_2O) and flow in liters per second (l/s). The vertical cursors numbered 1 to 4 indicate peak OP. Individual and mean measurements associated with these cursors are listed at the bottom of the figure. The mean data are also displayed in the box labeled "Means." Calculated velopharyngeal orifice area (A) are in square millimeters (mm^2). *(Courtesy of Dr. David J. Zajac, University of North Carolina.)*

with a flat tongue and the smaller opening with a humped tongue. Tongue posture and velopharyngeal opening also interact with oral port opening. Tongue posture had no influence on air flow through a velopharyngeal opening if the anterior oral port opening was small, but tongue humping "... caused ... [an] increase in nasal airflow with both small and large velopharyngeal ports when the anterior oral port was large ..." (p. 379). Velopharyngeal areas from 40 to 60 mm^2 were interpreted as a threshold value beyond which "the nose controls the flow." The nasal pathway resistance to air flow in this model differed from that of the Warren model, which offered resistance comparable to that observed in normal persons. To the extent that the resistance does not correspond to that of the human, findings may be in error.

Precautions Relative to Pressure-Flow Measurements

Pressure-flow measurements provide information about the coupling of the oral and the nasal cavities during speech and about resistance in the system. They are indirect measures of velopharyngeal function in that they describe the effects of velopharyngeal physiology. They do not describe either the movement of particular structures, such as the velum and lateral pharyngeal walls, or the location and configuration of any opening that is present. Direct measures such as fluoroscopy or endoscopy must be used to obtain that information.

High-frequency oscillations in pressure-flow waveforms are influenced by certain characteristics of the pressure-sensing tube. Tubes should be straight, short, and as large in internal diameter as possible. Very small tubes are easily clogged by mucus, whereas very large tubes do not allow tight lip closure. Pressure-sensing tubes should be positioned perpendicular to the air stream; false readings occur when air flow travels directly into the tube.

A concise description of several problems in aeromechanical assessment was presented by Müller and Brown (1980). They indicated that calculations of orifice areas for ports of the same size but of different geometric configurations may differ slightly from one another. Müller and Brown also pointed out that an area estimate is influenced by the shape of the entry and exit to the port, the presence or absence of a distinct periodic component to the flow, and the nature of the flow, that is, whether it is turbulent, laminar, or transitional. Other variables that may influence estimates of velopharyngeal area and nasal pathway resistance include the biomechanics of the tissues of the pertinent structures and changes in those tissues.

Warren (1989) responded to Müller and Brown by saying that the correction factor he uses works satisfactorily for the port configurations and air flows associated with speech and breathing. He agreed with them, however, that the hydrokinetic equation has limitations. He emphasized the importance of attention to detail in aerodynamic assessment of velopharyngeal area.

Warren (1989) recommended balancing transducers and calibration of equipment at the beginning of work with each patient. He would also calibrate the equipment against a tube with a known orifice. Since his report, pressure transducers have been designed that are more stable and require less frequent calibration. Kinks in tubing and leaks in the system including the juncture of cork with nose, will invalidate findings. Both nostrils should be patent. If one side is more open than the other, the more open side should be used for measuring flow (Riski and Warren, 1988). The catheter tubing selected for measurement of nasal air flow should fit the naris snugly. If one side is obstructed, the area will be incorrectly estimated. Placement of the oral catheter is not critical so long as it taps the stagnant oral air column and lip closure is airtight. Use of leak-resistant tubing connectors helps ensure the pressure-flow system is airtight.

Bumping a pressure-sensing tube will result in measurement of a pressure increase. Tubing may be obstructed by contact with tissue as well as by the accumulation of mucus. During strings of /pV/ syllables, the oral pressure trace should return to baseline each time the lips open. If it falls short of the baseline, something is wrong. Nasal air flow during utterance offset, nasal consonants, and respiration between test passages is normal.

Alternative Aeromechanical Procedures

Stuffins (1989) described the clinical use of nasal anemometry in Great Britain. The Exeter Nasal Anemometry equipment, which includes an anesthetist's nasal mask and a microphone, is used to record nasal air flow and speech.

Sandham and Solow (1987) described the use of anterior and posterior rhinomanometry (rhinometry) in measuring nasal respiratory resistance. Anterior and posterior rhinomanometry differ in placement of tubing used to measure differential air pressure across the nasal pathway. The anterior method is used to measure unilateral nasal respiratory resistance, and the posterior method is used to measure bilateral nasal respiratory resistance (see also Riski and Warren, 1988, and Smith and Guyette, 1993).

Measurement of Nasal Pathway Area and Mouth Breathing

The size of the velopharyngeal port is not the only factor influencing pressure-flow measures. Nasal airway size affects air flow: a constricted nasal air way offers high resistance to air flow. Interpretation of the influence of the velopharyngeal valve on a patient's speech depends on information about nasal pathway patency. Hairfield et al. (1987) referred to the nasal valve which they located ". . . in the region between the upper and lower lateral cartilages [of the nose] and the pyriform aperture just beyond the anterior ends of the inferior turbinates" (p. 184). The nasal valve includes the liminal valve, which is the most constricted portion of the nostril. It is located about 1 cm posterior to the nostril opening (Bateman and Mason, 1984).

Warren (1984) described the application of the pressure flow technique to the estimation of the cross-sectional area of the nasal passage. Hairfield et al. (1987) used posterior rhinomanometry to measure nasal valve area during nasal breathing. During nasal breathing the velopharyngeal port is open, and the narrowest constriction between an oral pressure-sensing tube and a nasal air flow mask is at the nasal valve. As shown in Fig. 10-25, to measure the smallest nasal cross-sectional area, Hairfield et al. placed a nasal mask over the nose and measured differential air pressure between the mask and the mouth and flow through the nose. Area was again calculated by use of the hydrokinetic equation.

Hairfield, Warren, and Seaton (1988) studied the prevalence of mouth breathing in patients with cleft palate. Mouth breathing was defined in terms of the ratio of nasal-to-tidal volume during respiration. Tidal volume was measured by means of inductive plethysmography, which senses movements of rib cage and abdomen; nasal volume was measured by use of a nose cap and pneumotachograph (Fig. 10-26).

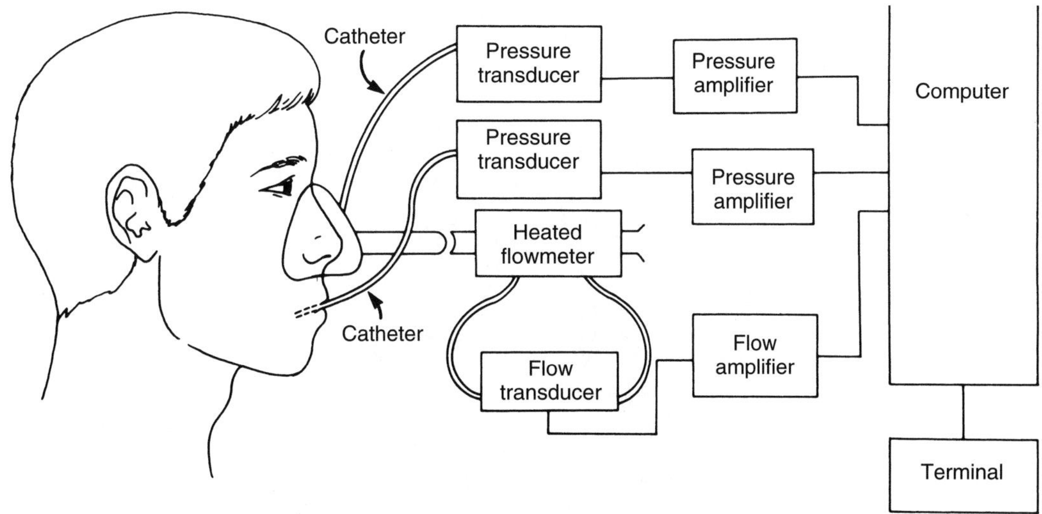

Figure 10-25 Schematic diagram of method used for measurement of nasal cross-sectional areas. *(From Hairfield WM, Warren DW, Hinton VA, and Seaton DL: Inspiratory and expiratory effects of nasal breathing.* Cleft Palate Journal *24:185, 1987.)*

Hairfield et al. wrote:

> Each [plethysmography] transducer measures changes in inductance that are proportional to changes in thoracic cage and abdominal volumes. Breathing changes the cross-sectional area of the transducer coils and the resulting inductance changes are converted to proportional voltages. The rib cage and abdominal signals are then calibrated against a known volume kv having the subjects breathe into a spirometer. The sum of the calibrated signals (i.e., thoracic and abdominal) is equivalent to tidal volume (p. 136).
>
> Breathing mode was defined by using the following classifications of percent nasal breathing: 80 to 100 percent, nasal; 60 to 79 percent, predominantly nasal, 40 to 59 percent, mixed oral-nasal; 20 to 39 percent, predominantly oral; 0 to 19 percent, oral (p. 135).

NASOMETER™

The Nasometer is a microcomputer-based acoustical instrument designed for use in assessment and treatment of patients with nasality problems (Instruction Manual. Kay Elemetrics Corp., Pine Brook, NJ). The Nasometer computes the ratio between acoustic energy detected by microphones positioned at the nose and the mouth. This ratio is termed nasalance. The result of this computation may be displayed in several ways, including statistical table, time history display or nasogram that shows nasalance for time periods from 2 through 100 seconds, and bar graph showing moment to moment nasalance peaks for feedback purposes. The Nasometer (Fig. 10-27) includes an input device consisting of headgear, a sound separator baffle, oral and nasal microphones, a Nasometer unit, a printed circuit board for use with personal computers, computer software, and a calibration stand. The Nasometer unit amplifies and filters signals from each microphone and converts them from analog to digital form. A calibration function is built into the device that enables the user to balance the oral and nasal microphones.

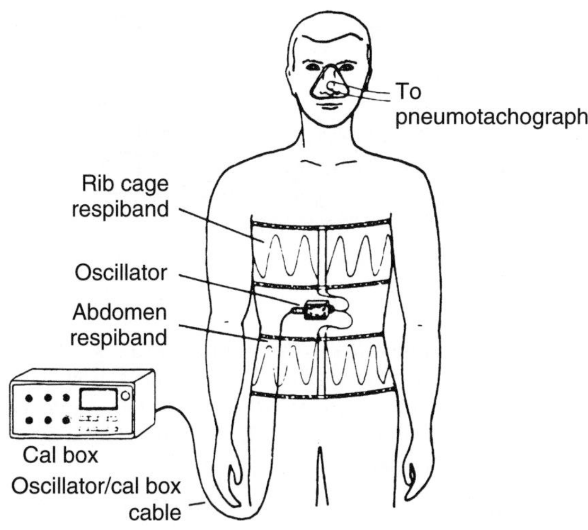

Figure 10-26 Schematic diagram of nasal cap placement and configuration of induction coils used for plethysmography. *(From Hairfield WM, Warren DW, Hinton VA, and Seaton DL: Prevalence of mouthbreathing in cleft lip and palate.* Cleft Palate Journal *25:136, 1987.)*

The Nasometer is based on an earlier instrument called Tonar (the oral nasal acoustic ratio), which was a similar acoustical device for the measurement of nasalance (Fletcher and Bishop, 1970). Fletcher reported that Tonar data correlated highly (Spearman $r = 0.91$) with psychophysical ratings of hypernasality (Fletcher, 1976), and some research was published relative to the effectiveness of Tonar as a biofeedback device for the reduction of hypernasality (Fletcher, Adams, and McCutcheon, 1989).

Nasometric data are usually obtained when the patient is repeating one of several standardized sets of sentences

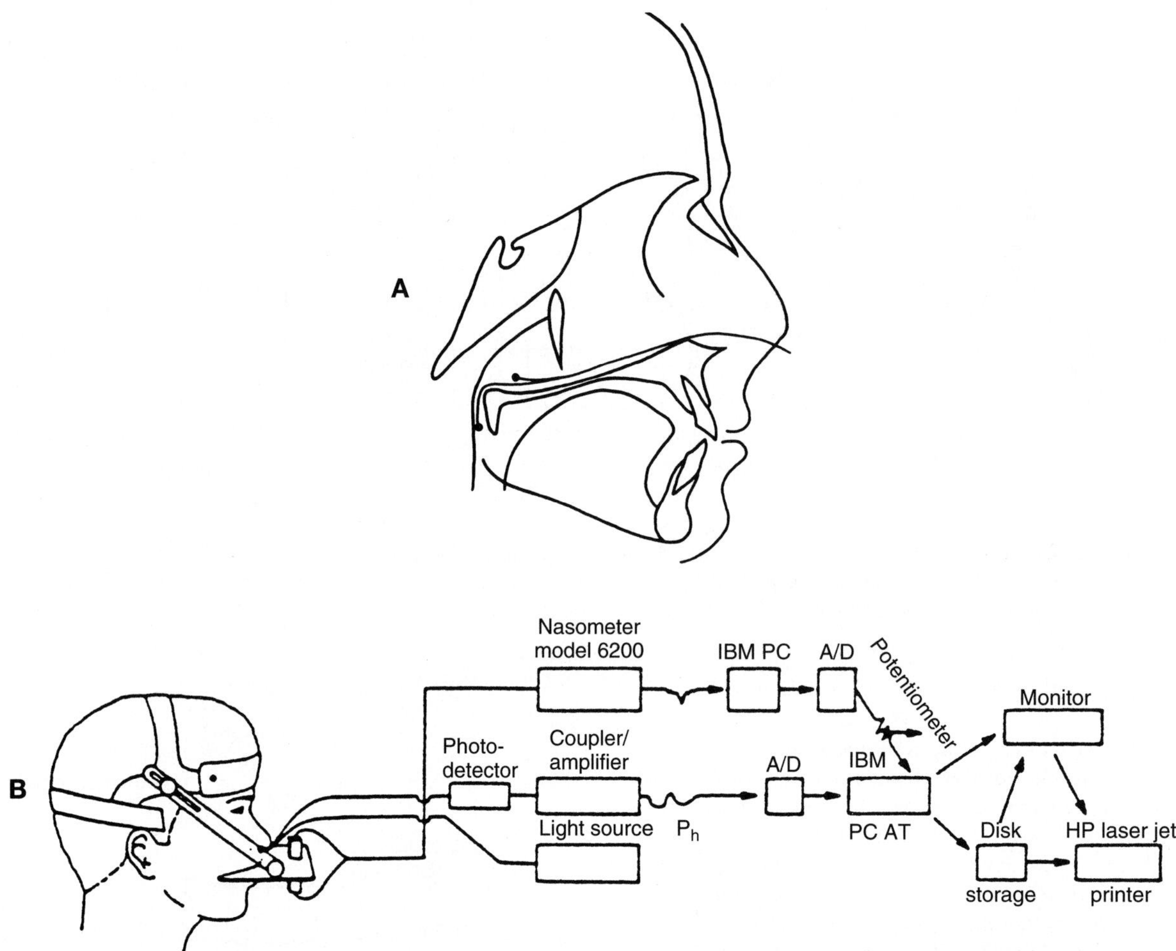

Figure 10-27 The photodetector: **A,** Placement of the photodetector probe. **B,** Schematic diagram of the photodetector system and Nasometer used in this study. *(From Dalston RM: Using simultaneous photodetection and nasometry to monitor velopharyngeal behavior during speech.* Journal of Speech and Hearing Research *32:195-202, 1989. © American Speech-Language-Hearing Association. Reprinted by permission.)*

provided with the unit. The Zoo Passage contains no nasal phonemes. It consists of a distribution of orally produced consonants and vowels. Watterson, Hinton, and McFarlane (1996) recommended the use of age appropriate stimuli for obtaining nasometry data. They introduced the Turtle Passage, which was found to yield nasalance measures similar to the Zoo Passage in the patients they examined. Dalston and Seaver (1992) reported that use of the Rainbow Passage offered no additional information beyond that obtained when the Zoo Passage and Nasal Sentences were used.

Dalston, Warren, and Dalston (1991) reported that Nasometer data correlated well with ratings of hypernasality (Pearson $r = 0.82$) but not with aerodynamic estimates of velopharyngeal orifice area (Pearson $r = 32$). These authors also found that audible nasal emission of air had a large impact on nasalance measures (Dalston et al. 1991). In a cross dialect interinstitutional study, Dalston, Neiman, and Gonzalez-Landa (1993) reported a Pearson correlation coefficient of 0.78 between nasalance and hypernasality ratings on the basis of analysis of 514 subjects. Mayo, Floyd, Warren, Dalston, and Mayo (1996) found no differences in nasalance measures due to race. Differences due to age and gender have not been found (van Doorn and Purcell, 1998) nor have differences due to vocal loudness (Watterson, York, and McFarlane, 1994).

An epidemiologic approach to assessing the value of nasalance measures was introduced by Dalston et al. (1991), who reported the sensitivity and specificity of Nasometer measures using a nasalance cutoff of .32. Sensitivity refers to the ability of the Nasometer to accurately identify patients as hypernasal when they were rated as such by trained listeners. Specificity refers to the ability of the Nasometer to identify as normal those patients who were not judged as hypernasal. Perfect sensitivity and specificity scores would be 1.0. The authors calculated nasometry sensitivity as 0.89 and specificity as 0.95. Hardin, Van Demark, Morris, and Payne (1992) found that a nasalance cutoff nasometry score of 0.27 resulted in a sensitivity of 0.76 and a specificity of 0.86.

The use of cutoff scores has greatly simplified interpretation of nasalance measures. However, variations in dialect and/or language spoken or differences in local standards for perceived nasality may have an impact on the preferred cutoff score used for nasalance measures (Anderson, 1996; Dalston, Neiman, and Gonzalez-Landa, 1993).

Karnell (1995) suggested that use of sentences devoid of pressure consonants, called low-pressure sentences, could eliminate the effects of audible nasal emission of air on nasalance measures. He found that some subjects scored differently relative to a nasalance cutoff score depending on whether they were measured with the low-pressure sentences or the Zoo Passage. Karnell further interpreted those findings as possible evidence that the low-pressure sentences may help identify a subgroup of patients with marginal velopharyngeal insufficiency. No perceptual data were provided, however, so it is not clear whether the nasalance differences reported were associated with perceivable differences in hypernasality. Watterson (1998) reported no statistical difference between measures obtained with the Zoo Passage and measures obtained with the low-pressure sentences in a group of 25 subjects. This may be expected, however, if the differential effect of the two sets of stimuli is more likely to have an impact only on a subgroup of patients with a specific type of marginal velopharyngeal inadequacy.

The Nasometer has proven to be a valuable clinical tool when used for the purpose of objectively documenting oral/nasal acoustic resonance balance. As such, it provides an objective means of tracking within subject changes over time. It must not be used as a measure of perceived hypernasality, however. Perceived judgments of hypernasality must be considered the clinical gold standard when the effects of velopharyngeal insufficiency on nasal resonance are assessed.

ACCELEROMETERS

Although they have not gained wide acceptance for routine clinical use, accelerometers have also been used in the study and treatment of nasalance (Lippman, 1981; Stevens, Kalikow, and Willemain, 1975). Horii (1983) has been prominent in this research. Accelerometers are sensitive to vibrations and are placed on the naris and larynx to study sound energy at the nose relative to that at the larynx. Vibrations picked up at a naris are amplified, filtered, rectified, and smoothed (Stevens, Kalikow, and Willemain, 1975). For sentences free from nasal consonants, Reich and Redenbaugh (1985) found statistically significant correlations from 0.85 to 0.92 between nasalance measured with accelerometers and ratings of hypernasality. Larson and Hamlet (1987) interpreted nasalance to reflect oral-nasal acoustical coupling but not necessarily physiological opening of the velopharyngeal port: the lower the frequency of the first formant of vowels the greater the nasalance will be. Because of this acoustical relationship, nasalance varies with vowel height. High vowels have greater nasalance than do low vowels. Moon (1990) examined the effects of nasal patency on accelerometric data. Smith, Hamlet, and Jones (1990) applied a pure tone sound source to the nose and used an accelerometer placed on the larynx to detect velopharyngeal closure during swallowing. They found that the period of attenuation of the accelerometric signal corresponded with the period of velopharyngeal closure observed by videofluoroscopy.

SPECTROGRAPHY

The spectrograph provides a visual display of changes in the frequency and intensity of speech over time. It has been used to identify the acoustical characteristics of hypernasality and of other forms of speech nasalization. Computer-based digital acoustic signal acquisition and display systems have replaced the older analog electrostatic drum-stylus systems of the 60s and 70s. Spectrography continues to play an important role in basic research and may help the clinician understand the nature of nasalized speech samples that puzzle the ear. Its use as a routine clinical tool is not widespread despite the work of Kent, Liss, and Philips (1989), who recommended spectrographic analysis for use in planning and evaluating therapy for velopharyngeal disability.

Haapanen and Iivonen (1992) examined spectrographic data from two groups of speakers who had received different types of pharyngeal flap surgery (Sanvenero-Rosselli [n = 4] and modified Honig [n = 4]) and a control group. They reported that the patients who received the modified Honig procedure produced spectrographic findings more similar to the control subjects than did the patients who received the Sanvenero-Rosselli procedure. Kataoka et al. (1996) described a spectrographic approach to evaluating hypernasality in vowels. In a similar study, Garnier et al. (1996) described spectral and cepstral[1] procedures that successfully discriminated between subjects who were and who were not hypernasal. Their procedure was successful for 59 of 60 patients tested.

PHOTODETECTION

Velopharyngeal function has been studied by measuring light reflected off of the velopharyngeal mechanism. Kunzel (1979) described the "velograph," which was used in that fashion. Another instrument, the photodetector (Dalston, 1982), measures the amount of light introduced into the mouth that can be detected above the velopharyngeal port. The photodetector (Fig. 10-27) includes a light source and a light detector (Dalston, 1982; Dalston and Keefe, 1987). Each is attached to a light-transmitting fiber. The fibers are coated for optical isolation and cemented together. The distal end of the transmitting fiber extends 30 mm beyond

[1]Cepstral analysis essentially applies Fourier analysis to a spectrum. A more complete analysis can be found in Noll (1967).

the end of the detecting fiber. They are passed through a naris and positioned so that the emitting fiber is in the oral cavity and the detector is in the nasal cavity. The two fibers are a constant distance from one another, and the light source does not vary in luminescence. Dalston (1982) reported a correlation coefficient of 0.91 between photodetector and aeromechanical measurement of velopharyngeal port size at the moment of peak oral-nasal differential air pressure for /p/ in syllable context. Dalston and Keefe (1987) described use of the photodetector with a personal computer and a means for its possible use in biofeedback therapy. It has been used to study timing of movement onset and offset.

Moon and Lagu (1987) described a second generation phototransducer. Data collected through use of a test box indicated that there is a strong linear relationship between aperture area and light output ($r = 0.998$). Jones and Moon (1989) noted that photodetection readings will vary with the proximity of the light source to orifice or cavity walls. Movement of photodetector fibers may confound timing studies. The phototransducers used by Dalston and by Moon and Lagu have response times more than adequate for study of speech movements. Karnell and Seaver (1993) described a photodetector integrated with a fiberoptic endoscope. They demonstrated that the range of photodetector response to velopharyngeal closure could be estimated by using a "light out" condition that would approximate a photodetector baseline indicative of complete velopharyngeal closure.

The photodetector is more intrusive than aeromechanical probes and does not show structural movement as does endoscopy. However, Dalston and Keefe (1987) stated that the photodetector has a capability for quantitative, real-time measurement of moment-to-moment changes in the velopharyngeal port opening area that spectrography, aeromechanics, and nasopharyngoscopy lack.

The photodetector appears to have promise as a means of examining in detail the patterns of oronasal coupling during dynamic speech production. These data could potentially facilitate identification of patients with inconsistent velopharyngeal closure. However, routine clinical use of the photodetector awaits further technological advances.

ELECTROMYOGRAPHY

Electromyography (EMG) is an instrumental technique for displaying electrical activity that accompanies muscle contraction (Cooper, 1965). When a neural impulse triggers muscle contraction, a depolarization wave passes along the muscle fibers as they contract. This wave is termed the action potential (Harris, 1970). The instrument has been used in the study of skilled movements to determine which muscles are contracting, when they contract, and the strength of contraction.

Minimal equipment for EMG studies includes electrodes to detect electrical activity, preamplifiers and amplifiers to allow display of electrical activity, and a recording and display device. The signals may be displayed on an oscilloscope or chart recorder, or broadcast through a loud speaker.

Different sorts of electrodes have been used to detect action potentials in EMG studies. Surface electrodes have been used to monitor the muscle underlying the skin upon which the electrodes are positioned, but it's frequently difficult or impossible to specify which muscle or muscles are responsible for the recorded signal. That problem is minimized when using needle electrodes which can be placed into the body of the muscle to be monitored, but they may be dislodged during the examination or may be impractical if the muscle (e.g., levator veli palatini) is difficult to reach (Harris, 1970). Consequently, hooked wire electrodes, inserted orally with a hyperdermic needle have been used most frequently for evaluation of the levator muscle (Seaver and Kuehn, 1980). A transnasal approach to insertion was described by Su et al. (1993).

It is desirable to study several muscles simultaneously because this affords information about interaction among muscles in the performance of skilled movements. A common practice in speech research is to have the subject repeat speech gestures several times and to average the EMG traces associated with those gestures.

Warren (1973) noted that in electromyography it is difficult to know exactly what muscle is being sampled, particularly in patients with cleft palate whose muscles have been affected by birth defect and surgery. Warren also noted that it is difficult to establish the relationship between observed electrical activity in a muscle and the actual muscle contraction. This issue has been addressed by investigators who have performed simultaneous electromyographic and cinefluorographic examinations (Fritzell, 1969a, 1969b; Lubker, 1968; Seaver and Kuehn, 1980).

There is a wide body of research literature involving EMG, and the studies have contributed greatly to our understanding of the velopharyngeal valving mechanism (Bell-Berti and Hirose, 1975; Fritzell, 1969a, 1969b; Kuehn, Folkins, and Cutting, 1982; Kuehn, Folkins, and Linville, 1988; Shelton et al., 1980). However, its invasiveness, discomfort, and complexity make it more appropriate for research than for clinical use in the study of cleft palate. It has been used to answer some questions that have clinical implications. For example, Trigos, Ysunza, Vargas, and Vasquez (1988) reported EMG data indicating that the salpingopharyngeus muscle is not affected by the Sanvanero-Roselli pharyngoplasty. They further suggested that salpingopharyngeus may be antagonistic to levator and, when present, may be useful for velar control. Moon and Canady (1995) found less EMG activity in subjects when they were reclined than when they were upright, suggesting that gravity may play a role in the control of the velopharyngeal mechanism. Tachimura, Hara, Koh, and Wada (1997) found that subjects with oronasal fistula produced greater levator EMG activity when the fistula was temporarily not occluded compared with when it was occluded. They interpreted their findings as evidence that levator muscle activity may be mediated by intraoral air pressure.

ACOUSTIC RHINOMETRY

The shape of a resonator directly influences the manner in which sound is transmitted and reflected as it travels through the resonator. Inversely, if one can measure characteristics of sound that have been transmitted through a resonator, it may be possible to estimate the cross sectional area of the resonator. This principle has been applied to the evaluation of nasal and velar anatomy in a device called the acoustic rhinometer. The rhinometer employs an electrical device positioned at the base of a hollow tube to produce a series of audible clicks that are introduced into the nasal cavity by coupling to tube to the nostril. The acoustic reflections caused by the shape of the nasal passage are recorded by a microphone in the tube and are simultaneously digitized and processed by a microcomputer. An output is produced that graphically and numerically displays the cross sectional area at various points along the length of the nasal cavity.

The rhinometer was first described as an instrument for assessing nasal septal deviations before and after rhinoplasty (Grymer et al., 1989). Dalston and Seaver (1992) suggested it might be useful for examination of the nasal airway and velopharyngeal port in children with cleft palate. It was applied to the evaluation of oral and nasal respiration in children by Zavras et al. (1994). Others have reported normative data (Corey et al., 1998) and data that document response to surgery (Muhler and Erler, 1997; Sipila and Suonpaa, 1997).

Seaver, Karnell, Gasparaitis, and Corey (1995) were the first to examine the acoustic rhinometer's potential for documenting velar movement (Fig. 10-28). They collected acoustic rhinometer data simultaneously with videofluorographic images of the nasal airway and velopharyngeal port from two healthy subjects while the velopharyngeal port was at rest and while it was elevated. The data indicated that acoustic rhinometer could provide valid measures of velar displacement (Fig. 10-29). Kunkel, Wahlmann, and Wagner (1998) reported similar data from 33 cleft palate subjects and 32 control subjects. They reported significant changes in acoustic rhinometric measures of epipharyngeal volume due to velar displacement. The authors suggested that the device may be clinically useful for evaluation of velopharyngeal mobility and for objectively evaluating effects of treatment.

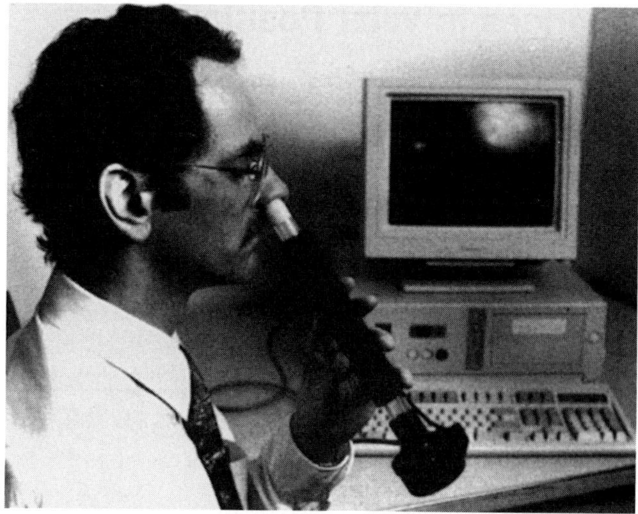

Figure 10-28 Instrumentation used to collect acoustic rhinometric data. *(From Seaver EJ, Karnell MP, Gasparaitis A, and Corey J: Acoustic rhinometric measurements of changes in velar positioning.* Cleft Palate–Craniofacial Journal *32:50, 1995.)*

ELECTROPALATOGRAPHY

Laboratories in the United Kingdom, Japan, and the United States are using electropalatography in the study and treatment of articulatory disorders in patients with speech disorders, including cleft palate (Fletcher, 1985; Hardcastle, Morgan Barry, and Nunn, 1989; Michi et al., 1986; Ohkiba and Hanada, 1989; Gibbon et al., 1999). To use this procedure, each subject is custom fitted with a palatal plate, and electrodes are positioned and embedded into the plate. Contacts between tongue and electrodes are fed into the computer. They may be displayed to the subject and compared with displays showing wanted articulatory patterns. Electropalatography has been shown to provide clinically useful feedback about performance to select patients with articulatory deficits. It has not enjoyed widespread use, however, because of the cost and complexity of the palatal plate.

RELATIONSHIPS AMONG MEASUREMENTS FROM DIFFERENT INSTRUMENTS

Of the instruments considered here, radiography, endoscopy, and pressure flow are regularly used to evaluate velopharyngeal competence. The Nasometer is used to obtain objective acoustic measures of nasalance that are correlated with the perception of hypernasal resonance, which is influenced by velopharyngeal adequacy. Knowledge of relationships among measures made with these devices is clinically important. Instruments differ in their strengths and weaknesses and consequently supplement one another in helping the clinician arrive at a valid understanding of the patient's velopharyngeal function. Orderly patterns in findings obtained with different instruments leads to confidence in our understanding of velopharyngeal function for speech. In this section we review research that reported relationships among measures made with these instruments.

Even findings obtained at different times with the same instrument and the same subject will not always agree. Where observations are made sequentially rather than

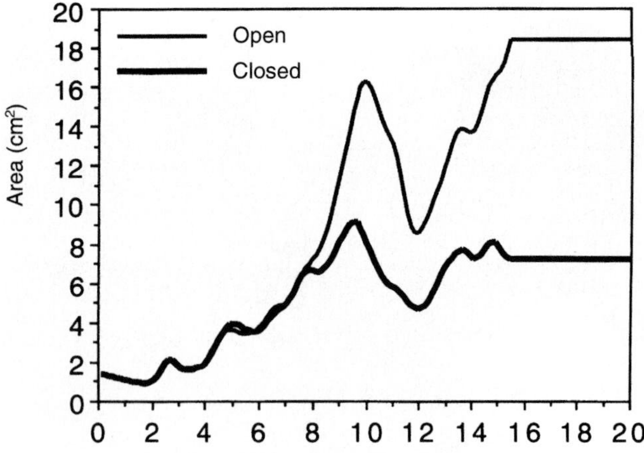

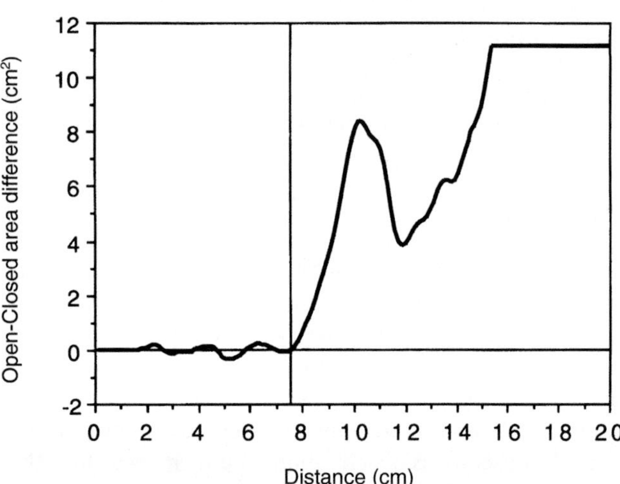

Figure 10-29 Area distance functions for subject 1. *Top,* The functions for the open and closed conditions. *Bottom,* The difference function derived by subtracting the closed area-distance function values from the open area-distance values. *(From Seaver EJ, Karnell MP, Gasparaitis A, and Corey J: Acoustic rhinometric measurements of changes in velar positioning.* Cleft Palate–Craniofacial Journal *32:50, 1995.)*

simultaneously, the differences may reflect variability in subject performance or differences attributable to the instrument or its application. When findings between two measures of the same variable differ, regardless of whether the measures are instrumental, it is difficult to know which, if either, measure is valid. This is a recurring problem in the evaluation of velopharyngeal function for speech because we have no single measure of velopharyngeal competence that can be used with confidence as a valid criterion for answering all clinical questions. Stringer and Witzel (1986) provided an example of the kinds of differences in findings that are frequently reported among measures. They compared lateral, Towne's, and basal videofluorographic views for effectiveness in identifying velopharyngeal insufficiency. The lateral view missed openings identified with basal and Towne's views, and the Towne view identified openings that were missed with the basal view when large adenoids were present.

Radiography and Aeromechanics

McWilliams et al. (1981) studied agreement among speech observations, videofluoroscopy, and pressure-flow data in the classification of patients' velopharyngeal adequacy. The pressure-flow data tended to classify as competent patients who were considered incompetent on the basis of fluorographic findings. This may have resulted because the aeromechanical observations were based on the study of /p/ sounds, and some individuals who closed the velopharyngeal port during those sounds did not close it during all other sounds. Such openings could be identified but not quantified for area by measuring nasal air flow as other obstruents are sampled.

Radiography and Nasendoscopy

Clinicians have reported disagreements in findings obtained with nasendoscopic and videofluorographic assessment of velopharyngeal function. Stringer and Witzel (1989) compared lateral, Towne's, and base views and nasopharyngoscopy for effectiveness in identifying velopharyngeal inadequacy in subjects who ranged in age from 4 to 41 years and who presented hypernasal speech. The authors concluded that the Towne view usually agreed with nasopharyngoscopy. However, there were enough disagreements to warrant further study and identification of reasons for the disagreements. The Towne view was said to be superior to the base view when adenoids were a problem. Skolnick (1989), in commenting on the Stringer and Witzel report, said that although the Towne oblique view may substitute for the base view, a frontal view is still needed for study of movement of the lateral walls in their full vertical extent.

Henningsson and Isberg (1988) reported that their use of an end-viewing endoscope failed to identify movements of the lateral walls in one third of a group of patients in whom such movement was seen in frontal videofluorography. They attributed the failure to the influence of adenoids or Passavant's ridge on the configuration of the nasopharynx. That is, in some patients the small angle formed by the palatal plane and a line tangent to the posterior nasopharyngeal wall was not conducive to positioning the endoscope for a satisfactory nasendoscopic examination of the velopharyngeal mechanism.

Radiography and Photodetector

Zimmerman et al. (1987) addressed relationships among photodetector and lateral cineradiographic indices to "opening and closing movements of the velum" and correspondence between the two indices over time. Cineradiography was done at 100 frames per second. Dependent variables were the times of occurrence of onset of velopharyngeal opening, maximum velopharyngeal opening, onset of velopharyngeal closure, and velopharyngeal contact. The authors concluded that output of the photodetector varied with opening and closing movements of the velopharyngeal port as observed in lateral cineradiography. "The majority of photodetector output changes occurred within 30 ms of corresponding changes in velar position measured by cineradiography" (p. 569). For 68 measures analyzed, photodetector output and velar displacement correlated 0.89 for subject 1 and 0.78 for subject 2. These results were statistically significant.

Photodetector and Nasendoscopy

Karnell and Seaver (1993), Karnell, Linville, and Edwards (1988a), and Karnell, Seaver, and Dalston (1988b) integrated a photodetection fiber to a flexible nasendoscope to permit their simultaneous insertion and use to study velopharyngeal function (Fig. 10-30). The nasendoscope was positioned to observe the velopharyngeal mechanism, and the light detector fiber was passed through the velopharyngeal port into the oral pharynx. This arrangement permitted the recording of an endoscopic image and of light from the endoscope as detected in the oral pharynx. Photodetector measurements were obtained from each video field (Fig. 10-31). Temporal measurement errors for repeated judgments by two observers were usually within 16.67 ms which was the time associated with one video field.

Findings obtained with the two instruments tended to agree within two video fields. Slight variations in closure identified by nasendoscopy were sometimes missed by the photodetector. Small movements observed endoscopically may not influence port size. In addition, some light may be photodetected because of tissue translucency and not because of velopharyngeal opening.

Aeromechanics and Tonar

Dalston and Warren (1986) used aeromechanical assessment to sort 124 consecutive patients into adequate, borderline, and inadequate velopharyngeal function categories. Subjects' speech was rated for hypernasality, and nasalance was measured with Tonar. Nasalance and hypernasality increased across velopharyngeal function categories. Area measures taken aeromechanically at the moment of peak oral-nasal differential air pressure during the /p/ in hamper correlated (Spearman $r = 0.80$) with listener judgments. Other correlations were 0.76 for Tonar and listener judgments and 0.74 for Tonar and area. Twenty-two of thirty subjects in the adequate closure category had some hypernasality. Variables such as degree of mouth opening may account for this. Nonetheless, the three measures tend to lead to the same treatment recommendations.

Photodetector and Nasometer

Dalston (1989) obtained photodetector and nasometric data simultaneously in the study of six normal adult subjects. The Nasometer data served as an index to voice onset and off-set as well as to nasalance (ratio of nasal energy to oral-plus-nasal energy), and the photodetector data provided an index to velopharyngeal opening. Voice onset and offset data were compatible with older research findings, which indicated that velopharyngeal closure is

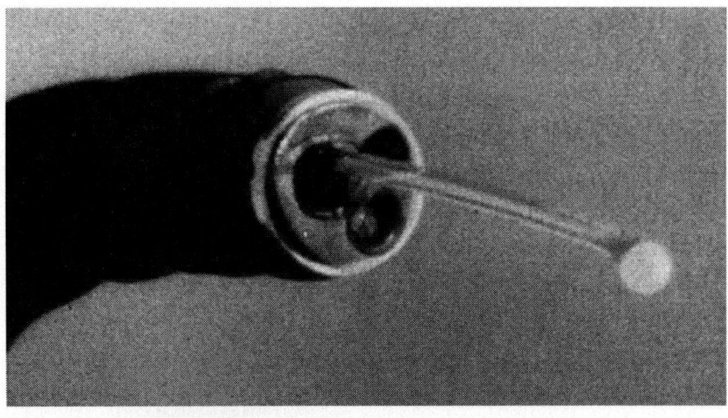

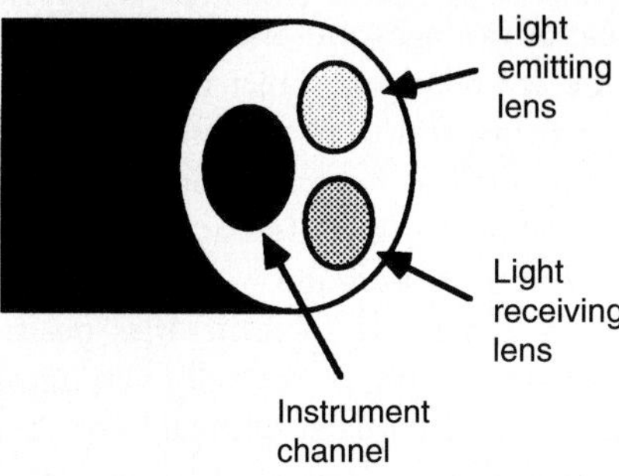

Figure 10-30 Olympus BF-3C20 endoscope with 3.7 mm light fiber placed through internal instrument channel. *(From Covello LV, Karnell MP, and Seaver EJ: Videoendoscopy and photodetection linearity of a new integrated system.* Cleft Palate–Craniofacial Journal *29:169, 1992.)*

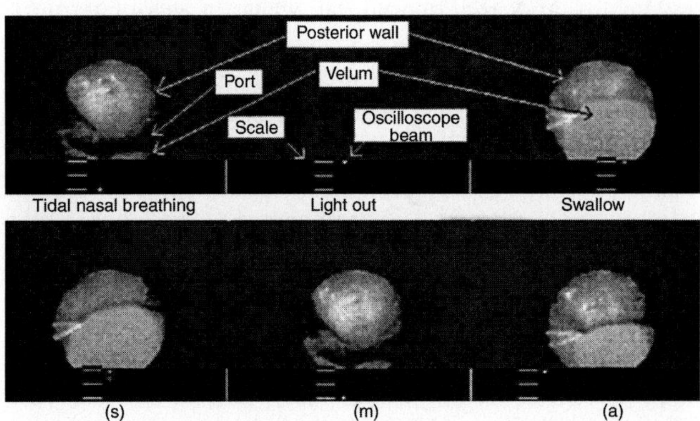

Figure 10-31 Samples of endoscopic images and photodetection recordings for the normal subject. The three horizontal lines on each oscilloscopic display are a scale representing the position of the photodetection beam during nasal tidal breathing *(bottom line),* the light-out condition *(top line),* and the halfway point between the bottom and top lines. *(From Karnell MP, and Seaver EJ: Integrated endoscopic photodetector evaluation of velopharyngeal function.* Cleft Palate–Craniofacial Journal *29:169, 1992.)*

achieved ahead of voice onset and maintained until voicing has ended. Closure led voicing and was maintained after voicing more strongly when sentences studied began with obstruents rather than with sonorants. Energy peaks associated with nasal consonants as measured by the two instruments were located closely together in time. That is, the data indicate that the maximum for nasal consonants obtained through the two instruments agreed within a mean of 1 ms (SD 16.4 ms).

DISCUSSION AND SUMMARY

Each instrument used for assessing the velopharyngeal mechanism has advantages and disadvantages. Radiography and endoscopy are relatively direct in that they provide a means for visual inspection of the mechanism at rest and during activities such as speech. Still radiographs can be used only for evaluating structures at rest or in production of a sustained sound in isolation.

Endoscopy is vulnerable to difficulties positioning the scope for adequate viewing of the velopharyngeal port and to impressionistic and perhaps unreliable or invalid interpretation of recordings. Oral endoscopy interferes with articulation, and topical anesthesia is usually needed for nasendoscopy.

Aerodynamic measures provide data about the area of the minimum velopharyngeal opening and nasal pathway resistance. They also provide data about nasal air leakage and about intraoral air pressure during speech. They do not provide information about the relative contributions of the velum and the pharyngeal walls to velopharyngeal function.

The very act of evaluating a patient's velopharyngeal function may influence that function, and it is always possible that the performance observed is not representative of the patient's usual performance or capability. There is little evidence that the instruments reviewed here offer precise prediction of future velopharyngeal function or speech behavior in any given individual. We are more successful anticipating group trends. For clinical decision making, we depend on the identification of patterns of velopharyngeal function across tasks, time, and instruments (Shelton and Trier, 1976). As indicated by Dalston and Warren (1986), listener judgment findings are better understood as the patient is evaluated with more than one additional measure. The appraisal of velopharyngeal function of patients and of research subjects is influenced by the examiner's conceptualization of velopharyngeal function.

The measures considered in this chapter are somewhat independent of one another in terms of how they relate conceptually to velopharyngeal function. That is, velopharyngeal function as studied radiographically is different from velopharyngeal function studied aerodynamically. In a statistical sense, different measures may account for different portions of velopharyngeal function variance. From either perspective, different measures of velopharyngeal function supplement rather than replace one another.

Research is continuing into the identification of variables that influence clinically relevant interpretations of instrumental measures. New insights into velopharyngeal function contribute to the use of instruments in patient evaluation. Karnell, Seaver, and Dalston (1988b) noted that in individuals with marginal velopharyngeal mechanisms the velopharyngeal port may open and close with the normal small upward and downward displacements of the velum associated with tongue height in running speech. At this time we are not sure of the predictive interpretations to be drawn from identification of this pattern.

In conclusion, we note that the use of instrumentation in the study of velopharyngeal structure and function is not necessarily more objective than is the study of speech by ear. If objective means freedom from observer bias, objectivity is not ensured simply because an instrument is used. Rather, objectivity depends on evidence that qualified observers working independently of one another arrive at similar findings (Guilford, 1954). The avoidance of observer bias in the interpretation of psychophysical or instrumental measures is enhanced when procedures for analysis of images or other stimuli are established and followed by clinicians using the instruments. For some instruments, satisfactory analysis protocols have yet to be widely accepted.

REFERENCES

American Speech-Language-Hearing Association: Vocal tract visualization and imaging. *ASHA* 34 (March, Suppl. 7):37-40, 1992.

American Speech-Language-Hearing Association: Roles of otolaryngologists and speech-language pathologists in the performance and interpretation of strobovideolaryngoscopy. *ASHA* 40 (Suppl. 18):32, 1998.

Anderson RT: Nasometric values for normal Spanish-speaking females: a preliminary report. *Cleft Palate Journal* 33:333-336, 1996.

Andreassen ML, Smith BE, and Guyette TW: Pressure-flow measurements for selected oral and nasal sound segments produced by normal adults. *Cleft Palate Journal* 28:398-406, 1991.

Bateman HE, and Mason RM: *Applied anatomy and physiology of the speech and hearing mechanism.* Springfield (IL): CC Thomas, 1984, p. 29.

Beery QC, Armany MA, and Katenberg B: Oral endoscopy in prosthodontic management of the soft palate defect. *Journal of Prosthetic Dentistry* 54:241-244, 1985.

Bell-Berti, and Hirose: Palatal activity in voicing distinctions: a simultaneous fiberoptic and EMG study. *Journal of Phonetics* 3, 69-74, 1975.

Bjork L: Velopharyngeal function in connected speech. *Acta Radiologica* Supplement 202, 1961a.

Bjork L: Velopharyngeal function in connected speech: studies using tomography and cineradiography synchronized with speech spectrography. Uppsala: Appelbergs Boktryckeri, 1961b.

Chen PK, Wu JT, Chen YR, and Noordhoff MS: Correction of secondary velopharyngeal insufficiency in cleft palate patients with the Furlow palatoplasty. *Plastic and Reconstructive Surgery* 94:933-941, 1994.

Cooper FS: Research techniques and instrumentation: EMG. ASHA Reports No. 1, 1965:153-168.

Corey JP, Gungor A, Nelson R, Xiling L, and Fredberg J: Normative standards for nasal cross-sectional areas by race as measured by acoustic rhinometry. *Otolaryngology–Head and Neck Surgery* 119:389-393, 1998.

Croft CB, Shprintzen RJ, Rakoff SJ: Patterns of velopharyngeal valving in normal and cleft palate subjects: a multi-view videofluoroscopic and nasendoscopic study. *Laryngoscope* 91:265-271, 1981.

Dalston RM: Photodetector assessment of velopharyngeal activity. *Cleft Palate Journal* 19:1-8, 1982.

Dalston RM: Using simultaneous photodetection and nasometry to monitor velopharyngeal behavior during speech. *Journal of Speech and Hearing Research* 32:195-202, 1989.

Dalston RM, and Keefe MJ: The use of a microcomputer in monitoring and modifying velopharyngeal movements. *Journal for Computer Users in Speech and Hearing* 3:159-169, 1987.

Dalston RM, Neiman GS, and Gonzalez-Landa G: Nasometric sensitivity and specificity: a cross-dialect and cross-culture study. *Cleft Palate–Craniofacial Journal* 30:285-291, 1993.

Dalston RM, Seaver EJ: Relative values of various standardized passages in the nasometric assessment of patients with velopharyngeal impairment. *Cleft Palate Journal* 29:17-21, 1992.

Dalston RM, and Warren DW: Comparison of Tonar II, pressure flow, and listener judgments of hypernasality in the assessment of velopharyngeal function. *Cleft Palate Journal* 23:108-115, 1986.

Dalston RM, Warren DW, and Dalston ET: A preliminary investigation concerning the use of nasometry in identifying patients with hyponasality and/or nasal airway impairment. *Journal of Speech and Hearing Research* 34:11-18, 1991.

D'Antonio LL, Achauer BM, and Vander Kam VM: Results of a survey of cleft palate teams concerning the use of nasendoscopy. *Cleft Palate Journal* 30:35-39, 1993.

D'Antonio L, Chiat D, Lotz W, and Netsell R: Pediatric videonasendoscopy for speech and voice evaluation. *Otolaryngology–Head and Neck Surgery* 94:578-583, 1986.

D'Antonio LL, Marsh JL, Province MA, Muntz HR, and Phillips CJ: Reliability of flexible fiberoptic nasopharyngoscopy for evaluation of velopharyngeal function in a clinical population. *Cleft Palate Journal* 26(3):217-225, 1989.

Engelke W, Hoch G, Bruns T, and Striebeck M: Simultaneous evaluation of articulatory velopharyngeal function under different dynamic conditions with EMA and videoendoscopy. *Folia Phoniatrica et Logopedica* 48:65-77, 1996.

Ericsson G: Analysis and treatment of cleft palate speech: some acoustic-phonetic observations [dissertation]. Linköping, Sweden: Linköping University, 1987.

Finkelstein Y, Shapiro-Feinberg M, Talmi YP, Nachmani A, DeRowe A, and Ophir D: Axial configuration of the velopharyngeal valve and its valving mechanism. *Cleft Palate Journal* 32:299-305, 1995.

Fletcher SG: "Nasalance" vs listener judgement of nasality. *Cleft Palate Journal* 13:31-44, 1976.

Fletcher SG: Speech production and oral motor skill in an adult with an unrepaired palatal cleft. *Journal of Speech and Hearing Disorders* 50:254-261, 1985.

Fletcher SG, and Bishop ME: Measurement of nasality with tonar. *Cleft Palate Journal* 7:610-621, 1970.

Fletcher SG, Adams LE, and McCutcheon MJ: Cleft palate speech assessment through oral-nasal acoustic measures. In Bzoch KR (ed.): *Communicative disorders related to cleft lip and palate.* 3rd ed. Boston: College-Hill, 1989.

Flexner SB: *The Random House dictionary of the English language.* 2nd ed. New York: Random House, 1987.

Fritzell B: *The velopharyngeal muscles in speech.* Goteborg: Orstadius Boktryckeri Aktiebolag, 1969a.

Fritzell B: The velopharyngeal muscles in speech. *Acta Otolaryngology* (Supplement) 250:1-81, 1969b.

Garnier S, Gallego S, Collet L, and Berger-Vachon C: Spectral and cepstral properties of vowels as means for characterizing velopharyngeal impairment in children. *Cleft Palate Journal* 33:507-512, 1996.

Gibbon F, Stewart F, Hardcastle WJ, Crampin L: Widening access to electropalatography for children with persistent speech sound disorders. *American Journal of Speech Pathology,* 8:319-334, 1999.

Gilbert STJ, and Piggott RW: The feasibility of nasalpharyngealscopy using the 70 degree Storz-Hopkins nasopharyngoscope. *British Journal of Plastic Surgery* 35:14-18, 1982.

Golding-Kushner KJ, Argamaso RV, Cotton RT, Grames LM, Henningsson G, Jones DL, Karnell MP, Klaiman PG, Lewin ML, Marsh JL, McCall GN, McGrath CO, Muntz HR, Nevdahl MT, Rakoff SJ, Shprintzen RJ, Sidoti EJ, Vallino LD, Volk M, Williams WN, Witzel MA, Dixon Wood VL, Ysunza A, D'Antonio L, Isberg A, Pigott RW, and Skolnick L: Standardization for the reporting of nasopharyngoscopy and multiview videofluoroscopy: a report from an international working group. *Cleft Palate Journal* 27:337-347, 1990.

Grymer LF, Hilberg O, Elbrond O, and Pedersen OF: Acoustic rhinometry: evaluation of the nasal cavity with septal deviations, before and after septoplasty. *Laryngoscope* 99:1180-1187, 1989.

Guilford JP: *Psychometric methods.* 2nd ed. New York: McGraw-Hill, 1954.

Guyette TW, and Carpenter MA: Accuracy of pressure-flow estimates of velopharyngeal orifice size in an analog model and human subjects. *Journal of Speech and Hearing Research* 31:537-548, 1988.

Haapanen ML, and Iivonen, A: Sound spectra in cleft palate patients with a Sanvenero-Rosselli and modified Honig secondary velopharyngeal flap. *Folia Phoniatrica* 44:291-296, 1992.

Hairfield WM, Warren DW, Hinton VA, and Seaton DL: Inspiratory and expiratory effects of nasal breathing. *Cleft Palate Journal* 24:183-189, 1987.

Hairfield WM, Warren DW, and Seaton DL: Prevalence of mouthbreathing in cleft lip and palate. *Cleft Palate Journal* 25:135-138, 1988.

Hardcastle W, Morgan Barry R, Nunn M. Instrumental articulatory phonetics in assessment and remediation: case studies with the electropalatograph. In Stengelhoffen J (ed.): *Cleft palate: the nature and remediation of communication problems.* Edinburgh: Churchill-Livingstone, 1989.

Hardin MA, Van Demark DR, Morris HL, and Payne MM: Correspondence between nasalance scores and listener judgements of hypernasality. *Cleft Palate Journal* 29:346-351, 1992.

Harris KS: Physiological measures of speech movements: EMG and fiberoptic studies. ASHA Reports No. 5, 1970:271-282.

Henrich DE, Hotson S, Drake AF, and Warren DW: Monitoring nasal and oral airway patency. *Cleft Palate Journal* 32:390-393, 1995.

Henningsson G, and Isberg A: A comparison between videofluoroscopic and nasopharyngoscopic registrations of velopharyngeal movements in hypernasal patients. In Henningsson G (ed.): *Impairment of velopharyngeal function in patients with hypernasal speech.* Stockholm: Department of Logopedics and Phoniatrics and the Department of Oral Radiology, Karolinska Institutet, 1988.

Henningsson G, and Isberg A: Comparison between multiview videofluoroscopy and nasendoscopy of velopharyngeal movements. *Cleft Palate Journal* 28:413-416, 1991.

Hirschberg J: Velopharyngeal insufficiency. *Folia Phoniatrica* 38:221-276, 1986.

Hixon TJ, Bless DM, and Netsell R: A new technique for measuring velopharyngeal orifice area during sustained vowel production: an application of aerodynamic forced oscillation principles. *Journal of Speech and Hearing Research* 19:601-607, 1976.

Honjo I, Mitoma T, Ushiro K, and Kawano M: Evaluation of velopharyngeal closure by CT scan and endoscopy. *Plastic and Reconstructive Surgery* 74(5):620-627, 1984.

Horii Y: An accelerometric measure as a physical correlate of perceived hypernasality in speech. *Journal of Speech and Hearing Research* 26:476-480, 1983.

Ibuki K, Karnell MP, and Morris HL: Reliability of the nasopharyngeal fiberscope (NPF) for assessing velopharyngeal function. *Cleft Palate Journal* 20:97-104, 1983.

Isberg A, Julin P, Kraepelien T, and Henrikson CO: Absorbed doses and energy imparted from radiographic examination of velopharyngeal function during speech. *Cleft Palate Journal* 26:105-109, 1989.

Isshiki N, Honjow I, and Morimoto M: Effects of velopharyngeal incompetence upon speech. *Cleft Palate Journal* 5:297-310, 1968.

Jones DL, and Moon JB: Response characteristics of the velopharyngeal photodetector to known orifice crosssectional areas. Proceedings of the annual convention of American Cleft Palate Association, San Francisco, 1989.

Karnell MP: *Videoendoscopy: from velopharynx to larynx.* San Diego: Singular Publishing Group, 1994.

Karnell MP: Nasometric discrimination of hypernasality and turbulent nasal airflow. *Cleft Palate Journal* 32:145-148, 1995.

Karnell MP, and Morris HL: Multiview videoendoscopic evaluation of velopharyngeal physiology in fifteen normal speakers. *Annals of Otology, Rhinology, and Laryngology* 94:361-365, 1985.

Karnell MP, and Seaver EJ: Integrated endoscopic/photodetector evaluation of velopharyngeal function. *Cleft Palate Journal* 30:337-342, 1993.

Karnell MP, Linville RN, and Edwards BA: Variations in velar position over time: a nasal videoendoscopic study. *Journal of Speech and Hearing Research* 31:417-424, 1988a.

Karnell MP, Seaver EJ, and Dalston RM: A comparison of photodetector and endoscopic evaluations of velopharyngeal functions. *Journal of Speech and Hearing Research* 31:503-510, 1988b.

Karnell MP, Ibuki K, Morris HL, and Van Demark DR: Reliability of the nasopharyngeal fiberscope (NPF) for assessing velopharyngeal function: analysis by judgment. *Cleft Palate Journal* 20:199-208, 1983.

Kataoka R, Michi K, Okabe K, Miura T, and Yoshida H: Spectral properties and quantitative evaluation of hypernasality in vowels. *Cleft Palate Journal* 33:43-50, 1996.

Keller E: Ultrasound measurements of tongue dorsum movements in articulatory speech impairments. In Ryalls JH (ed.): *Phonetic approaches to speech production in aphasia and related disorders.* Boston: College-Hill, 1987.

Kelsey CA, Minifie FD, and Hixon TJ: Applications of ultrasound in speech research. *Journal of Speech and Hearing Research* 12:564-575, 1969.

Kent RD, Liss JM, and Philips BJ: Acoustic analysis of velopharyngeal dysfunction in speech. In Bzoch KR (ed.): *Communicative disorders related to cleft lip and palate.* 3rd ed. Boston: College-Hill, 1989.

Kuehn DP, and Dalston RM: Cleft palate and studies related to velopharyngeal function. In Winitz H (ed.): *Human communication and its disorders, a review 1988.* Norwood (NJ): Ablex, 1988.

Kuehn DP, and Dolan KD: A tomographic technique of assessing lateral pharyngeal wall displacement. *Cleft Palate Journal* 12:200-209, 1975.

Kuehn DP, Folkins JW, and Cutting CB: Relationships between muscle activity and velar position. *Cleft Palate Journal* 19:25-35, 1982.

Kuehn DP, Folkins JW, and Linville RN: An electromyographic study of the musculus uvulae. *Cleft Palate Journal* 15:348-355, 1988.

Kunkel M, Wahlmann U, and Wagner W: Objective evaluation of velopharyngeal function by acoustic reflection measurements. *Mund-Kiefer-Und Gesichtschirurgie* 2(Suppl 1):S158-S162, 1998.

Kunzel HJ: Rontgenvideographische evaluierung eines photoelektrischen verfahrens zur registrierung der velumhole beim sprechen. *Folia Phoniatrica* 31:153-166, 1979.

Larson PL, and Hamlet SL: Coarticulation effects on the nasalization of vowels using nasal/voice amplitude ratio instrumentation. *Cleft Palate Journal* 24:286-290, 1987.

Leeper HA, Tissington ML, and Munhall KG: Temporal characteristics of velopharyngeal function in children. *Cleft Palate Journal* 35:215-221, 1998.

Lewis MB, and Pashayan HM: The effects of pharyngeal flap surgery on lateral pharyngeal wall motion: a videoradiographic evaluation. *Cleft Palate Journal* 17:301-304, 1980.

Lippman RP: Detecting nasalization using a low-cost miniature accelerometer *Journal of Speech and Hearing Research* 24:314-317, 1981.

Lotz WK, D'Antonio LL, Chait DH, and Netsell RW: Successful nasoendoscopic and aerodynamic examinations of children with speech/voice disorders. *International Journal of Pediatric Otorhinolaryngology* 26:165-172, 1993.

Lubker JF: An electromyographic-cinefluorographic investigation of velar function during normal speech production. *Cleft Palate Journal* 5:1-18, 1968.

Lubker JF: Velopharyngeal orifice area: a replication of analogue experimentation. *Journal of Speech and Hearing Research* 12:218-222, 1969.

Massengill RM Jr, Quinn G, Barry WF Jr, and Pickrell K: The development of rotational cinefluorography and its application to speech research. *Journal of Speech and Hearing Research* 9:254-265, 1966.

Mayo R, Floyd LA, Warren DW, Dalston RM, and Mayo CM: Nasalance and nasal area values: cross-racial study. *Cleft Palate Journal* 33:143-149.

McGowan JC III, Hatabu H, Yousem DM, Randall P, and Kressel HY: Evaluation of soft palate function with MRI: application to the cleft palate patient. *Journal of Computer Assisted Tomography* 16:877-882, 1992.

McWilliams BJ, and Bradley DP: Ratings of velopharyngeal closure during blowing and speech. *Cleft Palate Journal* 2:46-55, 1965.

McWilliams BJ, and Girdany B: The use of Televex in cleft palate research. *Cleft Palate Journal* 1:398-401, 1964.

McWilliams BJ, Glaser ER, Philips BJ, Lawrence C, Lavorato AS, Beery QC, and Skolnick ML: A comparative study of four methods of evaluating velopharyngeal adequacy. *Plastic and Reconstructive Surgery* 68:1-9, 1981.

McWilliams-Neely BJ, and Bradley DP: A rating scale for evaluation of videotape recorded x-ray studies. *Cleft Palate Journal* 1:88-94, 1964.

Michi K, Suzuki N, Yamashita Y, and Imai S: Visual training and correction of articulation disorders by use of dynamic palatography. *Journal of Speech and Hearing Disorders* 51:226-308, 1986.

Moll KL: Cinefluorographic techniques in speech research. *Journal of Speech and Hearing Research* 3:227-241, 1960.

Moll KL: "Objective" measures of nasality. *Cleft Palate Journal* 1:371-374, 1964.

Moon J: The influence of nasal patency on accelerometric transduction of nasal bone vibration. *Cleft Palate Journal* 27:266-269, 1990.

Moon JB, and Canady JW: Effects of gravity on velopharyngeal muscle activity during speech. *Cleft Palate–Craniofacial Journal* 32:371-375, 1995.

Moon JB, and Lagu RK: Development of a second-generation phototransducer for the assessment of velopharyngeal inadequacy. *Cleft Palate Journal* 24:240-243, 1987.

Muhler G, and Erler K: Comparative rhinomanometric measurements in children with cleft palate after cleft closure with and without velopharyngoplasty. *Folia Phoniatrica et Logopedica* 49:194-200, 1997.

Müller EM, and Brown WE Jr: Variations in the supraglottal air pressure waveform and their articulatory interpretation. *Speech and Language: Advances in Basic Research and Practice* 4:317, 1980.

Noll AM: Cepestrum pitch determination. *Journal of the Acoustical Society of America* 41:293-309, 1967.

Ohkiba T, and Hanada K: Adaptive functional changes in the swallowing pattern of the tongue following expansion of the maxillary dental arch in subjects with and without cleft palate. *Cleft Palate Journal* 26:21-30, 1989.

Osberg PE, and Witzel MA: The physiologic basis for hypernasality during connected speech in cleft palate patients: a nasendoscopic study. *Journal of Plastic and Reconstructive Surgery* 67:1-5, 1981.

Pannbacker MD, Lass NJ, Hansen GGR, Mussa AM, and Robison KL: Survey of speech-language pathologists' training, experience, and opinions on nasopharyngoscopy. *Cleft Palate Journal* 30:40-45, 1993.

Philips BJ, and Kent RD: Acoustic-phonetic descriptions of speech production in speakers with cleft palate and other velopharyngeal disorders. *Speech and Language: Advances in Basic Research and Practice* 11:113, 1984.

Piggott RW: The nasoendoscopic appearance of the normal palato-pharyngeal valve. *Plastic and Reconstructive Surgery* 43:19-24, 1969.

Piggott RW: Assessment of velopharyngeal function. In Edwards M, Watson ACH (eds.): *Advances in the management of cleft palate.* London: Churchill-Livingstone, 1980.

Piggott RW, Bensen JF, and White FD: Nasendoscopy in the diagnosis of velopharyngeal incompetence. *Plastic and Reconstructive Surgery* 43:141-147, 1969.

Piggott RW, and Makepeace AP: Some characteristics of endoscopic and radiologic systems used in elaboration of the diagnosis of velopharyngeal incompetence. *British Journal of Plastic Surgery* 35:19-32, 1982.

Ramamurthy L, Wyatt RA, Whitby D, Martin D, and Davenport P: The evaluation of velopharyngeal function using flexible nasendoscopy. *Journal of Laryngology and Otology* 111:739-745, 1997.

Reich AR, and Redenbaugh MR: Relation between nasal/voice accelerometric values and interval estimates of hypernasality. *Cleft Palate Journal* 22:237, 1985.

Riski JE, and Warren DW: Study session. American Cleft Palate Association Convention, Williamsburg, 1988.

Sandham A, and Solow B: Nasal respiratory resistance in cleft lip and palate. *Cleft Palate Journal* 24:278-285, 1987.

Scheier M: Die Bedeutung des Röntgenverfahrens fur die Physiologie der Sprache und der Stimme. *Archiv Laryngol Rhinol* 22:175, 1909.

Schneider E, and Shprintzen RJ: A survey of speech pathologist: current trends in the diagnosis and management of velopharyngeal. *Cleft Palate Journal* 17:249-253, 1980.

Schwartz MF: Developing a direct, objective measure of velopharyngeal inadequacy. *Clin Plast Surg* 2:305-308, 1975.

Seaver E, and Kuehn D: A cineradiographic and electromyographic investigation of velar positioning in non-nasal speech. *Cleft Palate Journal* 17:216-226, 1980.

Seaver EJ, Karnell MP, Gasparaitis A, and Corey J: Acoustic rhinometric measurements of changes in velar positioning. *Cleft Palate–Craniofacial Journal* 32:49-54, 1995.

Selley WG, Zananiri MC, Ellis RE, and Flack FC: The effect of tongue position on division of airflow in the presence of velopharyngeal defects. *British Journal of Plastic Surgery* 40:377-383, 1987.

Shelton RL, Beaumont K, Trier WC, and Furr ML: Videoendoscopic feedback in training velopharyngeal closure. *Cleft Palate Journal* 15:6-12, 1978.

Shelton R, Harris K, Sholes G, and Dooley P: Study of nonspeech voluntary palate movements by scaling and electromyographic techniques. In Bosma JF (ed.): *Second symposium on oral sensation and perception.* Springfield (IL): CC Thomas, 1980, pp. 432-441.

Shelton RL, and Trier WC: Issues involved in the evaluation of velopharyngeal closure. *Cleft Palate Journal* 13:127-137, 1976.

Shprintzen RJ: Nasopharyngoscopy. In Bzoch KR (ed.): *Communicative disorders related to cleft lip and palate.* 3rd ed. Boston: College-Hill, 1989.

Shprintzen RJ, and Bardach J: *Cleft palate speech management: a multidisciplinary approach.* St. Louis: Mosby, 1995.

Shprintzen RJ, McCall GN, and Skolnick ML: The effect of pharyngeal flap surgery on the movements of the lateral pharyngeal walls. *Journal of Plastic and Reconstructive Surgery* 66:570-573, 1980.

Siegel-Sadewitz VL, and Shprintzen RJ: Nasopharyngoscopy of the normal velopharyngeal sphincter: an experiment of biofeedback. *Cleft Palate Journal* 19:194-200, 1982.

Sipila J, and Suonpaa J: A prospective study using rhinomanometry and patient clinical satisfaction to determine if objective measurements of nasal airway resistance can improve the quality of septoplasty. *European Archives of Oto-Rhino-Laryngology* 254:387-390, 1997.

Skolnick ML: Videofluoroscopic examination of the velopharyngeal portal during phonation in lateral and base projections—a new technique for studying the mechanics of closure. *Cleft Palate Journal* 7:803-816, 1970.

Skolnick ML: Videofluoroscopic evaluation of the speech mechanism. Study session at the annual meeting of the American Cleft Palate Association, Denver, 1982.

Skolnick ML: Commentary. *Cleft Palate Journal* 26:91, 1989.

Skolnick ML, Shprintzen RJ, McCall GN, and Rakoff S: Patterns of velopharyngeal closure in subjects with repaired cleft palate and normal speech: a multi-view videofluoroscopic analysis. *Cleft Palate Journal* 12:369-376, 1975.

Smith BE, and Guyette TW: Component approach for partitioning nasal airway resistance: pharyngeal flap case studies. *Cleft Palate Journal* 30:78-81, 1993.

Smith BE, and Guyette TW: Pressure-flow differences in performance during production of the CV syllables /pi/ and /pa/. *Cleft Palate Journal* 33:74-76, 1996.

Smith BE, and Weinberg B: Prediction of velopharyngeal orifice area: a re-examination of model experimentation. *Cleft Palate Journal* 17:277-282, 1980.

Smith BE, and Weinberg B: Prediction of modeled velopharyngeal orifice areas during steady flow conditions and during aerodynamic simulation of voiceless stop consonants. *Cleft Palate Journal* 19:172-180, 1982.

Smith BE, Maddox CM, and Kostinski AB: Modeled velopharyngeal orifice area: prediction during simulated stop consonant production in the presence of increased nasal airway resistance. *Cleft Palate Journal* 22:149-153, 1985.

Smith D, Hamlet S, and Jones L: Acoustic technique for determining timing of velopharyngeal closure in swallowing. *Dysphagia* 5:142-146, 1990.

Stevens KN, Kalikow DN, Willemain TR: A miniature accelerometer for detecting glottal wave forms and nasalization. *Journal of Speech and Hearing Research* 18:594-599, 1975.

Stringer DA, and Witzel MA: Velopharyngeal insufficiency on video-fluoroscopy: comparison of projections. *AJR American Journal of Roentgenology* 146:15-19, 1986.

Stringer DA, and Witzel MA: Comparison of multi-view videofluoroscopy and nasopharyngoscopy in the assessment of velopharyngeal insufficiency. *Cleft Palate Journal* 26:88-92, 1989.

Stuffins GM: The use of appliances in the treatment of speech problems in cleft palate. In Stengelhofen J (ed.): *Cleft palate: the nature and remediation of communication problems.* Edinburgh: Churchill Livingstone, 1989.

Su CY, Hsu SP, and Chee EC: Electromyographic recording of tensor and levator veli palatini muscles: a modified transnasal insertion method. *Laryngoscope* 103(4 Pt 1):459-462, 1993.

Tachimura T, Hara H, Koh H, and Wada T: Effect of temporary closure of oronasal fistulae on levator veli palatini muscle activity. *Cleft Palate Journal* 34:505-511, 1997.

Taub S: The Taub oral panendoscope: a new technique. *Cleft Palate Journal* 3:328-346, 1966.

Trigos I, Ysunza A, Vargas D, and Vazquez MC: The San Venero Roselli pharyngoplasty: an electromyographic study of the palatopharyngeus muscle. *Cleft Palate Journal* 25:385-388, 1988.

Van Demark DR, Kuehn DP, Tharp RF: Prediction of velopharyngeal competency. *Cleft Palate Journal* 12:5-11, 1975.

van Doorn J, and Purcell A: Nasalance levels in the speech of normal Australian children. *Cleft Palate Journal* 35:287-292, 1998.

Warren DW: Instrumentation. ASHA Reports No. 9, 1973:26-33.

Warren DW: PERCI: a method for rating palatal efficiency. *Cleft Palate Journal* 16:279-285, 1979.

Warren DW: A quantitative technique for assessing nasal airway impairment. *American Journal of Orthodontics* 86:306-314, 1984.

Warren DW: Aerodynamic assessment of velopharyngeal performance. In Bzoch KR (ed.): *Communicative disorders related to cleft lip and palate.* 3rd ed. Boston: College-Hill, 1989.

Warren DW, and DuBois AB: A pressure-flow technique for measuring velopharyngeal orifice area during continuous speech. *Cleft Palate Journal* 1:52-57, 1964.

Warren DW: Aerodynamics of speech production. In Lass NJ (ed.): *Contemporary issues in experimental phonetics.* New York: Academic Press, 1976.

Watterson T: Nasalance and nasality in low pressure and high pressure speech. *Cleft Palate Journal* 35:293-298, 1998.

Watterson T, York SL, and McFarlane SC: Effects of vocal loudness on nasalance measures. *Journal of Communication Disorders* 27:257-262, 1994.

Watterson T, Hinton J, and McFarlane S: Novel stimuli for obtaining nasalance measures from young children. *Cleft Palate Journal* 33:67-73, 1996.

Willis CR, and Stutz ML: The clinical use of the Taub oral panendoscope in the observation of velopharyngeal function. *Journal of Speech and Hearing Disorders* 37:495-502, 1972.

Wilson FB II: The importance of laryngeal visualization in voice management. In Gerber SE, and Mencher GT (eds.): *International perspectives in communication disorders.* Washington: Gallaudet Press, 1988.

Witt PD, Marsh JL, Marty-Grames L, Muntz HR, and Gay WD: Management of the hypodynamic velopharynx. *Cleft Palate–Craniofacial Journal* 32:179-187, 1995.

Witt PD, O'Daniel TG, Marsh JL, Grames LM, Muntz HR, and Pilgram TK: Surgical management of velopharyngeal dysfunction: outcome analysis of autogenous posterior pharyngeal wall augmentation. *Plastic and Reconstructive Surgery* 99:1287-1296, discussion 1297-1300, 1997.

Witzel MA, and Stringer DA: Speech and language diagnosis and treatment. In Bardach J, and Morris HL (eds.): *Multidisciplinary management of cleft lip and palate.* Philadelphia: WB Saunders, 1990.

Yanagisawa E, Godley F, and Muta H: Selection of video cameras for stroboscopic videolaryngoscopy. *Annals of Otology Rhinology and Laryngology* 96:578-585, 1987.

Yamaoka M, Matsuya T, Muyazaki T, Nishio J, and Ibuki K: Visual training for velopharyngeal closure in cleft palate patients: a fibrescopic procedure. *Journal of Maxillofacial Surgery* 11:191-193, 1983.

Yamawaki Y, Nishimura Y, and Suzuki Y: Velopharyngeal closure and the longus capitis muscle. *Acta Oto-Laryngologica* 116:774-777, 1996.

Yates CC, McWilliams BJ, and Vallino LD: The pressure-flow method: some fundamental concepts. *Cleft Palate Journal* 27:193-197, 1990.

Zajac DJ, and Mayo R: Aerodynamic and temporal aspects of velopharyngeal function in normal speakers. *Journal of Speech and Hearing Research* 39:1199-1207, 1996.

Zajac DJ, and Yates CC: Accuracy of the pressure-flow method in estimating induced velopharyngeal orifice area: effects of the flow coefficient. *Journal of Speech and Hearing Research* 34:1073-1078, 1991.

Zavras AI, White GE, Rich A, and Jackson AC: Acoustic rhinometry in the evaluation of children with nasal or oral respiration. *Journal of Clinical Pediatric Dentistry* 18:203-210, 1994.

Zimmerman G, Dalston RM, Brown C, Folkins JW, Linville RN, and Seaver EJ: Comparison of cineradiographic and photodetection techniques for assessing velopharyngeal function during speech. *Journal of Speech and Hearing Research* 30:564-569, 1987.

Zwitman DH, Gyepes MT, and Sample F: The submentovertical projection in the radiographic analysis of velopharyngeal dynamics. *Journal of Speech and Hearing Disorders* 38:473-477, 1973.

Zwitman DH: Oral endoscopic comparison of velopharyngeal closure before and after velopharyngeal flap surgery. *Cleft Palate Journal* 19:40-46, 1982.

Zwitman DH, Sonderman JC, and Ward PH: Variations in velopharyngeal closure assessed by endoscopy. *Journal of Speech and Hearing Disorders* 39:366-372, 1974.

Chapter 11

Implications of Inadequate Velopharyngeal Function for Articulation, Resonance, and Voice

Speech is a complex phenomenon resulting from the interaction of many variables. However, there is consensus that velopharyngeal closure is the single most important factor that influences the quality and intelligibility of speech in most children with cleft palate after surgical closure of the cleft. After surgery, most children born with cleft palate will successfully develop normal, intelligible speech, primarily depending on their ability to achieve adequate velopharyngeal closure for speech. Inability to achieve velopharyngeal closure has a direct impact on speech learning, speech intelligibility, and speech quality. Moreover, inadequate velopharyngeal closure can have indirect implications for laryngeal and psychological health.

Earlier in this text we considered normal anatomy and physiology of the velopharyngeal system and how instrumentation is used to supplement perceptual judgments that lead to clinical assessments of adequacy of velopharyngeal closure for speech. Here, we consider abnormal velopharyngeal function, beginning with a discussion of the terminology used in descriptions of the complex phenomenon we think of as velopharyngeal inadequacy. We will then examine how inadequate velopharyngeal closure is reflected in assessment of physiology, articulation, resonance, voice production, and aerodynamics.

TERMINOLOGY OF VELOPHARYNGEAL INADEQUACY

Clinicians use slightly different terms for problems in the functioning of the velopharyngeal system, which may at times be confusing. Ironically, the inconsistency reflects efforts to segregate causes of these problems into separate categories. This chapter reviews the thinking on this semantic problem in some detail. In this book, however, the term "velopharyngeal inadequacy" is used as the umbrella term, and VPI (whether that means velopharyngeal inadequacy, incompetency, or insufficiency) as the umbrella abbreviation.

The term "velopharyngeal insufficiency" appears in much of the literature (e.g., Argamaso et al., 1994; Blakeley, 1969; Glaser et al., 1979; Kelsey et al., 1972; Levine and Goode, 1982; Motta and Cesari, 1996). Argamaso et al. (1994), using this as something of a generic term, pointed out that velopharyngeal problems were caused by a variety of craniofacial, neurological, and disease processes. Mechanical obstruction to closure was described by Shprintzen, Sher, and Croft (1987), regarding patients in whom hypertrophied tonsils prevented the velum from reaching the posterior pharyngeal wall, and by Warren, Bevin, and Winslow (1978), who documented posterior pillar webbing and palatopharyngeus displacement (abnormal insertion of the palatopharyngeus) as interfering with velopharyngeal closure.

Other clinical reports have used the terms "velopharyngeal incompetence" (Albery et al., 1982; Weber and Chase, 1970; Yules, 1970) and velopharyngeal inadequacy (Kipfmeuller and Lang, 1972; Mazaheri, Millard, and Erickson, 1964; Morr et al., 1989; Zwitman, Gyepes, and Ward, 1976) which are often used synonymously with velopharyngeal insufficiency. The term "palatopharyngeal insufficiency" has also been used (Bloomer, 1953; Shelton, Brooks, and Youngstrom, 1964; Yules and Chase, 1971). As we shall see, attempts to more narrowly define the terminology have not been very successful.

Loney and Bloem (1987) suggested the term "velopharyngeal insufficiency" be used as a general descriptor. They further proposed that the term "velopharyngeal incompetence" could be reserved to describe a velopharyngeal movement problem caused by neuromuscular involvement. Therefore, individuals with velopharyngeal incompetence would include those who are unable to move the palate adequately for speech regardless of whether the palatal structure is abnormal. Loney and Bloem would use the term "velopharyngeal inadequacy" to describe individuals who have difficulty with velopharyngeal closure for speech because of abnormal palatal structure. This group would include individuals with cleft palate or with palatal carcinoma who appear to have intact neuromotor systems for moving the palatal and pharyngeal structures but who, because of abnormal palatal structure, fail to achieve adequate velopharyngeal closure for speech.

Folkins (1988) cautioned against the nomenclature advised by Loney and Bloem on the grounds that, although the theoretical constructs described seemed straightforward, no operational definitions were identified that would enable straightforward categorization of individuals as having velopharyngeal incompetence, velopharyngeal inadequacy, or both. Without operational definitions and associated quantitative measurements that would clearly differentiate adequate movement from inadequate or perfect structure from imperfect, Loney and Bloem's nomenclature would only encourage the *illusion* that the chances of error and confusion would be reduced. Folkins agreed that misunderstanding can be reduced when there is only one meaning for clinical or scientific terms, but he contended that Loney and Bloem's approach merely substituted one set of poorly defined descriptors for another.

Trost-Cardamone (1989), like Folkins, agreed with the intent of the Loney and Bloem taxonomy but took issue with the details. She urged that "velopharyngeal inadequacy" be used as the general categorical term to describe velopharyngeal problems regardless of etiology. Trost-Cardamone suggested the use of "velopharyngeal insufficiency" to describe structural problems, "velopharyngeal incompetence" to describe neurogenic problems, and "velopharyngeal mislearning" to describe problems that fit in neither of the structural or neurogenic categories.

Here we take the position that accurate clinical description of behavior and structure is of central importance to the diagnostic process. The descriptive terms we use are helpful to the extent that they clearly reflect the condition and characteristics of the individual speaker. We consider velopharyngeal inadequacy a complex, subjective, descriptive concept, which is influenced by a wide variety of perceptual and physiologic observations. The structural and functional complexities of the velopharyngeal mechanism dictate the need for additional research before we consider adopting diagnostic terms that carry important treatment connotations.

CATEGORICAL DESCRIPTION OF VELOPHARYNGEAL INADEQUACY

Researchers and clinicians seem to have little difficulty discriminating among individuals who have normal or adequate velopharyngeal closure for speech from individuals who have severe velopharyngeal inadequacy. In fact, a noninvasive speech assessment and oral-peripheral examination will usually be enough to classify a patient as having adequate closure or severe velopharyngeal inadequacy. Physiologic assessments such as endoscopy or videofluoroscopy are performed in severe cases for the purpose of documenting physiologic details and treatment planning, not necessarily for diagnosis. If all patients could be categorized as either clearly adequate or clearly inadequate, diagnosis would be a relatively simple matter. Unfortunately, there are patients who do not fit neatly into either category.

Bzoch (1964) described four clinical studies in which use of pharyngeal flap and speech appliances were used to treat patients with velopharyngeal inadequacy. However, he reported, "some cases presented nasal emission distortion without obvious hypernasal resonance distortion, particularly if they had deviations of the nasal structures. Others presented hypernasal distortion without detectable nasal emission" (p. 277). The distribution of hypernasality among the groups studied was not reported, nor were ratings of severity of velopharyngeal inadequacy. However, it seems likely that some of these patients demonstrated what may be described as borderline or marginal velopharyngeal inadequacy.

Morris and Smith (1962) and McWilliams (1966) advanced the notion that some pathological speakers show velopharyngeal function that is barely adequate or that is adequate inconsistently. Koepp-Baker (1971) noted that a person may achieve sufficient approximation of velopharyngeal closure to achieve "weak or transient oral occlusives" in careful speech, but that with increased speech rate those sounds are omitted or replaced with glottal or pharyngeal sounds. Touch closure (McWilliams and Bradley, 1964; Van Demark, Kuehn, and Tharp, 1975) may be a form of borderline velopharyngeal incompetence. Powers (1986) and Hardin, Van Demark, and Morris (1990) suggested that patients with marginal velopharyngeal closure show performance that is variable.

Krause, Tharp, and Morris (1976) found that after primary cleft palate repair the prevalence and severity of velopharyngeal inadequacy varied on the basis of cleft type. Velopharyngeal incompetence was reported in 25% of patients with cleft palate only, 41% of patients with unilateral cleft lip and palate, and 43% of patients with bilateral cleft lip and palate. Marginal velopharyngeal inadequacy was found in 12% of patients with cleft palate without cleft lip, 15% of patients with unilateral cleft lip and palate, and 15% of those with bilateral cleft lip and palate. The group who had V-Y pushback surgery had a lower prevalence of velopharyngeal inadequacy (26%) after primary surgery than did the group who had the von Langenbeck procedure (44%). Both groups had a relatively low prevalence of marginal velopharyngeal inadequacy. The V-Y pushback group had a 16% incidence of marginal velopharyngeal inadequacy, whereas the von Langenbeck group had a 12% incidence.

Morris (1972, 1984) suggested terminology that he thought might be useful for patients who seemed neither to achieve adequate closure nor to demonstrate severe velopharyngeal inadequacy. He described so-called marginal or borderline cases as belonging to one of two categories: almost-but-not-quite (ABNQ) and sometimes-but-not-always (SBNA).

Morris' theory was that some patients with marginal velopharyngeal inadequacy nearly achieve closure but never actually do. They are consistently, but only moderately, hypernasal. Pressure consonant productions would be expected to be negatively affected as would ratings of speech intelligibility. These are the "ABNQ" patients.

Those patients who do achieve complete closure on some occasions but fail to do so consistently were described as "SBNA." These patients appear to have the physiological capability to achieve adequate closure but simply fail to do so consistently. They may give oral responses on single words but have nasalized connected speech, or they may give oral responses on speech tasks containing no nasal consonants but show moderate or severe nasalization when required to include one or more nasal consonants.

It is important to note that Morris' predictions about the ABNQ and SBNA subgroups were based solely on his interpretation of the patient's speech characteristics as perceived by the clinician and not on the basis of observed velopharyngeal physiology. He extended his observations of perceived speech characteristics to predict velopharyngeal physiology. Speech science has repeatedly shown us, however, that it is hazardous, at best, to map perceived speech quality to observed speech physiology. A given speech percept can be produced by more than one pattern of articulatory function.

In the only attempt to date to directly test Morris' theory of marginal velopharyngeal inadequacy, Hardin, Morris, and Van Demark (1986) attempted to determine the extent to which the ABNQ subgroup might consist of those who demonstrated touch closure or a slight velopharyngeal gap on a lateral still cephalograph. They found that nearly half of the 50 subjects examined had better speech than the model would have predicted. They concluded that their selection criteria were too restrictive or the model was too simplistic. Both possibilities seem likely. This report will be considered in greater detail later in this chapter.

On a purely conceptual level, it seems likely that additional borderline or marginal categories exist beyond the ABNQ and SBNA categories suggested by Morris. There may be additional subcategories that are identifiable when velopharyngeal closure capability is estimated from speech examined at a phonemic-segmental level. For example, Massengill and Brooks (1973) reported that 29 of 143 (20%) patients with repaired clefts were observed with cinefluorography achieving complete velopharyngeal closure for isolated /p/ productions and for /s/ productions in sentence context ("Susie saw the silly sisters") but not during production of isolated vowel /i/. Four other patients achieved closure for /p/ but not for /i/ or /s/, and three others achieved closure for /s/ but not for /i/ or /p/. Certainly, a more direct approach to addressing questions regarding the physiological character of marginal velopharyngeal inadequacy would be to examine the physiology and the perceived speech characteristics together.

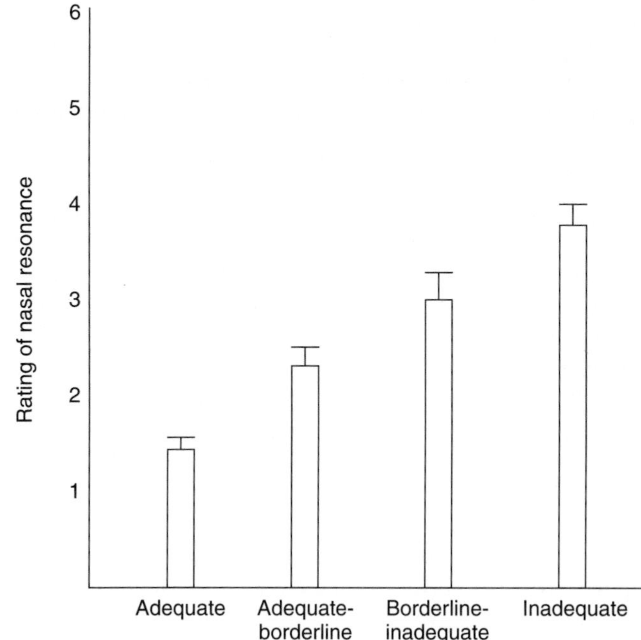

Figure 11-1 Ratings of nasal resonance balance across categories of velopharyngeal closure for 124 subjects with cleft lip, cleft palate, or both. T bars indicate SE above and below the means. *(Redrawn from Warren DW, Dalston RM, and Mayo R: Hypernasality and velopharyngeal impairment.* Cleft Palate Journal *31:257-262, 1994.)*

Laine et al. (1988) and Warren, Dalston, and Mayo (1994) used aerodynamic estimates of velopharyngeal orifice area and perceptual judgments of speech quality to categorize patients as adequate, adequate/borderline, borderline/inadequate, and inadequate. Fig. 11-1 (Warren, Dalston, and Mayo, 1994) shows how nasality ratings for a group of patients with cleft palate were distributed across each of these categories. Table 11-1 (Laine et al., 1988) shows associated aerodynamic measurements. This categorization scheme appeared to evolve from earlier work by Warren (1979) and Dalston and Warren (1986) in which adequate, borderline, and inadequate categories were described. This approach differs substantially from that described by Morris in that a physiologic aerodynamic measure was used to assist patient categorization.

Hardin, Van Demark, and Morris (1990) reported that many children judged to have marginal velopharyngeal inadequacy at an early age are no longer classified as marginal when they are older. They found that 14 of 48 subjects who were categorized as having marginal velopharyngeal inadequacy at age 6 years were judged as competent by age 18 years. Another 17 subjects became inadequate and the remaining 17 did not change. The authors further reported that articulation performance and nasality ratings at age 6 years were the best predictors of later velopharyngeal function. However, given that their predictive analysis

Table 11-1 **Mean Airflow Rates and Nasal Pressures in Subjects with Different Degrees of Velopharyngeal Inadequacy**

	Airflow Rate (cc/s)		*Nasal Pressure (cm H_2O)*			
Velopharyngeal Closure	*M*	*SE*	*M*	*SE*	*Spearman Correlation Coefficients*	*P-Values for Spearman Correlation Coefficients*
Adequate	26.8	2.5	0.2	0.0	.55	.0001
Adequate/borderline	101.0	9.4	1.3	0.4	.06	.7892
Borderline/inadequate	167.5	13.4	1.9	0.4	.20	.3942
Inadequate	308.2	33.2	2.6	0.3	.28	.1239
All groups	89.9	8.8	0.9	0.1	.75	.0001

From Laine T, Warren DW, Dalston RM, Hairfield WM, and Morr KE: Intraoral pressure, nasal pressure and airflow rate in cleft palate speech. *Journal of Speech and Hearing Research* 31:432-437, 1988.

was incorrect for 20 of 48 patients (42%), the authors reported that the power of the analysis was inadequate. The important message from this investigation is that variability in velopharyngeal adequacy may be expected from a substantial portion of patients with marginal classification.

Patients have been observed who, during videoendoscopic examinations, appear to achieve adequate velopharyngeal closure for oral pressure consonants but fail to achieve velopharyngeal closure during vocalic segment productions (Karnell, 1994) within an utterance. One example of this type of marginal velopharyngeal inadequacy is demonstrated by the patient presented in Fig. 11-2. Physiologically, it appears that this individual may belong to the SBNA category described by Morris. However, the most direct interpretation of Morris' SBNA group would involve an individual who could achieve complete closure throughout an utterance on one occasion but who failed to achieve adequate closure for the same utterance on another occasion. This could be described as "inter-utterance closure variability." The subject demonstrated in Fig. 11-2 demonstrates "intra-utterance closure variability" because she achieves closure for consonants but not for vowels within a single utterance.

An example of interutterance variability is demonstrated in Fig. 11-3. This individual appeared to achieve complete closure for pressure consonants and for vowels in context with pressure consonants ("Popeye plays baseball"). However, when pressure consonants were removed ("Where were you"), incomplete velopharyngeal closure was observed.

These observations lead to more questions than answers. For example, are other intra-utterance closure inconsistencies identifiable? Is it possible that some patients who may be considered SBNA or ABNQ on the basis of observed physiology have perceived speech characteristics consistent with adequate velopharyngeal closure, whereas others are perceived as demonstrating marginal or severe VPI?

There is clearly a need for studies that examine the characteristics of patients who may be considered part of the borderline or marginal velopharyngeal inadequacy group. Patients in this group are often difficult to manage. Although they may not be severely affected, they frequently seek treatment. Is surgical management too much for such problems? Does speech therapy play a role? These questions deserve to be fully answered.

This discussion of the terminology used to describe velopharyngeal inadequacy illustrates how clinicians evaluate the perceived correlates of the velopharyngeal mechanism with concern for structure and movement and how those evaluations contribute to decisions about treatment. As we have seen from examination of normal velopharyngeal movements, the goal is not a simple binary, on or off, open or closed issue. Both large and small velopharyngeal movements take place (Moll, 1964) that result in more or less complete velopharyngeal closure for speech (Karnell et al., 1995).

The picture may be further complicated by the presence of tonsil and adenoid tissue. The relative position of tonsillar and adenoid tissue to the velopharyngeal port requires close consideration of the possible influence on velopharyngeal closure. Kummer, Billmire, and Myer (1993) described a patient whose hypertrophic tonsillar tissue extended into the nasopharynx, preventing complete velopharyngeal closure and creating a partial obstruction to nasal airflow and resonance. The patient was described as having a mixture of hypernasality, cul-de-sac resonance, and hyponasality. Tonsillectomy resulted in elimination of all of these abnormal resonant characteristics.

Some velopharyngeal movements serve to permit clearly identifiable alterations in oral nasal coupling, whereas other movements do not appear to alter oral-nasal coupling at all. When this is considered within the context of an individual who continuously varies oral impedance during speech and whose anterior nasal passages may become more occluded (e.g., upper respiratory obstruction because of upper respiratory congestion) or less occluded (e.g., elimination of upper respiratory congestion) over time, our ability to fully understand how the velopharyngeal mechanism influences

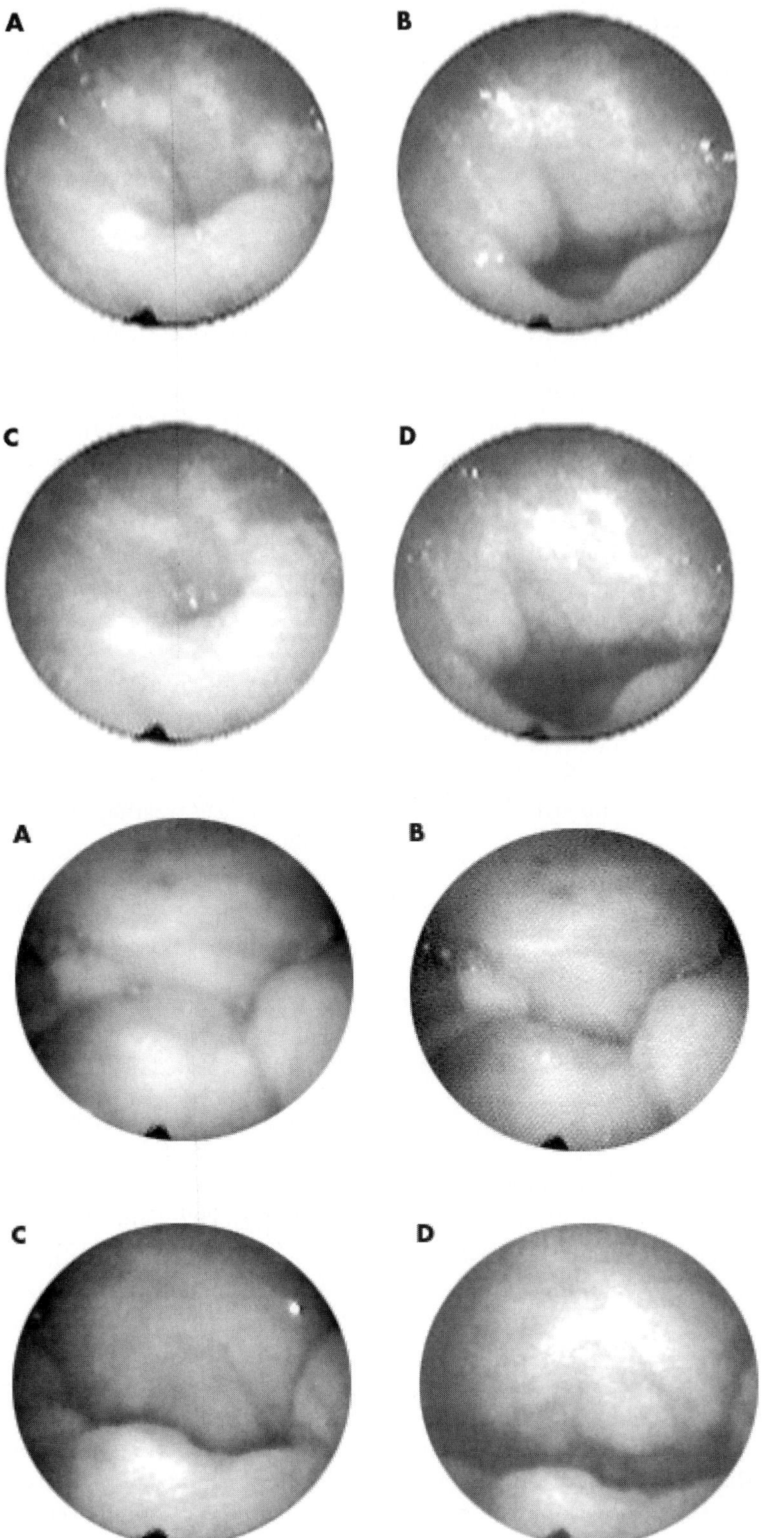

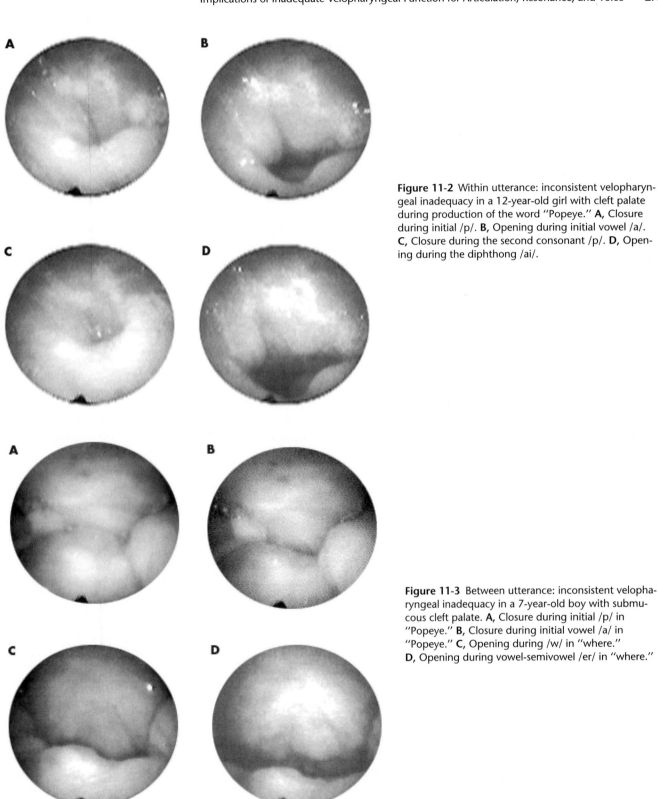

Figure 11-2 Within utterance: inconsistent velopharyngeal inadequacy in a 12-year-old girl with cleft palate during production of the word "Popeye." **A,** Closure during initial /p/. **B,** Opening during initial vowel /a/. **C,** Closure during the second consonant /p/. **D,** Opening during the diphthong /ai/.

Figure 11-3 Between utterance: inconsistent velopharyngeal inadequacy in a 7-year-old boy with submucous cleft palate. **A,** Closure during initial /p/ in "Popeye." **B,** Closure during initial vowel /a/ in "Popeye." **C,** Opening during /w/ in "where." **D,** Opening during vowel-semivowel /er/ in "where."

perceived speech is seriously challenged. Yet that is what clinicians are faced with every day and, in spite of the difficulties, we seem to do a reasonably good job of it.

Clinical skill develops in part as the clinician begins to appreciate the range of function expected from the patients to be evaluated. Each patient stimulates clinical hypotheses that, after testing, are either accepted, rejected, or modified. The review that follows will include a summary of some findings that are associated with various degrees of velopharyngeal inadequacy.

MARGINAL VELOPHARYNGEAL INADEQUACY

Physiology

As stated previously, nasal videoendoscopy and videofluorography demonstrate considerable variability of velopharyngeal performance in individuals with marginal velopharyngeal inadequacy. Some children may achieve closure for brief periods of time but not for all oral speech sounds. When closure is approximated, it may not occur for sufficient duration or with sufficient force to prevent audible nasal emission of air during pressure consonant production. In other children adequate closure may be achieved during some pressure consonant productions, but closure for vowels and semivowels may be incomplete.

For example, Massengill and Brooks (1973) described 143 patients with repaired cleft palate who had lateral view cinefluorography of the velopharyngeal port. Twenty-nine of these 143 (20%) were described as having complete closure during /p/ production but incomplete closure during /i/. The mean midsagittal distance from the palate to the posterior pharyngeal wall during /i/ was 7.62 mm (range 1-18 mm). Four patients (3%) achieved closure during /p/ but not during /i/ or /s/. The mean midsagittal gap was 7.0 mm (range 1-11) and 8.25 mm (range 3-14), respectively. Three patients (2%) achieved closure during /s/ but not during /p/ or /i/. The mean midsagittal distance was 8.33 (range 3-14 mm) during /p/ and 10.66 (range 7-17) during /i/. A similar subject was described by Karnell, Folkins, and Morris (1985).

Hardin, Morris, and Van Demark (1986) examined Morris' (1984) model of marginal velopharyngeal closure/ velopharyngeal inadequacy by attempting to determine whether the ABNQ group could be identified on the basis of "touch closure" observed on lateral still x-ray films of 52 patients with cleft palate. The authors maintained that if the speech characteristics of these subjects were consistent with the characteristics of those expected in the ABNQ group, they would have to demonstrate (1) mild-moderate nasal escape of air during production of pressure consonants, (2) incorrect production of pressure consonants during the Iowa Pressure Articulation Test and during stimulability testing, (3) clinical ratings of 3 to 4 for articulation defectiveness (1 = normal, 7 = severe), and (4) nasality ratings of 3 to 4 (1 = normal, 7 = severe). The majority of the 52 subjects met fewer than three of these criteria. Most subjects appeared to have speech that was better than the model would have predicted. The authors suggested that the ABNQ model as described by Morris (1984) may be too simplistic or their experimental design was flawed by the use of two-dimensional lateral cephalograms.

Velopharyngeal ports greater in estimated area than 20 mm^2 are insufficient for impounding oral air pressure for articulation, whereas lesser areas may permit build-up of the needed air pressures (Warren and Devereux, 1966). Research by Isshiki et al. (1968) provided support for the contention that velopharyngeal ports greater than 20 mm^2 are incompatible with normal speech. These authors sought to identify the degree of velopharyngeal closure essential to speech by introducing velopharyngeal openings into normal speakers. They inserted 4.5-cm tubes through the velopharyngeal port and studied oral air pressure, nasal air flow, articulation, and nasality. The tubes were 0, 5, 7, 9, and 12 mm in internal diameter; the cross-sectional area of the 5-mm tube was 19.6 mm^2. The critical degree of closure was to be defined in terms of observed alteration of speech as larger openings were introduced.

Peak oral air pressures of 9 and 8 cm H_2O were recorded with the 5- and 7-mm tubes. These oral air pressures are ample for articulation. However, the pressures measured with the 5-mm tube in use were accompanied by nasal air flows of between 200 and 300 ml/s. The pressures seem high considering the amount of flow measured; however, information about rate of respiratory air flow was not reported. Nasal flow was observed with open tubes of each size, and larger flows were observed with progressively larger tubes. Misarticulation and hypernasality were associated with the 5-mm tube, and they became worse from tube to tube.

Isshiki et al. concluded that a port created by insertion of an open tube with a 5-mm diameter was sufficient to interfere with speech; consequently, a larger opening would not be acceptable. Because speech was somewhat hypernasal and articulation was affected in subjects wearing the 5-mm tube, it also seems unreasonable to accept 5-mm diameter openings (19.6 mm^2 area) as satisfactory for speech production. Openings between 0 and 5 mm in diameter were not studied. It is possible that the pressure-sensing tube was partially collapsed by the velopharyngeal muscles. However, this seems unlikely considering the large nasal flows observed. Nasal leaks around the outside of the catheter were possible. The authors stated that the tubes were sufficiently long (4.5 cm) to prevent tissue from occluding either end of the tube.

Aerodynamic Measures

Aerodynamic measures in individuals with borderline velopharyngeal inadequacy will usually appear in the abnormal range. Intraoral air pressure will typically range from 1 to 5 cm H_2O and nasal air flow will approximate 100 to 250 ml/s during plosive productions.

Sapienza et al. (1996) described an adult male subject with an unrepaired bilateral cleft palate who produced /pa/ repetitions with and without a palatal obturator that was modified to approximate oronasal coupling areas similar to what may be expected in borderline or marginal velopharyngeal inadequacy. Intraoral air pressure decreased from 7 cm H_2O with the obturator in place to 4.56 cm H_2O and 3.72 cm H_2O as 10 mm^2 and 20 mm^2 openings were introduced into the obturator. Nasal airflow increased from 28.6 L/s to 105.92 and 203 L/s under these conditions.

Dalston and Warren (1986) described patients as having borderline velopharyngeal closure if pressure-flow estimates of velopharyngeal orifice area were 10 to 19.9 mm^2. Laine et al. (1988) examined the sensitivity and specificity of aerodynamic measures for identifying velopharyngeal inadequacy in 211 patients with cleft palate or suspected velar dysfunction. They found that nasal air flow rates of 125 ml/s were frequently associated with velar dysfunction (sensitivity 0.85; specificity 0.96). They reported that errors occurred most frequently in subjects with borderline velopharyngeal inadequacy.

Warren, Dalston, and Mayo, (1993) examined 11 patients who were perceived as hypernasal despite having aerodynamic pressure-flow findings that suggested normal velopharyngeal closure. They found that these patients demonstrated a delay of about 50 ms in achieving closure, a longer interval of nasal emission, and a shorter duration of actual closure compared with control groups. They speculated that hypernasality may be associated with the actual time the velopharyngeal mechanism is open, rather than the volume of air escaping from the nasal chamber.

Warren et al. (1985) studied temporal relationships between oral air pressure and nasal air flow in the word "hamper" as produced by groups of persons differing in velopharyngeal competency. You may recall from Chapter 10, "hamper" was used because the /mp/ phonemes require rapid movement of the velopharyngeal structures from a "port-open" to a "port-closed" posture. Within a subgroup of patients presenting borderline velopharyngeal adequacy, the occurrence of hypernasality was associated with overlap between nasal flow associated with /m/ and the pressure peak associated with /p/.

Nasalance

Fletcher (1976) reported median nasalance measures of 18 for subjects with mild hypernasality and 24 for subjects with moderately hypernasal speech. These hypernasality ratings are consistent with borderline velopharyngeal adequacy, as will be described in greater detail below.

Dalston and Warren (1986) reported a mean nasalance measure of 34 for patients with borderline velopharyngeal adequacy. This measure was consistent with the 33.73 mean nasalance measure reported by Valino-Napoli and Montgomery (1997) for their mildly hypernasal group. They also reported a nasalance measure of 27.43 for the group they described as having inconsistent hypernasality.

Hypernasality

Fortunately, thanks to improvements in cleft care, relatively few patients demonstrate severe hypernasality after initial palatal closure (Bardach et al., 1984, 1992; Morris et al., 1993; Peterson-Falzone, 1995). However, some patients who are not severely hypernasal nonetheless have clinically significant hypernasality. Clinicians rate these patients in the middle to lower end of hypernasality scales. Nasal mirror fogging may be inconsistent. These individuals are frequently described as exhibiting borderline or marginal velopharyngeal inadequacy. Children in this category may be quite variable in their speech characteristics.

Leanderson et al. (1974) reported that eight of 24 (33%) patients who were younger than age 25 years and who received pharyngeal flap surgery had "slight" or "moderate" nasality before surgery (1 = strong, 2 = slight, 3 = moderate, and 4 = none). Eight of 19 (42%) patients older than 25 years had "slight" or "moderate" nasality before surgery. Mean group ratings were not reported.

McWilliams et al. (1981) categorized patients as having borderline velopharyngeal inadequacy if they had mild hypernasality. Patients with more severe ratings of hypernasality were categorized as having velopharyngeal inadequacy without specific nominal reference to severity.

Van Demark and Morris (1983) reported nasality ratings (1 = normal and 7 = hypernasal) for a group of patients with cleft palate who were judged to have marginal velopharyngeal closure between the ages of 3 and 6 years. These data were compared with similar data for a group of 51 patients with clefts who had adequate velopharyngeal closure. The marginal group performed worse (mean 3.12) compared with the velopharyngeal closure group (mean 2.50) through age 14 years. From age 15 through 16 years the two groups' mean ratings were identical (1.65). The authors argued that patients who have adequate closure from ages 3 to 6 years tend to maintain adequate closure over time, but patients who are judged as marginal at an early age may be expected to vary between marginal or competent categories as they grow older.

Hardin, Van Demark, and Morris (1990) described how articulation performance varied from age 4 to 18 years for a group of 48 patients who were judged to have marginal velopharyngeal inadequacy at age 6 years. To examine how speech performance varies in this marginal group, the authors subcategorized these 48 patients according to their later velopharyngeal adequacy ratings assigned to them at age 18 years. Fig. 11-4 graphically demonstrates how mean ratings of hypernasal resonance were poorer from ages 4 through 7 years for the 17 subjects who were judged to have inadequate velopharyngeal closure at age 18 years compared with the two groups who remained marginal or became adequate by age 18 years. The mean articulation test scores for the three groups became quite similar from ages 8 through 16 years but by age 15 years the patients who performed poorest at an early age again began to perform poorly. These data demonstrate how the changing nature of speech performance in the population with marginal velopharyngeal inadequacy complicates our ability to make treatment decisions for them when they are young.

Audible Nasal Emission

Audible nasal emission may well occur in cases of marginal velopharyngeal inadequacy when there is sufficient closure to generate intraoral air pressure for speech but inadequate closure to prevent nasal escape of air. In fact, some patients with relatively little hypernasality may demonstrate audible nasal emission of air because of inadequate force of closure

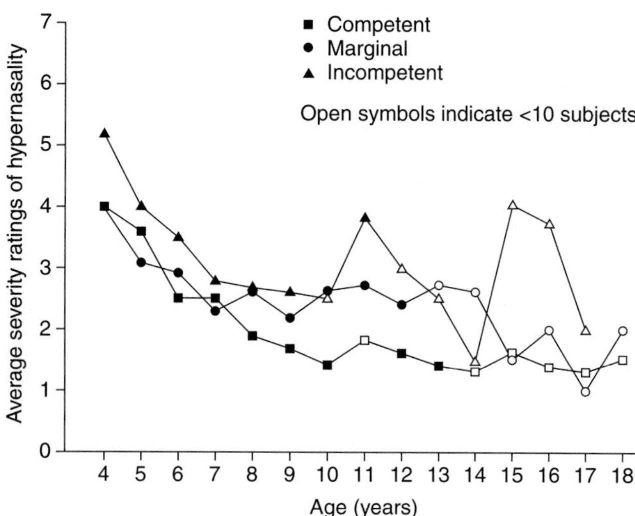

Figure 11-4 Average severity ratings of hypernasality in connected speech for the three adolescent groups (7-point severity scale: 1= normal; 7= extremely severe). *(Redrawn from Hardin MA, Van Demark DR, and Morris HL: Long-term speech results of cleft palate speakers with marginal velopharyngeal competence.* Journal of Communication Disorders *19:461-473, 1990. With permission of Elsevier Science.)*

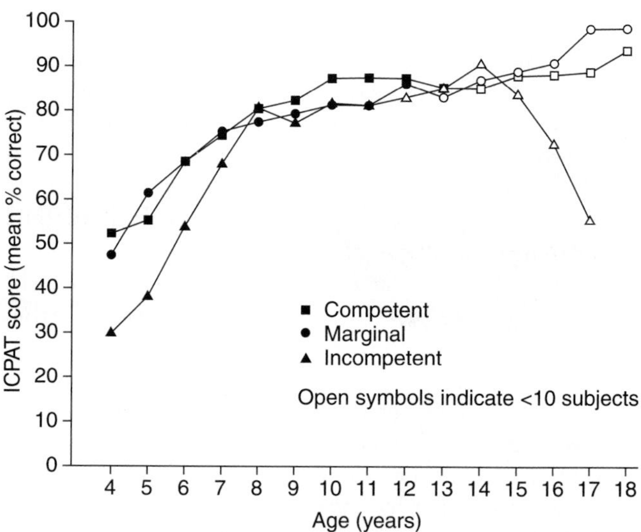

Figure 11-5 Average percentage of elements correct on the ICPAT for the three adolescent groups. *(Redrawn from Hardin MA, Van Demark DR, and Morris HL: Long-term speech results of cleft palate speakers with marginal velopharyngeal competence.* Journal of Communication Disorders *19:461-473, 1990. With permission of Elsevier Science.)*

to prevent oral air pressure from breaching the velopharyngeal sphincter.

Kummer et al. (1992) examined eight patients with hypernasal resonance alone, 10 patients with hypernasal resonance and "nasal rustle" (audible nasal emission of air), and 10 patients with nasal rustle without hypernasality (n = 10). They examined each patient by multiview videofluorographic records obtained near the time when a complete speech evaluation was completed. The group with nasal rustle without hypernasality was found to have significantly greater velopharyngeal contact and lateral pharyngeal wall movement than the groups with hypernasal resonance. The two groups with hypernasal resonance did not significantly differ from each other regarding any of the physiological measures obtained. The authors interpreted these findings as evidence that nasal rustle is usually found in patients with a small velopharyngeal opening. The authors further suggested that such patients be considered for a trial period of speech therapy before physical management is considered, particularly when the nasal rustle is inconsistent, phoneme specific, or related to articulation errors. Ruscello, Shuster, and Sandwisch (1991) reported that speech therapy was indeed effective in eliminating context-specific nasal emission in an adult patient.

Articulation and Intelligibility

Oral articulation may or may not be affected by marginal or borderline velopharyngeal inadequacy. Patients who are able to achieve adequate or nearly adequate velopharyngeal closure will be able to generate sufficient intraoral air pressure to enable appropriate development of articulatory placement for oral consonants. The sounds may not be perceptually normal, however, because mild-moderate hypernasality or audible nasal emission of air may occur with speech in individuals with borderline velopharyngeal inadequacy.

In the Van Demark and Morris (1983) report articulation scores for the marginal group were an average of 14% lower (mean 52%) than for the velopharyngeal closure group (mean 66%) through age 11 years. From ages 12 through 16 years, there was little difference between the two (marginal 83%, velopharyngeal closure 81%).

In the Hardin, Van Demark, and Morris report (1990) articulation test scores at an early age helped to predict which patients who were considered marginal at age 6 years would ultimately become inadequate by age 17 years. Fig. 11-5 shows how articulation test scores were lower on average from ages 4 to 7 years for the patients who were later considered to have inadequate closure compared with the patients who ultimately remained marginal or became adequate. Articulation and nasality observations made at an early age were the factors that were found to be the best predictors of velopharyngeal inadequacy later. These data suggest that those patients who may be considered to have marginal mechanisms at an early age but who score poorly (less than 50% correct) on articulation tests by age 5 years may ultimately require physical management.

Hoarseness

It is unlikely that hoarseness will develop as a result of marginal velopharyngeal inadequacy. As discussed above, patients with marginal velopharyngeal inadequacy are capable of nearly achieving velopharyngeal closure, or do achieve closure inconsistently. This enables the patient to

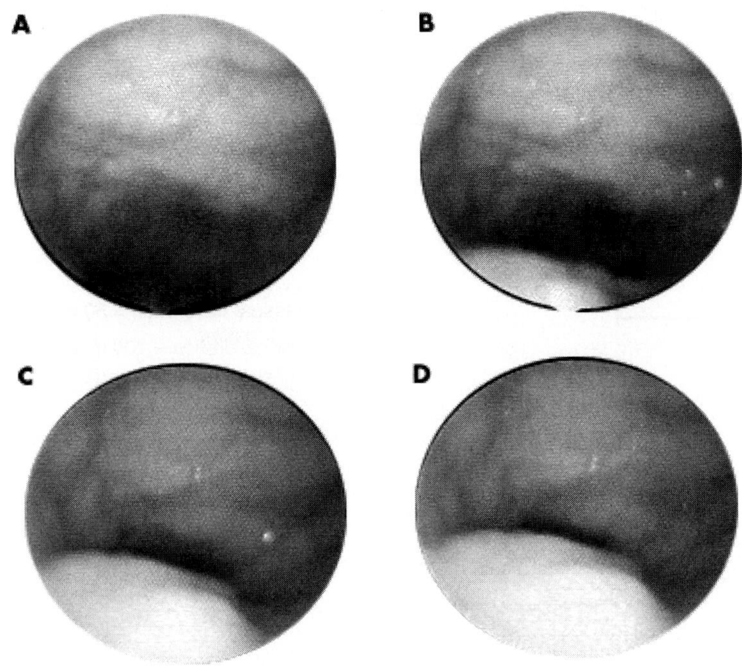

Figure 11-6 Velopharyngeal inadequacy in a 3-year-old girl with a repaired cleft of the hard and soft palate only. **A,** Maximum velopharyngeal opening at rest. **B,** Beginning of velar elevation toward closure. **C,** Continued velopharyngeal movement toward closure. **D,** Maximum velopharyngeal closure.

achieve increased intraoral air pressure for production of consonant sounds without resorting to laryngeal valving as a compensatory maneuver. Dysphonia that is sometimes associated with such laryngeal compensation would be unlikely to occur. The clinician should bear in mind, however, that dysphonia is common in preadolescent children as a result of vocal abuse. The presence of dysphonia in this age group may co-occur with marginal velopharyngeal inadequacy, but one must not assume the marginal velopharyngeal inadequacy is the cause of the dysphonia. Such an assumption could lead to the erroneous decision to treat the velopharyngeal inadequacy with the expectation the dysphonia would subsequently resolve. Dysphonia caused by vocal abuse unrelated to velopharyngeal inadequacy deserves direct attention by an otolaryngologist and speech-language pathologist knowledgeable about voice disorders in children.

SEVERE VELOPHARYNGEAL INADEQUACY

Physiology

Velopharyngeal inadequacy may be considered severe when speech is severely hypernasal from lack of velopharyngeal closure. Perception of severe hypernasal speech alone is sufficient evidence for a diagnosis of severe velopharyngeal inadequacy, provided no evidence of oral/nasal coupling anterior to the intact velum is present (such as an oronasal fistula). Physiological examination should be completed to describe in detail the velopharyngeal physiology before consideration of treatment options.

In patients with severe velopharyngeal inadequacy, nasal videoendoscopic (Fig. 11-6) and videofluoroscopic evaluations most likely will show failure of the velopharyngeal mechanism to achieve velopharyngeal closure at any time during oral speech attempts. Some movements of the velopharyngeal structures (velum, lateral pharyngeal walls, and posterior pharyngeal wall) may be observable depending on the speech sample. Movements that do occur will likely be most noticeable during attempts to produce pressure consonants. Velopharyngeal closure will not be achieved or will occur so infrequently as to have little positive impact on speech.

In patients with severe velopharyngeal inadequacy the residual velopharyngeal gap is usually relatively large. Massengill and Brooks (1973) reported a mean cinefluorographic midsagittal distance from the palate to the posterior pharyngeal wall of 12.33 mm (range 4-29 mm) during production of the vowel /i/ for 24 patients who they described as having ". . . failed to obtain velopharyngeal closure during the entire evaluation" (p. 316). During production of /p/, the mean midsagittal distance for these patients was 10.95 mm (range 2 to 23 mm), similar to the mean reported during production of /s/, which was 10.66 (range 1 to 30 mm). It is not clear from this report whether all the patients in this group would be rated as having "severe" velopharyngeal inadequacy or whether some might be considered to have "marginal" or "borderline" velopharyngeal inadequacy.

Severe velopharyngeal inadequacy may also occur in individuals with no history of palatal clefting, such as those who have palatal paralysis, craniofacial disorders such as hemifacial microsomia, disease processes such as palatopharyngeal carcinoma, congenital palatal inadequacy, or learning disorders. Warren, Bevin, and Winslow (1978) described three patients with congenital palatal inadequacy related to abnormalities of the posterior faucial pillars.

It is likely that many patients with velopharyngeal

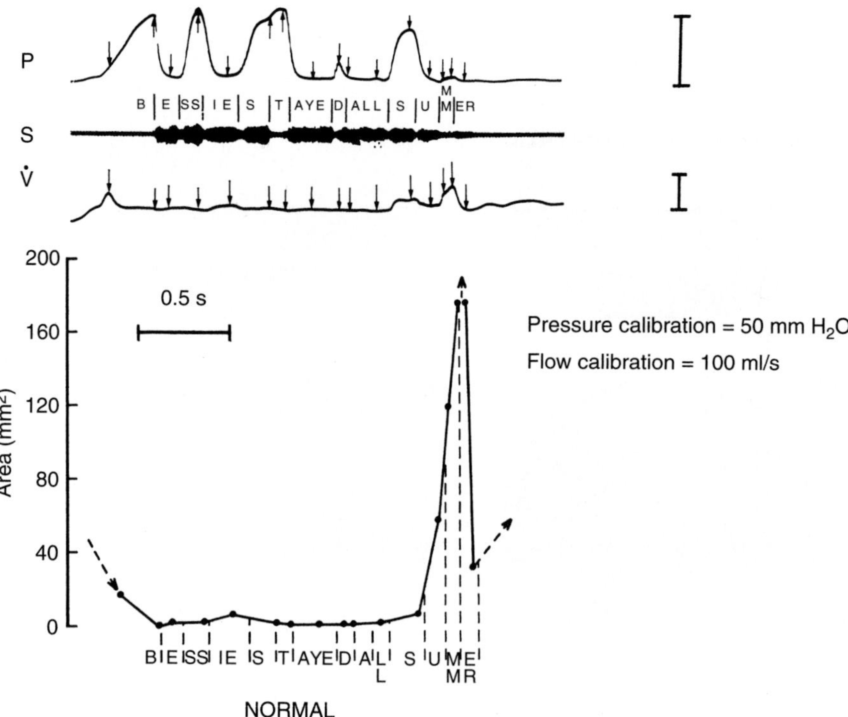

Figure 11-7 Pressure *(P),* sound *(S),* and airflow *(V)* patterns of normal speech. The area graph demonstrates that closure is nearly complete until the vowel preceding the nasal consonant. At this point, as the velum relaxes, air passes through the orifice and the pressure drops. *Arrows,* Points of measurement. *(From Warren DW: A physiologic approach to cleft palate prosthesis.* Journal of Prosthetic Dentistry *15:770-778, 1965.)*

inadequacy who require secondary surgical management are considered preoperatively to be severely affected, but most reports do not clearly indicate severity of preoperative velopharyngeal inadequacy. For example, Shprintzen et al. (1979) reported that 29 of 60 subjects (48%) who had received pharyngeal flap surgery had poor or no lateral wall motion before surgery. Of the remaining 31, nine (15%) had excellent lateral wall movement and 22 (37%) had moderate lateral wall movement. No data were reported about velar or posterior wall movement, however, nor were observations about extent, timing, or consistency of velopharyngeal closure described.

Osberg and Witzel (1981) used nasendoscopy to study velar and pharyngeal wall motion in patients with cleft palate who had had primary palatal surgery. One group consisted of six patients with ratings of 3 to 6 on a 6-point hypernasality scale; the other group consisted of 13 persons whose ratings were 1 or 2. The subjects free from hypernasality moved toward closure with velar elevation; there was little lateral wall motion. The hypernasal subjects, on the other hand, approximated closure through medial movement of the lateral walls. One patient was able to shift from hypernasal to nonhypernasal speech; in doing so, he shifted from lateral wall to velar movement, and the shape of the opening changed from "a circular midline defect to a transverse slit-like gap." The authors offered an interpretation that slit-like openings associated with velar motion allow less air flow than circular openings with similar cross-sectional areas. The latter openings were associated with medial movement of the lateral pharyngeal walls. No reliability information about the endoscopic data were provided.

Rolnick and Hoops (1971) studied plosive phoneme duration spectrographically in 20 subjects with and without obturators. Duration was increased on removal of the prosthesis. The increase in duration was seen as an attempt at compensation for poor velopharyngeal closure.

Zimmerman, Karnell, and Rettaliata (1984) observed an association between hypernasality and the tardiness of velopharyngeal closure relative to voice onset and achievement of maximum vocal tract constriction. They inferred that lowering of the mandible and tongue may constrain movement of the velum.

Aerodynamic Measures

Warren (1965) reported aerodynamic estimates of velopharyngeal orifice size in several patients with normal (Fig. 11-7), acceptable (Fig. 11-8), and hypernasal (Fig. 11-9) speech. These data clearly show the impact that velopharyngeal inadequacy can have on intraoral air pressure, nasal air flow, and estimates of velopharyngeal orifice area.

Intraoral air pressure during oral consonant attempts will be markedly reduced to less than 1 cm H_2O. Nasal airflow during the same attempts to produce oral speech will exceed 300 ml/s (Warren, Dalston, and Mayo, 1994). Investigators have reported oral air pressures in the ranges of 3 to 8 cm H_2O are needed for normal stop plosives and 3 to 7 cm H_2O for fricatives (Arkebauer et al., 1967). Moderately higher values were reported by Subtelny et al. (1966). The data provided by Warren and his colleagues indicate that oral air pressure peaks of this magnitude can be developed with velopharyngeal ports as large as 20 mm^2 if sufficient respiratory flow is used and the mouth is closed. However,

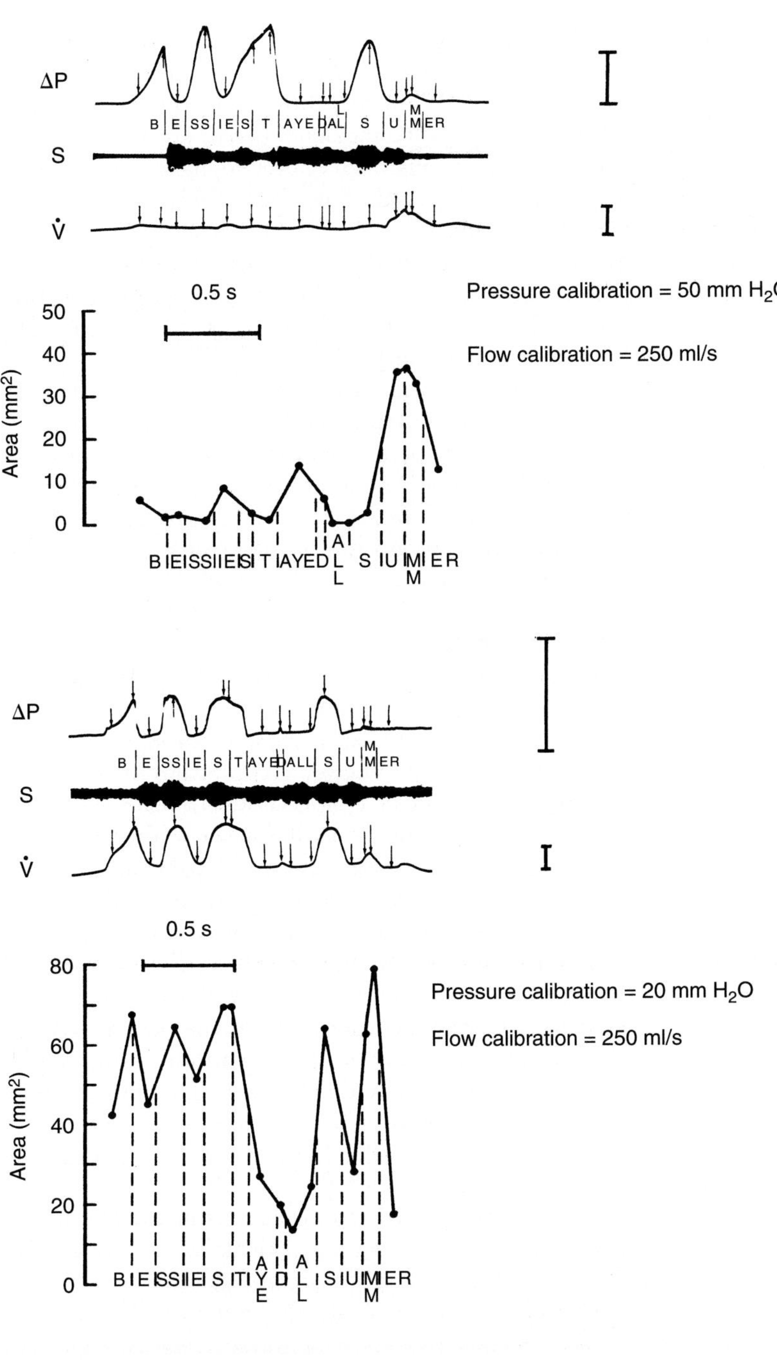

Figure 11-8 Speech patterns of a prosthetically treated patient whose voice quality was rated acceptable as normal. Note the similarity in pressure and air flow patterns with those of the normal subject. Although muscle valving against the appliance is not as tight as normal velopharyngeal closure, it is within adequate limits for normal voice quality. *(From Warren DW: A physiologic approach to cleft palate prosthesis.* Journal of Prosthetic Dentistry *15:770-778, 1965.)*

Figure 11-9 Speech patterns of velopharyngeal insufficiency. This subject, although wearing an appliance, was rated as having moderately nasal speech. The area graph discloses inadequate muscle valving. Low orifice differential pressure and high nasal air flow are associated with sphincter inadequacy. *(From Warren DW: A physiologic approach to cleft palate prosthesis.* Journal of Prosthetic Dentistry *15:770-778, 1965.)*

turbulence across the velopharyngeal orifice and nasal airway would probably cause noise at those flow rates.

Subtelny et al. (1970) reported a mean intraoral pressure measure of 4.28 cm H_2O for 46 patients who later received pharyngeal flap surgery. This improved to 7.57 cm H_2O postoperatively. They reported preoperative mean nasal airflow measures of 670 ml/s, which improved to "less than 100 ml/s" after surgery. The preoperative severity of velopharyngeal inadequacy was not clearly specified in their report, however.

Sapienza et al. (1996) recorded a variety of aerodynamic measures in a 38-year-old man with unrepaired bilateral cleft palate. The subject produced /pa/ repetitions with and without a palatal obturator, which enabled him to produce normal speech, and also while wearing an altered obturator, which permitted various amounts of oral nasal coupling. Intraoral air pressure decreased from 7 cm H_2O with the obturator in place to 3.42 when a 30 mm^2 opening was introduced into the obturator. When the obturator was removed, intraoral air pressure further decreased to 3.21 cm

H_2O. Nasal air flow increased from 28.6 L/s with the obturator in place to 546.0 L/s when a 30 mm^2 opening was introduced and further to 671 L/s when the obturator was completely removed. Not surprisingly, when the speaker increased vocal loudness under each of these conditions, the effects of nasal coupling on intraoral air pressure and nasal air flow were magnified. Also, larger lung volumes were expended as the degree of oral/nasal coupling increased. The authors suggested that their findings were evidence of active laryngeal and respiratory compensatory adjustments made on-line during speech.

Any theory that endeavors to explain velopharyngeal function must account for timing phenomena. Central programing of the coordinated movements involved in velopharyngeal closure will be a topic of future research, as will the extent to which timing problems can be modified, at least in part, by behavioral management.

Warren and Mackler (1968) observed that the duration of oral port constriction for voiceless consonants is increased in subjects with cleft who have good closure compared with those with poor closure. Normal speakers used shorter durations for voiceless consonants than did either of the two groups with cleft palates. Duration was determined from measurements of intraoral pressure. Oral port constriction was greatest for voiceless fricative consonants. The authors hypothesized that speakers with cleft palate who had good closure extend the duration of oral port constriction to provide more acoustic cues and thus increase intelligibility. The speakers with poor closure do not use this compensatory phenomenon, presumably because it would be accompanied by an increase in nasal escape of air.

Nasalance

Fletcher (1976) reported that persons with speech rated as severely hypernasal yielded median nasalance measures of 52. Median nasalance for speakers rated as having very severe hypernasality was 49.

Dalston and Warren (1986) reported judged nasality ratings and nasalance measures (from Tonar II) for 124 patients with various degrees of velopharyngeal adequacy on the basis of pressure-flow data (Table 11-2). Patients who were judged to have inadequate velopharyngeal mechanisms were found to have mean nasalance measures of 38.9 (SD 13.7). Perceived mean nasality for these same patients was 3.4 (SD 0.7), where 1 = normal resonance and 5 = severe hypernasality.

Valino-Napoli and Montgomery (1997) reported nasalance values for 13 speakers who were judged to have moderate/severe hypernasality defined as "consistent nasality greater in degree than mild hypernasality, weak pressure consonants, greater frequency of facial grimacing." Mean nasalance during production of the Zoo Passage for these speakers was 50.31.

Hypernasality

Skilled clinicians rate the severity of hypernasality in patients with severe velopharyngeal inadequacy at the middle to severe end of perceptual rating scales. For example, in a study by Warren, Dalston, and Mayo (1994), hypernasality ratings (1 = normal nasality and 6 = severe nasality) for 11 patients under the age of 15 years who were categorized as having severe velopharyngeal inadequacy was 3.3 (SE 0.4). They reported that patients aged 15 years and above who were categorized as having velopharyngeal inadequacy received mean hypernasality ratings of 4.1 (SE 0.3). In this study patients were assigned to velopharyngeal inadequacy categories on the basis of aerodynamic measurement of velopharyngeal orifice size, not on the basis of perceived speech ratings. The limitations of the aerodynamic approach to assessing velopharyngeal inadequacy orifice area described in Chapter 10 could explain,

Table 11-2 **Comparison of Patient Assessments Made by Pressure-Flow, Tonar II (Nasalance), and Listener Judgments (Nasality)***

	Pressure-Flow Area Measurement Categories											
	Adequate (0–9.9 mm²)				*Borderline (10–19.9 mm²)*				*Inadequate (20+ mm²)*			
Patient Assessments	*N*	*$\bar{X}$*	*SD*	*MAX*	*N*	*$\bar{X}$*	*SD*	*MAX*	*N*	*$\bar{X}$*	*SD*	*MAX*
Nasalance	63	10.7	6.9	31.6	27	33.9	14.5	73.9	34	38.9	13.7	64.2
Nasality	61	1.4	0.5	3.0	25	2.8	0.7	4.0	32	3.4	0.7	4.0
Age	63	11.7	3.8	25.4	27	13.0	4.3	22.8	33	18.9	10.1	44.0

*Listener judgments were missing for two subjects in each of the three pressure-flow categories. MAX represents the maximum value obtained within each pressure-flow category by each of the other two assessment techniques.

From Dalston RM, and Warren DW: Comparison of Tonar II, pressure-flow, and listener judgements of hypernasality in the assessment of velopharyngeal function. *Cleft Palate Journal* 23:108-115, 1986.

in part, why the nasality judgments for some patients in the velopharyngeal inadequacy group averaged in the middle of the scale.

In a study of early versus late primary hard palate closure, Henningsson, Karling, and Larson (1990) reported that hypernasality was significantly worse for the late closure group than for the early closure group. Although eight of 24 (33%) were rated as 2 or higher on a scale where 0 = no hypernasality and 4 = severe hypernasality, 19 of 21 (90%) of the late-closure group was rated as 2 or higher. These findings clearly demonstrate that late palate closure tends to result in greater severity of velopharyngeal inadequacy.

McWilliams et al. (1981) categorized patients as having velopharyngeal incompetence if they demonstrated moderate to very severe hypernasality, but additional characteristics were also described. These included visible to audible nasal escape, sibilant or affricate distortions resulting from reduced intraoral pressure, or phonemes produced pharyngeally or laryngeally. Patients who had lesser symptoms of velopharyngeal inadequacy were categorized as borderline.

Van Demark and Morris (1983) reported nasality ratings (1 = normal, 7 = severe) for 30 patients who from the age of 3 through 6 years were judged to have inadequate velopharyngeal closure. From age 3 through age 16 years, the mean rating for this group was 3.5. Interestingly, this was only 1.1 point higher than the mean rating for a group of 51 patients judged to have adequate closure. The differences were greatest from age 3 through 9 years (mean 1.7) but reduced substantially from age 10 through 16 years (mean 0.6). The authors emphasized that 28 of the 30 incompetent patients received pharyngeal flaps, management that likely contributed to the improvement observed in this group after age 9 years.

Dalston and Warren (1986) reported mean nasality ratings of 3.4 (SD 0.7) on a scale where 1 = normal and 5 = severe nasality for 32 subjects categorized as having inadequate velopharyngeal closure on the basis of aerodynamic measures. Similar findings were reported by Warren (1979).

In a later study, Shprintzen (1988) described "ratings of velopharyngeal inadequacy" that were obtained for the purposes of determining the need for pharyngeal flap surgery in 300 patients with hypernasal speech. Although no actual preoperative or postoperative ratings of velopharyngeal inadequacy were reported in this study, patients were categorized as normal, mildly hypernasal, moderately hypernasal, severely hypernasal, or hyponasal. Results of pharyngeal flap surgery were described in terms of postoperative nasality, but with the exception of those patients who received obstructive pharyngeal flaps no postoperative physiologic data were described.

Finkelstein et al. (1991) reported that of 40 patients with velopharyngeal inadequacy eight (20%) were considered as having severe hypernasality. It was not clear from this report, however, whether the patients described represent a randomly selected group.

Audible Nasal Emission

A cold mirror placed under the nares during speech fogs clearly and consistently during attempts at oral speech production for patients with severe velopharyngeal inadequacy. Nasal air flow may or may not be audible in these patients. McWilliams et al. (1981) associated the presence of nasal emission with velopharyngeal inadequacy only when audible and only when associated with moderate to very severe hypernasality. When there is a consistent large velopharyngeal opening during pressure consonants, children may develop compensatory articulatory patterns (glottal stops, pharyngeal fricatives, etc.) rather than attempt to create pressure consonants with sufficient effort to result in audible nasal emission of air.

Zajac et al. (1996) described an adult patient with mild mental retardation and no cleft palate who had severe velopharyngeal inadequacy with audible nasal emission of air. Production of the audible nasal emission during /s/ phonemes was accompanied by visible nares constriction, which was credited with enabling this patient to achieve higher intraoral air pressures for /s/ than for /p/ when no such nares constriction occurred. The authors speculated that the patient used increased respiratory effort to compensate for the velopharyngeal inadequacy during production of /p/ but such efforts were insufficient for the longer duration /s/ production. Hence, they suggested that the nares constriction was an additional attempt by the patient to achieve adequate oral pressures.

Articulation and Intelligibility

Oral articulation will likely be severely impaired unless speech therapy has been offered early and often. When therapy has not been received, compensatory articulation errors will likely be prevalent and speech intelligibility will be severely impaired. Audible nasal emission of air may not be as apparent in patients with compensatory articulation errors because the air stream will be valved below the level of the velopharyngeal port, preventing nasal escape of air even though the velopharyngeal mechanism does not close. Except when overriding health concerns are involved, there is little debate among clinicians that children with such severe hypernasal speech require physical management.

Subtelny et al. (1969) reported perceptual and aerodynamic data for a group of patients they described as having "rather gross palatopharyngeal defects" before and after pharyngeal flap surgery. It is not clear from this description whether all the patients in their study should be considered as exhibiting severe velopharyngeal inadequacy, but we will make that assumption here. They reported a preoperative articulation mean error rate of 24% before surgery for the 58 patients examined. Preoperative mean intelligibility rating for this group was 59%. These numbers improved to 12% and 73% postoperatively.

Data reported by Van Demark and Morris (1983) demonstrated that mean Iowa Pressure Articulation Test scores from age 4 through 16 were 56.8% correct for 30 patients who were judged to have inadequate closure between ages 3 and 6 years. This compared with 71.5% correct for 51 patients who had adequate closure. Differences were greatest between the two groups through age 10 years (velopharyngeal inadequacy 38.69%, velopharyngeal closure 63.57%), after which the differences became minimal (velopharyngeal inadequacy 77.93%, velopharyngeal closure 80.73%). The great majority of the velopharyngeal inadequacy group (28 of 30) received pharyngeal flaps, which may account, in large part, for the improvement in that group.

Hoarseness

Hoarseness has been reported in some patients with velopharyngeal inadequacy (Brooks and Shelton, 1963; D'Antonio et al., 1988; Hess, 1959; Leder and Lerman, 1985; McDonald and Baker, 1951; McWilliams, Bluestone, and Musgrave, 1969; Zajac and Linville, 1989). If the association exists, it seems most likely that velopharyngeal inadequacy would have to be severe to cause hoarseness. Bernthal and Beukelman (1977) noted that increases in velopharyngeal opening resulted in acoustic damping, which may lead to increased vocal effort in patients with velopharyngeal inadequacy and associated increased risk for vocal abuse. Leder and Lerman (1985) suggested that velopharyngeal inadequacy resulted in increased laryngeal adduction as an effort to provide a constriction inferior to the inadequately functioning velopharyngeal port (p. 840). Such compensatory laryngeal adduction would be unlikely to occur unless velopharyngeal inadequacy was consistent and severe enough to make supraglottic management of speech aerodynamics impossible for the patient. Such patients would be more likely to use glottal valving substitutions for articulation (glottal stops), which could further contribute to dysphonia.

SUMMARY

Both perceived speech characteristics and the physiologic effects of various degrees of velopharyngeal inadequacy have been reviewed. Clearly, much is known about these characteristics, but much has yet to be learned. For example, more research is needed that clarifies the various manifestations of what we clinically refer to as marginal velopharyngeal inadequacy. Data are also needed that speak to the efficacy of speech therapy designed to address velopharyngeal inadequacy. This issue is addressed in the chapter on treatment of speech and language problems (Chapter 12). What role surgical management should play remains a source of continuous clinical debate. As more information becomes available we may find we can improve our ability to treat marginal velopharyngeal inadequacy conservatively yet effectively.

REFERENCES

Albery EH, Bennett JA, Pigott RW, and Simmons RM: The results of 100 operations for velopharyngeal incompetence—selected on the findings of endoscopic and radiological examination. *British Journal of Plastic Surgery* 35:118-126, 1982.

Argamaso RV, Levandowski GJ, Golding-Kushner KJ, and Shprintzen RJ: Treatment of asymmetric velopharyngeal inadequacy with skewed pharyngeal flap. *Cleft Palate Journal* 31:287-294, 1994.

Arkebauer HJ, Hixon TJ, and Hardy JC: Peak intraoral air pressures during speech. *Journal of Speech and Hearing Research* 10:196-209, 1967.

Bardach J, Morris HL, Olin WJ, Gray SD, Jones DL, Kelly KM, Shaw WC, and Semb G: Results of multidisciplinary management of bilateral cleft lip and palate at the Iowa Cleft Palate Center. *Plastic and Reconstructive Surgery* 89:419-432, 1992.

Bardach J, Morris HL, Olin WH, McDermott-Murray J, Mooney M, and Bardach E: Late results of multidisciplinary management of unilateral cleft lip and palate. *Annals of Plastic Surgery* 12:235-242, 1984.

Bernthal JE, and Beukelman DR: The effect of changes in velopharyngeal orifice area on vocal intensity. *Cleft Palate Journal* 14:63-77, 1977.

Blakeley RW: The rationale for a temporary speech prosthesis in palatal inadequacy. *British Journal of Disorders of Communication* 4:134-139, 1969.

Bloomer HH: Observations on palatopharyngeal movements in speech and deglutition. *Journal of Speech and Hearing Disorders* 18:230-246, 1953.

Brooks A, and Shelton R: Voice disorders other than nasality in cleft palate children. *Cleft Palate Bulletin* 13:63-64, 1963.

Bzoch KR: Clinical studies of the efficacy of speech appliances compared to pharyngeal flap surgery. *Cleft Palate Journal* 1:275-286, 1964.

Dalston RM, and Warren DW: Comparison of Tonar II, pressure-flow, and listener judgements of hypernasality in the assessment of velopharyngeal function. *Cleft Palate Journal* 23:108-115, 1986.

D'Antonio LL, Muntz H, Providence M, and Marsh J: Laryngeal/voice findings in patients with velopharyngeal dysfunction. *Laryngoscope* 98:432-438, 1988.

Finkelstein Y, Talmi YP, Kravitz K, Bar-Ziv J, Nachmani A, Hauben DJ, and Zohar Y: Study of the normal and insufficient velopharyngeal valve by the "forced sucking test." *Laryngoscope* 101:1203-1212, 1991.

Fletcher SG: "Nasalance" vs. listener judgement of nasality. *Cleft Palate Journal* 13:31-44, 1976.

Folkins JW: Velopharyngeal nomenclature: incompetence, inadequacy, insufficiency, and dysfunction. *Cleft Palate Journal* 25:413-416, 1988.

Glaser ER, Skolnick ML, McWilliams BJ, and Sprintzen RJ: The dynamics of Passavants ridge in subjects with and without velopharyngeal inadequacy—a multi-view video fluoroscopic study. *Cleft Palate Journal* 16:24-33, 1979.

Hardin MA, Morris HL, and Van Demark DR: A study of cleft palate speakers with marginal velopharyngeal competence. *Journal of Communication Disorders* 19:461-473, 1986.

Hardin MA, Van Demark DR, and Morris HL: Long-term speech results of cleft palate speakers with marginal velopharyngeal competence. *Journal of Communication Disorders* 23:401-416, 1990.

Henningsson G, Karling J, and Larson O: Early or late surgery of the hard palate? A preliminary report on comparison of speech results. In Huddart AG, and Ferguson MWJ (eds.): *Cleft lip and palate: long-term results and future prospects.* Vol 1. New York: Manchester University Press, 1990.

Hess DA: Pitch, intensity, and cleft palate voice quality. *Journal of Speech and Hearing Research* 2:113-125, 1959.

Isshiki N, Honjow I, Morimoto M: Effects of velopharyngeal incompetence upon speech. *Cleft Palate Journal* 5:297-310, 1968.

Isshiki N, Honjow I, and Morimoto M: Cineradiographic analysis of movement of the lateral pharyngeal wall. *Plastic and Reconstructive Surgery* 44:357-363, 1969.

Karnell MP: *Videoendoscopy: from velopharynx to larynx.* San Diego: Singular Publishing Group, 1994.

Karnell MP, Folkins JW, and Morris HL: Relationships between perceived and kinematic aspects of speech production in cleft palate speakers. *Journal of Speech and Hearing Research* 28:63-72, 1985.

Karnell, MP: Nasometric discrimination of hypernasality and turbulent nasal airflow. *Cleft Palate Journal* 32:145-148, 1995.

Kelsey CA, Ewanowski SJ, Crummy AB, and Bless DM: Lateral pharyngeal-wall motion as a predictor of surgical success in velopharyngeal insufficiency. *New England Journal of Medicine* 287:64-68, 1972.

Kipfmeuller LJ, and Lang BR: Treating velopharyngeal inadequacies with a palatal lift prosthesis. *Journal of Prosthetic Dentistry* 27:63-72, 1972.

Koepp-Baker H: Orofacial clefts: their forms and effects. In Travis LE (ed.): *Handbook of speech pathology and audiology.* 2nd ed. New York: Appleton-Century-Crofts, 1971.

Krause CM, Tharp RF, and Morris HL: A comparative study of results of the Von Langenbeck and the V-Y pushback palatoplasties. *Cleft Palate Journal* 13:11-19, 1976.

Kummer AW, Billmire DA, and Myer CM III: Hypertrophic tonsils: the effect on resonance and velopharyngeal closure. *Plastic and Reconstructive Surgery* 91:608-611, 1993.

Kummer AW, Curtis C, Wiggs M, Lee L, and Strife JL: Comparison of velopharyngeal gap size in patients with hypernasality, hypernasality and nasal emission, or nasal turbulence (rustle) as the primary speech characteristic. *Cleft Palate Journal* 92:152-156, 1992.

Laine T, Warren DW, Dalston RM, Hairfield WM, and Morr KE: Intraoral pressure, nasal pressure and airflow rate in cleft palate speech. *Journal of Speech and Hearing Research* 31:432-437, 1988.

Leder SB, and Lerman JW: Some acoustic evidence for vocal abuse in adult speakers with repaired cleft palate. *Laryngoscope* 95:837-840, 1985.

Levine PA, and Goode RL: The lateral port control pharyngeal flap: a versatile approach to velopharyngeal inadequacy. *Otolaryngology–Head and Neck Surgery* 90:310-314, 1982.

Loney RW, and Bloem TJ: Velopharyngeal dysfunction: recommendations for use of nomenclature. *Cleft Palate Journal* 24:334-335, 1987.

Massengill R Jr, and Brooks R: A study of the velopharyngeal mechanism in 143 repaired cleft palate patients during production of the vowel /i/, the plosive /p/, and a /s/ sentence. *Folia Phoniatr* 25:312-322, 1973.

Mazaheri M, Millard RT, and Erickson DM: Cineradiographic of normal to noncleft subjects with velopharyngeal inadequacy. *Cleft Palate Journal* 1:199-210, 1964.

McDonald ET, and Baker HK: An integration of research and clinical observation *Journal of Speech and Hearing Disorders* 16:9-20, 1951.

McWilliams BJ: Speech and language problems in children with cleft palate. *Journal of the American Medical Womens Association* 21:1005-1015, 1966.

McWilliams BJ, Bluestone CD, and Musgrave MD: Diagnostic implications of vocal cord nodules in children with cleft palate. *Laryngoscope* 79:2072-2080, 1969.

McWilliams BJ, Glaser ER, Philips BJ, Lawrence CL, Lavorato AS, Beery QC, and Skolnick ML: A comparative study of four methods of evaluating velopharyngeal adequacy. *Plastic and Reconstructive Surgery* 68:1-9, 1981.

McWilliams-Neely BJ, and Bradley DP: A rating scale for evaluation of video tape recorded x-ray studies. *Cleft Palate Journal* 1:88-94, 1964.

Moll KL: Objective measures of nasality. Letter to the editor. *Cleft Palate Journal* 1:371-374, 1964.

Morr KE, Warren DW, Dalston RM, and Smith LR: Screening of velopharyngeal inadequacy by differential pressure measurements. *Cleft Palate Journal* 26:42-44, 1989.

Morris HL: Cleft palate. In Weston AJ (ed.): *Communicative disorders: an appraisal.* Springfield (IL): CC Thomas, 1972.

Morris HL: Types of velopharyngeal incompetence. In Winitz H (ed.): *Treating articulation disorders: for clinicians by clinicians.* Baltimore: University Park Press, 1984.

Morris HL, Bardach J, Ardinger H, Jones D, Kelly KM, Olin WH, and Wheeler J: Multidisciplinary treatment results for patients with isolated cleft palate. *Cleft Palate-Craniofacial Journal* 92:842-851, 1993.

Morris HL, and Smith JK: A multiple approach for evaluating velopharyngeal competency. *Journal of Speech and Hearing Disorders* 27:218-226, 1962.

Motta S, and Cesari U: Aerodynamic study of velopharyngeal inadequacy before and after logopedic treatment. *Folia Phoniatrica et Logopedica* 48:11-21, 1996.

Osberg PE, and Witzel MA: The physiologic basis for hypernasality during connected speech in cleft palate patients: a nasendoscopic study *Journal of Plastic and Reconstructive Surgery* 67:1-5, 1981.

Peterson-Falzone SJ: Speech outcomes in adolescents with cleft lip and palate. *Cleft Palate Journal* 32:125-128, 1995.

Powers GR: *Cleft palate.* Austin: Pro-Ed, 1986.

Rolnick MI, and Hoops HR: Plosive phoneme duration as a function of palato-pharyngeal adequacy. *Cleft Palate Journal* 8:65-76, 1971.

Ruscello DM, Shuster LI, and Sandwisch A: Modification of context-specific nasal emission. *Journal of Speech and Hearing Research* 34:27-32, 1991.

Sapienza CM, Brown WS, Williams WN, Wharton PW, and Turner GE: Respiratory and laryngeal function associated with experimental coupling of the oral and nasal cavities. *Cleft Palate Journal* 33:118-126, 1996.

Shelton RL Jr, Brooks AR, and Youngstrom KA: Articulation and patterns of palatopharyngeal closure. *Journal of Speech and Hearing Research* 29:390-408, 1964.

Shprintzen RJ: Pharyngeal flap surgery and the pediatric upper airway *International Anesthesiology Clinics* 26:79-88, 1988.

Shprintzen RJ, Sher AE, and Croft CB: Hypernasal speech caused by tonsillar hypertrophy. *International Journal of Pediatric Otorhinolaryngology* 14:45-56, 1987.

Shprintzen RJ, Lewin ML, Croft CB, Daniller AI, Argamaso RV, Ship AG, and Strauch B: A comprehensive study of pharyngeal flap surgery: tailor made flaps. *Cleft Palate Journal* 16:46-55, 1979.

Subtelny JD, Worth JH, and Sakuda M. Intraoral pressure and rate of flow during speech. *Journal of Speech and Hearing Research* 9:498-518, 1966.

Subtelny JD, Kho GH, and McCormack RM: Multidimensional analysis of bilabial stop and nasal consonants: Cineradiographic and pressured-flow analysis. *Cleft Palate Journal* 6:263-289, 1969.

Trost-Cardamone JE: Coming to terms with VPI: a response to Loney and Bloem. *Cleft Palate Journal* 26:68-70, 1989.

Valino-Napoli LD, and Montgomery AA: Examination of the standard deviation of mean nasalance scores in subjects with cleft palate: implications for clinical use. *Cleft Palate Journal* 34:512-519, 1997.

Van Demark DR, and Morris HL: Stability of velopharyngeal competency. *Cleft Palate Journal* 20:18-22, 1983.

Van Demark DR, Kuehn DP, and Tharp RA: Prediction of velopharyngeal competency. *Cleft Palate Journal* 12:5-11, 1975.

Warren DW: A physiologic approach to cleft palate prosthesis. *Journal of Prosthetic Dentistry* 15:770-778, 1965.

Warren DW: Perci: a method for rating palatal efficiency. *Cleft Palate Journal* 16:279-285, 1979.

Warren DW, and Devereux JL: An analog study of cleft palate speech. *Cleft Palate Journal* 3:103-114, 1966.

Warren DW, and Mackler SB: Duration of oral port constriction in normal and cleft palate speech. *Journal of Speech and Hearing Research* 11:391-401, 1968.

Warren DW, Bevin AG, and Winslow RB: Posterior pillar webbing and palatopharyngeus displacement: possible causes of congenital palatal incompetence. *Cleft Palate Journal* 15:68-72, 1978.

Warren DW, Dalston RM, and Mayo R: Hypernasality in the presence of "adequate" velopharyngeal closure. *Cleft Palate Journal* 30:150-154, 1993.

Warren DW, Dalston RM, and Mayo R: Hypernasality and velopharyngeal impairment. *Cleft Palate Journal* 31:257-262, 1994.

Warren DW, Dalston RM, Trier WC, and Holder MB: A pressure-flow technique for quantifying temporal patterns of palatopharyngeal closure. *Cleft Palate Journal* 22:11-19, 1985.

Weber J Jr, and Chase RA: Stress velopharyngeal incompetence in an oboe player. *Cleft Palate Journal* 7:858-861, 1970.

Yules RB: Secondary correction of velopharyngeal incompetence *Journal of Plastic and Reconstructive Surgery* 45:234-244, 1970.

Yules RB, and Chase RA: Secondary techniques for correction of palatopharyngeal incompetence. In Grabb WC, Rosestein SW, and Bzoch KR (eds.): *Cleft lip and palate: surgical dental, and speech aspects.* Boston: Little, Brown, 1971.

Zajac DJ, and Linville RJ: Voice perturbations of children with perceived nasality and hoarseness. *Cleft Palate Journal* 26:226-232, 1989.

Zajac DJ, Mayo R, Kataoka R, and Kuo JY: Aerodynamic and acoustic characteristics of a speaker with turbulent nasal emission: a case study. *Cleft Palate Journal* 33:440-444, 1996.

Zimmerman GN, Karnell MP, and Rettaliata P: Articulatory coordination and the clinical profile of two cleft palate speakers. *Journal of Phonetics* 12:297-306, 1984.

Zwitman DH, Gyepes MT, and Ward PH: Assessment of velar and lateral wall movement by oral telescope and radiographic examination in patients with velopharyngeal inadequacy and in normal subjects. *Journal of Speech and Hearing Disorders* 41:381-389, 1976.

Chapter 12

TREATMENT OF SPEECH-LANGUAGE PROBLEMS

A large percentage of children with cleft palate ultimately require speech-language intervention. Estimates vary across reports (Albery, 1989; Blakeley and Brockman, 1995; Bzoch, 1997a; Dalston, 1990; Hardin-Jones and Jones, 1997; Grames et al., 1999; Van Demark, 1997), but on average it would appear that at least 50% of these children will require the services of a speech-language pathologist at some point in their lives. Bzoch (1997a) estimated that up to 25% to 30% of children with cleft palate *who receive team management* demonstrate speech problems related to the cleft throughout the preschool years.

The majority of children referred for therapy typically require intervention to enhance their articulation or phonological development or general expressive language functioning. Although the course of speech-language therapy will be very straightforward for some children, it will be far more complex for others who demonstrate articulation and resonance problems associated with velopharyngeal inadequacy. You must know when it is appropriate to initiate speech therapy, when it is appropriate to refer for physical management, and when it is prudent to defer management of all kinds. The initial assessment will not always provide the information needed to develop a long-term course of management. Frequently, the therapy process itself must provide the information needed to arrive at a diagnosis.

EARLY INTERVENTION PROGRAMING

Initially the primary role of a speech-language pathologist working on a cleft palate team will be one of parent education. Parents are often unsure of what the impact of the cleft will be and thus are uncertain of what they should expect of the child. It is not uncommon for parents to report that other professionals have advised them "not to worry" about speech until the palate is repaired. Presumably, such advice is delivered with the concern that a child who begins talking before palatal repair may develop compensatory articulations in response to velopharyngeal inadequacy. Although some children who undergo late palatal surgery certainly do develop aberrant articulations, it is important to remember that the majority of children we see do not develop them at all. We should never discourage a parent's efforts to foster good communication skills in a baby with cleft palate. Instead, we should encourage their efforts by providing them with appropriate information. As Hahn (1989) stated, "Parents are going to teach speech and language consciously or unconsciously, whether or not they are advised; they need direction, information on normal language development, and specific suggestions on practical ways to start" (p. 313). If parents are not involved in the management process early on, they may inadvertently assign all responsibility for management to the professionals involved with their child. Instead of actively stimulating good communicative behaviors, some parents may simply sit back and wait for surgery to occur, assuming that normal speech will then emerge spontaneously. Others may adopt a different but equally casual attitude toward the child's speech and language development, passively accepting the delays in the child's speech as a natural consequence of the "clefting" experience. Parents need to get the message early on that the goal for the child is normal speech and that their participation is needed to foster that goal.

First and foremost, parents of babies with cleft palate should be informed of the impact that a cleft has on a child's oropharyngeal mechanism and how this may be expected to affect the child's early communicative efforts as well as speech production performance after palatoplasty. In addition to counseling parents about the expected impact of the cleft on speech, the clinician will also want to encourage aggressive language stimulation. As indicated in Chapter 7, it is not uncommon for these children to experience delays in speech sound development and expressive language. Before palatal surgery, parents should be encouraged to engage the child in vocal play and babbling games (just as they would with any infant). They should be informed that nasal consonants and glides will be more easily and perhaps more readily produced than pressure consonants. However, approximations of pressure consonants should always be accepted despite any distortion that may be present. Compensatory articulations, particularly aberrant glottal behaviors, should be described and the parents counseled to avoid reinforcing them (as happens when they are repeated to a baby). Instead of repeating that "cute" growl to the baby, parents should be encouraged to simply ignore these undesired behaviors when they are produced but reinforce the baby's efforts to vocalize by producing a babble or word that contains desired consonants (e.g., mamama). Parents should also be encouraged to monitor the different consonants that the child produces while babbling.

Along these same lines of thought, parents and professionals alike often ignore the quality of a child's early vocalizations in anticipation of identifying that long-awaited first word. Absence of plosive articulations as well as anterior tongue tip and labial sounds during the advanced stages of prelinguistic development should always alert the clinician to possible delays in later speech development (Albery and Russell, 1994). During the early stages of language development, the goal of phonological therapy should be to increase consonant inventory and range of syllable shapes. When a child's expressive vocabulary consists of less than 50 words, babbling games can be used to stimulate production of new consonants. Paul (1995) recommended that initial efforts to expand a child's consonant inventory focus first on nasals and stops. She summarized a number of contexts previously described by Bleile and Miller (1993) that may facilitate consonant production during the early stages of speech development. These contexts are shown in Box 12-1. In addition to encouraging the production of a wider range of sounds, Albery and Russell (1994) recommended that activities be incorporated into a child's daily routine to increase oral sensitivity and awareness (to increase oral air flow), encourage imitation, and increase auditory awareness. Specific activities to stimulate early speech-language development can be found in Stengelhofen (1990) and Lynch, Brookshire, and Fox (1993).

It is important to recognize that intervention directed toward enhancing early vocabulary development may also facilitate expansion of a child's phonetic repertoire. Scherer (1999) examined the results of a vocabulary intervention program administered to three 2-year-old children with repaired cleft lip and palate. Milieu intervention[1] was provided using a multiple baseline design across two conditions: vocabulary comprehended and vocabulary not comprehended. The treatment facilitated both word use and phonological performance for all three children. Scherer noted that although there was a weak trend for the children to acquire more target words containing consonants that were present in the children's pretreatment repertoire, a large percentage of acquired words contained consonants that were not present in the pretreatment inventory. One child increased his consonant inventory by nine consonants and the other two added six consonants to their repertoire.

[1]Milieu teaching techniques include strategies such as modeling and incidental teaching that are incorporated into routine activities to elicit child responses.

Box 12-1 **Contexts for Facilitating Consonant Production in Early Speech**

1. Stressed syllables facilitate consonant production (*baby* to facilitate /b/).
2. Velar consonants are facilitated at the ends of syllables (*talk* to facilitate /k/) and when they come before a back vowel (*good* to facilitate /g/).
3. Alveolar consonants are facilitated when they precede a front vowel (*tea* to facilitate /t/).
4. To facilitate production of a consonant at a new place of articulation, use a word that contains another consonant at the same place of articulation (*toss* to facilitate /s/).
5. Position facilitates the production of voicing distinctions. Use beginning contexts to facilitate production of voiced consonants (*dough* to facilitate /d/) and ending contexts to facilitate production of voiceless consonants (*eat* to facilitate /t/).
6. Fricatives are facilitated in contexts between vowels (*taffy* to facilitate /f/).

From Paul R: *Language disorders from infancy through adolescence.* St. Louis: Mosby, 1995. Modified from Bleile K, and Miller S: Infants and toddlers. In Bernthal J (ed.): *Articulatory and phonological disorders in toddlers with medical needs.* New York: Thieme, 1993, pp. 81-109.

Bzoch (1997a) noted that although strategies have been identified to prevent and/or treat the speech disorders associated with cleft palate early on, they are frequently unavailable or simply provided too late for some children. He estimated that 95% of all infants born with cleft lip and palate could demonstrate speech and language comparable to their peers by 5 to 6 years of age if optimal management were provided by the cleft palate team. According to Bzoch, an optimal program would include:

- Parent counseling regarding language development
- Home speech and language stimulation program
- Direct speech therapy when indicated
- Team management approach involving the plastic surgeon and a dental specialist *in each community*

The results of one such program were recently reported. Blakeley and Brockman (1995) described the results of a 4-year project designed to ensure age-appropriate articulation, normal resonance, and normal hearing by age 5 years for 90% of a group of children with cleft lip and palate. Forty-one children 12 to 24 months of age were enrolled in the project and were provided speech and hearing assessments every 3 to 4 months. During these visits, parents were provided with information regarding normal development, speech-language stimulation, and specific sound–facilitating techniques and were asked to provide both direct and indirect stimulation for the child. During the project, eight children were fitted with temporary speech appliances and one child received secondary surgical management for velopharyngeal inadequacy. Twenty-seven children (66%) received direct articulation therapy with a speech pathologist. When re-evaluated at 5 years of age, 93% of the children demonstrated age-appropriate articulation and 93% had normal oral-nasal resonance balance. Eighty-eight percent of the children demonstrated both normal articulation and resonance. Normal receptive and expressive language were reported for 95% and 88% of the subjects, respectively. Finally, by the end of the program, 98% of the participants had normal hearing.

The results reported by Blakeley and Brockman are impressive and serve to remind us of the potential impact that early intervention *with parental involvement* can have. Early intervention programing will not circumvent delays in communication for all of the children we see, but it can facilitate acquisition of normal speech and language behaviors and encourage parents to assume an active role in the child's development.

The impact of earlier intervention and advances in surgical management are evident in the speech production skills of children with cleft palate seen today. The incidence of children with cleft palate who demonstrate severe articulation and resonance disorders appears to have declined throughout the years. Bzoch (1997a) compared the percentage of children in his population who had demonstrated speech disorders during the past 40 years: Although approximately 75% of 1000 children studied in the 1960s had "cleft palate speech disorders," only 20% of 50 children he studied in the 1970s to 1980s demonstrated such problems. He also pointed out that the majority of the latter children demonstrated mild developmental or dental-related articulation disorders. In contrast to these samples, Bzoch further reported that only one or two of the 20 children in his 1990s sample produced any of the articulation and resonance disorders he studied.

DIRECT ARTICULATION-PHONOLOGICAL THERAPY

The majority of older children with cleft palate who are referred for direct speech-language therapy require intervention to establish correct phonetic placements. Regardless of whether the child demonstrates poor consonant development, developmental substitution errors, compensatory articulation errors, hypernasality or nasal emission, or some combination of these errors, the initial goal of therapy for the majority of children we see will be correct articulatory placement. As the child acquires the appropriate phonetic patterns, the focus of therapy may then shift to mastery of phonemic patterns (Trost-Cardamone and Bernthal, 1993).

The principles of therapy are essentially the same for children with cleft palate as they are with any other child, but the impact of the cleft must always be considered. If the child demonstrates developmental articulation or phonological errors and has normal resonance, then therapy will proceed as it would for any other child. Emphasis is initially placed on establishing production of stops and fricatives on the assumption that establishing stopping and frication in a few sounds will contribute to generalization of those features in other sounds. Traditionally, bilabial stops have been taught before linguadental and linguapalatal stops or fricatives because their place of articulation is more visible. However, you should not feel constrained by the developmental literature when selecting sounds to target in therapy, particularly when a child demonstrates articulation or resonance problems related to the cleft. It is important to recognize, as Bzoch (1997a) pointed out, that not all speech problems are equally handicapping. Although stops are typically introduced before fricatives for noncleft children, it is sometimes easier to stimulate a fricative consonant than a stop consonant in some young children with velopharyngeal inadequacy. This is particularly true for young children with poor consonant development who may be producing only nasals, glides, and glottals. They often find it easier to comprehend the idea of "moving" air through the mouth than "stopping" air in the mouth. It is also easier at times to break up glottal articulation by establishing correct placement of voiceless fricatives before initiating therapy for stops because the vocal folds are abducted for a longer period of time before onset of voicing for the vowel and a glottal stop is less likely to be triggered. Thus, the normal developmental sequence of "voiced" before "voiceless" cognates needs to be reversed.

The type and frequency of therapy delivered to some children with cleft palate is a growing concern in smaller communities and school systems with limited resources. It is not uncommon to find that a preschooler with cleft palate and a severe phonological delay has been enrolled in classroom-based therapy or provided individual, direct intervention for only 20 to 30 minutes once a week. Such practice may be economically expedient but is rarely efficacious and thus not in the child's best interest. The type of therapy and the frequency of therapy should be based on each child's individual needs. A child who is demonstrating a general delay in language development may well benefit from enrollment in a classroom-based intervention program. A child with intelligible speech who demonstrates developmental substitution errors may indeed benefit from direct speech therapy provided only once a week. However, a child with cleft palate who demonstrates poor consonant development or compensatory articulation errors will likely require more intensive intervention (typically at least two times a week) to establish normal oral articulation in a reasonable period of time.

In general, we recommend use of long-standing therapy techniques for teaching children to produce sounds in syllables and words and then establishing automatic use of those sounds in conversation. Therapy should include use of auditory and visual models for imitation, practice, and reinforcement of responses in age-appropriate speech material and should be organized to encourage generalization from that which is taught in therapy to speech units not used in therapy and to situations outside the clinic.

Initiating articulation therapy for some young children with cleft palate who demonstrate evidence of velopharyngeal inadequacy can be difficult when they make no effort to use their oral articulators to create labial and lingual constrictions to stop or modulate air flow. Requests to imitate a prolonged fricative in isolation may result in a child closing the mouth while producing a nasal grimace and simply forcing air through the velopharyngeal port into the nose. Requests to say /pɑ/ may result in /ʔɑ/, /hɑ/ or /mɑ/. (Note: The latter production is likely a learned behavior, not an obligatory consequence of velopharyngeal inadequacy, especially when audible nasal emission precedes the /m/.) Velopharyngeal inadequacy can certainly prevent a child from producing a consonant with adequate oral pressure, but it should not prevent a child from attempting to create an oral constriction to begin with. Some young children need to spend time discovering their mouth and all the interesting things it can do before consonants sounds can be produced in a purposeful way.

Blowing tasks are useful with young children in teaching the *concept* of oral air flow. However, they are not very useful in teaching consonant production. It is important to incorporate the idea of oral air flow into tasks that directly involve production of consonant sounds. For example, a child might initially be asked to feel the air stream as the clinician produces a series of /p/ sounds and then be asked to produce the sound himself. The productions may then be directed to a tissue, allowing the child to observe the displacement of the tissue. A young child might also be engaged in a cotton ball race with the clinician. Instead of blowing the cotton ball across the table, however, the child might be stimulated to move it across the table by placing his mouth next to it and saying /pʌ/. Excessive oral pressure should not encouraged. In cases where the child simply opens his mouth to "blow" air, /p/ can be shaped by asking the child to compresses his lips tightly and release only "pops" of air (e.g., sustained /ppppppp/ or "raspberry").

Although blowing tasks can be used to heighten awareness of oral air flow, they should never be considered a therapy *goal.* These tasks should simply represent one of many activities that can be used to teach a consonant sound. It is important when using these activities with young children that everyone (clinician and parents alike) understand their purpose. Blowing activities are designed to teach the concept of oral air flow; they are not useful as exercises for the soft palate and, in and of themselves, do not improve velopharyngeal function.

A word about oral motor exercises. Young children who demonstrate a restricted consonant inventory and those who produce compensatory articulations are frequently enrolled in therapy designed to increase strength of the oral musculature. Oral motor "exercises" are introduced on the assumption that lack of oral articulation reflects an underlying problem with muscle strength. Unfortunately, the majority of children with cleft palate who are subjected to these treatment strategies do not benefit from them because there is no underlying neuromotor problem to begin with. Golding-Kushner (1995, p. 335) pointed out that, ". . . most patients with very severe glottal stop speech disorders have normal tongue tip activity during production of nasal /n/ and normal bilabial closure for nasal /m/. It should be obvious that if tongue movement/elevation is sufficient for /n/, it is sufficient for the oral cognates /t,d,s,l/." She argued that therapy to "strengthen" the tongue is a waste of time because the problem is not a lack of strength but rather what the tongue has (or has not) been taught to do. We agree.

Poor Consonant Development

Children with cleft palate who demonstrate poor consonant development in the absence of significant cognitive and receptive language delays, hearing loss, or neurological problems are challenging management cases for the speech-language pathologist who serves on a cleft palate team. When a child's consonant inventory is limited to nasals, glottals, and glides, speech may sound very hypernasal (because of the preponderance of nasal and glottal productions). Although an underlying inadequacy of the velopharyngeal mechanism may be present, it cannot be properly evaluated (and thus properly managed) until the child is *attempting* to produce some pressure consonants. The appropriate management in cases like this is therapy to eliminate the nasal and glottal substitutions and establish oral articulations (i.e., oral place features). Surgical management should not be considered until the child is *attempting* production of pressure consonants and there is evidence of velopharyngeal inadequacy.

What must a child do to demonstrate that he or she is attempting production of pressure consonants? The answer here is not always as straightforward as the question would suggest. Broen, Doyle, and Bacon (1993) described the results of a diagnostic, home-based therapy program that was developed for a 2-year, 9-month-old child with repaired cleft palate. Before therapy, the child demonstrated poor consonant development, substituting /h/ or glottal stops for word initial consonants. Intervention was provided by the child's mother one or two times a day for an average of 18 minutes per session, 5 days a week, for approximately 1 year. Four groups of consonants were taught, including labials (/p/, /b/, /m/), alveolars, (/t/, /d/, /n/), palatal alveolar (/ʃ/), and velars (/g/, /ŋ/). The mother was instructed to reinforce correct place of articulation "regardless of manner, voicing, or nasality" (e.g., /p/, /b/, /f/, /v/ produced as /m/ would be considered correct).

The authors reported that, although the frequency of word-initial consonant omissions and /h/ substitutions decreased throughout the treatment period, nasal substitutions and glottalized oral productions increased. This finding was not necessarily surprising because the latter productions were considered correct and thus were being reinforced. A speech bulb fitting was initiated when the child was 3 years 7 months of age. The authors reported that once the bulb was completely fitted 2 months later, the child's nasal substitutions and glottalized oral productions "almost disappeared." They noted, however, that little change occurred in the frequency of glottal stops. Broen, Doyle, and Bacon suggested that, although the former two articulation patterns might have represented accurate articulations to the child, the glottal stops represented true substitutions for oral consonants and thus were retained after physical management. They argued that it might have been more appropriate to terminate therapy after the second phase of the program (teaching alveolar placement) because the child was attempting production of labial and alveolar consonants (albeit in the form of nasal substitutions and glottalized oral productions) and the frequency of glottal stops was increasing. It might also be argued that the child should have been enrolled in direct therapy with a speech-language pathologist to enhance oral articulations.

Several points should be made about these findings. First, the authors' assumption that the nasal substitutions produced by this child reflected her attempt to produce the appropriate place features for oral consonants is an assumption that is not applicable to all children. Some children with velopharyngeal inadequacy produce oral articulations such as /b/ and /d/ that are accompanied by severe audible nasal emission, and these productions are perceptually different from the nasal consonants /m/ and /n/. It cannot be assumed that a child who substitutes an /m/ for a /b/ is exhibiting an error that is *obligatory* to velopharyngeal inadequacy. It seems likely that nasal consonants are initially produced as substitutions for other consonants simply because they are one of the few consonants that a toddler with velopharyngeal inadequacy can correctly produce. Although they may initially develop as a result of velopharyngeal inadequacy, they probably persist as a learned behavior for many children. As indicated above, we believe that these types of errors should be minimized before surgical management is considered so that the functional potential of the velopharyngeal mechanism can be more accurately assessed.

The rapid elimination of nasal substitutions and coarticulated glottal stops reported by Broen, Doyle, and Bacon (1993) after placement of a speech bulb was very impressive. Unfortunately, not all centers offer prosthetic management as an adjunct to treatment. The findings reported by these authors, however, certainly support the use of speech bulbs to control velopharyngeal inadequacy in young children. By controlling velopharyngeal inadequacy early on, it may be possible to more quickly eradicate the atypical substitution errors that prevent both the early study and treatment of the problem.

Dental Malocclusion and Oral Distortions

Dental-occlusal problems frequently compromise articulatory precision in children with cleft palate and result in oral distortion. Children in the early grades frequently have mixed dentition, including missing or partially erupted teeth. Children born with clefts of the secondary palate may also present with maxillary arch collapse that precludes positioning of the tongue within the maxillary arch, resulting in lateralization of some fricatives and affricates. Rotated anterior teeth and ectopic teeth may also contribute to oral distortion of these sounds. Some children can benefit from traditional placement therapy techniques and will eliminate distortion errors despite the dental-occlusal problems present. Other children will not be able to eliminate the distortion until their dental status is improved either through orthognathic or orthodontic management. Because we have no way of predicting who will benefit from speech therapy and who will not, therapy to correct these errors should always be conducted on a trial basis and is probably best initiated with school-aged children (not young preschoolers who may have difficulty identifying these errors). Therapy may be deferred if the dental status is expected to improve relatively soon.

Bear in mind that some children with severe malocclusions will simply not be capable of producing certain consonants using standard articulatory placements. For these children, adaptive strategies may already be evident or may need to be established. Children with a severe Class II malocclusion may be unable to approximate the lips for adequate production of bilabial consonants, so production of these consonants must be accomplished by labiodental articulation. Children with a severe Class III malocclusion may also have difficulty approximating the lips for bilabial production. In addition, these children may be forced to produce an inverted /f/ and /v/ (e.g., lower teeth–upper lip articulation) and may be obligated to produce some lingua-alveolar consonants using an interdental placement (because the tongue would otherwise have to retract for adequate lingua-alveolar placement). Finally, it is important to note that children with missing upper anterior teeth or a retruded maxilla may also use bilabial fricatives as substitutes for labiodental fricatives.

Phoneme-Specific Nasal Emission

Most clinicians address the problem of phoneme-specific nasal emission by using a facilitating sound to elicit oral production of the target sound. For example, /t/ is a sound that shares the same place of production as /s/. When a child who produces a /t/ (that is free of nasal emission) is instructed to produce a series of /t/s and prolong the last one (e.g., "t...t...t...tsssssss), the result will be an oral /s/. A word of caution here: the target sound in this example is a "long" /t/, not an /s/. It is important to instruct the child to produce a long /t/ not an /s/ because the latter sound is associated with nasal emission in the child's mind. Referring to the target sound as "s" can, and initially probably will, elicit nasal emission. Occasionally, a child with phoneme-specific nasal emission may be seen who cannot produce /t/ or is unable to transition from an oral /t/ to an oral /s/. In such cases, other nonaffected fricatives can be used to facilitate /s/, such as /ʃ/ and /θ/. These strategies are further described in the compensatory articulation section below.

Riski (1984) recommended placing a straw in front of the patient's mouth (so that air passes through it during production of /tsss/) to increase perceptual awareness of oral turbulence. Some children may also initially benefit from having their nares occluded while attempting to sustain an /s/. Although this strategy may result in immediate oral air flow for /s/ in some children (and thus provide useful sensory information), it is not uncommon for a child to attempt to continue to force air into the nose during this task. In such cases the oral cavity is generally obstructed by the tongue, and no frication (either oral or nasal) is heard until the nares are unoccluded. This type of strategy, when successful, should be used sparingly during therapy to ensure that the child does not become reliant on it. Other types of auditory and visual feedback that may be helpful in eliminating phoneme-specific nasal emission include the use of simple devices such as a See-Scape (Pro-Ed) and a listening tube–stethoscope.

At times, a patient is encountered who demonstrates hypernasality and audible nasal emission resulting from velopharyngeal inadequacy and who also demonstrates phoneme-specific nasal emission in the form of posterior nasal fricatives. In cases of mild velopharyngeal inadequacy, it is often advisable to eliminate the posterior nasal fricatives first before surgical management is considered. This is because the severe nasal "snorting" that characterizes these learned behaviors can easily inflate perceptual judgments of nasality. Once the functional nasal emission has been eliminated, the severity of nasality should be re-evaluated. In some cases the nasalization may not be severe enough to actually warrant surgical management.

Clinical findings. Witzel, Tobe, and Salyer (1988) described the use of nasopharyngoscopy as a biofeedback tool to eliminate phoneme-specific nasal emission in a 10-year-old girl. The child had received 4 years of speech therapy at school to improve articulation of /s/ but continued to demonstrate audible nasal emission on this sound. The child received one biofeedback session where she was instructed to monitor velopharyngeal movements as she produced a /t/ followed by an /s/. According to the authors the child successfully closed the velopharyngeal port on /s/ during connected speech after this session and was referred for traditional therapy. Maintenance of closure was evident on follow-up examination the following year.

Ruscello, Shuster, and Sandwisch (1991) described a program to eliminate context-specific nasal emission with a combination of biofeedback and articulation therapy. An adult patient who demonstrated nasal frication during production of /s/ in consonant clusters and in postvocalic singletons received nine 50-minute therapy sessions over a period of 10 weeks. During the initial five sessions the patient practiced words containing the /s/ target in words while monitoring nasal air flow on a computer screen (using PERCI-PC). Thereafter, nasal air pressure was monitored with a water manometer. The authors reported that their patient could successfully differentiate between correct and incorrect productions of /s/ after practice at the word level; however, visual feedback was provided until the patient "had successfully completed practice with sentence items." A 40-item sampling task containing /s/ items at the word, phrase, sentence, and conversational level was administered during five baseline assessments and after each of the nine treatment periods. Results indicated that by the final session only one item on the sampling task was considered perceptually unacceptable. It is significant to note that Ruscello and his colleagues provided their patient with visual feedback because the patient did not hear the errors in his speech.

Although visual feedback can facilitate identification of nasal emission for patients who do not demonstrate auditory awareness, traditional articulation therapy alone is sufficient in the majority of cases. Because procedures such as nasopharyngoscopy are relatively costly and may be difficult to carry out with young children, they should probably be introduced only when conventional therapy procedures have failed to assist a child in eliminating this particular type of error. We would add, however, that biofeedback therapy of this type can, for some patients, be far more cost-effective than uneventful speech therapy that is delivered over a number of years, as demonstrated in the report of Witzel, Tobe, and Salyer.

Compensatory Articulation

Glottal and pharyngeal articulations are often difficult to eliminate in young children. This is true whether they occur in an individual with past or present velopharyngeal inadequacy. Because these maladaptive patterns are atypical and do not simply reflect a delay in normal phonological development, they can have more serious consequences for speech intelligibility than other developmental substitutions that the child may be producing. Thus, it is often advisable to address these errors in therapy before addressing other substitution errors.

Historically, clinicians believed that surgical management for velopharyngeal inadequacy should be performed before therapy to eliminate compensatory articulations was initiated. Because these aberrant articulation patterns develop in response to velopharyngeal inadequacy, it was assumed that they could not be eliminated until the velopharyngeal inadequacy was resolved. As indicated in Chapter 7, however, several investigators have demonstrated that an increase in oral articulations is generally accompanied by an increase in velopharyngeal movements (Golding-Kushner, 1981; Henningsson and Isberg, 1986; Shprintzen, 1986, as cited by Hoch et al., 1986; Ysunza, Pamplona, and Toledo, 1992). This has led most experienced clinicians to defer surgery until glottal and pharyngeal substitutions have been eliminated, or at least substantially reduced. Although reducing hypernasality is not a goal of therapy, it is certainly not uncommon for perceived hypernasality to diminish as oral articulation improves. The overall improvement in velopharyngeal function may not alter the need for surgical management, but it can minimize the need for a wide, obstructive pharyngeal flap. In addition, better velopharyngeal function increases the odds of a successful surgical result. When confronted with a highly unintelligible child who demonstrates pervasive glottal or pharyngeal substitutions, there is little to be gained by rushing into surgical management. As Hoch et al. (1986, p. 316) pointed out, "If there are pervasive glottal stop substitutions preoperatively, the postoperative result will be severe unintelligibility regardless of whether hypernasality was eliminated or not."

General principles of therapy that should be considered when planning treatment for compensatory articulations were outlined in earlier reports by Trost-Cardamone (1990, 1995). She advised the use of visual aids (e.g., lateral-view diagram of head and tongue) to contrast the desired articulatory placements with faulty placements and recommended the use of a large mirror for visual monitoring because the use of auditory feedback alone is rarely sufficient. She also recommended that therapy focus on establishing the place of articulation only. Once place is established, traditional therapy approaches are applicable. Finally, she recommended initially selecting treatment targets that are (1) produced with anterior placements, (2) visible, and (3) unvoiced. Additional criteria that should be considered when selecting a sound for treatment include how stimulable a child is for correctly producing the sound and how developmentally appropriate it is.

Bzoch (1997a) recommended the use of *multiple sound articulation training* to eliminate gross sound substitution patterns. In this type of training program, four or more sound elements are taught then quickly reinforced during home practice activities. Additional sounds are taught each session until all sounds involved in the gross substitution pattern (e.g., glottal or pharyngeal substitutions) have been included. According to Bzoch, it is preferable to work on the entire pattern of behavior because when only selected consonants are targeted for remediation, the other gross substitution errors inhibit change in speech behavior. Hoch et al. (1986) argued that although it might be advantageous to work on two or more sounds simultaneously, success should be demonstrated at the phrase level for one sound before introducing another. Van Demark and Hardin (1986) also cautioned that although establishing correct place of articulation might be a relatively easy task in some patients, maintaining the new behavior and generalizing it to conversational speech is far more difficult and requires close observation, perhaps for a longer period of time.

Glottal stops. Several authors have described strategies used to eliminate glottal stop substitutions (Bzoch, 1997b; Golding-Kushner, 1995; Hoch et al., 1986; Trost-Cardamone, 1990). These laryngeal productions are generally addressed by having a patient whisper the target sound and produce an aspirate /h/ after it (and before the vowel) to break up the glottal pattern. It is typically recommended that voiceless stops be addressed before voiced stops. In addition, labial and lingual stops are often more easily modified than velar stops are (and thus are typically addressed first in therapy). When attempting to eliminate glottal stop substitutions for labial and lingual stops, the patient is generally instructed to sustain /h/ as lips open and close for production of /p/ or /t/. The patient is instructed to overaspirate the stop consonant before gradually adding voicing for the vowel. When attempting to eliminate glottal stop substitutions for velar stops, instruct the patient to produce the velar nasal (ŋ) while you occlude their nares. The result will be a velar stop. The patient can be encouraged to overaspirate the stop consonant using /h/. Golding-Kushner (1995) noted that it is more difficult for some patients to produce oral stops in the initial position than the medial or final position of a syllable/word. Table 12-1 shows the sample sequence of trials using successive approximation that Golding-Kushner described for eliminating glottal stops in the initial and medial position of words.

It is often easier to eliminate compensatory articulation and establish an oral stop by first training a voiceless homorganic oral fricative (Trost, 1981). Hoch et al. (1986) suggested that, when appropriate for the child's needs, a voiceless fricative would be a good initial target to work on because the vocal folds will be abducted for a lengthy time before onset of voicing for the subsequent vowel. They also recommended the use of nasal consonants to facilitate the production of target sounds having the same (or similar) place of articulation (e.g., /n/ facilitates /t/ in "fun time").

Pharyngeal fricatives or stops. These atypical patterns of articulation can be eliminated by use of anterior facilitating sounds to elicit the target sound. For example, if a child substitutes a voiceless pharyngeal fricative for an /s/, /s/ can be elicited by having the child produce a series of /t/s followed by a prolonged /t/ (e.g., t...t...tssssssss). When a pharyngeal fricative is coarticulated with an oral articulation, either an unaspirated continuant or a stop can be used to stimulate the target sound (Trost-Cardamone, 1995). Other articulatory postures that have been recommended to facilitate production of /s/ include /Θ/ and /ʃ/ (Riski, 1984). The patient is instructed to initiate oral airflow for /Θ/ and then gradually retract the tongue to a postdental position while maintaining oral air flow. Riski reported that in his experience this strategy was the most successful one for facilitating /s/. Alternatively, the patient can be instructed to produce /ʃ/ first with normal lip rounding and then with lips retracted. Retracting the lips often results in the lingual-palatal constriction for /ʃ/ moving anteriorly to form /s/ (Riski, 1984). Trost-Cardamone (1995) noted that the high, front vowel /i/ can also facilitate anterior placement. She recommended the use of ortho elastics and cereal bits placed on the tongue to facilitate phonetic placements. Anecdotal reports suggest that pharyngeal fricatives are often more easily eliminated than glottal stops

Table 12-1 Sample Sequence of Trials Used to Eliminate Glottal Productions and Establish Oral Stop Consonants

Training Oral Stop in Initial Word Position		*Training Initial Oral Stop from Medial Word Position*	
Trial	*Comments*	*Trial*	*Comments*
$T^{hhhhhh}UUUUUU$	Fully whispered	$^{hhhhhh}AAAAAA$	Fully whispered
$T^{hhhhhh}UU\underline{UUUU}$	Voicing is introduced after the vowel onset	$^{hhhhhh}AAAP^{hhhhhh}AAAAA$	Fully whispered, bilabial closure overlaid
$T^{hhhhhh}\underline{UUUUUU}$	Voicing is introduced at the vowel onset	$^{hhhhhh}AAP^{hhhhhh}AA\underline{AAAA}$	Voicing is introduced after the vowel onset
$T^{hhh}\underline{UUUUUU}$	The duration of aspiration is decreased	$^{hhhhhh}AAP^{hhhhhh}\underline{AAAAAA}$	Voicing is introduced at the vowel onset
$T^{h}\underline{U}$	Normal production of /t/	$^{hhhhhh}AAP^{hhh}\underline{AAAAAA}$	Duration of /p/, release aspiration decreased
		$^{hhhhhh}AAP^{h}\underline{A}$	Normal duration of /p/, release aspiration for medial position
		$^{hh}AP^{h}\underline{A}$	Decreased duration of "carrier aspiration"
		$P^{h}\underline{A}$	Normal production of /p/ in initial position

NOTE: repeated letters represent elongation of a sound, and underlined segments are voiced.
Adapted from Golding-Kushner K: Treatment of articulation and resonance disorders associated with cleft palate and VPI. In Shprintzen RJ, and Bardach J (ed.): *Cleft palate speech management: a multidisciplinary approach.* St. Louis: Mosby, 1995.

(Morley, 1970) and thus are typically addressed first in therapy when both types of compensatory articulations are present.

Middorsum palatal stops. The goal of therapy when eliminating middorsum palatal stops is to establish the linguaalveolar place of production and/or the velar place of production. As with other atypical articulations, the place feature should be established first before the stop manner is addressed. Trost-Cardamone (1995) observed that homorganic /n,l/ and /s,z/ can be helpful in teaching the appropriate placement for linguaalveolar stops. A word of caution: when a palatal fistula is present, these substitution errors may be more easily eliminated after surgical closure or obturation of the fistula (Hoch et al., 1986).

Therapy for Older Patients

The speech pathologist who specializes in cleft palate and craniofacial disorders probably has fewer adolescent and adult patients with cleft palate than was once the case. The services that patients receive earlier in life are effective, and many patients now speak normally by the time they reach adolescence. Nonetheless, there are still patients in this age category who do not speak well. The initial cleft may have been severe, velopharyngeal inadequacy may persist, and the patient may have especially severe facial disfigurement and dental-occlusal problems. Some of these patients will have had previous speech therapy as a child and will report that the therapist "did as much as he or she could do" before dismissing them for lack of progress. These patients present a great challenge to the speech pathologist and merit special consideration. Unfortunately, the passage of time for many older patients frequently results in articulatory gestures that are firmly entrenched and highly resistant to therapy.

Some adolescent and adult patients have made remarkable adjustments to existing physiological deficits and have better articulation patterns than could be predicted from assessment of their mechanism. Perhaps in attempts to compensate for velopharyngeal deficits, dental malocclusion, midface deficiency, or a combination, they have learned adaptive or compensatory articulations that result in intelligible but different speech. The speech-language pathologist must decide whether speech therapy is likely to be effective in modifying these behaviors or whether the patient's speech is as proficient as can reasonably be expected.

Reports describing the efficacy of articulation therapy in adolescents and adults with cleft palate are rare, and those that do exist typically reflect the response of a patient to some type of biofeedback therapy. The results of these clinical investigations (described on p. 308) as well as anecdotal clinical reports suggest that abnormal speech patterns in adult patients are often times so entrenched and automatic that their modification is difficult, if not impossible to accomplish. For patients who do not achieve velopharyngeal closure, the task of acquiring and automating satisfactory articulatory placement is arduous, time consuming, and expensive. Failure can be expected in a number of patients and there are times when it will be best to accept speech as it is. For patients who are highly motivated to change their speech behaviors, a trial period of therapy may be warranted to examine their commitment to the therapy process and their response to treatment. It seems doubtful that most adults will be able to modify their articulatory behaviors with conventional articulation strategies alone. Modification is more likely to occur if some type of biofeedback therapy is provided, such as electropalatography or nasopharyngoscopy.

Older patients with poor speech remind us of the importance of early diagnosis and treatment. An important goal for all cleft palate specialists is the prevention of such severe speech disorders.

Electropalatography

Electropalatography (EPG)[2] is a procedure that has been used to study lingual articulation and treat articulatory disorders in children and adults with cleft palate. The instrumentation involves an acrylic palatal plate that is fabricated for each patient. Electrodes are embedded throughout the plate and exposed on the lingual surface. When the electrodes are contacted by the tongue, a signal is sent to an external processing unit through lead-out wires. Real-time visual feedback of the location and timing of tongue contacts with the hard palate is provided on a computer monitor.

Compared with other types of treatment procedures, EPG might be considered a somewhat expensive intervention tool. The device is commercially available but requires use of a palatal plate custom fitted for each individual patient. Although the expense would be considered negligible for a patient who has received years of unproductive speech therapy, it would be unnecessary for many patients with articulation problems who have responded to more conventional therapy procedures.

Stengelhofen (1990) noted that electropalatography may be particularly useful for children whose misarticulations are deeply entrenched and unresponsive to conventional therapy procedures. Several investigators have examined EPG as a biofeedback tool for children with cleft palate. A summary of their findings follows.

Clinical findings. Michi et al. (1986) used dynamic palatography to correct palatalized and lateralized articulations in a 6-year-old girl with a repaired unilateral cleft lip and palate and an anterior oronasal fistula 2 mm in diameter. The child demonstrated adequate velopharyngeal closure on nasendoscopic assessment. Audible nasal emission and hypernasality were not evident; however, the posterior articulatory contacts produced by the child could have masked nasal emission that otherwise might occur because of an anterior fistula. The authors described a therapy plan that included teaching the child (1) to identify palatographic patterns and to associate them with awareness of tongue position, (2) to understand information on the palatographic display, and (3) to learn correct articulatory movements. The therapy was intended to terminate unwanted articulatory contacts and then to replace them with correct places of articulation. The authors followed a progression from phonemes produced in isolation and syllables to production in words, sentences, and paragraphs, and then conversation was followed. They offered evidence that in the course of 49 hourly sessions over a period of 1 year the child made and maintained substantial articulatory improvement, including the elimination of tongue backing and air stream lateralization. Neither of those misarticulations was likely to self-correct. Progress was more rapid than that made by other children who had therapy that did not involve dynamic palatography.

Hardcastle, Barry, and Nunn (1989) described the use of electropalatography to modify articulation in two boys ages 7 and 5 years who demonstrated velopharyngeal adequacy. Both children demonstrated persistent articulatory problems affecting mostly fricatives and affricates and had received previous speech therapy. Before therapy, both children were provided with a "trainer plate" that did not contain electrodes and were instructed to wear it for increasingly longer periods of time before the first EPG recording session. The first child received 15 hours of therapy "initially given on an intensive basis." Although he achieved "reasonable alveolar and palatoalveolar fricatives" during single word production and during "careful speech and reading in the clinic situation," he did not maintain these behaviors outside of the clinical setting nor carry them over to conversational speech. The other child received five 1-hour sessions of therapy over a period of 2 weeks. He, too, achieved adequate production of his target sounds in "carefully controlled speech situations" but was unable to carryover these productions in conversational speech. Nonetheless, both children demonstrated improvement with the EPG procedure and were able to continue their improvement even when the visual feedback was withdrawn.

The efficacy of electropalatographic therapy was further examined by Whitehill, Stokes, and Yonnie (1996) using a multiple baseline approach. They described treatment results for an 18-year-old Cantonese-speaking woman with bilateral cleft lip and palate and velopharyngeal inadequacy who had received a combined palatoplasty and pharyngeal flap at 13 years of age. The subject had previously received 13 sessions of conventional speech therapy directed toward improving place of articulation for velar and alveolar stops and reducing nasalance, but the results had been disappointing. At the onset of electropalatography treatment the subject demonstrated velopharyngeal inadequacy (with "touch" closure for fricatives and affricates), moderate hypernasality, audible nasal emission, and posterior articulation of obstruents. Twenty-three 1-hour treatment

[2]Two commercially available EPG instruments that have been described in previous reports include the Palatometer manufactured by Kay Elemetrics (Fletcher, 1989; Fletcher, McCutcheon, and Wolf, 1975) and the British EPG system developed at the University of Reading (Gibbon, Stewart, Hardcastle, and Crampin, 1999).

sessions were provided over a 4-month period. According to the authors, "rapid and dramatic" improvement was evident for the two therapy targets (/s/ and /t/) and generalization to nontarget phonemes occurred. Production of /s/ was considered "acceptable" in conversational speech, although the authors acknowledged that it was produced with "slight palatalization." The subject produced /t/ correctly at the single word level and achieved 55% accuracy in conversational speech. Nasal emission/plosion was eliminated for these consonants as well; however, a significant reduction in hypernasality was not noted.

Whitehill, Stokes, and Yonnie stated that electropalatography may be particularly useful in treating the articulation problems of individuals with cleft palate for two reasons. First, the posterior articulations demonstrated by this group may be particularly responsive to the real-time visual feedback provided by EPG. Second, if patients with cleft palate demonstrate a reduction in oral sensation, then the use of visual feedback may be particularly valuable in establishing alveolar place targets.

The particular appeal of EPG for children and adults with cleft palate who produce intractable articulation errors is that it offers an alternative feedback system for patients who are otherwise unable to modify their behavior by auditory or kinesthetic feedback. Children with compensatory articulation patterns and adolescents and adults who demonstrate persistent articulation problems would appear to be good candidates for this type of intervention. Because of the expense involved in such a system, it should probably be introduced to a patient only after an uneventful course of speech therapy. The treatment results to date are promising but limited in scope. Additional studies are needed that document not only change in target behaviors but also long-term maintenance of that change.

Gibbon and her colleagues (1999) recently described an EPG network set up in Scotland to increase patient accessibility to this type of treatment. Four centers were equipped with EPG systems including portable training units that could be sent out on loan. Speech-language pathologists working at the centers were trained to use the equipment by EPG specialists who provided hands-on demonstrations of the equipment and provided suggestions for treatment. EPG data obtained during treatment sessions are transferred electronically from the centers to EPG specialists who assist with data analysis and interpretation. This ambitious project should, as Gibbon et al. anticipate, facilitate treatment efficacy research by making EPG available to a substantially larger number of children.

MODIFICATION OF HYPERNASALITY AND NASAL EMISSION IN PATIENTS WITH BORDERLINE VELOPHARYNGEAL INADEQUACY

Children who demonstrate clinically significant hypernasality and audible nasal emission associated with velopharyngeal inadequacy will generally require surgical management to establish normal resonance. In an ideal world, surgical correction of velopharyngeal inadequacy would be accomplished before initiation of articulation therapy so that a child would have the advantage of learning correct sound placements with an adequate velopharyngeal system. However, it is often the case that young children are referred for therapy before an adequate objective assessment of velopharyngeal function can be performed. In such cases, it is appropriate to initiate therapy with a goal of establishing correct place of articulation. *Velopharyngeal inadequacy will not prevent a child from learning correct articulatory placements in therapy! Therapy should never be withheld until surgical management of velopharyngeal inadequacy has been performed when a delay in speech sound development is present.*

A number of authors (Hardin, 1991; Kummer and Lee, 1996; Morris, 1972; Van Demark and Hardin, 1990) have advocated a period of trial speech therapy for children who demonstrate borderline/marginal velopharyngeal inadequacy. Although speech therapy alone is unlikely to totally eliminate nasalization of speech in any patient (except in functional cases), it may minimize the perception of hypernasality and/or audible nasal emission for patients who demonstrate

- Mild hypernasality and audible nasal emission
- Inconsistent hypernasality and audible nasal emission
- A small velopharyngeal opening
- Nasalization of speech only in certain contexts or when fatigued
- A reduction of nasalization during stimulability tasks
- Compensatory articulation patterns.

Therapy can be effective in reducing nasalization of speech when it is associated with oral-motor dysfunction or dysarthria and when it persists after pharyngoplasty (Kummer and Lee, 1996; Peterson-Falzone, 1988). Finally, it may be appropriate to initiate a trial period of therapy in certain cases where the patient is unable to receive either surgical or prosthetic management.

Although therapy to establish age-appropriate articulation is frequently a long-term venture, therapy to reduce perceived nasality should always be conducted on a short-term trial basis. When efforts to modify nasality are unsuccessful after 6 to 8 weeks of intervention, this treatment should be abandoned and alternative treatments should be considered. Therapy should continue only when other articulation or language goals can be addressed.

Traditional Strategies

Strategies commonly recommended in the literature to minimize the perception of hypernasality or audible nasal emission all have one thing in common: they attempt to manipulate the oral cavity in an effort to change oral resonance. This is an important point to remember in therapy and when counseling patients and their family. We are not attempting to directly alter what is happening at the velopharyngeal port because *behavioral strategies cannot alter structural problems.* Our goal is to encourage oral resonance and articulation through modification of oral activity. The activities listed below have been described by many authors (Hardin, 1991; Hoch et al., 1986; Kummer and Lee, 1996; Van Demark, 1997; Van Demark and Hardin, 1990); however, most reports are tutorial or anecdotal. Data regarding the effectiveness of these procedures in minimizing nasalization of speech are needed.

Increasing mouth opening. A number of authors have recommended increasing mouth opening to promote an increase in oral resonance (Boone and McFarlane, 1994; Coston, 1986; McDonald and Koepp-Baker, 1951; Shelton et al., 1968; Van Demark and Hardin, 1990). As a speaker increases mouth opening, oral resistance decreases and a subsequent increase in oral air flow is expected. As oral air flow increases, nasal air flow should decrease and thus result in speech that is perceived as less nasal. One means of attaining an increased mouth opening during vowels, glides, and liquids is simply to call the patient's attention to that goal and to practice it with visual feedback. A mirror or television monitor may be useful for this purpose. Another technique is to teach exaggerated articulatory movements that lead to greater range of mouth opening and vice versa. Although this procedure may be useful in minimizing listener perception of hypernasality for patients with a small velopharyngeal gap who speak with a restricted oral opening, it is probably not a useful strategy for many patients who are already using appropriate labial and mandibular movements during speech. Indeed, increasing mouth opening too much runs the risk of increasing perceived nasality because muscular connections between the tongue or mandible and velum could act to open the velopharyngeal port (Peterson-Falzone, 1982).

Light articulatory contacts. Several authors (Coston, 1986; Shelton, Hahn, and Morris, 1968; Van Demark and Hardin, 1990) have also recommended the use of light articulatory contacts to decrease listener perception of audible nasal emission. Golding-Kushner (1995) advised against the use of light articulatory contacts (as well as rate reduction) to improve speech intelligibility. She argued that although strong contacts may increase the perception of nasal turbulence, they are associated with increased velopharyngeal movements and better speech intelligibility (Hoch et al., 1986). Golding-Kushner regarded the use of light articulatory contacts and rate reduction strategies as a "poor and inefficient use of time." We would agree with her arguments when normal articulation and resonance are considered a reasonable goal for the patient. At times, however, a child may have mild nasalization of speech that is not considered severe enough to warrant surgical intervention. In such cases the use of light articulatory contacts may be warranted to decrease the perception of nasal emission.

Decreasing rate of speech. Reducing speech rate is a commonly used yet controversial technique for reducing perceived nasality. Clinicians have assumed that because the position of the velum is constrained by the position of other articulators during connected speech, reducing the rate of articulation would allow a sluggish velum more time to elevate and achieve closure against the posterior pharyngeal wall. Although this notion is an attractive one, data to support a strong relationship between speaking rate and nasality have not been reported. In fact, studies that have manipulated speech rate (D'Antonio, 1982; Jones and Folkins, 1985) and word-level production time (Jones, Folkins, and Morris, 1990) have failed to identify any systematic effects on perceived nasality.

Despite the lack of experimental support, clinicians continue to use rate reduction strategies in therapy. Because there is little to lose (and perhaps something to gain) by introducing such a strategy in therapy, it may be appropriate to investigate on a trial basis the impact of rate reduction for specific patients. Remember, however, that the speech production characteristics of the patient should always drive the therapy that is administered. Actively manipulating the speaking rate of a patient who is already speaking at an appropriate rate is not appropriate. Rate reduction strategies should be used only when rate itself is a problem.

Programs Related to Phonetic Context

Several authors have developed programs designed to systematically decrease hypernasality. Lang (1974) developed and tested a program designed to eliminate hypernasality. Sommers (1983) said that Lang's program was based on the assumption that there is a hierarchy for degree of perceived nasality for both consonants and vowels (Moore and Sommers, 1973, 1975). According to Lang, the hierarchy of vowels from least to most nasal is /ɔ/, /a/, /ɛ/, /æ/, /u/, and /i/. Consonants, in the same order, are glides and glottal fricatives, plosives, fricatives, affricates, and /z/. This latter part of the hierarchy is difficult to understand because /s/ has been found in many studies to be most difficult for speakers with cleft palate (see Chapter 7).

Lang's therapy program is summarized in Box 12-2. The program is highly specific and quite rigid in that 100% nasal-free speech must be produced at each level before moving to the next. Careful programing has also been developed to ensure self-monitoring at 100% agreement with the speech pathologist. Lang tested this program with 11 children ages 9 to 13 years at an 8-week summer camp at Duke University. All subjects had repaired cleft palates, and hypernasality was present in their spontaneous speech. No information was provided about velopharyngeal valving, although reference was made to valving in the results. One child "whose velopharyngeal valving was very poor" successfully completed only step 1 of the program; three completed step 2; three completed step 4; one, step 5; and two, step 9. Lang thought that the children's progress was directly related to their degrees of velopharyngeal adequacy (Sommers, 1983). Another way to put it is that the lack of significant progress for most of the children during the 8 weeks of intensive therapy was related to their *inadequacy.*

Another systematic approach to remediating hypernasality was developed by Ray and Baker (1990). The *Hyperna-*

Box 12-2 Thirteen Steps for the Elimination of Hypernasality in Phonetic Contexts

1. Correct production of the following vowels. Practice in the order listed: /ɔ/, /e/, /ɛ/, /æ/, /u/, /i/.
2. Correct production of VCV combinations utilizing each vowel (from least to most nasal) in combination with each consonant (from least to most nasal).
3. Correct production of CVC combinations utilizing each vowel (from least to most nasal) in combination with each consonant (from least to most nasal).
4. Correct production of the varied vowel and consonant combinations (from least to most nasal) in the initial and final positions of monosyllabic words.
5. Correct production of the varied vowel and consonant combinations (from least to most nasal) in bisyllabic words.
6. Correct production of the 10 short phrases and sentences loaded with the following phonemes in combination with all of the vowels: /r/, /w/, /h/, /l/, /j/.
7. Correct production of 10 short phrases and sentences loaded with the following consonants in combination with all of the vowels: /t/, /p/, /k/, /g/, /b/, /d/.
8. Correct production of 10 short phrases and sentences loaded with the following consonants in combination with all of the vowels: /v/, /f/, /ð/, /θ/, /s/.
9. Correct production of 10 short phrases and sentences loaded with the following consonants in combination with all of the vowels: /ʤ/, /ʒ/, /ʧ/, /ʃ/, /z/.
10. Correct production of all consonant and vowel combinations in long sentences.
11. Correct production of all consonant and vowel combinations while reading a short paragraph. (If the child does not read, poems or nursery rhymes can be substituted at this step.)
12. Correct production of all consonant and vowel combinations in a structured conversational task.
13. Correct production of all vowel and consonant combinations in a spontaneous conversational task.

From Sommers RK: *Articulations disorders.* Englewood Cliffs (NJ): Prentice-Hall, 1983.

sality Modification Program was designed for patients who demonstrate hypernasality due to velopharyngeal inadequacy but who have received surgical management (when indicated) and are able to produce consonants without nasal emission. The program consists of a resonance evaluation that systematically analyzes the influence of phonetic context on nasality. Treatment stimuli that have been phonetically controlled and arranged in a hierarchical fashion from least to most influential are provided and include

- Voiceless consonant + vowel + voiceless consonant
- Vowel + voiceless consonant
- Voiceless consonant + vowel
- Voiced consonant + vowel + voiceless consonant
- Voiceless consonant + vowel + voiced consonant
- Voiced consonant + vowel
- Vowel + voiced consonant
- Voiced consonant + vowel + voiced consonant
- Isolated vowels
- Nasal + vowel + voiceless consonant
- Nasal + vowel
- Nasal + vowel + voiced consonant
- Voiceless consonant + vowel + nasal
- Voiced consonant + vowel + nasal
- Vowel + nasal
- Nasal + vowel + nasal.

Therapy begins by addressing hypernasality in the least nasal phonetic context. By focusing on what the patient is "doing right," appropriate feedback cues can be provided for oral resonance. The standard techniques for reducing hypernasality that were described above (e.g., increasing mouth opening) are used to promote oral resonance.

Hierarchical approaches to modifying hypernasality such as those described above are useful in helping clinicians develop a systematic program of intervention. However, the efficacy of such resonance programs for individuals with cleft palate has not been examined. Such programs are probably useful for only a select group of patients with borderline velopharyngeal inadequacy who demonstrate mild hypernasality.

THERAPY FOR PERSONS WITH VELOPHARYNGEAL INADEQUACY

We are reluctant to initiate therapy to reduce nasalization of speech for patients with gross velopharyngeal inadequacy. However, patients are seen who refuse physical management that is needed or for whom management is not available. The health of some patients may also preclude surgery that could enhance speech. Some patients show so little movement of the velopharyngeal structures that they are poor candidates for surgery or obturation (although one or the other will probably still be provided). Any speech therapy provided to these patients is not expected to establish normal speech; rather, the goal is to help the patient do as well as possible.

As is true when working with patients who demonstrate borderline velopharyngeal inadequacy, the primary goal of therapy will be to establish correct articulatory placement. The speech pathologist should avoid asking these patients to produce sounds with good oral air pressure because such efforts may encourage the gross substitutions that therapy is intended to correct. Strategies to reduce perceived nasalization that were previously described, including use of a greater mouth opening, rate reduction, and light articulatory contacts, may also be used.

There are two important warnings to be considered. One is that the patient, the family, and other specialists involved in patient care must be well informed about the restricted goals for therapy. It may be necessary to repeat this information. Otherwise these individuals may infer that the speech pathologist continues to be optimistic and that therapy is expected to result in normal speech. There is a danger that its continued use will serve to delay consideration of additional physical management.

The second warning relates to the first. There is a danger that ineffective therapy will be continued for prolonged periods. Bzoch (1997a) referred to patients who had had up to 8 years of speech therapy with little improvement. Continuation of therapy in the absence of improvement is irresponsible. The speech pathologist must be careful to resist providing therapy beyond the time when no further improvement is to be expected. There are limits to our capabilities, and once we have done our best, within the limits presented by the patient and our resources, we must withdraw from the case with careful explanations to all concerned. The continuation of any therapy is contingent on evidence of its effectiveness.

THERAPY FOLLOWING SECONDARY SURGICAL MANAGEMENT

Parents and professionals alike expect a dramatic shift in resonance after secondary surgical management for velopharyngeal inadequacy and are frequently alarmed when that does not immediately occur. Although secondary management should result in elimination of hypernasality and audible nasal emission for most of the children we see, nasalization can persist in some young children for a variety of reasons. Before assuming that surgery has failed, the clinician should examine the child's speech production patterns for alternative explanations. For example, the persistence of nasalization immediately after surgery would not be an unexpected finding in a child who presented with pervasive nasal substitutions or glottal and pharyngeal articulations preoperatively. When children with these error patterns are referred for surgery (Note: We believe that surgery should be deferred when possible until these atypical patterns are minimized and oral articulatory gestures established), parents and professionals should be counseled about the expected postoperative result. If elimination of these atypical errors occurs after therapy with little to no improvement in resonance, then referral to the plastic surgeon is appropriate. Children with essentially no movement of the velopharyngeal structures before surgical management may also demonstrate some degree of hypernasality after surgery. This is not an unexpected finding in some children because some movement is needed to close the ports lateral to a pharyngeal flap or the central port after a sphincter pharyngoplasty. Children who present with velopharyngeal inadequacy and coexisting phoneme-specific posterior nasal fricatives will also demonstrate persistence of the latter errors after surgery even when the velopharyngeal inadequacy has been totally eliminated. In other cases a dramatic decrease in hypernasality and audible nasal emission will be evident after surgery, but some degree of nasalization persists. As a general rule of thumb, most children should be given an adequate period of time (6 to 12 months in most cases) to adjust to the new mechanism before a surgical revision is considered.

Occasionally, a child who receives secondary surgical management will demonstrate essentially no change in resonance and audible nasal emission. When that occurs and there is no obvious explanation, the child should be referred for direct visualization of the mechanism to rule out the possibility of flap inadequacy or dehiscence.

A REVIEW OF THE EFFECTIVENESS OF ARTICULATION AND RESONANCE THERAPY

A question that is frequently asked by clinicians treating children with cleft palate is whether changes in articulation can reasonably be expected when velopharyngeal inadequacy is present. Although studies examining this issue are limited in both quantity and design, the data indicate that children do benefit from articulation therapy even when velopharyngeal valving problems are present. Chisum et al. (1969) evaluated articulation therapy delivered to children who had hypernasality, audible nasal emission, or both and who were thought to have a borderline-adequate velopharyngeal mechanism. To serve as a subject, an individual was required to have articulation errors on at least three different speech sounds. Eleven children ages 6 to 12 years served as experimental subjects and received 30-minute articulation therapy sessions twice each week over an average period of 7.2 months. The control group, which included 12 children with cleft palate or velopharyngeal inadequacy, did not receive treatment. Differences in pretreatment and posttreatment articulation test scores revealed that the experimental subjects significantly reduced their articulation errors, whereas the control subjects did not.

Harrison (1969) evaluated a language and speech stimulation program devised for preschool children with cleft palate. Subjects with velopharyngeal inadequacy and their mothers were taught to accept nasal air flow in the production of speech sounds. The stimulation procedures used were directed to consonant placement regardless of the child's ability to imitate a particular sound. Articulation was tested with the Miami Imitative Ability Test and the Bzoch Error Pattern Articulation Test, which samples 24 consonants in 100 test items. Both experimental and control subjects made gains on each test, but the experimental group made statistically greater gains on the Bzoch test. Harrison (1969) thought the gains might have been greater had the stimulation been directed to sounds the children could imitate. However, it is also possible that training directed to sounds the children could not imitate may have helped to make the necessary articulation gestures available for incorporation into the children's phonology.

Shelton et al. (1969) used sagittal cinefluorography to determine whether articulation improvement with therapy was accompanied by changes in velopharyngeal function. They studied size of the velopharyngeal gap, forward

the patient even if surgery or prosthesis proves necessary. He noted that the individual's velopharyngeal structures and function will influence the success of muscle training (e.g., the person whose palate is short is a poor candidate). However, the patient who demonstrates motion in some activities, including gagging or blowing, but not during speech, may benefit. The person who sometimes achieves closure during speech is more likely to establish normal closure patterns than are individuals who do not achieve closure. He noted that any gains that are achieved will usually occur early. Increased velopharyngeal motion should be seen within a month, and if no gain has been made in 3 months, additional work will likely be ineffective.

Research evidence. One goal of therapeutic exercise has been to elicit movement or greater range of movement through the triggering of reflexes, to bring that increased range of motion under conscious control, and then to establish it in automatic, skilled speech performance (Yates, 1980). Tactile and electrical stimulation were used in a number of early studies to enhance voluntary control of the palatopharyngeal musculature (Peterson, 1974; Tash et al., 1971; Weber, Jobe, and Chase, 1970; Yules and Chase, 1969; Yules et al., 1968). Although some of these studies showed a reduction in nasal air flow and an increase in velar elevation and pharyngeal wall movement during simple tasks, generalization to conversational speech was not demonstrated.

The efficacy of blowing, sucking, and swallowing exercises in improving velopharyngeal closure was evaluated in several early studies. Massengill et al. (1968) used blowing exercises with five subjects, sucking exercises with four, and swallowing exercises with four subjects. The subjects, who ranged in age from 8 to 18 years, received articulation training during the study period. Subjects who performed the swallowing exercise reduced velopharyngeal gaps as determined by cephalometric films made before and after treatment; however, the authors made no attempt to evaluate the influence of this change on speech.

Powers and Starr (1974) also used palatal exercises with four children who were between 8 and 11 years of age and who had surgically repaired cleft palates. The exercises involved blowing, sucking, swallowing, and gagging. Each task was performed to specified criteria a designated number of times over a 6-week period. Nasality ratings and cephalometric measurements of the velopharyngeal gap observed during the production of a prolonged /i/ were made before and after the therapy program and again 6 weeks later. No gains were made in either velopharyngeal function or hypernasality. The authors noted that their procedures were comparable to those that Massengill et al. (1968) reported as successful.

Other techniques for enhancing velopharyngeal function have also been studied. Lubit and Larsen (1969) described an appliance intended to serve as a palatal exerciser. It consisted of a maxillary-retention segment and an attached inflatable bag. Inflation of the bag displaced the velum superiorly and posteriorly and exerted pressure against the posterior wall of the larynx. The authors claimed that 28 patients benefited from use of the exerciser. However, the only data reported were selected radiographs, speech ratings, oral manometer readings, and spectrograms from one individual. In a second report (Lubit and Larsen, 1971), two of four subjects treated continued to show velopharyngeal openings during test sounds even after treatment. The authors offered several conjectures about the physiological mechanisms whereby their exerciser might bring about improved velopharyngeal function. However, the data reported are not adequate to support their conclusion that benefit actually occurred. Also, as Peterson (1974) pointed out, the device would offer resistance to muscles that would serve to depress the velum, not elevate it.

In his discussion of behavioral approaches to treating velopharyngeal closure and nasality, Starr (1993) concluded that there was not enough evidence to support the use of muscle exercises in therapy to modify hypernasality. "If they have a role in therapy, three things must occur before their value can be established. First, procedures must be devised that will allow measurement of the adequacy of specific muscle function. . . . Second, exercise programs must be developed to treat the specific muscle deficiencies that are identified. . . . Third, researchers must determine how to train patients to use new muscle competencies, if they are created" (p. 340). He noted that efforts to use general exercises without first determining their effects on specific muscles would be unlikely to either help patients or increase our understanding.

We must conclude that the bulk of the evidence regarding the effectiveness of muscle training is negative. The better the controls and measurements in these studies, the more negative the results. No one to date has demonstrated in sizable samples that muscle training can be used to develop velopharyngeal movements that are as remarkable in range of movement and skill of execution as those required for normal speech production. Perhaps improved technology and methods will give a more favorable result in the future. Until then, we consider therapeutic exercise for velopharyngeal function to be experimental and do not recommend it for routine clinical practice.

The failure of palatal exercises to improve velopharyngeal closure during speech is probably related to many factors. It is well known that the pattern of velopharyngeal closure achieved during nonspeech tasks is different from those seen during speech. Therefore, any attempt to *exercise* the velopharyngeal musculature to increase muscle strength or endurance must occur within the context of speech itself if changes in closure during speech are the expected result. Also, if the goal of the therapy is to *exercise* the muscles of the velum to increase muscle strength or endurance, then some type of resistance training is needed.

Kuehn and Moon (1994) found that levator muscle activity during speech for their normal subjects "tended to occur in the lower region of its operating range as determined in relation to the blowing task" (p. 1269). They hypothesized that maximum activation of the musculature during nonspeech activities such as swallowing might be needed to ensure the tight velopharyngeal closure needed to oppose any nasal regurgitation. Lower muscle activity would likely occur for speech and other repetitive or sustained activities to prevent fatigue. Kuehn and Moon speculated that patients who demonstrate evidence of adequate velopharyngeal closure during single words or sustained consonants (e.g., /s/) but who break down in connected speech may have adopted a pattern of velopharyngeal movement that allows them to avoid muscle fatigue. "Perhaps because of weaker velopharyngeal muscles, these individuals may have a lower threshold of fatigue than individuals having normal strength and they may have developed a pattern of neuromotor control to remain below the fatigue threshold" (p. 1270). They reasoned that the velopharyngeal muscles of patients with hypernasality might be functioning closer to the threshold for fatigue than is the case in speakers with normal speech. The authors concluded that strengthening the muscles might extend a patient's operating range, thereby increasing "the difference between the functional range for speech and the threshold of fatigue." A promising treatment technique to strengthen the velopharyngeal musculature and reduce the effects of fatigue is continuous positive air pressure (CPAP) therapy.

CPAP Therapy

In 1991, Kuehn described a muscle resistance training program that used a CPAP device. The CPAP device is a commonly used clinical tool for patients with obstructive sleep apnea. It generates a continuous positive air pressure that is transmitted to a patient through a nasal mask and prevents collapse of the airway during sleep. Kuehn reasoned that the CPAP device could be used in a muscle resistance training program for speakers with velopharyngeal inadequacy because the muscles of the soft palate must work against CPAP's positive pressure to close the velopharyngeal port.

The 8-week CPAP therapy program described by Kuehn appears both time and cost-effective because the patient can take the device home and simply follow a preestablished protocol. The basic therapy procedure consists of the following steps:

- CPAP mask is placed over nose
- Appropriate pressure is set for current session
- Patient produces 50 VNCV utterances
- Patient produces six sentences
- Steps 3 and 4 are repeated until session time expires.

A starting pressure is determined for each patient (typically ~3 cm H_2O) and is gradually increased throughout the therapy period. The amount of time devoted to each session also increases each week. During week 1 the patient may spend 10 minutes producing the VNCV utterances and sentences comprising the CPAP materials. By week 8 the patient is devoting 24 minutes to the task. When the VNCV utterances are produced, stress is placed on the second syllable. As the velum elevates forcefully (from its lowered position for the nasal consonant), the velopharyngeal musculature presumably must "contract forcefully, not only because of the particular phonetic sequencing, but also against the resistance provided by the positive air pressure in the nasal cavities" (p. 963).

A potential advantage of CPAP therapy compared to other muscle training exercises is that it is conducted *during* speech production. According to Kuehn, the neurophysiologic control mechanisms used are probably more appropriate than would be the case if nonspeech activities were used.

Kuehn described the preliminary results of CPAP therapy for four patients. Two of the patients were 8-year-old girls (one with Klippel-Feil syndrome and one with unilateral cleft lip and palate) who demonstrated moderate hypernasality. Both demonstrated a reduction in hypernasality after the 8-week therapy program as determined by listener judgment. The third subject was a 14-year-old adolescent with velopharyngeal inadequacy who demonstrated severe hypernasality. No improvement was evident after 1 month of therapy, so CPAP therapy was terminated. The fourth patient was a 20-year-old adult with moderate hypernasality resulting from a closed head injury. A reduction in hypernasality (from a rating of 4 to a rating of 2 on a 7-point severity scale) was also evident for this patient at the end of the therapy program.

Kuehn and his associates (2000) examined the efficacy of CPAP therapy for 43 patients with repaired cleft palate who demonstrated hypernasal speech. Speech recordings were obtained before and after 8 weeks of home-based CPAP therapy. Six judges independently rated the tape-recorded speech samples for hypernasality (without knowledge of the pre- and post-CPAP recording conditions) using "protocol-guided comparisons" with reference recordings. On average, the decrease in mean hypernasality score was small (approximately 0.2 points on a 7-point scale) but statistically significant. Although some patients showed a more substantial decrease in hypernasality (approximately 1 point), others demonstrated no change at all. It is important to note that none of the subjects were severely impaired, and so the potential for improvement was limited. The authors noted that while CPAP therapy may be beneficial in reducing hypernasality for some patients, considerable variability exists across patients in their response to the treatment.

Additional research is needed to determine who the appropriate candidates for CPAP therapy are and to determine whether the short-term gains reported by Kuehn are maintained over time. Kuehn, Moon, and Folkins (1993) identified four assumptions underlying CPAP therapy that should be examined in future research. The first assumption, that the muscles of velopharyngeal closure are actually subjected to a resistive load, was examined in their 1993 report. They found greater levator veli palatini muscle activity during conditions where positive pressure was introduced to the nasal cavities than during atmospheric pressure conditions. Their findings support the use of CPAP therapy as a resistance exercise to strengthen the muscles of velopharyngeal closure. The second and third assumptions underlying CPAP therapy are that the resistive loading "can be used in a systematic program of progressive resistance exercise" (p. 361) and that the resistance exercise will eventually strengthen the velopharyngeal musculature. The final assumption discussed by Kuehn, Moon, and Folkins was that strengthening the velopharyngeal musculature will actually result in reduced hypernasality.

Whistling-Blowing Technique

Shprintzen, McCall, and Skolnick (1975) described and evaluated a therapy intended to develop velopharyngeal closure during speech from velopharyngeal closure present during blowing and whistling. The authors hypothesized that subjects who close the velopharyngeal port during blowing and whistling but not during speech probably learned to leave the velopharyngeal muscles turned off as they developed speech before surgical provision of a structurally adequate mechanism.

Four subjects, ranging in age from 4 to 19 years, were taught to phonate while whistling or blowing. Nasal emission was monitored with a scape-scope. Once each subject could successfully phonate and whistle (or blow) simultaneously, the latter nonspeech activity was gradually eliminated. Treatment duration ranged from 22 sessions administered over 13 weeks to 36 sessions administered over 15 weeks.

All four subjects improved their velopharyngeal function during speech as indicated by the velopharyngeal pattern observed from the videofluorographic tape and evidence of reduced nasal air leakage. One subject, an individual with hearing loss, retained mild hypernasality and nasal snorting. The other three subjects achieved essentially normal function. Unfortunately, despite these encouraging results, follow-up investigations have not been reported. More important, however, is the fact that videofluoroscopic and nasoendoscopic evaluations performed after the original report was published revealed that patients who demonstrated velopharyngeal closure during blowing and whistling *also* achieved closure during sustained production of /s/ and /f/ (Shprintzen, 1989). That finding led Shprintzen and his colleagues to revise their therapeutic approach for such patients, eliminating the nonspeech tasks and basing therapy on speech tasks alone.

Information Feedback

Biofeedback was defined by Davis and Drichta (1980) as "an intervention technique that uses electronics to monitor and amplify body functions that may be too subtle for normal awareness" (p. 283). Instruments provide the learner with information about subliminal body functions in a direct and rapid manner. According to Davis and Drichta, biofeedback differs from other techniques in that information is provided directly to the patient during performance and the information is available to the patient to use as he or she chooses.

The term biofeedback is used here to refer to the use of information derived from performance about performance to improve performance. However, departing from the definition of Davis and Drichta, we accept descriptive information provided by a clinician as a form of biofeedback therapy. The emphasis is on providing the patient with information about performance rather than on reinforcement. Usually the learner watches or listens to information obtained through endoscopy, aeromechanical measures, auditory recordings, electromyography, or other instruments.

Procedures intended to improve velopharyngeal function by supplying information to the patient about that function are found in the early attempts at speech habilitation for the patient with cleft palate. Moser (1942) discussed use of cold mirrors, water manometers, and stethoscopes for this purpose. Kantner (1937) noted that in therapy these devices work best with individuals who sometimes achieve velopharyngeal closure even though they do not do so in automatic speech. In a landmark study, Masland (1946) coupled pneumoscopes to the nose and mouth of patients and used the devices in conjunction with a kymograph to record and display oral and nasal air pressure. Masland's patients wore prosthetic speech appliances, and it was hoped that they would learn to close the velopharyngeal sphincter against the pharyngeal segments of the appliances. The patients were to accomplish this by monitoring their pressure traces during the production of /pV/ syllables. Four case studies were presented. The subjects were variable in their success at reducing nasal emission; two eliminated the nasal air leakage on oral consonants and two reduced the frequency of occurrence of the leakage.

Endoscopic feedback. Numerous clinical investigators have examined the use of endoscopic feedback in treating velopharyngeal valving disorders. Shelton and his colleagues described the results of oral endoscopic training in a series of early reports. In the first study, Shelton et al. (1975) used an oral panendoscope attached to a videorecorder to provide feedback in teaching velopharyngeal movements. Three normal subjects learned to position themselves on an endoscope and observe their velopharyngeal ports displayed on a television screen. Each subject attempted closure on 10 nonspeech trials initiated by fixation of the larynx and then on 10 additional trials wherein reflexive movements elicited by touch pressure cues were to be imitated. The subjects readily learned to use the feedback system to perform the task under investigation.

In a subsequent report, Shelton et al. (1978) used oral endoscopy as a biofeedback tool for two adolescent subjects—one with a surgically repaired cleft palate who had received a pharyngeal flap and another who had velopharyngeal insufficiency. Both subjects were taught to position themselves on an oral endoscope coupled to a video camera and playback system and were instructed to attempt to increase the range of velopharyngeal motion during production of syllables while monitoring their velopharyngeal structures on the television screen. The subjects approximated closure frequently as the study progressed; however, performance gains were not established on an automatic level, and the subjects' clinical speech problems were not resolved.

Shelton and Ruscello (1979) summarized the treatment results for several patients with hypernasality, audible nasal emission, or both. With one exception, these patients all had cleft palate or velopharyngeal inadequacy. One adolescent had a 50 dB bilateral, congenital, neural hearing loss. Attempts were made to improve velopharyngeal function by having the subjects monitor their performance either by oral videoendoscopy or by the pen trace of an oscillograph displaying nasal air flow. When misarticulation was also a problem, subjects were given articulation training. One subject with cleft palate who had normal hearing was taught to monitor his nasal air flow through a hearing aid with the microphone placed under his nose.

Shelton and Ruscello reported that their patients did not benefit from the biofeedback therapy. The child with the hearing loss reduced nasal air flow during training sessions but at the cost of unwanted change in other speech behaviors. Other subjects were reported to have reduced the production of nasal noises during /sk/, /st/, and other clusters as they participated in articulation training. The nasal snort or fricative seems more amenable to elimination than does audible nasal emission. This is perhaps because the snort involves an articulatory maneuver.

It seems likely that the inability of Shelton's subjects to generalize their performance in some cases and demonstrate no change in others was related, at least in part, to the limitations associated with oral endoscopy. The use of an oral endoscope does not permit monitoring of movements *during* connected speech tasks. In fact, observation of the mechanism is only possible during production of low, back vowels, and that observation is limited in vertical extent once the velum elevates or velopharyngeal closure occurs. Other investigators have used a nasoendoscope during biofeedback therapy. Because the scope is passed through the nose instead of the mouth, it does not interfere with articulation. The patient can monitor movements of the velopharyngeal structures during connected speech.

Investigators in Japan have reported success using nasoendoscopic feedback to develop velopharyngeal closure in patients with palatal clefts. Miyazaki et al. (1974) described change in subjects' velopharyngeal function from pretraining to posttraining observations. Initially, the subjects were classified as having one of four closure patterns: complete closure only during swallowing; complete closure on swallowing and blowing; complete closure during swallowing, blowing, and nonnasal consonants; and complete closure during swallowing and blowing and on plosives, fricatives, and some vowels. Patients were treated once or twice monthly for more than 6 successive months. The subjects differed in their pretreatment closure patterns, but none had the most adequate pattern of closure. At the end of the study, 16 of 37 patients had closure that was considered to be the best or most adequate, and the others had improved their patterns. The authors concluded that patients who achieve closure during blowing can also easily achieve closure during phonation. Unfortunately, no experimental control features were reported for this study, so the findings must be interpreted with some caution.

Nishio et al. (1976) described a study related to that of Miyasaki et al. Most of their subjects initially achieved velopharyngeal closure during swallowing but had to learn to close the velopharynx during blowing and phonation. On average, it took 3.4 months for nine "visually trained" subjects to develop velopharyngeal closure during blowing. It took 5.6 months for 11 subjects who had received both secondary management and visual training to develop closure during blowing. Once closure was present in blowing, the authors found that it took less than 1 month to develop closure for plosives and fricatives.

Similar findings were reported by Yamaoka et al. (1983). Fifty-nine hypernasal speakers with repaired cleft palate ages 8 to 45 years received nasoendoscopic therapy. Therapy was provided every 2 weeks for approximately 1 year. According to the investigators, 59% (35 of 59) of the patients demonstrated improved velopharyngeal function after the treatment period and 15% demonstrated velopharyngeal closure during all experimental tasks (e.g., blowing and production of sustained vowels and CV combinations). Ten of the 12 patients who had originally achieved complete velopharyngeal closure during blowing and swallowing (but not speech) tasks demonstrated marked improvement after the treatment period. Two of these subjects achieved closure in all experimental tasks, whereas seven others had developed the ability to close the velopharyngeal port during production of pressure consonants as well as some vowels. Of particular interest was the finding that 8 of the 32 patients who had originally achieved velopharyngeal closure only during swallowing demonstrated velopharyngeal closure during blowing and production of pressure consonants after nasoendoscopic feedback.

This latter finding was unexpected. Because velopharyngeal closure in swallow involves a different mechanism than that used in speech, generalization of closure from swallow to speech is not anticipated.

Nasendoscopy was also used successfully by Siegel-Sadewitz and Shprintzen (1982) to modify the first author's pattern of velopharyngeal closure. She originally demonstrated a circular pattern of closure successfully inhibited lateral pharyngeal wall motion over six 20-minute sessions. She was able to produce the new coronal closure pattern "at will" during short connected speech samples (without visual feedback during the sixth session) and reportedly switched back and forth between the two closure patterns with no change in vocal quality and only a slight decrease in speech rate. Starr (1993) noted that although the findings reported by Shelton et al. (1975) and Siegel-Sadewitz and Shprintzen (1982) suggest that speakers can learn to control the velopharyngeal musculature with visual feedback, ". . . the limits of available voluntary control have not been defined" (p. 345).

Hoch et al. (1986, p. 322) reported the results of nasoendoscopic therapy for nine patients with velopharyngeal inadequacy. Biofeedback therapy was provided once a week. Traditional speech therapy was also initiated once each "patient was able to manipulate the velopharyngeal sphincter so that there was an audible change." Six of the nine subjects demonstrated velopharyngeal closure after four to nine therapy sessions. Two of these patients demonstrated inconsistent velopharyngeal inadequacy of structural origin, two had arrhythmic velopharyngeal valving patterns, and two had phoneme-specific nasal emission. Of particular interest was the authors' report that these subjects continued to achieve velopharyngeal closure during follow-up examination 1 to 3 years after treatment. Hoch et al. reported that two of the remaining three subjects improved velopharyngeal valving and received a pharyngeal flap. Only one subject who demonstrated arrhythmic velopharyngeal valving failed to benefit from nasoendoscopic feedback. Although the subjects with phoneme-specific nasal emission might have benefited equally well from traditional therapy procedures alone, the success reported by Hoch et al. for their other subjects was particularly encouraging.

Successful biofeedback results were also reported by Witzel et al. (1989). In their study, three adult patients who demonstrated persistent velopharyngeal inadequacy after pharyngeal flap surgery received videonasopharyngoscopic biofeedback therapy. Two subjects also received articulation therapy between biofeedback sessions. Initially, the subjects were asked to observe their velopharyngeal ports on a television monitor as they produced nonspeech tasks (e.g., blowing, whistling, swallowing) that resulted in closure of the ports. They were instructed to attend to movement of the lateral pharyngeal walls as well as the sensations associated with that movement and then to attempt to purposefully move the structures. Once each subject could voluntarily move the lateral pharyngeal walls without speech, sounds that were associated with the greatest range of lateral pharyngeal wall motion were introduced. Therapy progressed from production of consonants (± vowel) to conversational speech. Two of the three patients completed the therapy program. Both demonstrated substantial improvement in velopharyngeal function and in speech. One was reexamined a year after treatment and was observed to close the ports on each side of a pharyngeal flap completely and "appropriately" during connected speech. Follow-up data were not reported for the other subject, but the authors reported normal articulation and resonance at discharge.

The results of these investigations indicate that some patients can modify velopharyngeal function and maintain that function using visual feedback provided by nasoendoscopy. Witzel, Tobe, and Salyer (1988) noted that although nasopharyngoscopic feedback may be more expensive than other therapy techniques and requires both patient motivation and cooperation, it is a valuable adjunct to therapy because it provides important visual information that is missing in other more traditional techniques. In their 1989 report the authors noted that the visual feedback provided by nasoendoscopy should outweigh its disadvantages ". . . particularly in the older patient whose speech patterns are long-standing and ingrained" (p. 134). They urged additional study of the procedure as a biofeedback tool for patients with velopharyngeal inadequacy and stressed the need for investigations involving experimental controls and precise treatment protocols. Although the ideal candidate for nasoendoscopic feedback therapy has yet to be identified, the collective findings from the aforementioned studies would suggest that patients who achieve velopharyngeal closure during blowing and production of some pressure consonants are most likely to benefit from this intervention.

Nasometer feedback. The nasometer and its instrumental predecessor, Tonar II, have also been used in biofeedback research with individuals with clefts. Recall from Chapter 10 that the nasometer is a microcomputer-based tool that measures the relative amount of nasal acoustic energy as a patient talks. That information is provided to the user in the form of a "nasalance" score.[3] For purposes of therapy, a visual trace of the information can be displayed in real time with use of either a time history or bar thermometer display. The nasalance threshold is set approximately 10% above the mean nasalance score obtained during production of a nonnasal passage and then reduced in 5% to 10% decrements as the individual successfully produces treatment stimuli at or below the target threshold.

The use of Tonar II in nasalance reduction therapy was first described by Fletcher (1972). In his initial report he described treatment results for two adult patients. The first patient, a 23-year-old woman with hypernasality from a tonsilloadenoidectomy, received seven therapy sessions and reduced her nasalance from 70% to below 15%. According to Fletcher, she maintained this nasalance level on 3-month follow-up. The other patient was a woman with repaired cleft palate who wore a speech bulb. She reportedly reduced her nasalance from 85% to 5%; information regarding maintenance was not provided.

In a follow-up study, Fletcher (1978) described results of biofeedback using the Tonar II for 19 subjects ages 5 to 15 years who had a repaired cleft palate. The goal in this study was to determine whether subjects could modify their nasalance scores on specific stimulus sentences during a

[3]Results of investigations conducted throughout the past decade suggest that nasalance scores in the high 20s or above obtained on passages devoid of nasal consonants (e.g., Zoo Passage) are probably associated with at least mild to moderate hypernasality (Dalston, 1997, p. 339).

1-week intensive therapy program. A reduction in the average nasalance score from 40% to 31% was reported for the total group. According to Fletcher, eight subjects achieved and maintained normal levels of nasalance (15%) on two sentence groups, five subjects reached normal nasalance levels but were unable to maintain that performance level, five subjects reduced their nasalance but not to normal levels, and one subject did not demonstrate any appreciable change in nasalance.

Starr (1993) described an interesting study by Burrell (1989) that examined the effects of nasometer therapy on two patients who demonstrated mild, inconsistent hypernasality. The first patient, an 11-year-old boy, received therapy 1 hour a day for 8 days. His nasalance scores for each of three lists of therapy sentences decreased from 40% to 48% to less than 20%. Listener judgments revealed a significant reduction in hypernasality and lateral videofluoroscopy indicated an improvement in palatal function (palatal-pharyngeal contact had been evident on one of nine test sentences before therapy and was evident across all sentences after therapy). The second patient, an 18-year-old woman with repaired cleft palate, demonstrated a reduction in nasalance scores from 31% to 26% before therapy to less than 15% after treatment. Although listener judgments suggested a significant reduction in hypernasality, no modifications in velopharyngeal function were evident on posttherapy lateral and frontal videofluoroscopic films.

Starr noted that although the results obtained by Burrell did not address the long-term maintenance of changes observed during the therapy period, they did provide "evidence that changes in velopharyngeal function occur in conjunction with decreases in nasality associated with behavioral therapy" (p. 344). Presumably, patients who successfully reduce their nasalance score by nasometer feedback can do so either through a modification of velopharyngeal function or through the use of oral articulatory adjustments that decrease oral resistance.

It is somewhat surprising that, despite its user friendliness and relative low cost, the nasometer has not been the focus of more treatment efficacy studies. The preliminary reports described above suggest that patients with mild, inconsistent hypernasality are good candidates for such a treatment program. Until additional supportive data are reported, however, nasometer therapy should be considered experimental and initiated only after careful consideration of patient candidacy issues (e.g., age, severity of velopharyngeal inadequacy, and adequacy of speech sound development) and establishment of a short-term, measurable goal. Appropriate treatment stimuli are provided in the nasometer manual.

Other feedback tools. The usefulness of other procedures as biofeedback tools has also been examined. Moller et al. (1973) used a strain-gauge transducer to monitor and train velar movement during /u/ in a 12-year-old boy with perceptual and radiographic evidence of velopharyngeal insufficiency and a short velum. The transducer was cemented to a maxillary molar so that a sensor tip touched the middle third of the velum in the midline and followed its movement. Additional instrumentation was used to record the subject's responses, to display them to the subject, to compare them with a criterion level set by the investigators, and to reward correct responses. Training was provided three times a week for a total of 15 sessions. Sagittal cephalometric radiographs indicated that although the child increased velar movement during phonation of /u/, the size of the velopharyngeal gap was not reduced. The configuration of the boy's posterior pharyngeal wall changed during treatment apparently because adenoid atrophy was occurring at the same time. The authors noted that information about motion of the lateral pharyngeal walls might have been useful.

Tudor and Selley (1974) attached a U-shaped orthodontic wire to an acrylic base plate. It was positioned to touch and lift the resting soft palate. The authors inferred that the wire provided patients with information about the location of the palate and contributed to their development of voluntary velar movement. They also made an electrical visual aid in which two electrodes connected to a control box replaced the wire loop used in the earlier appliance. When the soft palate elevated, breaking contact with the electrodes, a light went out. The authors had the patient wear the palatal training appliance all day. The purpose of the electrical visual aid was to replace speech therapy and practice. The patient was asked to feel the appliance and to lift the velum away from it. The authors recommended this procedure for patients of all ages if they fail to achieve velopharyngeal closure because of weakness or poor coordination. Five of eleven patients who had had dysarthria for 2 years ceased to drool and established intelligible speech within 3 weeks of using this procedure. The authors presented this information as a preliminary report and included neither pretreatment nor posttreatment data.

Later Selley et al. (1987) stated that use of the U-shaped palatal training appliance results in resensitization of the velum-to-tongue contact and consequently reduced tongue humping. That in turn results in a more open oral tract and increased opportunity for air and sound to exit orally. Stuffins (1989) described use of the palatal training appliance with 26 patients and reported substantial success.

Dalston and Keefe (1987) described use of a microcomputer in conjunction with the photodetector for monitoring and modifying velopharyngeal movements. They cited unpublished preliminary evidence from a small number of normal and cleft palate speakers and asserted ". . . that the computer-based biofeedback treatment approach described in this paper enables subjects to modify velopharyngeal behaviors and, where appropriate, reduce or eliminate hypernasality and nasal emission of air. . . ." (p. 167).

Discussion

Skeletal muscle is subject to conscious control, and it should be possible to teach skilled motion of the velopharyngeal structure within any limitations imposed by tissue deficiency, impaired innervation, or both. It is evident that some patients with cleft palate do learn remarkable velopharyngeal motions and that a few apparently can reduce, but not eliminate, both nasal emission and hypernasality. Noncleft persons and some patients with cleft palates readily learn to make movements of the velum and perhaps of the pharyngeal walls. However, demonstrations of increased velopharyngeal movements are not often associated with resolution of the patient's clinical problem. At present, no standard criteria have been established for identifying potential candidates for biofeedback training or for performing such training. The speech pathologist would be hard pressed to predict with any precision the response of individual patients to biofeedback treatments.

If biofeedback is to be useful, it must be used with techniques capable of establishing skilled patterns of opening and closing the velopharyngeal port during connected speech. Unless normal velopharyngeal function in automatic speech is achieved, the patient will continue to have disordered speech. Even if the size of the velopharyngeal opening is reduced, an opening large enough to impair speech may remain.

As indicated earlier, another objective of biofeedback may be to increase range of motion of the velopharyngeal structures to enhance the patient's response to some other treatment such as a pharyngeal flap (Cole, 1979; McGrath and Anderson, 1990). Although intuitively appealing, there are no reported data to support the contention that increasing velopharyngeal movements improves the long-term surgical result.

A number of variables should be considered in further development and evaluation of biofeedback methods. For example, the way in which biofeedback information is presented to the patient may influence treatment effectiveness. Yates (1980) wrote that feedback may be presented continuously or noncontinuously, during a trial or at the end of a trial. The information may be binary, or it may reflect gradations of performance. The choice of a response unit for use in therapy is an important consideration. Should feedback monitoring use nonspeech activities, words, sentences, or something else? If possible, response units should be chosen that do not trigger old, unwanted responses. These variables have not been studied relative to velopharyngeal function training.

Choices about feedback mode must also be made. The literature reviewed earlier does not offer clear guidance regarding choice of feedback display for teaching velopharyngeal function. Some authors appear to assume that direct observation of the velopharyngeal mechanism with a nasopharyngoscope is necessarily the form of feedback most likely to be effective. However, Hixon (1990) has suggested that a display reflecting a parameter controlled by the velopharyngeal mechanism, such as resistance or air flow, might be more effective than display of the structures themselves or electrical activity of the muscles. We suspect that different modes of biofeedback are not mutually substitutable for use in rehabilitation of the cleft palate patient.

As indicated earlier, duration of therapy may also be an important treatment variable. Shprintzen, McCall, and Skolnick (1975) and Miyazaki et al. (1974) reported success in treatment periods ranging from roughly 3 to 6 months. Reports of increased velopharyngeal motion with obturator reduction have involved even longer periods of time. As a rough rule of thumb, we might expect biofeedback to be effective within a 6-month period, if at all. However, investigators might consider use of longer study periods.

Finally, there are important choices to be made in patient selection for biofeedback therapy. Patients who demonstrate inconsistent velopharyngeal closure would appear to be the best candidates because they demonstrate the ability to close the velopharyngeal port at times. The nature of the inconsistency (e.g., velopharyngeal timing problem), however, may limit a patient's ability to generalize closure achieved during one task/sound to others. Still less certain, on the basis of current knowledge, is whether patients with consistent borderline velopharyngeal inadequacy can be expected to benefit. Ruscello (1997) considered subject selection the primary factor limiting research in treatment of velopharyngeal inadequacy. He recommended that future research address subject variables that may influence response to treatment (e.g., potential for velopharyngeal closure) and advised investigators to strive to understand the mechanisms involved in subject response to such therapy.

SUMMARY

Children with cleft palate require surgical and dental management to establish a mechanism that is adequate for normal speech production. For some children, these treatments alone are sufficient and normal speech develops; other children demonstrate disordered speech. As a group, these children can be expected to exhibit a wide range of speech production problems and thus require different types of intervention. Even children who produce speech characteristics that are seemingly identical (e.g., audible nasal emission) may have very different etiological components and require totally different management. The goals and procedures of therapy for children who demonstrate developmental errors are no different than those used with noncleft children. Children with cleft palate who demonstrate articulation or resonance problems associated with velopharyngeal inadequacy may require both behavioral and surgical management to establish normal speech production. The goal of speech therapy for these children should be to establish appropriate articulatory placements. Establishing normal resonance for a child who demonstrates severe hypernasality and audible nasal emission because of velopharyngeal inadequacy is an appropriate surgical goal. Efforts to eliminate excessive nasalization of speech using behavioral strategies should only be attempted on a trial basis when the adequacy of the velopharyngeal mechanism is questioned or a patient demonstrates borderline inadequacy.

Clinical research and clinical reports suggest that strategies such as CPAP therapy and biofeedback hold promise as treatment options for select patients. Unfortunately, the data are not compelling enough at this time to justify routine application of any one of these procedures. Some patients appear to improve their velopharyngeal function with these procedures; however, the degree of improvement for many is not great enough to avoid the need for surgical management. Additional study is needed to determine who the appropriate treatment candidates are. Because we cannot always be certain that an individual patient is making the best possible use of the speech mechanism, there is no precise way to distinguish between those who might acquire adequate use of the velopharyngeal mechanism through training and those who cannot. Individuals who sometimes close the velopharyngeal port during speech or during blowing or whistling would appear to be the most likely candidates for velopharyngeal valving therapy. However, even they may differ from each other in the extent to which they achieve closure and will surely differ in their prognoses for response to training. Until additional research is carried out, we remain skeptical about the benefits of therapy directed at improving velopharyngeal valving for speech.

REFERENCES

Albery L: Approaches to the treatment of speech problems. In Stengelhofen J (ed.): *Cleft palate: the nature and remediation of communication problems.* Edinburgh: Churchill Livingston, 1989.

Albery L, and Enderby P: Intensive speech therapy for cleft palate children. *British Journal of Disorders of Communication* 19:115-124, 1984.

Albery L, and Russell J: *Cleft palate sourcebook.* Bicester: Winslow Press Limited, 1994.

Blakeley RW, and Brockman JH: Normal speech and hearing by age 5 as a goal for children with cleft palate: a demonstration project. *American Journal of Speech-Language Pathology* 4:25-32, 1995.

Bleile K, and Miller S: Articulation and phonological disorders in toddlers with medical needs. In Bernthal J (ed.): *Articulatory and phonological disorders in special populations.* New York: Thieme, 1993.

Boone DR, and McFarlane SC: *The voice and voice therapy.* Englewood Cliffs (NJ): Prentice-Hall, 1994.

Broen PA, Doyle SS, and Bacon CK: The velopharyngeally inadequate child: phonologic change with intervention. *Cleft Palate–Craniofacial Journal* 30:500-507, 1993.

Burrell K: The modification of nasality using nasometer feedback [thesis]. Minneapolis: University of Minnesota, 1989.

Bzoch KR: Rationale, methods, and techniques of cleft palate speech therapy. In Bzoch KR (ed.): *Communicative disorders related to cleft lip and palate.* Austin: Pro-Ed, 1997a.

Bzoch KR: Clinical assessment, evaluation, and management of 11 categorical aspects of cleft palate speech disorders. In Bzoch KR (ed.): *Communicative disorders related to cleft lip and palate.* Austin: Pro-Ed, 1997b.

Chisum L, Shelton RL, Arndt WB, and Elbert M: The relationship between remedial speech instruction activities and articulation change. *Cleft Palate Journal* 6:57-64, 1969.

Cole RM: Direct muscle training for the improvement of velopharyngeal activity. In Bzoch KR (ed.): *Communicative disorders related to cleft lip and palate.* 2nd ed. Boston: Little, Brown, 1979.

Coston GN: Therapeutic management of speech disorders associated with velopharyngeal inadequacy. *Journal Childhood Communication Disorders* 10:75-85, 1986.

D'Antonio LL: An investigation of speech timing in individuals with cleft palate [dissertation]. San Francisco: University of California, 1982.

Dalston RM: Communication skills of children with cleft lip and palate: a status report. In Bardach J, and Morris HL (eds.): *Multidisciplinary management of cleft lip and palate.* Philadelphia: WB Saunders, 1990.

Dalston RM: The use of nasometry in the assessment and remediation of velopharyngeal inadequacy. In Bzoch KR (ed.): *Communicative disorders related to cleft lip and palate.* Austin: Pro-Ed, 1997.

Dalston RM, and Keefe MJ: The use of a microcomputer in monitoring and modifying velopharyngeal movements. *Journal of Computer Users in Speech and Hearing* 3:159-169, 1987.

Davis SM, and Drichta CE: Biofeedback: theory and application to speech pathology. In Lass NJ (ed.): *Speech and language: advances in basic research and practice.* Volume 3. New York: Academic Press, 1980.

Fletcher SG: Contingencies for bioelectric modification of nasality. *Journal of Speech and Hearing Disorders* 37:329-346, 1972.

Fletcher SG: *Diagnosing speech disorders from cleft palate.* New York: Grune and Stratton, 1978.

Fletcher SG: Palatometric specification of stops, affricate, and sibilant sounds. *Journal of Speech and Hearing Research* 32:736-748, 1989.

Fletcher SG, McCutcheon MJ, and Wolf MB: Dynamic palatometry. *Journal of Speech and Hearing Research* 18:812-819, 1975.

Gibbon F, Stewart F, Hardcastle WJ, and Crampin L: Widening access to electropalatography for children with persistent sound system disorders. *American Journal of Speech-Language Pathology* 8:319-334, 1999.

Golding-Kushner K: The effect of articulation therapy on velopharyngeal closure. Proceedings of the Fourth International Congress on Cleft Palate and Related Craniofacial Anomalies, Acapulco, Mexico, 1981.

Golding-Kushner KJ: Treatment of articulation and resonance disorders associated with cleft palate and VPI. In Shprintzen RJ, and Bardach J (eds.): *Cleft palate speech management: a multidisciplinary approach.* St. Louis: Mosby, 1995.

Grames LM, Marsh JF, Pilgram T, Muntz HR, and Karzon RK: Speech therapy outcome and duration in children with cleft lip and palate. Poster presentation, proceedings of the American Cleft Palate–Craniofacial Association annual meeting, Scottsdale, 1999.

Hahn E: Directed home stimulation program for infants with cleft lip and palate. In Bzoch KR (ed.): *Communicative disorders related to cleft lip and palate.* 3rd ed. Boston: Little, Brown, 1989.

Hardcastle W, Barry RM, and Nunn M: Instrumental articulatory phonetics in assessment and remediation: case studies with the electropalatograph. In Stengelhofen J (ed.): *Cleft palate: the nature and remediation of communication problems.* New York: Churchill Livingstone, 1989.

Hardin MA: Cleft palate: intervention. *Clinics in Communication Disorders* 1:12-18, 1991.

Hardin-Jones MA, and Jones DL: Age at palatoplasty and speech in children with cleft palate. Poster presentation, proceedings of the American Speech-Language-Hearing Association annual convention, Boston, 1997.

Harrison RJ: A demonstration project of speech training for the preschool cleft palate child: final report. Project No. 6-1167, grant No. OEG-2-6-061101-1553. US Office of Education, Bureau of the Handicapped, HEW, 1969.

Henningsson GE, and Isberg AM: Velopharyngeal movement patterns in patients alternating between oral and glottal articulations: a clinical and cine radiological study. *Cleft Palate Journal* 23:1-9, 1986.

Hixon TJ: Personal communication, 1990.

Hoch L, Golding-Kushner K, Siegel-Sadewitz VL, and Shprintzen RJ: Speech therapy. *Seminars in Speech and Language* 7:313-326, 1986.

Jones DL, and Folkins JW: Effect of speaking rate on judgments of disordered speech in children with cleft palate. *Cleft Palate Journal* 22:246-252, 1985.

Jones DL, Folkins JW, and Morris HL: Speech production time and judgments of disordered nasalization in speakers with cleft palate. *Journal of Speech and Hearing Research* 33:458-466, 1990.

Kantner CE: Four devices in the treatment of rhinolalia aperta. *Journal of Speech and Hearing Disorders* 2:73-76, 1937.

Kantner CE: The rationale of blowing exercises for patients with repaired cleft palates. *Journal of Speech Disorders* 12:281-286, 1947.

Kantner CE: Diagnosis and prognosis in cleft palate speech. *Journal of Speech and Hearing Disorders* 13:211-222, 1948.

Kuehn DP: New therapy for treating hypernasal speech using continuous positive airway pressure (CPAP). *Plastic and Reconstructive Surgery* 88:959-966, 1991.

Kuehn DP, Imrey PB, Tomes L, Jones DL, O'Gara MM, Seaver EJ, Smith BE, Van Demark DR, and Wachtel JM: Efficacy of continuous positive airway pressure (CPAP) in the treatment of hypernasality. Paper presented at the annual meeting of the American Cleft Palate Association, Atlanta, 2000.

Kuehn DP, and Moon JB: Levator veli palatini muscle activity in relation to intraoral air pressure variation. *Journal of Speech and Hearing Research* 37:1260-1270, 1994.

Kuehn DP, Moon JB, and Folkins JW: Levator veli palatini muscle activity in relation to intranasal air pressure variation. *Cleft Palate–Craniofacial Journal* 30:361-368, 1993.

Kummer A, and Lee L: Evaluation and treatment of resonance disorders. *Language Speech and Hearing Services in Schools* 27:271-281, 1996.

Lang M: Program for the elimination of hypernasality. Unpublished manuscript, Kent State University, 1974.

Lubit EC, and Larsen RE: The Lubit palatal exerciser: a preliminary report. *Cleft Palate Journal* 6:120-133, 1969.

Lubit EC, and Larsen RE: A speech aid for velopharyngeal incompetency. *Journal of Speech and Hearing Disorders* 36:61-70, 1971.

Lynch JI, Brookshire BL, and Fox DR: *A curriculum for infants and toddlers with cleft palate: developing speech and language.* Austin: Pro-Ed, 1993.

Masland MW: Testing and correcting cleft palate speech. *Journal of Speech and Hearing Disorders* 11:309-314, 1946.

Massengill R Jr, Quinn GW, Pickerell KL, and Levinson C: Therapeutic exercise and velopharyngeal gap. *Cleft Palate Journal* 5:44-47, 1968.

McDonald ET, and Koepp-Baker H: Cleft palate speech: an integration of research and clinical observation. *Journal of Speech and Hearing Disorders* 16:9-20, 1951.

McGrath CO, and Anderson MW: Prosthetic treatment of velopharyngeal incompetence. In Bardach J, and Morris HL (eds.): *Multidisciplinary management of cleft lip and palate.* Philadelphia: WB Saunders, 1990.

Michi K, Suzuki N, Yamashita Y, and Imai S: Visual training and correction of articulation disorders by use of dynamic palatography: serial observation in a case of cleft palate. *Journal of Speech and Hearing Disorders* 51:226-238, 1986.

Miyazaki T, Matsuya T, Yamaoka M, and Nishio J: *A nasopharyngeal fiberscope (film).* Boston: American Cleft Palate Association, 1974.

Moller KT, Path M, Werth LJ, and Christiansen RL: The modification of velar movement. *Journal of Speech and Hearing Disorders* 38:323, 1973.

Moore WH, and Sommers RK: Phonetic contexts: their effects on perceived nasality in cleft palate speakers. *Cleft Palate Journal* 10:72-83, 1973.

Moore WK, and Sommers RK: Phonetic contexts: their effects on perceived intelligibility in cleft palate speakers. *Folia Phoniatrica* 27:410-422, 1975.

Morley ME: *Cleft palate and speech.* 7th ed. Baltimore: Williams & Wilkins, 1970.

Morris HL: Cleft palate. In Weston AJ (ed.): *Communicative disorders.* Springfield (IL): CC Thomas, 1972.

Moser HM: Diagnostic and clinical procedures in rhinolalia. *Journal of Speech and Hearing Disorders* 7:1-4, 1942.

Nishio J, Yamaoka M, Matsuya T, and Miyazaki T: How to exercise the velopharyngeal movement by the velopharyngeal fiberscope. *Japanese Journal of Oral Surgery* 20:450, 1974. Abstracted in *Cleft Palate Journal* 13:310, 1976.

Paul R: *Language disorders from infancy through adolescence: assessment and intervention.* St. Louis: Mosby, 1995.

Peterson SJ: Electrical stimulation of the soft palate. *Cleft Palate Journal* 11:72-86, 1974.

Peterson-Falzone SJ: Resonance disorders in structural defects. In Lass NJ, McReynolds LV, Northern JL, and Yoder DE (eds.): *Speech, language, and hearing.* Vol 2. Philadelphia: WB Saunders, 1982.

Peterson-Falzone SJ: Speech disorders related to structural defects: part 1. In Lass NJ, McReynolds LV, Northern JL, and Yoder DE (eds.): *Handbook of speech-language pathology and audiology.* Philadelphia: Decker, 1988.

Philips BJ, and Harrison RJ: Articulation patterns of preschool cleft palate children. *Cleft Palate Journal* 6:245-253, 1969.

Powers GL, and Starr CD: The effects of muscle exercises on velopharyngeal gap and nasality. *Cleft Palate Journal* 11:28-35, 1974.

Prins D, and Bloomer HH: A word intelligibility approach to the study of speech change in oral cleft patients. *Cleft Palate Journal* 2:357-368, 1965.

Ray B, and Baker BM: *Hypernasality modification program: a systematic approach.* Tucson: Communication Skill Builders, 1990.

Riski JE: Functional velopharyngeal incompetence: diagnosis and management. In Winitz H (ed.): *Treating articulation disorders: for clinicians by clinicians.* Baltimore. University Park Press, 1984.

Ruscello DM: Considerations for behavioral treatment of velopharyngeal closure for speech. In Bzoch KR (ed.): *Communicative disorders related to cleft lip and palate.* 4th ed. Boston: Little, Brown, 1997.

Ruscello DM, Shuster LI, and Sandwisch A: Modification of context-specific nasal emission. *Journal of Speech and Hearing Research* 34:27-32, 1991.

Schendel LL, and Bzoch KR: Advantages of intensive summer training programs. In Bzoch KR (ed.): *Communicative disorders related to cleft lip and palate.* Boston: Little, Brown, 1970.

Scherer N: The speech and language status of toddlers with cleft lip and/or palate following early vocabulary intervention. *American Journal of Speech-Language Pathology* 8:81-93, 1999.

Selley WG, Zananiri M-C, Ellis RE, and Flack FC: The effect of tongue position on division of airflow in the presence of velopharyngeal defects. *British Journal of Plastic Surgery* 40:377-383, 1987.

Shelton RL, and Ruscello DM: Palatal and articulation training in patients with velopharyngeal closure problems. Proceedings of the annual meeting of the American Cleft Palate Association, San Diego, 1979.

Shelton RL, Hahn E, and Morris H: Diagnosis and therapy. In Spriestersbach DC, and Sherman D (eds.): *Cleft palate and communication.* New York: Academic Press, 1968.

Shelton RL, Beaumont K, Trier WC, and Furr ML: Videoendoscopic feedback in training velopharyngeal closure. *Cleft Palate Journal* 15:6-12, 1978.

Shelton RL, Chisum L, Youngstrom KA, Arndt WB, and Elbert M: Effect of articulation therapy on palatopharyngeal closure, movement of the pharyngeal wall, and tongue posture. *Cleft Palate Journal* 6:440-448, 1969.

Shelton RL, Lindquist AF, Chisum L, Arndt WB, Youngstrom KA, and Stick SL: Effect of prosthetic speech bulb reduction on articulation. *Cleft Palate Journal* 5:195-204, 1968.

Shelton RL, Paesani A, McClelland KD, and Bradfield SS: Panendoscopic feedback in the study of voluntary velopharyngeal movements. *Journal of Speech and Hearing Disorders* 40:232-244, 1975.

Shprintzen RJ: Surgery for speech: the planning of operations for velopharyngeal insufficiency with emphasis on the preoperative assessment of both pharyngeal physiology and articulation. Proceedings of the British Craniofacial Society, Manchester University Press, 1986.

Shprintzen RJ: Research revisited. *Cleft Palate Journal* 26:148, 1989.

Shprintzen R, McCall GM, and Skolnick L: A new therapeutic technique for the treatment of velopharyngeal incompetence. *Journal of Speech and Hearing Disorders* 40:69-83, 1975.

Siegel-Sadewitz VL, and Shprintzen RJ: Nasopharyngoscopy of the normal velopharyngeal sphincter: an experiment of biofeedback. *Cleft Palate Journal* 19:194-200, 1982.

Sommers RK: *Articulation disorders.* Englewood Cliffs (NJ): Prentice-Hall, 1983.

Starr CD: Treatment by therapeutic exercises. In Bardach J, and Morris HL (eds.): *Multidisciplinary management of cleft lip and palate.* Philadelphia: WB Saunders, 1990.

Starr CD: Behavioral approaches to treating velopharyngeal closure and nasality. In Moller KT, and Starr CD (eds.): *Cleft palate: interdisciplinary issues and treatment.* Austin: Pro-Ed, 1993.

Stengelhofen J: *Working with cleft palate.* Bicester: Winslow Press, 1990.

Stuffins GM: The use of appliances in the treatment of speech problems in cleft palate. In Stengelhofen J (ed.): *Cleft palate the nature and remediation of communication problems.* Edinburgh: Churchill Livingstone, 1989.

Tash EL, Shelton RL, Knox AW, and Michel JF: Training voluntary pharyngeal wall movements in children with normal and inadequate velopharyngeal closure. *Cleft Palate Journal* 8:277-290, 1971.

Tomes LA, Kuehn DP, and Peterson-Falzone SJ: Behavioral treatments of velopharyngeal impairment. In Bzoch KR (ed.): *Communicative disorders related to cleft lip and palate.* Austin: Pro-Ed, 1997.

Trost JE: Articulatory additions to the classical description of the speech of persons with cleft palate. *Cleft Palate Journal* 18:193-203, 1981.

Trost-Cardamone JE: The development of speech: cleft palate misarticulations. In Kernahan DE, and Rosenstein SW (eds.): *Cleft lip and palate: a system of management.* Baltimore: William & Wilkins, 1990.

Trost-Cardamone JE, and Bernthal JE: Articulation assessment procedures and treatment decisions. In Moller KT, and Starr CD (eds.): *Cleft palate: interdisciplinary issues and treatment.* Austin: Pro-Ed, 1993.

Trost-Cardamone JE: Diagnosis and management of speakers with craniofacial anomalies. Short course presented at the American Speech-Language-Hearing Association Annual Convention, Orlando (FL), 1995.

Tudor C, and Selley WG: A palatal training appliance and a visual aid for use in the treatment of hypernasal speech. *British Journal of Disorders of Communication* 9:117-122, 1974.

Van Demark DR: Some results of intensive speech therapy for children with cleft palate. *Cleft Palate Journal* 11:41-49, 1974.

Van Demark DR: Speech and voice therapy techniques for school-age and adult patients with remaining cleft palate speech disorders. In Bzoch KR (ed.): *Communicative disorders related to cleft lip and palate.* Austin: Pro-Ed, 1997.

Van Demark DR, and Hardin M: Effectiveness of intensive articulation therapy for children with cleft palate. *Cleft Palate Journal* 23:215-224, 1986.

Van Demark DR, and Hardin MA: Speech therapy for the child with cleft lip and palate. In Bardach J, and Morris HL (eds.): *Multidisciplinary management of cleft lip and palate.* Philadelphia: WB Saunders, 1990.

Weber J Jr, Jobe RP, and Chase RA: Evaluation of muscle stimulation in the rehabilitation of patients with hypernasal speech. *Plastic and Reconstructive Surgery* 46:173-174, 1970.

Whitehill TL, Stokes SF, and Yonnie MYH: Electropalatography treatment in an adult with late repair of cleft palate. *Cleft Palate–Craniofacial Journal* 33:160-168, 1996.

Witzel MA, Tobe J, and Salyer K: The use of nasopharyngoscopy biofeedback therapy in the correction of inconsistent velopharyngeal closure. *International Journal of Pediatric Otorhinolaryngology* 15:137-142, 1988.

Witzel MA, Tobe J, and Salyer KE: The use of videonasopharyngoscopy for biofeedback therapy in adults after pharyngeal flap surgery. *Cleft Palate Journal* 26:129-134, 1989.

Yamaoka M, Mastuya T, Miyazaki T, Nishio J, and Ibuki K: Visual training for velopharyngeal closure in cleft palate patients: a fiberscopic procedure (preliminary report). *Journal of Maxillofacial Surgery* 11:191-193, 1983.

Yates AI: *Biofeedback and the modification of behavior.* New York: Plenum Press, 1980.

Yules RB, and Chase RA: A training method for reduction of hypernasality in speech. *Plastic and Reconstructive Surgery* 43:180-185, 1969.

Yules RB, Welch J, Urbani J, and Elliott R: Untraining nasality. Proceedings of the annual meeting of the American Cleft Palate Association, Miami Beach, 1968.

Ysunza A, Pamplona C, and Toledo E: Change in velopharyngeal valving after speech therapy in cleft palate patients. *International Journal of Pediatric Otorhinolaryngology* 24:45-54, 1992.

Chapter 13

Physical Management of Velopharyngeal Inadequacy

When the initial palatoplasty does not provide adequate velopharyngeal closure, or when closure appears adequate for speech in early childhood but then changes to inadequate closure as a result of natural growth of the craniofacial skeleton or adenoid involution, the team needs to consider how best to reestablish good velopharyngeal function. The surgical approaches consist of augmentation of the velum itself (repositioning of velar muscles to increase velar length or improve the effectiveness of the muscular motion) and a variety of procedures for altering the position and the function of pharyngeal musculature. As in treatment of noncleft velopharyngeal inadequacy, the choice of surgical procedure is usually based on the appearance of the velopharyngeal port as seen on nasopharyngoscopic or radiographic studies; the same imaging is used in assessment of results (Albery et al., 1982; Crockett, Bumsted, and Van Demark, 1988; Peat et al., 1994; Pigott, 1974, 1979; Shprintzen, 1979; Shprintzen et al., 1979). The prosthetic approaches to this problem consist of obturators to cover palatal defects, palatal lifts, and obturators or "speech bulbs" to close off the velopharyngeal port during speech.

SURGICAL MANAGEMENT OF VELOPHARYNGEAL INADEQUACY

Velar Augmentation Procedures

As mentioned previously, many of the surgical maneuvers used in initial palatoplasties to produce a soft palate with maximum possible length or the closest approximation to normal muscle orientation are also used for those same purposes in patients for whom the first surgery did not produce the optimum result. Currently, these include intravelar veloplasty (levator reconstruction), various modifications of the V-Y pushback, and the Furlow Z-plasty, all described in Chapter 4 (Chen et al., 1994; Coston et al., 1986; D'Antonio, 1997; Furlow, 1994; Hudson et al., 1995; Kriens, 1970; Witt and D'Antonio, 1993). The Millard island flap was popular for a while as a secondary procedure in cleft palate surgery (Dijkstra, 1969; Hoge, 1966; Millard, 1962; Millard et al., 1970; Noordhoff, 1970) but is now rarely mentioned in the surgical literature. Pigott (1987) designed what he called a "fish flip flap" that was also an attempt to create a "normal velar knee" or eminence of the musculus uvulae, but a follow-up study of his patients (Peat et al., 1994) revealed only a 50% success rate, and he ceased recommending it. Pigott's experience with this procedure is a good reminder of the necessity of *long-term* follow-up of patients.

Several clinical researchers using the Furlow Z-plasty as a secondary procedure have attempted to measure the preoperative velopharyngeal deficit with the goal being to estimate the maximum velopharyngeal gap size that this procedure may be expected to "cure" (Fig. 13-1). Lindsey and Davis (1996) stated that gaps of 6 to 8 mm could be corrected by the Z-plasty, but they had operated on only four cases. Chen et al. (1994) felt that the Furlow procedure was best recommended for cases with velopharyngeal gaps of 5 mm or less. One study found that patients could gain as much as 10 mm in velar length from the Z-plasty (Peterson-Falzone et al., 1997), but of course the full length of the velum is not an indication of the effective length (posterior nasal spine to the velar eminence) in speech. Furlow (1997) commented that his double opposing Z-plasty was successful because it "construct[ed] a functioning palatal muscle sling," not just because it lengthened the velum.

The advantage of all the velar augmentation procedures is that, when they work, they do so by approximating or reproducing the velopharyngeal physiology that would have been in place if the cleft had not occurred. In contrast, most forms of pharyngoplasty—particularly centrally placed pharyngeal flaps—attempt to achieve closure by mechanisms that are not as physiologically natural. In addition, if a velar augmentation procedure does not achieve the

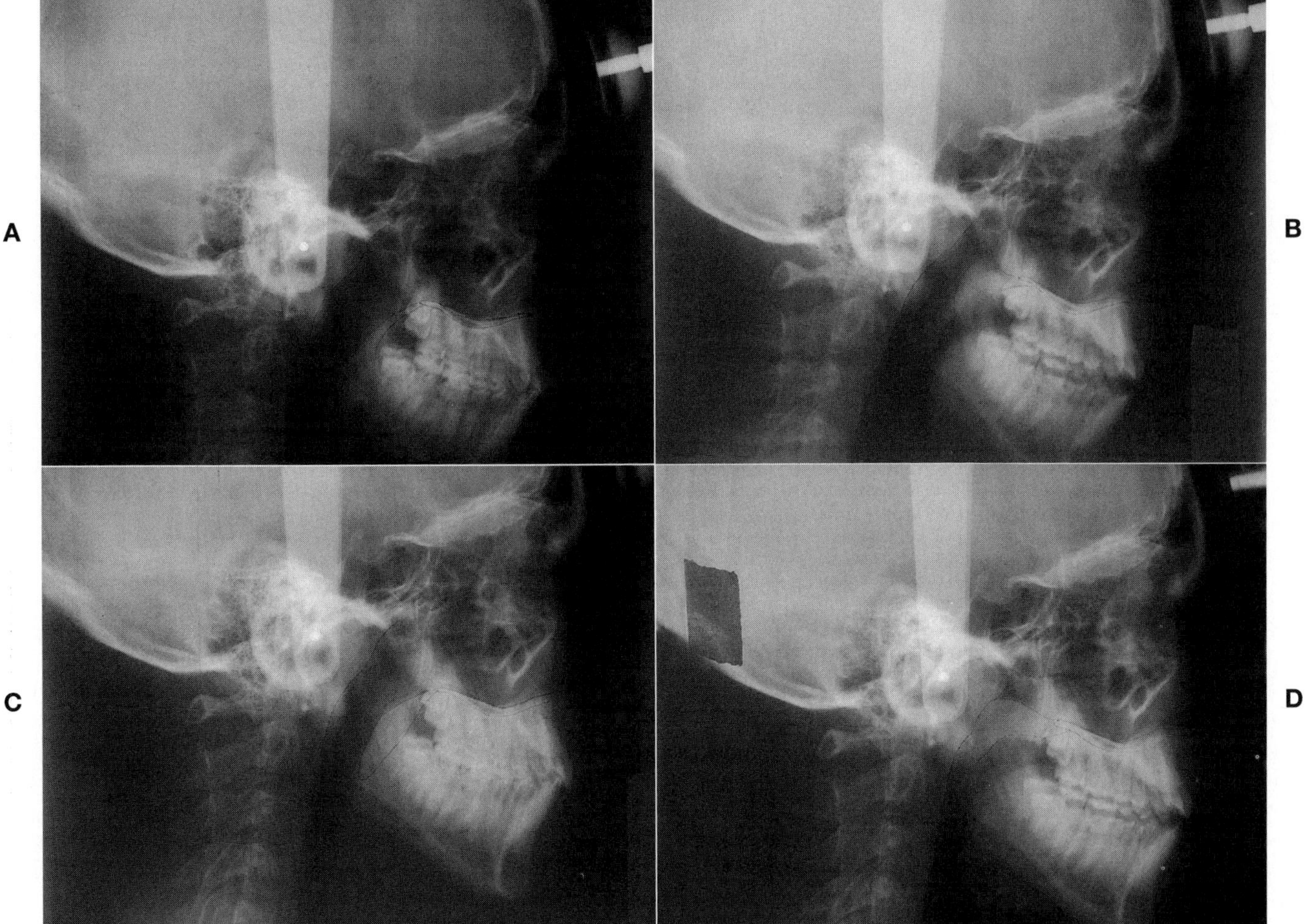

Figure 13-1 Increase in the length and thickness of the soft palate (compare **A** with **C**) and improvement in contact of the velum with the posterior pharyngeal wall during production of a sustained fricative (compare **B** with **D**) in a patient who underwent a Furlow double-reversing Z-plasty.

desired result, the surgeon and team have the option of trying a structural rearrangement of the pharyngeal musculature, as discussed in the following section.

Pharyngeal Flap

In terms of the history of secondary velopharyngeal surgery, centrally placed[1] pharyngeal flaps have the longest standing and thus the greatest cumulative number of patients. The first pharyngeal flap was an inferiorly based design by Schoenborn in 1876 (see Bernstein, 1967). In 1886, Schoenborn published a superiorly based version. Sanvenero-Roselli (1934) also designed a superiorly based flap, and by the 1950s this started to become the most common approach to velopharyngeal inadequacies. Superiorly based flaps (Fig. 13-2) have been used in the majority of clinical reports, but in the 1970s there was a revival of interest in inferiorly based flaps (Fig. 13-3), which are technically easier for the surgeon to perform but limited in the size of velopharyngeal opening that can be covered in comparison with superiorly based flaps (Randall et al., 1978; Whitaker et al., 1972). There has been a steady flow of studies on these two operations and their variations (Albery et al., 1982; Bernstein, 1967, 1975; Brondsted et al., 1984; Buchholz et al., 1967; Crockett, Bumsted, and Van Demark, 1988; Dibbell et al., 1965; Dixon, Bzoch, and Habal, 1979; Engstrom, Fritzell, and Johanson, 1970; Honig, 1967; Isshiki and Morimoto, 1975; Johns et al., 1994; Marsh and Wray, 1980; McCoy and Zahorsky, 1972; Morris and Spriestersbach, 1967; Morris et al., 1995; Peat et al., 1994; Pensler and Reich, 1991; Pigott, 1974, 1979; Sadove and Eppley, 1996; Seyfer, Prohazka, and Leahy, 1988; Shprintzen, 1979; Shprintzen, McCall, and Skolnick, 1980; Shprintzen et al., 1979; Skoog, 1965; Trier, 1994; Van Demark and Hardin, 1985; Yules and Chase, 1969; Zwitman, 1982).

The endoscopic studies of Pigott (Pigott, Bensen, and White, 1969; Pigott, 1974, 1979) and later of Shprintzen

[1]Meaning in the midsagittal plane, in the middle of the velopharyngeal port.

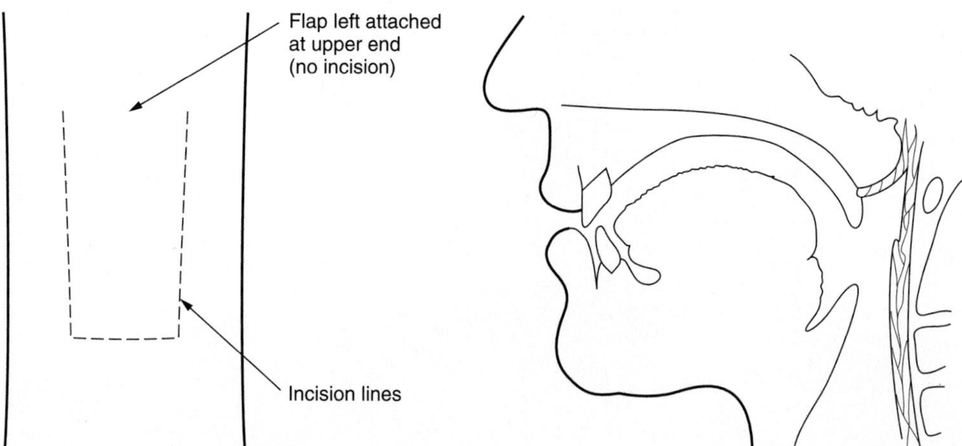

Figure 13-2 How a superiorly based pharyngeal flap is outlined by the surgeon on the posterior pharyngeal wall. The incisions are made on the left, right, and bottom, leaving the flap attached to the posterior pharyngeal wall on the top.

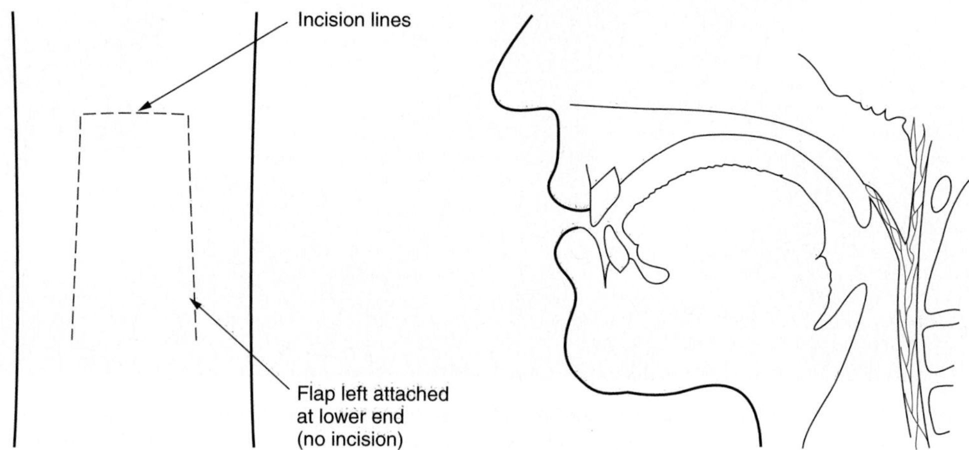

Figure 13-3 For an inferiorly based pharyngeal flap, the incisions are made on the left, right, and top, leaving the flap attached to the posterior pharyngeal wall at the bottom.

et al. (1979), together with multiview videofluorographic studies (Argamaso et al., 1980; Skolnick and McCall, 1972, 1973), revolutionized treatment decisions (e.g., what type of pharyngeal flap to perform) and methods for assessing surgical outcome. Earlier reports had demonstrated that flaps were essentially tissue obturators, not structures that were active in closing the velopharyngeal port as had once been postulated.[2] Morris and Spriestersbach (1967), for example, reported that a good speech result from a flap was dependent on either mesial movement of the lateral pharyngeal walls or superoposterior movement of the flap (the latter being a result of the movement of the velum, not of the flap), and that the mesial movement of the lateral walls was a more accurate predictor of success of the operation. The same conclusion was reached by other clinicians studying pharyngeal flaps (Kelsey et al., 1972). Fig. 13-4 shows the lateral walls and a centrally placed flap at rest and during speech production, as viewed endoscopically.

The width of a pharyngeal flap is ultimately dependent not only on how broad a flap is designed on the posterior pharyngeal wall, but also to some extent on how it is sutured into the soft palate and how well the raw surface is lined with mucosa (after flap insertion) to minimize postoperative shrinkage or "tubing." The flap may be sutured to the upper surface of the velum, interposed into the velum through a sagittal slit (midline cut), or interposed

[2]Kapetansky (1975) designed what he called "a dynamic repair for velopharyngeal insufficiency" using "bilateral transverse pharyngeal flaps." This was actually just a way of raising two pedicles from an S-shaped incision in the pharyngeal wall and transposing them into the posterior of the soft palate, with one flap on the oral surface of the velum and the other on the nasal surface. The result was a midline bridgelike structure between the posterior pharyngeal wall and the velum, and subsequent endoscopic assessment of his patients revealed that it was not the flap itself that was "dynamic." Rather, as with other midline pharyngeal flaps, closure was dependent on mesial movement of the lateral pharyngeal walls (Kapetansky, 1990). Thus, Kapetansky's flaps were neither bilateral nor dynamic.

into a longitudinal (horizontal) incision in the posterior border of the velum.

Shprintzen et al. (1979) used endoscopic and multiview videofluorographic information to select the specific type of pharyngeal flap to be used for patients, greatly improving their success rates in comparison to random assignment of patients to procedures.[3] Flaps could be "tailored" (preselected) to be wide, medium, or rather thin (see the article for the surgical details). In addition, the site of base of the flap on the posterior pharyngeal wall could be selected on the basis of the vertical level of greatest lateral pharyngeal wall motion. (The insertion site of the flap can migrate inferiorly over time as a result of contracture, particularly if the raw surface of the flap is not lined with mucosa at the time of surgery. Scarring and contracture also means the flap will become narrower as it heals, and Shprintzen et al. [1979] purposefully selected a procedure that would end up as a narrower "obturator" when the velopharyngeal gap as seen on endoscopy or base-view videofluoroscopy was small.) When movement toward velopharyngeal closure was asymmetrical, as it often is in patients with hemifacial microsomia, the site of insertion could be altered accordingly (Shprintzen et al., 1980).[4,5]

Two companion papers on the width of centrally placed pharyngeal flaps at rest and in speech and on the postoperative effects of that width on pharyngeal wall movement toward the flap recently expanded substantially on earlier studies (Karling et al., 1999a, 1999b) but also partially refuted those studies. As in the Shprintzen et al. study of 1979, the type of procedure was selected to fit what the clinicians saw on preoperative endoscopic and videofluorographic studies. If they saw little inward movement of the lateral pharyngeal walls preoperatively, they used a type of pharyngeal flap insertion (into a transverse or sandwich-type opening cut along the posterior edge of the velum) that presumably would result in a wider flap. If they saw good inward movement of the pharyngeal walls on imaging studies, they used a "midline split" of the velum to provide the housing for the flap. They tried to protect their study from the other factors they knew could affect pharyngeal wall movement, including oronasal fistulae, predominant glottal articulations, large tonsils, and neurological deficiencies or "mental handicaps." The postoperative evaluations were no less than 1 year after the procedure. The authors found that (1) the method of insertion of the flap did not affect width at rest but did affect width during speech, in that the transverse flaps widened but the flaps inserted in the midline did not and that (2) the narrower "midline-split" insertion flaps resulted in a subsequent increase in medial pharyngeal wall motion to meet the flap, whereas the pharyngeal wall motion decreased after the placement of a wider flap. The authors felt that the decrease was caused by the flap forming an obstacle to medial motion and that the conflicting results of Shprintzen, McCall, and Skolnick (1980) might have been attributable to the fact that the earlier study did not attempt to relate the amount of movement in the pharyngeal walls *after* the flap to the amount of movement required for them to meet the flap

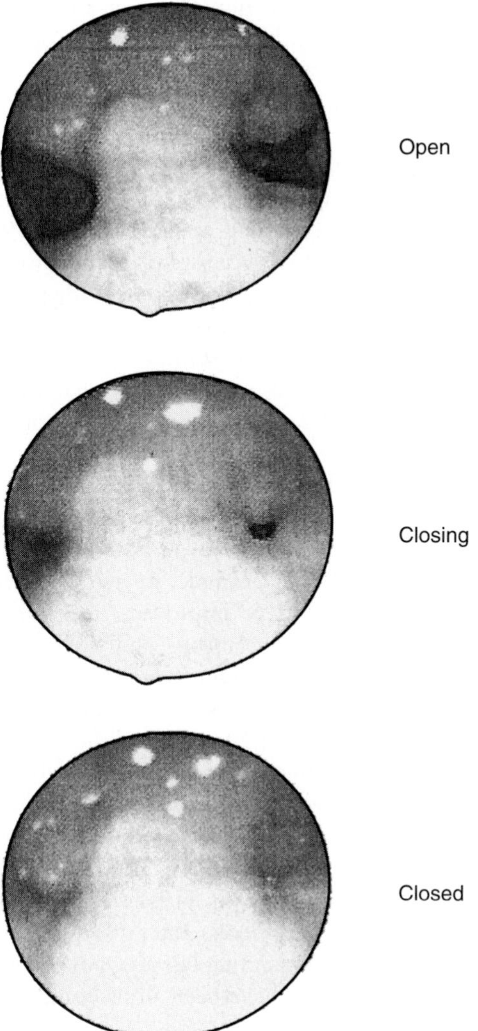

Figure 13-4 Endoscopic view of a centrally placed pharyngeal flap, with open ports on each side that are closed, during speech, by inward movement of the lateral pharyngeal walls.

[3]Shprintzen, McCall, and Skolnick (1980) also showed that the amount of movement in the lateral pharyngeal walls could increase or decrease after pharyngeal flap surgery, presumably due at least in part to the width of the flap.

[4]Witzel and Stringer (1990) recommended adding the Waters view and the Towne's view to videofluoroscopic studies when the adenoids or the tonsils might be blocking a portion of the view of the velopharyngeal system: the Waters view is essentially a slanted view from above (sneaking past the adenoid pad), and the Towne view is a slanted view from below (sneaking past the tonsils). See the article for a schematic of how these views are obtained.

[5]An additional concern in the planning of any surgery involving incisions on the posterior pharyngeal wall is the abnormal course of the carotid arteries in patients with velocardiofacial syndrome, which is the most common syndrome of clefting. Diagnostic imaging of the arteries (e.g., by magnetic resonance imaging scans) should be done before surgery in all patients with velocardiofacial syndrome (Mitnick et al., 1996).

and seal the ports. They noted that if the majority of patients in their study had a combination of moderate preoperative lateral wall activity and a wide flap, no significant change in adduction would be expected, which would explain the finding of predominantly consistent lateral wall activity in the preoperative versus postoperative comparisons. Although it was not the main point of the companion studies of Karling et al. (1999a, 1999b), it is worth noting that their success rate in bringing "speech resonance" up to either a normal or "adequate" level was 92%.

It is difficult to compare studies or to draw general conclusions about success rates with pharyngeal flaps because the reported rates have varied as much with the stringency of the clinicians' criteria for success as with any other factor (type of patients, specific type of flap, length of follow-up, etc.). Too many authors have used only vague categories of speech outcome (e.g., "normal" versus "improved" speech). For example, Seyfer, Prohazka, and Leahy (1988) reported 92% "improved" speech in patients receiving primary pharyngeal flaps and 90% in patients receiving secondary flaps. Although success rates of 90% or higher would seem to be impressive, they operated on only 39 patients over a period of 10 years, and their test for nasal emission consisted of fogging of a mirror held beneath the nares. Most reports over the last few decades have indicated pharyngeal flap success rates somewhere between 60% and 100%, if these numbers are even meaningful in view of all the known and unknown pitfalls in drawing such conclusions. In general, success rates have gone *up* as a result of better surgical planning but *down* in proportion to how stringent clinicians have been in assessing their own results.

In many reports, patients with hyponasal speech postoperatively were included in the groups with desirable outcomes. Hyponasality and other signs of airway obstruction in the immediate postoperative period after a pharyngeal flap are not unusual because of the effects of edema (Crockett, Bumsted, and Van Demark, 1988; Graham et al., 1973; Lesavoy et al., 1996; Morris and Spriestersbach, 1967). This is one reason why judgments about outcome should not be made in the first few weeks after surgery. In fact, Lesavoy et al. (1996) reported that patients who showed signs of airway obstruction immediately after surgery were more apt to have a good speech result in the long term. However, persistent hyponasality is not desirable, particularly if it is accompanied by persistence of other symptoms indicating an obstructed airway (e.g., oronasal breathing with a constant mouth-open posture, snoring, reduced exercise tolerance, daytime sleepiness, interrupted nighttime breathing in the supine position). In a recent study by Morris et al. (1995), more than 89% of patients who had had pharyngeal flaps snored. This is not as benign a symptom as one might initially assume because snoring may be one indicator of the presence of sleep apnea.

Hyponasality and other signs of airway obstruction were particularly frequent in reports on primary pharyngeal flaps and on the "lateral port control" flaps (Hogan, 1973, 1975; Hogan and Schwartz, 1977). In the case of primary pharyngeal flaps, it is possible that the airway became increasingly obstructed as the adenoid pad grew. Another possibility is that this early attachment of the velum to the posterior pharyngeal wall interfered with the normal downward-and-forward growth of the face, thus restricting the size of the upper airway. The "LPC" flap was constructed so as to leave lateral ports the size of catheters totaling 0.20 cm^2 in cross-sectional area, leaving the catheters in place until the tissue healed. The 0.20 cm^2 was based on Warren's aerodynamic data indicating that a velopharyngeal opening greater than this number would result in the perceptual stigmata of inadequate closure for speech (see Chapter 10 for a review of aerodynamic assessments of velopharyngeal closure). However, subsequent reports indicated a disturbingly high incidence of airway obstruction, indicating either that further tissue contracture was taking place after the catheters were removed or that a space of 0.20 cm^2 was not a large enough airway for normal resonance balance in some speakers. The "LPC" flap is not as popular as it was when first reported, and, as indicated earlier, primary flaps decreased in popularity as palatoplasty techniques expanded and improved in ability to provide good velopharyngeal function without pharyngeal flaps.

Reports of persistent airway obstruction, including obstructive sleep apnea in some patients, have grown in number as more clinicians have become aware of the possible dangers (Ruddy, Stokes, and Pearman, 1991; Shprintzen, 1988; Shprintzen et al., 1992; Sirois et al., 1994; Ysunza et al., 1993). Of particular concern in this regard are patients with abnormally crowded upper airways such as found in Robin sequence (Abramson, Marrinan, and Mulliken, 1997; Shprintzen, 1988; Shprintzen et al., 1992; Thurston et al., 1980) or patients with neurologic problems (Cadieux et al., 1984.) In all the reports on potential complications after pharyngeal flaps or other types of pharyngoplasty, concerns about the upper airway have matched or exceeded concerns about persistent speech problems. Most surgeons and teams have had some patients in whom it was necessary to completely remove the flap, even if it meant a relapse into velopharyngeal inadequacy: breathing is more important than speech.

The relationship between pharyngeal flaps and other sources of possible airway obstruction deserves special consideration, particularly in growing children. You will remember that the adenoid pad may be helpful in providing "velopharyngeal" closure when the velum is foreshortened. However, the pad may still be increasing in size after a flap is performed, adding to obstruction of the airway. Thus, when clinicians are attempting to document the effect of a flap on speech or on growth (see below), they may not be studying the effect of the flap alone. Tonsils may also serve as a source of obstruction, particularly of the lateral ports on each side of a flap (Shprintzen, 1988). Reath, LaRossa, and Randall (1987) recommended removing the tonsils at the time of flap surgery, a recommendation that stimulated a vehement response directed to the points that (1) removal of the tonsils alone may be all that is necessary in treating velopharyngeal inadequacy if they are mechanically in the way of velar movement and (2) simultaneous tonsillectomy and pharyngeal flap could result in unnecessary complications such as excessive edema, scarring, and bleeding (Argamaso et al., 1988).

In attempts to "re-do" pharyngeal flaps that either failed to eliminate velopharyngeal inadequacy or resulted in an overcorrection with hyponasality and an obstructed airway, good results have been difficult to obtain (Barot, Cohen, and LaRossa, 1986; Cosman and Falk, 1975; Friedman et al., 1992; Hirshowitz and Bar-David, 1976; Hoffman, 1985; Owsley and Chierici, 1976; Owsley, Creech, and Dedo, 1972). Barot, Cohen, and LaRossa (1986) and Hoffman (1985) both offered techniques for trying to enlarge lateral ports that had stenosed, causing airway obstruction, but neither gave objective speech data. Caouette-Laberge et al. (1992) divided the flap at its base in eight cases, but the flap readhered in five. Speech results were mixed: Some patients had normal resonance; some were still hyponasal; and some, hypernasal (the speech results are difficult to follow in the article because the numbers of patients are inconsistent in the postoperative clinical evaluations). When velopharyngeal inadequacy persists after a flap and surgeons try to improve speech by transposing additional tissue into the lateral ports or by taking down the old flap and replacing it with a larger one, there is the danger of more scar tissue and stenosis. Owsley and Chierici (1976) stated that "re-do" pharyngeal flaps improved speech only about 50% of the time.

In addition to the effects of pharyngeal flaps on speech and breathing, clinicians have been concerned about the possible effect of flaps on facial growth. There are two possible mechanisms for flaps to affect growth. First, the flap could theoretically "tether" the maxilla, holding it in a posterior position instead of letting it grow forward. Second, if there is significant airway obstruction, the patient may adopt a constant mouth-open posture, changing the way the mandible grows. One relatively small study (Keller et al., 1988) on 16 patients who had either cleft palate only or unilateral cleft lip and palate showed a significant reduction in maxillary arch width and length in patients who had flaps in comparison to matched controls with clefts but no flaps. However, two larger studies (Semb and Shaw, 1990a, 1990b; Subtelny and Pinedo Nieto, 1978) yielded essentially negative results, failing to substantiate a significant effect of pharyngeal flaps on midfacial growth. Long and McNamara (1985) reported significant differences in some facial angles and linear measurements in patients with flaps compared with nonflap controls, especially in the size and position of the mandible (presumably because of the effects of partial obstruction of the airway). However, in a study offering longitudinal data, Isberg et al. (1993) reported what appeared to be *temporary* changes in the growth pattern and position of the mandible in 20 cleft lip and palate patients with flaps, similar to what was seen in children with enlarged adenoids; these changes were no longer identifiable in the same patients four years after the surgery. A slightly later article on children with cleft palate only (Ren, Isberg, and Henningsson, 1994) reported differences in mandibular position and increased anterior face height (a reflection of an habitual mouth-open posture) but found these changes to be temporary, stating, "We suggest that the influence of a pharyngeal flap on facial growth has no long term clinical importance" (p. 28). The authors felt that a more normal position and growth pattern for the mandible was re-established over time, as the remainder of the craniofacial complex grew. Ren, Isberg, and Henningsson (1993) also documented the interactive effect of a flap and a large adenoid pad, reporting that children with both sources of airway obstruction showed significantly more retrusion of the maxilla and increased mandibular inclination with a steeper mandibular plane than found in children who had the flap only, without an adenoid pad. In general, the clinical data on the topic of pharyngeal flaps and facial growth suggest that changes in mandibular position and growth pattern are likely to be temporary unless there is continued interference with breathing even as the craniofacial complex increases in size. The data sets on maxillary retrusion are not entirely consistent, but the bulk of the evidence does not substantiate a significant effect.

Augmentation Pharyngoplasty

Augmentation pharyngoplasties are attempts to bring the posterior pharyngeal wall forward, creating the equivalent of an adenoid pad. The techniques that have been used include (1) rearranging adjacent soft tissue, (2) implanting cartilage, and (3) injecting or implanting various types of synthetic materials.[6]

Soft tissue advancement. Passavant (1862) tried to advance the soft tissues of the posterior pharyngeal wall by suturing the two palatopharyngeal muscles in the midline to accentuate the ridge that carries his name. By 1878, he was attempting to create this ridge by folding a flap of pharyngeal mucosa upon itself (cited in Dorrance, 1933). Hynes (1950) created an elevation on the wall by dissecting the salpingopharyngeus and its overlying mucosa, lifting these two lateral flaps and suturing them into a pocket he created on the posterior pharyngeal wall by making an

[6]In the early 1900s, one surgeon tried fat grafts, one tried paraffin, and one tried petroleum jelly, all of which melted. See Peterson-Falzone (1988) or Witt and D'Antonio (1993) for a brief history of the early techniques.

incision just below the eustachian tube orifice (Fig. 13-5).[7] He later modified this procedure to include the palatopharyngeus, salpingopharyngeus, and a portion of the superior constrictor (Hynes, 1953, 1967). He surgically closed the large lateral defects created by the lifting of the lateral flaps, a maneuver that he felt helped to decreased the overall size of the velopharynx. None of his articles contained objective data on speech outcome. Calnan (1976) decried his own results with the Hynes procedure, and Harding concluded in 1979 that the procedure had fallen into disrepute.[8]

A recent report by Witt et al. (1997) on "autogenous posterior pharyngeal wall augmentation" involved the use of a rolled, superiorly based myomucosal flap to create extra thickness on the posterior pharyngeal wall for patients with small velopharyngeal defects. The results obtained on their 14 patients led them to conclude that the procedure "[did] not result in speech improvement." In his commentary on the article, Furlow (1997) offered several instructive criticisms, one of which was (p. 1297), "Witt et al. should have limited [their conclusion] to the rolled flap procedure rather than to 'autogenous posterior pharyngeal wall augmentation,' since there are other methods of augmenting the posterior pharynx with autologous tissue. Autogenous costal cartilage implants and those sphincter pharyngoplasties in which the transferred posterior pillars turn out to be statis are examples of autogenous posterior pharyngeal wall augmentations to which the authors' conclusions do not pertain."[9] More disturbing was the fact that the authors subjected their perceptual judgments to statistical testing for probability (a highly questionable procedure with only 14 patients), rather than reporting the results on a case-by-case basis.

Cartilage implants. Autogenous cartilage (usually from the patient's rib) was used to create an anterior projection or pad on the pharyngeal wall in a series of studies in the 1960s and 1970s (Calnan, 1971; Hagerty and Hill, 1961; Hagerty, Hess, and Mylin, 1968; Hagerty, Mylin, and Monat, 1974; Hess, Hagerty, and Mylin, 1968). Although the reports were initially optimistic, Hagerty, Hess, and Mylin (1968) found that no patient reached a normal level of nasal resonance, and Hess et al. (1968) found that midsagittal velopharyngeal gaps averaging 5 mm persisted in more than one fourth of the patients. In general, surgeons had difficulty getting a large enough transplant of cartilage into the posterior pharyngeal wall and getting it to remain in place: the size of the cartilage transplants diminished over time, and also they tended to migrate downward. Better results were obtained by Trigos et al. (1988). Limiting their selection of patients to those in whom the velopharyngeal deficit was less than 5 mm^2 as estimated from nasopharyngoscopy and videofluoroscopy,

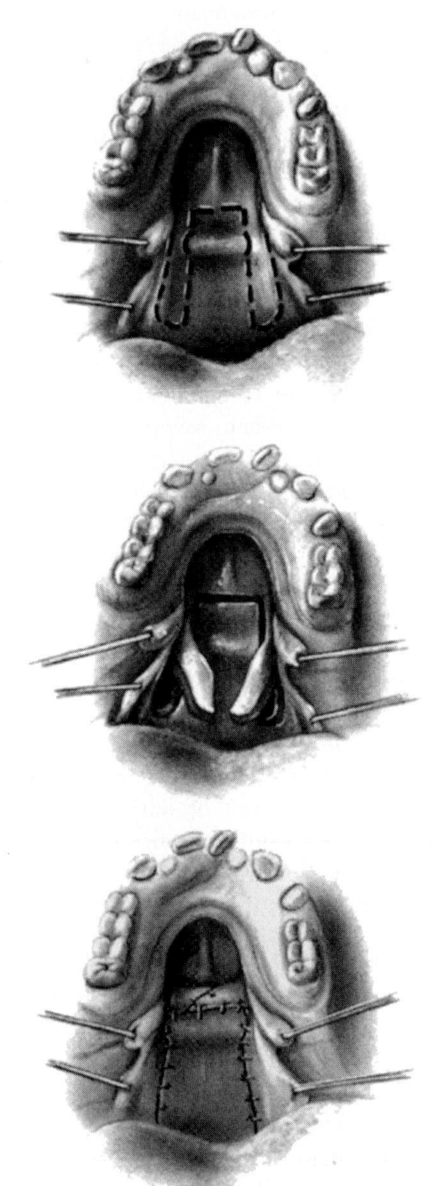

Figure 13-5 Schematic representation of the Hynes pharyngoplasty. *(From Millard DR:* Cleft craft: the evolution of its surgeries. *Volume 3:* Alveolar and palatal deformities. *Boston: Little, Brown, 1980, pp. 653-654.)*

[7]Note that the description of this operation makes the assumption that both the salpingopharyngeus muscles and Passavant's ridge are constant anatomical landmarks. Neither is the case: the salpingopharyngeus is a variable finding in human cadavers, and Passavant's ridge is not seen in all speakers either with or without clefts.

[8]There were a few other inventive methods of "muscle transplantation" that were short-lived. Kiehn et al. (1965) tried transplanting the temporalis or masseter muscle to suspend nonfunctioning velums, but the speech results were uninterpretable and the procedure never gained popularity. The same was true for the "bilateral pharyngoplasty" of Sullivan (1961), in which lateral superior constrictor flaps were raised from both sides of the pharynx and sutured into the superior surface of the velum. Gold and Song (1980) transplanted the tendon of the palmaris longis to the velopharynx; no speech results were given and no further reports appeared. Meyer, Failat, and Kelly (1981) designed what they called a "bilateral Z-flap pharyngoplasty," which transposed the posterior faucial pillars in a fashion that may have been similar to Hynes, but the their diagrams were simplistic; the procedure, if it was actually a "new" one, did not appear in any subsequent literature or reports.

[9]The term "autogenous" means self-generated; originated within the body. "Autologous" means occurring naturally or normally in a structure or tissue, normal to the part. These terms are often used interchangeably in medical literature.

they eliminated hypernasality and audible nasal emission in 10 cases. They had followed their patients for at least 1 year and found good stability of the implants and the speech results. However, less stable results were reported by Denny, Marks, and Oliff-Carneol (1993), who used cartilage implants in 20 patients with gaps measuring only 1 to 3 mm on radiographic studies. They reported obtaining "normal resonance and articulation" in five of 20, "some improvement" in 11, and no change in four. There were several methodological problems in their study, among them the fact that at least seven of the 20 patients were syndromic and postoperative follow-up was only 8 weeks. The authors stated that the implants had to be about three times the size of the measured gap in order to have any effect. This suggestion is consistent with the earlier studies in which cartilage implants did not seem to hold their size or position over time, the report by Trigos et al. (1988) being an exception.

Synthetic materials. Other materials that have been used in attempts to move the posterior pharyngeal wall forward include

- Injectable or implantable forms of silicone or Silastic (Blocksma, 1963, 1964; Brauer, 1973)
- Teflon implants or injections (Bluestone, Musgrave, and McWilliams, 1968; Bluestone et al., 1968; Furlow et al., 1982; Janeke, 1982; Kuehn and Van Demark, 1978; Lewy, Cole, and Wepman, 1965; Smith and McCabe, 1977; Sturim and Jacob, 1972; Ward, Goldman, and Stoudt, 1966; Ward, Stoudt, and Goldman, 1967)
- Proplast implants (Wolford, Oelschlaeger, and Deal, 1989)
- Most recently, injectable collagen (Remacle et al., 1990).

As summarized by Witt and D'Antonio (1993), many of these techniques were abandoned because of unpredictable results, postoperative complications, or restrictions imposed by the Food and Drug Administration. The reports on silicone or Silastic implants (solid or gel forms) contained no data on outcome other than percentages of patients who were said to have "improved." Reports on the use of injectable Teflon were promising, although some patients required second or third injections to reach the desired effect on speech or to maintain that effect over time. Clinicians were particularly enthusiastic about Teflon injection because it could be carried out under a topical anesthetic, allowing immediate judgment of the effect on speech. Also, obturation of the velopharyngeal deficit could be observed by simultaneous endoscopy. However, in 1978 the Food and Drug Administration withdrew approval of the use of injectable Teflon in the velopharynx after a fatality. Proplast in a mesh form was implanted in the posterior pharyngeal wall in only one published report (Wolford, Oelschlaeger, and Deal, 1989), and there were subsequent problems with extrusion.

Collagen is part of the natural composition of the skin in mammals, including humans. The injectable collagen used by Remacle et al. (1990) was a purified form of bovine dermal collagen suspended in saline solution. They injected it into the posterior pharyngeal wall of four patients with postpalatoplasty velopharyngeal inadequacy, and one with presumably noncleft velopharyngeal inadequacy. They did no imaging studies (e.g., nasopharyngoscopy) before surgery. Results were assessed by rhinomanometric testing (instrumentation not specified), subjective evaluation of voice recordings, and cineradiographic studies. They did not indicate the size of the increase in bulk on the posterior pharyngeal wall. Hypernasality was reportedly eliminated in three patients but only partially improved in the other two. The authors did not state how long after surgery the results were assessed. There were no subsequent published studies of collagen injection either by these authors or others, which may indicate that the procedure was found to be less than desirable in the long term.

Sphincter Pharyngoplasty

Hynes (1953, 1967) stated that his pharyngoplasty could work in any of three ways: by advancing the posterior pharyngeal wall, by reducing the overall diameter (specifically the lateral dimensions) of the pharynx in a static manner, or by producing an active sphincter. Although he did not use the word "sphincter" in his publications, he described the ridge he created as "very prominent and *often contractile*" (Hynes, 1950), and his work served as the foundation for later innovators who tried to get the velopharynx to work in a sphincteric fashion.

Orticochea (1968, 1970) is the name most frequently associated with sphincter pharyngoplasty. He dissected the posterior faucial pillars from their inferior attachments and the lateral pharyngeal wall and sutured them to an inferiorly based pharyngeal flap (Fig. 13-6). In the immediate postoperative period this procedure creates lateral defects where the posterior pillars were detached from the lateral pharyngeal wall. When these have healed, there is in theory one small central sphincter that closes during speech (Fig. 13-7).[10] In 1983 Orticochea reported an 89% success rate on 236 cases with a variety of etiological bases for their velopharyngeal inadequacy. Speech was simply categorized by broad perceptual categories, and movement of the newly created sphincter was assessed *only* by what he saw on the intraoral view. In his comments on the article, Jackson (1983) pointed out that the failure rate was really closer to 50%, considering all the patients who still had signs of velopharyngeal inadequacy. Stradoudakis and Bambace (1984) reported only modest success in 16 patients operated by Orticochea's procedure: five still had evidence of velopharyngeal inadequacy and three were hyponasal when evaluated from 6 months to 4 years after surgery (yielding a success rate of 50% unless the hyponasal patients are counted as successes).

[10]Millard (1980, p. 659) commented that he found ". . . several of [Orticochea's] ideas lacking in principle. . . ." Among the questions is how often the surgically created lateral defects actually heal spontaneously.

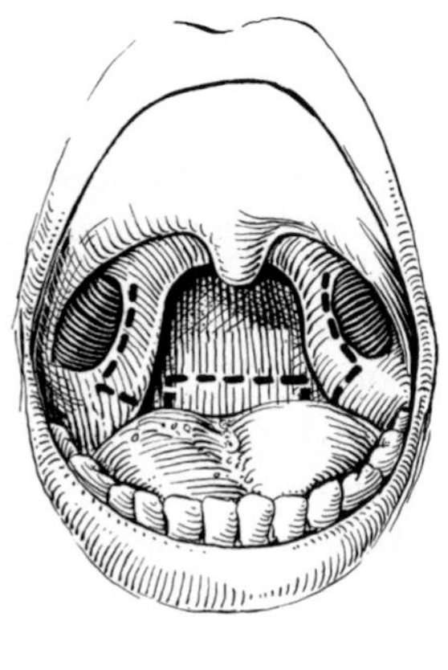

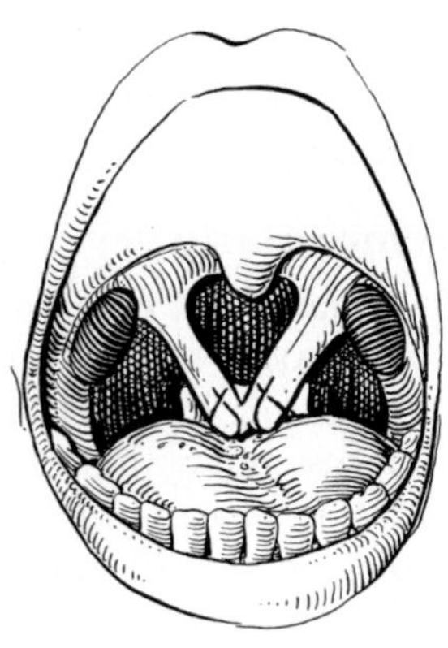

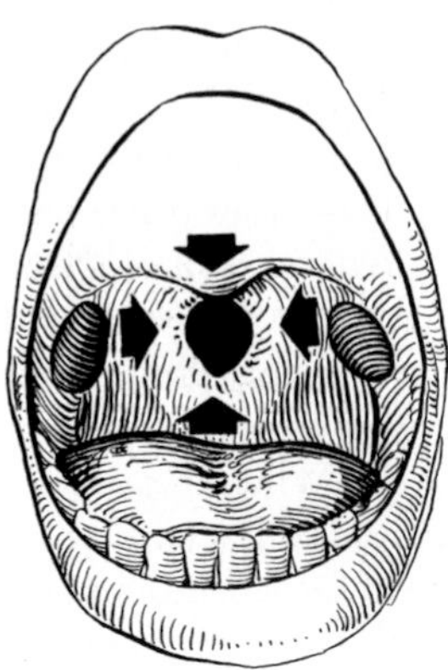

Figure 13-6 Schematic representation of the Orticochea pharyngoplasty. *(From Millard DR:* Cleft craft: the evolution of its surgeries. *Volume 3:* Alveolar and palatal deformities. *Boston: Little, Brown, 1980, pp. 653-654.)*

Jackson (Huskie and Jackson, 1977; Jackson, 1977, 1985; Jackson and Silverton, 1977) substituted a superiorly based midline flap for the inferiorly based flap used by Orticochea. In the first report on 26 patients (Huskie and Jackson, 1977), severe nasal escape was found in two, moderate escape in six, and mild escape in eight, meaning that some degree of velopharyngeal inadequacy persisted in 62% up to 1 year postoperatively. In the Jackson and Silverton report (1977), there was persistence of some degree of velopharyngeal inadequacy in 49% of cases.

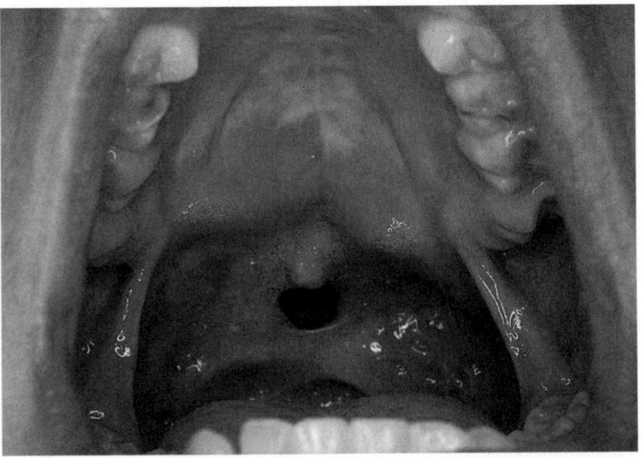

Figure 13-7 An intraoral photo of a patient who has had an "Orticochea" pharyngoplasty, demonstrating the central sphincter that is supposed to close during speech.

Lendrum and Dhar (1984) reported "improvement" in nasal escape in 47/53 patients (88.7%) but complete elimination of nasal escape in 20 (37%). They had no objective speech data, but some of their observations were instructive: they remarked that the central sphincter could remain incompetent for up to *3 years* after surgery. The pattern of motion of the two palatopharyngeal flaps toward closure was usually like "an iris diaphragm" (which would be a fully circumferential sphincter, the anterior arc being the velum itself) but sometimes "with a side-to-side shutter action." (Because muscles can only pull, and cannot push, one assumes that the "side-to-side shutter action" would be the result of the pull on the anterior and posterior insertions of the flaps, much like pulling a rubber band suspended over a thumb and forefinger.)

Moss, Pigott, and Albery (1987) modified the Hynes pharyngoplasty somewhat, altering the way the dissection of the musculature was carried out and the way the lateral flaps were sutured together and into the posterior pharyngeal wall. They had used their version of a sphincter pharyngoplasty on 40 patients with velopharyngeal inadequacy of varying etiologies. The speech results were given only in rather general terms but were impressive if the subjective judgments were valid: 38 of the 40 patients had "no or variable nasal escape," whereas 33 had normal or "slight" hyponasal resonance 6 months postoperatively. The authors concluded that their procedure was suitable for patients with a mobile palate and a velopharyngeal gap 5 mm or less in the anteroposterior dimension. The anterior projection of the posterior pharyngeal wall in their patients ranged from 2 to 12 mm, with an average of 6.22 mm.

Pigott (1993) critiqued the work of Hynes (1950, 1953, 1967), placing it into historical perspective and pointing out the aspects that still seemed to have valid applications. He criticized Jackson's substitution (Jackson and Silverton, 1977) of a "trap-door of mucosa [and] muscle" for the simple incision on the posterior pharyngeal wall used by

Hynes. Pigott (1993) did comment that the transverse incision had to be placed "as high as possible," a comment that seems to ignore the fact that the velum in some speakers may not reach toward a level on the posterior pharyngeal wall that is "as high as possible" but actually toward a lower point (see Chapter 3 on velopharyngeal physiology). Overall, Pigott (1993) concluded that the Hynes procedure as described in 1953 and 1967 "rarely produces symptoms of velopharyngeal obstruction and should be considered as a relatively physiological operation" (p. 441).

Subsequent teams devising their own versions of the Orticochea procedure moved the site of insertion of the palatopharyngeal flaps (onto the posterior pharyngeal wall) upward from what had first been described (Riski et al., 1984; Roberts and Brown, 1983).[11] Riski et al. (1984) reported "successful resolution of nasality" in 43 of 55 patients (78%), including 16 of the 26 patients in whom the ultimate height of flap insertion was still below the level at which velopharyngeal closure was attempted (as viewed radiographically) before surgery. As the work on the sphincter pharyngoplasty progressed with the work of Riski et al. (1992a, 1992b) and that of Witt et al. (1994, 1995a), the success rates began to increase over the one half to two thirds rates reported in earlier studies. In the report of Riski et al. (1992a) the sphincter pharyngoplasty was used only in patients with active velar elevation. Their procedure was actually a modified Hynes rather than an Orticochea procedure, using a single transverse incision on the posterior pharyngeal wall to house the insertion of the lateral flaps and also closing the bilateral defects inherent in the Orticochea procedure. They reported improving their success rate from 67% with the Orticochea to 84% with the modified Hynes procedure.

Another relatively recent study on the Orticochea procedure (James et al., 1996) lacked objective speech data but reported "lessening of nasal escape" in 49 of 54 patients (91%) and complete elimination of nasal escape in 40 (74%). These numbers are fairly high, if valid. All the patients had had both preoperative and postoperative speech therapy, but the authors did not specify the aims of that therapy or how the behavioral intervention might have influenced the outcome of their surgical intervention.

Riski et al. (1992a, 1992b) evaluated the causes of failures in sphincter pharyngoplasty procedures. They divided these into (1) problems in patient selection and (2) problems with surgical planing and technique. In the first category the culprits leading to failure were large velopharyngeal gaps and residual speech deficits (pre-existing and persistent compensatory articulations). The second category included low flap placement (insertion of the lateral flaps migrating downward from the desired site), flap dehiscence (separating spontaneously from their attachment[s]), and "flaps not approximated in the midline," meaning persistence of a central opening akin to the rubber band not being pulled sufficiently for the two sides to approximate. Witt et al. (1995a) derived similar answers in their failed cases but also echoed the all-important factor of the surgeon's "learning curve" (experience).

Pensler and Reich (1991) reported that their own success rate with the Jackson version of the sphincter pharyngoplasty (1985) was 75%, whereas that with traditional pharyngeal flaps was 70%. However, they had (1) no objective speech data and (2) grossly uneven numbers of patients (75 with pharyngeal flaps, 10 with sphincter pharyngoplasties), invalidating their chi-square analysis of their results. They did report a 4% occurrence of sleep apnea in the flap group, without specifying the time of postoperative follow-up. Perioperative or postoperative upper airway dysfunction, including sleep apnea, has also been reported in some cases of sphincter pharyngoplasties (Witt et al., 1996).

Current versions of sphincter pharyngoplasties remain popular and can be an important part of the team's or surgeon's repertoire of techniques, particularly when patients are carefully selected with regard to the size of the velopharyngeal deficit and behavior of the velar and pharyngeal musculature as seen on radiographic and endoscopic views.[12] As with all other surgical approaches to secondary management of velopharyngeal inadequacy, success of sphincter pharyngoplasty is first and foremost dependent on accurate diagnosis of the problem.

PROSTHODONTIC MANAGEMENT OF VELOPHARYNGEAL INADEQUACY

Speech Bulbs

When surgical repair has not provided a velum of sufficient length for velopharyngeal closure in speech, a prosthetic device usually called a "speech bulb" may be used.[13] The oral portion of the device clasps to the teeth, although prosthodontists experienced in the treatment of patients with clefts will attempt a combination denture + speech bulb or palatal obturator when necessary (Fig. 13-8) (Adisman, 1971; Duthie, 1983; Mazaheri, 1979; Mazaheri and Mazaheri, 1976; McKinstry and Aramani, 1985; Moore, 1976; Rosen and Bzoch, 1997). In fact, Mazaheri (1979) stated, "The edentulous condition is not a

[11]Riski et al. (1987) also described combining an Orticochea pharyngoplasty with primary palatoplasty.

[12]Bonawitz, Conley, and Denny (1995) described the use of a "unilateral Orticochea" for two patients with an asymmetric deficit in velopharyngeal closure.

[13]In a retrospective report on the types of prosthetic treatment sought from their cleft palate team and Department of Dentistry and Maxillofacial Prosthetics, Delgado, Schaaf, and Emrich (1992) noted that, over a 21-year time period, the number of "speech aid" prostheses has dropped significantly, the number of palatal obturators (meaning devices to cover fistulae or incompletely closed clefts) had stayed about the same, and the number of feeding devices fabricated for infants had increased.

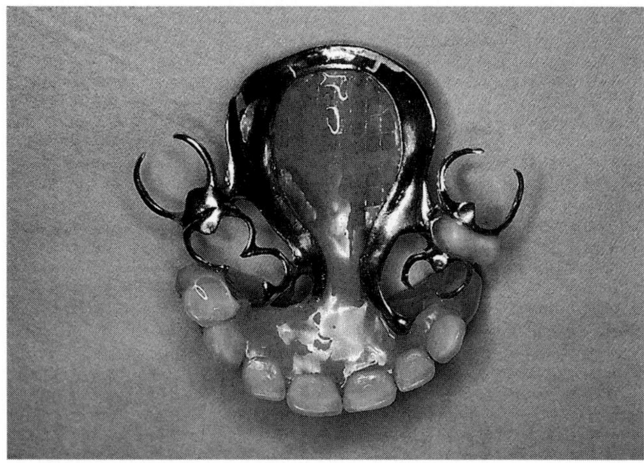

Figure 13-8 A combination denture + palatal obturator.

contraindication for a speech aid appliance." Usually an obturator for a patient with a repaired cleft has an "under-and-up" design (Fig. 13-9), the posterior extension from the anterior oral plate being directed somewhat inferiorly beneath the velum and the pharyngeal bulb being placed up behind the velum to make contact with the pharyngeal walls. The success of treatment depends primarily on the correct design and placement of the bulb, which in turn depends on adequate visualization of the velopharyngeal port at rest and during speech and swallowing. The prosthodontist on the cleft palate–craniofacial team looks to such studies—usually nasopharyngoscopy, sometimes videofluoroscopy—to determine the optimum size, vertical height, and shape of the speech bulb (Beery, Rood, and Schramm, 1983; Karnell, Rosenstein, and Fine, 1987; Riski, Hoke, and Dolan, 1989; Walter, 1981). In general, the success of a speech bulb depends on the amount and the vertical level of motion of the pharyngeal walls, a fact that has been known to clinicians for many decades (Curtis and Chierici, 1964; Mazaheri and Millard, 1965). In fact, some clinicians have used temporary speech bulbs to help identify the best size and placement for planned pharyngeal flaps (Curtis and Chierici, 1964; Marsh and Wray, 1980).

Palatal Lifts

In contrast to speech bulbs that fill the velopharyngeal space, palatal lifts are essentially horizontal, rigid arms[14] designed to lift the velum into a position from which velopharyngeal closure can be more easily obtained (Fig. 13-10). These devices are not meant to be an acrylic substitution for the velum itself. They have occasionally been described in the treatment of individuals with clefts, but either as part of combination lift-and-bulb appliances or for cases in whom the repaired palate is intact but deficient in movement. Palatal lifts are most frequently used for patients with neurological impairment of velar movement,[15,16] and there is an extensive body of literature on this topic (Adisman, 1971; Curtis and Chierici, 1964; Dalston, 1977; Enderby, Hathorn, and Servant, 1984; Gonzalez and Aronson, 1970; Holley, Hamby, and Taylor, 1973; Kerman, Singer, and Davidoff, 1973; Kipfmueller and Lang, 1972; Johns, 1985; Lang, 1967; Lang and Kipfmueller, 1969; LaVelle and Hardy, 1979; Lawshe et al., 1971; Marshall and Jones, 1971; Mazaheri, 1979; Mazaheri and Mazaheri, 1976; Millard, 1971; Netsell and Daniel, 1979; Posnick, 1977; Rosen and Bzoch, 1997; Schweiger, Netsell, and Sommerfeld, 1970; Valauri, 1977; Wedin, 1972; Witt et al., 1995a, 1995c; Yules et al., 1971).

In practical terms, an optimum effect on speech with the use of a palatal lift is still dependent on having at least some degree of movement in either the velum itself or portions of the pharyngeal musculature. When there is absolutely no movement, speech outcome is necessarily a compromise, falling somewhere along the continuum between (1) complete obstruction of the velopharyngeal port by pushing the velum backward and upward to the posterior pharyngeal wall and making the device wide enough to also push the velum laterally or posterolaterally against the lateral pharyngeal walls and (2) incomplete closure of the velopharyngeal system, leaving some degree of opening that does not vary with the speech task. As with speech bulbs, in cases when the optimum result cannot be achieved, a "middle-of-the-road" compromise is reached in which the velopharyngeal port is neither sufficiently closed for completely nonnasal production of pressure consonants nor adequately open for normal nasal resonance on nasal consonants and vocalic segments.

Two relatively recent reports by Witt et al. (Witt and Marsh, 1997; Witt et al., 1995b) illustrate the difficulties in obtaining satisfactory speech results in this population: Even with the benefits of a multidisciplinary team for treatment planning and execution and use of nasoendoscopy for the fitting and subsequent modifications of palatal lifts, satisfactory results were obtained in only five of 18 patients.

A Special Topic: Palatal Speech Aids (Lifts and Obturators) as Speech Training Devices

A portion of the literature on palatal lifts creates some confusion by presenting lifts as "palatal training" devices or devices for "velopharyngeal stimulation." Mazaheri (1979) and Mazaheri and Mazaheri (1976), for example, viewed palatal lifts as a means of stimulating velopharyngeal

[14]Spratley, Chenery, and Murdoch (1988) designed a palatal lift with the posterior portion attached to the oral portion with a hinge with the idea that the movable portion would allow more comfortable breathing and swallowing for the patient. However, they offered scant information on their results and no long-term follow-up. There were no subsequent reports on this device.

[15]See Chapter 2 for a discussion of the question as to whether there can truly be neurological impairment of the velopharyngeal system alone or only as part of a more generalized dysarthria.

[16]In the older literature there were occasional case reports of patients with palatal paresis being treated with a speech bulb (e.g., Wedin, 1972).

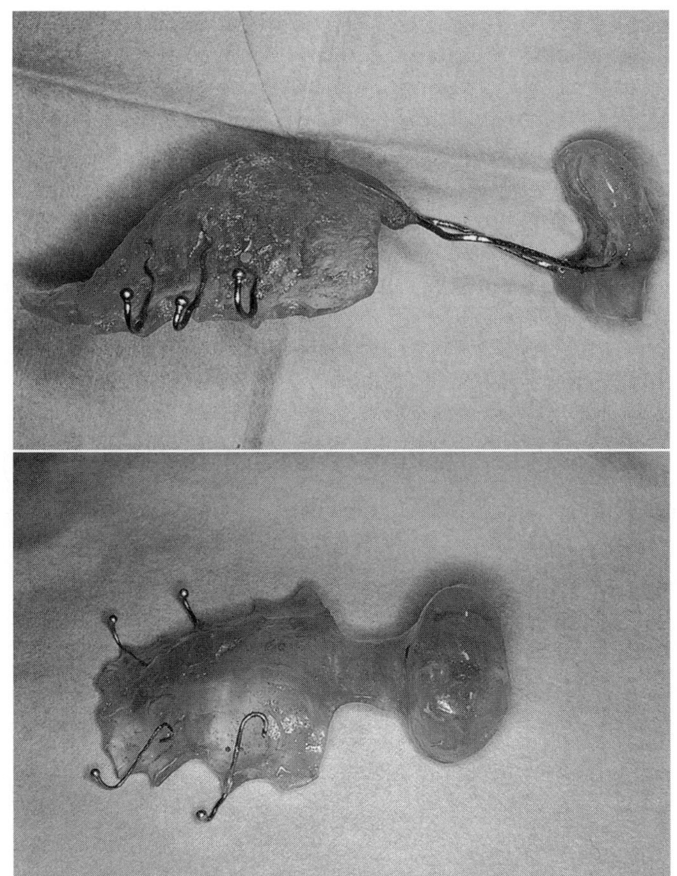

A

B

Figure 13-9 **A** and **B,** Two "under-and-up" prostheses fabricated for patients with repaired palates but inadequate velopharyngeal closure.

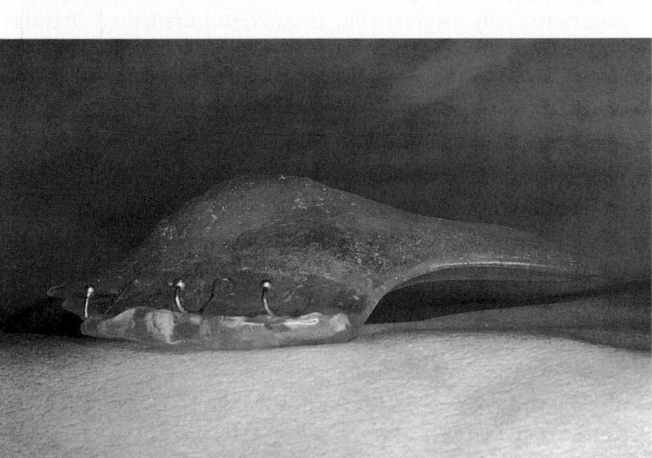

A

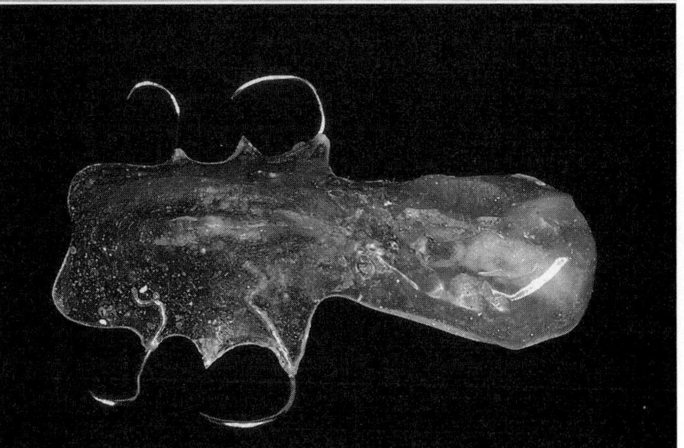

B

Figure 13-10 **A** and **B,** Two palatal lift prostheses.

motion, but they had no experimental or control data to support this view. Millard (1971) had the same view with regard to both palatal lifts and speech bulbs. Clinicians in England inconsistently used the term "palatal lift" to refer to a wire loop extended under the velum from an oral acrylic plate, but they then labeled the device a "palatal training appliance" (Duxbury and Graham, 1985, 1986; Selley, 1979; Thompson, Ferguson, and Barton, 1985; Tudor and Selley, 1974). The basic tenet of the treatment was that the patient could learn to lift the velum upward off the wire loop, gradually increasing the muscular action of the velum. Selley (1979) wrote of the "palatal training appliance" being used in patients with "complaints of drooling, stroke, feeding in-coordination, and hypernasal speech." The diagnostic categories for the patients with hypernasal speech included repaired clefts, "in-coordination" or "lazy palate," submucous cleft palate, and palatopharyngeal disproportion. He described the appliance as being a "U-shaped wire loop with open ends embedded in an acrylic base plate. The closed end of the loop is bent . . . to conform to the shape of the resting soft palate. The wire is adjusted so that it only just touches the palate, without applying any pressure" (p. 53). The thought was that the training appliance would "encourage development of movements of the soft palate" because it would "produce a tactile feedback of soft palate movements" (presumably because the patient would be able to feel the velum lose contact with the loop), "stimulate sensory neurological development, and encourage dorsal tongue relaxation." The clinicians who used this device felt that encouraging "dorsal tongue relaxation" could reduce hypernasality "by increasing oral patency." However, all the articles written on the "palatal training appliance" were hypothetical in nature, without evidence supporting the principles put forth by the authors. The articles did state that velopharyngeal closure for speech was improved through use of the device, but did not report actual data (e.g., the percentage of patients in whom speech improved, over what period of time, etc.). It seems likely that improvement in velopharyngeal function did in fact occur in at least some patients, but we have no scientific evidence pertaining to the actual mechanism(s) by which the results were achieved.

Reporting on the same patients and same treatment as in Witt et al. (1995b), Witt et al. (1995c) concluded they had no proof that palatal lift prostheses altered neuromuscular patterning of the velopharynx. One problem with their report might have been that the average length of time between the fitting of the palatal lift and the postfitting evaluation was only 4.4 months, although no one has derived a standard for the amount of time over which such an appliance should be tried before drawing conclusions about effects on speech. Witt et al. (1995c) reported that velopharyngeal closure was unchanged in 69% of their patients. Speech improved in 15% and deteriorated in 15%. They decided their results (no change in 69%, improvement in 15%, deterioration in 15%) "neither support[ed] the concept that palatal lift prostheses alter[ed] the neuromuscular patterning of the velopharynx, nor provide[d] objective documentation of the feasibility of prosthetic 'weaning' (gradual reduction of the device)" (p. 469).

There is a long history in the literature of speech bulbs or obturators gradually producing changes in the movement of the velopharyngeal mechanism. By far the largest percentage of these reports or studies were purely empirical, and it is very difficult to use the information they offered to help one decide whether an obturator as a potential stimulator of activity could be a reasonable treatment approach for a given patient. However, over a period of 35 years or more, enough clinicians have made similar observations of increased activity in the velopharyngeal mechanism to warrant a review of the topic.

In 1960, Blakeley presented the idea of using a velopharyngeal obturator to completely close off the nasopharynx so that oral productions of pressure consonants would be "obligatory." He was originally seeking to simply force oral emission of air instead of nasal emission (although he did not deal with the possibility that a child could persist in glottal and pharyngeal placements even with complete blockage of the nasopharynx). In one case in which he used this approach, he noticed "during the third year of speech training" that the appliance had apparently stimulated additional pharyngeal activity to the extent that it was "too large and had to be removed." This was the beginning of a surge of interest in "obturator reduction programs," an interest that is actively pursued to this day.

A few years later, Blakeley (1964) described gradual reduction of the size of a prosthetic speech bulb in response to (or possibly as a prompt for) increased inward motion of pharyngeal musculature. He also suggested that the eventual placement of a (centrally based) pharyngeal flap should be considered only when it had been determined that further increases in velopharyngeal movement were no longer possible. A follow-up report by Blakeley (1969) presented more clinical observations about the initial use of a large velopharyngeal obturator leading to increased velopharyngeal movement, reduction of the obturator, and further increases in movement. In fact, Blakeley (1969) considered such a program to be a "must" for a successful pharyngoplasty, feeling that the obturator and its subsequent reduction led to improvements in velopharyngeal movement that were needed before a successful pharyngoplasty could be performed. Obturator reduction as a means of increasing velopharyngeal movement was also reported by Millard (1971) and Weiss (Weiss, 1971; Weiss and Louis, 1972; Wong and Weiss, 1972). Clinicians continue to explore and advocate obturator reduction programs (Golding-Kushner, Cisneros, and LeBlanc, 1995; McGrath and Anderson, 1990).

What is unclear in the reports on obturator reduction programs is what the mechanism(s) for the changes in velopharyngeal activity may actually be. Does "forcing" oral direction of the air stream by blocking the velopharyngeal port provide some form of feedback (auditory, tactile, proprioceptive) that gives enough unconscious or conscious information to the speaker to be able to increase velopharyngeal activity in speech? Does the stimulation of the pharyngeal section against the musculature somehow stimulate that musculature to work against the resistance of the bulb? The latter is one of the standard tenets of physical therapy for other parts of the body but has been difficult to prove or use in therapy for velopharyngeal closure (Dalston, 1977; Ruscello, 1997). If the increased movement of the velopharyngeal musculature is not the result of working against resistance but in some other way a direct result of reducing the size of the bulb, what causes the musculature to respond? The musculature cannot "look over there" and decide to make a stronger movement to meet the bulb. What is it that "tells" the musculature to make the additional effort? With so little possibility for conscious feedback of velopharyngeal activity (Dalston, 1977; Ruscello, 1997; Tomes, Kuehn, and Peterson-Falzone, 1997), even if the speaker hears increased nasal emission when the bulb is reduced, how does he or she trigger increased movement of the velopharyngeal mechanism? Despite all the clinical observations that have been made over more than 30 years on results of obturator reduction, we still lack a sound theoretical construct for this therapeutic approach.

One further note about obturator reduction programs is that this form of therapy for altering behavior of the velopharyngeal mechanism must be quite aggressive, that is, the clinician must make clear to the patient or parents that frequent and regular visits to the treating facility will be necessary. In addition, if the treating team uses nasopharyngoscopy to monitor the status of the patient and design changes in the bulb, the patient will have to undergo repeated examinations (Golding-Kushner, Cisneros, and LeBlanc, 1995). However, if the result of the program is that the patient either will not have to undergo additional surgery or may be able to have a smaller, less obstructive pharyngeal flap, it may well be worth all the time and effort.

REFERENCES

Abramson DL, Marrinan EM, and Mulliken JB: Robin sequence: obstructive sleep apnea following pharyngeal flap. *Cleft Palate–Craniofacial Journal* 34:256-260, 1997.

Adisman IK: Cleft palate prosthetics. In Grabb WC, Rosenstein SW, and Bzoch KR (eds.): *Cleft lip and palate: surgical, dental and speech aspects.* Boston: Little, Brown, 1971, pp. 617-642.

Albery E, Bennett J, Pigott R, and Simmons R: The results of 100 operations for velopharyngeal incompetence—selected on the findings of endoscopic and radiological examination. *British Journal of Plastic Surgery* 35:118-126, 1982.

Argamaso RV, Bassila M, Bratcher GO, Brodsky L, Cotton RT, Croft CB, Greenberg LM, Laskin R, MacKenzie-Stepner K, Meyer CM, Rakoff SJ, Ruben RJ, Sher AE, Shprintzen RJ, Sidoti EJ, Singer L, Strauch B, Stringer D, and Witzel MA: Tonsillectomy and pharyngeal flap operation should not be performed simultaneously [letter]. *Cleft Palate Journal* 25:176-177, 1988.

Argamaso RV, Shprintzen RJ, Strauch B, Lewin M, Daniller A, Ship A, and Croft C: The role of lateral pharyngeal wall movement in pharyngeal flap surgery. *Plastic and Reconstructive Surgery* 66:214-219, 1980.

Barot LF, Cohen MA, and LaRossa D: Surgical indications and techniques for posterior pharyngeal flap revision. *Annals of Plastic Surgery* 16:527-531, 1986.

Beery Q, Rood S, and Schramm V: Pharyngeal wall motion in prosthetically managed cleft palate adults. *Cleft Palate Journal* 20:7-17, 1983.

Bernstein L: Treatment of velopharyngeal incompetence. *Archives of Otolaryngology* 85:67-74, 1967.

Bernstein L: A modified pharyngeal flap operation. *Transactions of the American Academy of Ophthalmology and Otolaryngology* 80:514-518, 1975.

Blakeley R: Temporary speech prosthesis as an aid in speech training. *Cleft Palate Bulletin* 10:63-65, 1960.

Blakeley R: The complementary use of speech prostheses and pharyngeal flaps in palatal insufficiency. *Cleft Palate Journal* 1:194-198, 1964.

Blakeley R: The rationale for a temporary speech prosthesis in palatal insufficiency. *British Journal of Disorders of Communication* 4:134-139, 1969.

Blocksma R: Correction of velopharyngeal insufficiency by silastic pharyngeal implant. *Plastic and Reconstructive Surgery* 31:268-274, 1963.

Blocksma R: Silicone implants for velopharyngeal incompetence: a progress report. *Cleft Palate Journal* 1:72-81, 1964.

Bluestone CD, Musgrave RH, and McWilliams BJ: Teflon injection pharyngoplasty. *Cleft Palate Journal* 5:558-564, 1968.

Bluestone CD, Musgrave RH, McWilliams BJ, and Crozier PA: Teflon injection pharyngoplasty. *Cleft Palate Journal* 5:19-22, 1968.

Bonawitz SC, Conley SF, and Denny AD: Modified Orticochea pharyngoplasty for treatment of unilateral velopharyngeal incompetence. *Annals of Plastic Surgery* 35:607-611, 1995.

Brauer RO: Retropharyngeal implantation of silicone gel pillows for velopharyngeal incompetence. *Plastic and Reconstructive Surgery* 51:254-262, 1973.

Brondsted K, Liisberg W, Orsted B, Prytz S, and Fogh-Andersen P: Surgical and speech results following palatopharyngoplasty operations in Denmark 1959-1977. *Cleft Palate Journal* 21:170-179, 1984.

Buchholz R, Chase R, Jobe R, and Smith H: The use of the combined palatal pushback and pharyngeal flap operation: a progress report. *Plastic and Reconstructive Surgery* 39:554-561, 1967.

Cadieux RJ, Kales A, McGlynn TJ, Jackson D, Manders EK, and Simmonds MA: Sleep apnea precipitated by pharyngeal surgery in a patient with myotonic dystrophy. *Archives of Otolaryngology* 110:611-613, 1984.

Calnan JS: Congenital large pharynx. *British Journal of Plastic Surgery* 24:263-271, 1971.

Calnan JS: Surgery for speech. In Calnan JS (ed.): *Recent advances in plastic surgery, I.* Edinburgh: Churchill Livingstone, 1976, pp. 39-57.

Caouette-Laberge L, Egerszegi EP, de Remont A-M, and Ottenseyer I: Long-term follow-up after division of a pharyngeal flap for severe nasal obstruction. *Cleft Palate Craniofacial Journal* 29:27-31, 1992.

Chen PK-T, Wu J, Chen Y-R, and Noordhoff MS: Correction of secondary velopharyngeal insufficiency in cleft palate patients with the Furlow palatoplasty. *Plastic and Reconstructive Surgery* 94:933-941, 1994.

Cosman B, and Falk AS: Pharyngeal flap augmentation. *Plastic and Reconstructive Surgery* 55:149-155, 1975.

Coston GN, Hagerty RF, Jannarone RJ, McDonald V, and Hagerty RC: Levator muscle reconstruction: resulting velopharyngeal competency—a preliminary report. *Plastic and Reconstructive Surgery* 77:911-918, 1986.

Crockett DM, Bumsted RM, and Van Demark DR: Experience with surgical management of velopharyngeal incompetence. *Otolaryngology–Head and Neck Surgery* 99:1-9, 1988.

Curtis T, and Chierici G: Prosthetics as a diagnostic aid in pharyngeal flap surgery. *Cleft Palate Journal* 1:95-98, 1964.

Dalston RM: Prosthodontic management of the cleft-palate patient: a speech pathologist's view. *Journal of Prosthetic Dentistry* 37:190-195, 1977.

D'Antonio LL: Correction of velopharyngeal insufficiency using the Furlow double opposing Z-plasty. *Western Journal of Medicine* 102:101-102, 1997.

Delgado AA, Schaaf NG, and Emrich L: Trends in prosthodontic treatment of cleft palate patients at one institution: a twenty-one year review. *Cleft Palate–Craniofacial Journal* 29:425-428, 1992.

Denny AD, Marks SM, and Oliff-Carneol S: Correction of velopharyngeal insufficiency by pharyngeal augmentation using autologous cartilage: a preliminary report. *Cleft Palate–Craniofacial Journal* 30:46-54, 1993.

Dibbell D, Laub D, Jobe R, and Chase R: A modification of the combined pushback and pharyngeal flap operation. *Plastic and Reconstructive Surgery* 36:165-171, 1965.

Dijkstra R: Secondary lengthening of the soft palate using Millard's island flap technique. *British Journal of Plastic Surgery* 22:113-118, 1969.

Dixon V, Bzoch KR, and Habal M: Evaluation of speech after correction of rhinophonia with pushback palatoplasty combined with pharyngeal flap. *Plastic and Reconstructive Surgery* 64:77-83, 1979.

Dorrance GM: *The operative story of cleft palate.* Philadelphia: WB Saunders, 1933.

Duthie N: Prosthetic treatment of a cleft palate. *British Dental Journal* 155:57-58, 1983.

Duxbury JT, and Graham SM: Palatal training aids for velopharyngeal insufficiency: an interdisciplinary approach. *Dental Update* 12:609-614, 1985.

Duxbury JT, and Graham SM: Velopharyngeal insufficiency: a joint approach. *Middle East Dentistry* January-February:32-34, 1986.

Enderby P, Hathorn IS, and Servant S: The use of intra-oral appliances in the management of acquired velopharyngeal disorders. *British Dental Journal* 157:157-159, 1984.

Engstrom K, Fritzell B, and Johanson B: A study of speech improvement following palatopharyngeal flap surgery. *Cleft Palate Journal* 7:419-431, 1970.

Friedman HI, Haines PC, Coston GN, Lett ED, and Edgerton MT: Augmentation of the failed pharyngeal flap. *Plastic and Reconstructive Surgery* 90:314-318, 1992.

Furlow LT: Correction of secondary velopharyngeal insufficiency in cleft palate patients with the Furlow palatoplasty. *Plastic and Reconstructive Surgery* 94:942-943, 1994.

Furlow FT: Discussion of Witt et al. Surgical management of velopharyngeal dysfunction: outcome analysis of autogenous posterior pharyngeal augmentation. *Plastic and Reconstructive Surgery* 99:1297-1300, 1997.

Furlow LT, Williams W, Eisenbach D, and Bzoch KR: A long-term study on treating velopharyngeal insufficiency by Teflon injection. *Cleft Palate Journal* 19:47-61, 1982.

Gold A, and Song I: A tendon transplant pharyngoplasty. *Cleft Palate Journal* 17:283-290, 1980.

Golding-Kushner KJ, Cisneros GJ, and LeBlanc EM: Speech bulbs. In Bardach J, and Shprintzen RJ (eds.): *Cleft palate speech management.* St. Louis: Mosby, 1995, pp. 352-363.

Gonzalez J, and Aronson A: Palatal lift prosthesis for treatment of anatomic and neurologic palatopharyngeal insufficiency. *Cleft Palate Journal* 7:91-104, 1970.

Graham WP, Hamilton R, Randall P, Winchester R, and Stool S: Complications following posterior pharyngeal flap surgery. *Cleft Palate Journal* 10:176-180, 1973.

Hagerty RF, and Hill MJ: Cartilage pharyngoplasty in cleft palate patients. *Surgery, Gynecology, and Obstetrics* 112:350-356, 1961.

Hagerty RF, Hess D, and Mylin W: Velar motility, velopharyngeal closure, and speech proficiency in cartilage pharyngoplasty: the effect of age at surgery. *Cleft Palate Journal* 5:317-326, 1968.

Hagerty RF, Mylin W, and Monat R: Augmentation pharyngoplasty. In Georgiade NG (ed.): *Symposium on management of cleft lip and palate and associated deformities.* St. Louis: Mosby, 1974, pp. 192-194.

Harding R: Surgery. In Cooper H, Harding R, Krogman W, Mazaheri M, and Millard DR (eds.): *Cleft palate and cleft lip: a team approach to clinical management and rehabilitation of the patient.* Philadelphia: WB Saunders, 1979, pp. 163-262.

Hess D, Hagerty R, and Mylin W: Velar motility, velopharyngeal closure, and speech proficiency in cartilage pharyngoplasty: an eight year study. *Cleft Palate Journal* 5:153-162, 1968.

Hirshowitz B, and Bar-David D: Repeated superiorly based pharyngeal flap operation for persistent velopharyngeal incompetence. *Cleft Palate Journal* 13:45-53, 1976.

Hoffman S: Correction of lateral port stenosis following a pharyngeal flap operation. *Cleft Palate Journal* 22:51-55, 1985.

Hogan VM: A clarification of the surgical goals in cleft palate speech and the introduction of the lateral port control (L.P.C.) pharyngeal flap. *Cleft Palate Journal* 10:331-345, 1973.

Hogan VM: A biased approach to the treatment of velopharyngeal incompetence. *Clinics in Plastic Surgery* 2:319-325, 1975.

Hogan VM, and Schwartz MF: Velopharyngeal incompetence. In Converse JM (ed.): *Plastic and reconstructive surgery: cleft palate and craniofacial anomalies.* Philadelphia: WB Saunders, 1977, pp. 2268-2283.

Hoge J: Millard's island flap in secondary lengthening of cleft soft palates. *British Journal of Plastic Surgery* 19:317-321, 1966.

Holley LR, Hamby GR, and Taylor PP: Palatal lift for velopharyngeal incompetence: report of a case. *Journal of Dentistry for Children* 40:467-470, 1973.

Honig CA: The treatment of velopharyngeal insufficiency after palatal repair. *Archivum Chirurgicum Neerlandicum* 19:71-81, 1967.

Hudson DA, Grobbelaar AO, Fernandes DB, and Lentin R: Treatment of velopharyngeal incompetence by the Furlow Z-plasty. *Annals of Plastic Surgery* 34:23-26, 1995.

Huskie C, and Jackson I: The sphincter pharyngoplasty—a new approach to the speech problems of velopharyngeal incompetence. *British Journal of Disorders of Communication* 12:31-35, 1977.

Hynes W: Pharyngoplasty by muscle transplantation. *British Journal of Plastic Surgery* 3:128-135, 1950.

Hynes W: The results of pharyngoplasty by muscle transplantation in "failed cleft palate" cases, with special reference to the influence of the pharynx on voice production. *Annals of the Royal College of Surgeons of England* 13:17-35, 1953.

Hynes W: Observations on pharyngoplasty. *British Journal of Plastic Surgery* 20:244-256, 1967.

Isberg A, Ren Y-F, Henningsson G, and McWilliam J: Facial growth after pharyngeal flap surgery in cleft palate patients: a five-year longitudinal study. *Scandinavian Journal of Plastic and Reconstructive Surgery* 27:119-126, 1993.

Isshiki N, and Morimoto M: A new folded pharyngeal flap. *Plastic and Reconstructive Surgery* 55:461-465, 1975.

Jackson IT: The sphincter pharyngoplasty as a secondary procedure in cleft palates. *Plastic and Reconstructive Surgery* 59:518-524, 1977.

Jackson IT: Discussion of Orticochea M: A review of 236 cleft palate patients treated with dynamic muscle sphincter. *Plastic and Reconstructive Surgery* 71:189-190, 1983.

Jackson IT: Sphincter pharyngoplasty. *Clinics in Plastic Surgery* 12:711-718, 1985.

Jackson IT, and Silverton F: The sphincter pharyngoplasty as a secondary procedure in cleft palates. *Plastic and Reconstructive Surgery* 59:518-524, 1977.

James NK, Twist M, Turner MM, and Milward TM: An audit of velopharyngeal incompetence treated by the Orticochea pharyngoplasty. *British Journal of Plastic Surgery* 49:197-201, 1996.

Janeke J: Teflon paste injection for velopharyngeal incompetence [letter]. *South African Medical Journal* 62:547, 1982.

Johns DF: Surgical and prosthetic management of neurogenic velopharyngeal incompetency in dysarthria. In Johns DF (ed.): *Clinical management of neurogenic communicative disorders.* 2nd ed. Boston: Little, Brown, 1985, pp. 153-177.

Johns DF, Cannito MP, Rohrich RJ, and Tebbetts JB: The self-lined superiorly based pull-through velopharyngoplasty: plastic surgery–speech pathology interaction in the management of velopharyngeal insufficiency. *Plastic and Reconstructive Surgery* 94:436-445, 1994.

Kapetansky DI: Transverse pharyngeal flaps: a dynamic repair for velopharyngeal insufficiency. *Cleft Palate Journal* 12:44-50, 1975.

Kapetansky DI: Bilateral transverse pharyngeal flaps for hypernasal speech. In Bardach J, and Morris HL (eds.): *Multidisciplinary management of cleft lip and palate.* Philadelphia: WB Saunders, 1990, pp. 392-400.

Karling J, Henningsson G, Larson O, and Isberg A: Adaptation of pharyngeal wall adduction after pharyngeal flap surgery. *Cleft Palate–Craniofacial Journal* 63:166-172, 1999a.

Karling J, Henningsson G, Larson O, and Isberg A: Comparison between two types of pharyngeal flap with regard to configuration at rest and function and speech outcome. *Cleft Palate–Craniofacial Journal* 63:154-165, 1999b.

Karnell MP, Rosenstein H, and Fine L: Nasal videoendoscopy in prosthetic management of palatopharyngeal dysfunction. *Journal of Prosthetic Dentistry* 58:479-484, 1987.

Keller BG, Long RE, Gold ED, and Roth MD: Maxillary dental arch dimensions following pharyngeal flap surgery. *Cleft Palate Journal* 25:248-257, 1988.

Kelsey C, Ewanowski S, Crummy A, and Bless D: Lateral pharyngeal wall motion as a predictor of surgical success in velopharyngeal insufficiency. *New England Journal of Medicine* 287:64-68, 1972.

Kerman P, Singer L, and Davidoff A: Palatal lift and speech therapy for velopharyngeal incompetence. *Archives of Physical Medicine and Rehabilitation* 54:271-276, 1973.

Kiehn CL, DesPrez JD, Tucker A, and Malone M: Experiences with muscle transplants to incomplete soft palates. *Plastic and Reconstructive Surgery* 35:123-130, 1965.

Kipfmueller LJ, and Lang BR: Treating velopharyngeal inadequacies with a palatal lift prosthesis. *Journal of Prosthetic Dentistry* 27:63-72, 1972.

Kriens OB: Fundamental anatomic findings for an intravelar veloplasty. *Cleft Palate Journal* 7:27-36, 1970.

Kuehn D, and Van Demark DR: Assessment of velopharyngeal competency following Teflon pharyngoplasty. *Cleft Palate Journal* 15:145-149, 1978.

Lang GR: Modification of the palatal lift speech aid. *Journal of Prosthetic Dentistry* 17:620-626, 1967.

Lang BR, and Kipfmueller LJ: Treating velopharyngeal inadequacy with the palatal lift concept. *Plastic and Reconstructive Surgery* 46:467-477, 1969.

LaVelle WE, and Hardy J: Palatal lift prostheses for treatment of palatopharyngeal incompetence. *Journal of Prosthetic Dentistry* 42:308-315, 1979.

Lawshe BS, Hardy JC, Schweiger JW, and Van Allen MW: Management of a patient with velopharyngeal incompetency of undetermined origin: a clinical report. *Journal of Speech and Hearing Disorders* 36:547-551, 1971.

Lendrum J, and Dhar BK: The Orticochea dynamic pharyngoplasty. *British Journal of Plastic Surgery* 37:160-168, 1984.

Lesavoy MA, Borud LJ, Thorson T, Riegelhuth ME, and Berkowitz CD: Upper airway obstruction after pharyngeal flap surgery. *Annals of Plastic Surgery* 36:27-30, 1996.

Lewy R, Cole R, and Wepman J: Teflon injection in the correction of velopharyngeal insufficiency. *Annals of Otology, Rhinology, and Laryngology* 74:874-879, 1965.

Lindsey WH, and Davis PT: Correction of velopharyngeal insufficiency with Furlow palatoplasty. *Archives of Otolaryngology–Head and Neck Surgery* 122:881-884, 1996.

Long R, and McNamara J: Facial growth following pharyngeal flap surgery: skeletal assessment on serial lateral cephalometric radiographs. *American Journal of Orthodontics* 87:187-196, 1985.

Marsh J, and Wray R: Speech prosthesis versus pharyngeal flap: a randomized evaluation of the management of velopharyngeal incompetency. *Plastic and Reconstructive Surgery* 5:592-594, 1980.

Marshall R, and Jones J: Effects of a palatal lift prosthesis upon the speech intelligibility of a dysarthric patient. *Journal of Prosthetic Dentistry* 25:327-333, 1971.

Mazaheri M. Prosthodontic care. In Cooper HK, Harding R, Krogman W, Mazaheri M, and Millard R (eds.): *Cleft palate and cleft lip: a team approach to clinical management and rehabilitation of the patient.* Philadelphia: WB Saunders, 1979, pp. 268-357.

Mazaheri M, and Mazaheri E: Prosthodontic aspects of palatal elevation and palatopharyngeal stimulation. *Journal of Prosthetic Dentistry* 35:319-326, 1976.

Mazaheri M, and Millard RT: Changes in nasal resonance related to differences in location and dimension of speech bulbs. *Cleft Palate Journal* 2:167-175, 1965.

McCoy F, and Zahorsky C: A new approach to the elusive dynamic pharyngeal flap. *Plastic and Reconstructive Surgery* 49:160-164, 1972.

McGrath CO, and Anderson MW: Prosthetic treatment of velopharyngeal incompetence. In Bardach J, and Morris HL (eds.): *Multidisciplinary management of cleft lip and palate.* Philadelphia: WB Saunders, 1990, pp. 809-815.

McKinstry R, and Aramany M: Prosthodontic considerations in the management of surgical compromised cleft palate patients. *Journal of Prosthetic Dentistry* 53:827-831, 1985.

Meyer R, Failat A, and Kelly T: Bilateral Z-flap pharyngoplasty in the treatment of rhinolalia. *Head and Neck Surgery* 3:366-370, 1981.

Millard DR: The island flap in cleft palate surgery. *Surgery, Gynecology, and Obstetrics* 116:297-300, 1962.

Millard DR: *Cleft craft: the evolution of its surgeries.* Volume 3: *Alveolar and palatal deformities.* Boston: Little, Brown, 1980.

Millard DR, Batstone J, Heycock M, and Bensen J: Ten years with the palatal island flap. *Plastic and Reconstructive Surgery* 46:540-547, 1970.

Millard RT: Training for optimal use of the prosthetic speech appliance. In Grabb WC, Rosenstein SW, and Bzoch KR (eds.): *Cleft lip and palate: surgical, dental and speech aspects.* Boston: Little, Brown, 1971, pp. 861-867.

Mitnick RJ, Bello JA, Golding-Kushner KJ, Argamaso RV, and Shprintzen RJ: The use of magnetic resonance angiography prior to pharyngeal flap surgery in patients with velocardiofacial syndrome. *Plastic and Reconstructive Surgery* 97:908-919, 1996.

Moore DJ: The continuing role of the prosthodontist in the treatment of patients with cleft lip and palate. *Journal of Prosthetic Dentistry* 36:186-192, 1976.

Morris HL, and Spriestersbach DC: The pharyngeal flap as a speech mechanism. *Plastic and Reconstructive Surgery* 39:66-70, 1967.

Morris HL, Bardach J, Jones D, Christiansen JL, and Gray SD: Clinical results of pharyngeal flap surgery: the Iowa experience. *Plastic and Reconstructive Surgery* 95:652-662, 1995.

Moss ALH, Pigott RW, and Albery EH: Hynes pharyngoplasty revisited. *Plastic and Reconstructive Surgery* 79:346-355, 1987.

Netsell R, and Daniel B: Dysarthria in adults: physiologic approach to rehabilitation. *Archives of Physical Medicine and Rehabilitation* 60:502-508, 1979.

Noordhoff MS: The island flap in secondary cleft palate surgery. *Plastic and Reconstructive Surgery* 46:463-467, 1970.

Orticochea M: Construction of a dynamic muscle sphincter in cleft palates. *Plastic and Reconstructive Surgery* 41:323-327, 1968.

Orticochea M: Results of the dynamic muscle sphincter operation in cleft palates. *British Journal of Plastic Surgery* 23:108-114, 1970.

Orticochea M: A review of 236 cleft palate patients treated with dynamic muscle sphincter. *Plastic and Reconstructive Surgery* 71:180-188, 1983.

Owsley JQ, and Chierici G: The re-do pharyngeal flap. *Plastic and Reconstructive Surgery* 57:180-185, 1976.

Owsley JQ, Creech B, and Dedo H: Poor speech following the pharyngeal flap operation: etiology and treatment. *Cleft Palate Journal* 9:312-318, 1972.

Passavant G: Zweiter Artikel uber die Operation der angeborenen Spalten des harten Gaumens und der damit complicirten Hasenscharten. *Archiv der Heilkunde* 3:305-338, 1862.

Peat BG, Albery EH, Jones K, and Pigott RW: Tailoring velopharyngeal surgery: the influence of etiology and type of operation. *Plastic and Reconstructive Surgery* 93:948-953, 1994.

Pensler JM, and Reich DS: A comparison of speech results after the pharyngeal flap and the dynamic sphincteroplasty procedures. *Annals of Plastic Surgery* 26:441-443, 1991.

Peterson-Falzone SJ: Speech disorders related to craniofacial structural defects: part 2. In Lass NJ, McReynolds LV, Northern JL, and Yoder DE (eds.): *Speech-language pathology and audiology.* Toronto: BC Decker, 1988, pp. 477-547.

Peterson-Falzone SJ, Kaloust SW, Ferrari C, Hoffman WY, and Ousterhout DK: Changes in velar dimensions consequent to the Furlow double-reversing Z-plasty. Proceedings of the 54th annual meeting of the American Cleft Palate–Craniofacial Association, New Orleans, April, 1997.

Pigott R: The results of nasopharyngoscopic assessment of pharyngoplasty. *Scandinavian Journal of Plastic and Reconstructive Surgery* 8:148-152, 1974.

Pigott R: The results of pharyngoplasty by muscle transplantation by Wilfred Hynes. *British Journal of Plastic Surgery* 46:440-442, 1993.

Pigott RW: An assessment of some surgical techniques used in the management of palatal incompetence. In Ellis R, and Flack R (eds.): *Diagnosis and treatment of palato glossal malfunction.* London: College of Speech Therapists, 1979, pp. 67-60.

Pigott RW: Objectives for cleft palate repair. *Annals of Plastic Surgery* 19:247-259, 1987.

Pigott RW, Bensen JF, and White FD: Nasendoscopy in the diagnosis of velopharyngeal incompetence. *Plastic and Reconstructive Surgery* 43:141-147, 1969.

Posnick W: Prosthetic management of palatopharyngeal incompetency for the pediatric patient. *Journal of Dentistry for Children* March-April: 117-121, 1977.

Randall P, Whitaker L, Noone R, and Jones W: The case for inferiorly based posterior pharyngeal flap. *Cleft Palate Journal* 15:262-265, 1978.

Reath DB, LaRossa D, and Randall P: Simultaneous posterior pharyngeal flap and tonsillectomy. *Cleft Palate Journal* 24:250-253, 1987.

Remacle M, Bertrand B, Eloy P, and Marbaix E: The use of injectable collagen to correct velopharyngeal insufficiency. *Laryngoscope* 100:269-274, 1990.

Ren Y-F, Isberg A, and Henningsson G: Interactive influence of a pharyngeal flap and an adenoid on maxillofacial growth in cleft lip and palate patients. *Cleft Palate–Craniofacial Journal* 30:144-149, 1993.

Ren Y-F, Isberg A, and Henningsson G: The influence of pharyngeal flap on facial growth. *Scandinavian Journal of Plastic and Reconstructive Surgery* 29:63-68, 1994.

Riski JE, Hoke JA, and Dolan EA: The role of pressure flow and endoscopic assessment in successful palatal obturator revision. *Cleft Palate Journal* 26:56-62, 1989.

Riski JE, Georgiade N, Serafin D, Barwick WJ, Georgiade GS, and Riefkohl R: The Orticochea pharyngoplasty and primary palatoplasty: an evaluation. *Plastic and Reconstructive Surgery* 18:303-309, 1987.

Riski JE, Ruff GL, Georgiade GS, and Barwick WJ: Evaluation of failed sphincter pharyngoplasties. *Annals of Plastic Surgery* 28:545-553, 1992a.

Riski JE, Ruff GL, Georgiade GS, Barwick WJ, and Edwards PD: Evaluation of the sphincter pharyngoplasty. *Cleft Palate–Craniofacial Journal* 29:254-261, 1992b.

Riski J, Serafin D, Riefkohl R, Georgiade G, and Georgiade NG: A rationale for modifying the site of insertion of the Orticochea pharyngoplasty. *Plastic and Reconstructive Surgery* 73:882-890, 1984.

Roberts T, and Brown B: Evaluation of a modified sphincter pharyngoplasty in the treatment of speech problems due to palatal insufficiency. *Annals of Plastic Surgery* 10:209-213, 1983.

Rosen MS, and Bzoch KR: Prosthodontic management of the individual with cleft lip and palate for speech habilitation needs. In Bzoch KR (ed.): *Communicative disorders related to cleft lip and palate.* 4th ed. Austin: Pro-ed, 1997, pp. 153-167.

Ruddy J, Stokes M, and Pearman K: Pharyngoplasty surgery and obstructive sleep apnea. *Journal of Laryngology and Otology* 105:195-197, 1991.

Ruscello DM: Considerations for behavioral treatment of velopharyngeal closure for speech. In Bzoch KR (ed.): *Communicative disorders related to cleft lip and palate.* 4th ed. Austin: Pro-ed, 1997, pp. 509-562.

Sadove AM, and Eppley BL: Surgical repair of the cleft palate and velopharynx. In Berkowitz S (ed.): *Cleft lip and palate: perspectives in management.* Volume II: *An introduction to other craniofacial anomalies.* San Diego: Singular, 1996, pp. 99-109.

Sanvenero-Roselli G: Divisione palatina, sua cura chirurgica. In Sanvenero-Roselli G (ed.): *La divisione congenital del labio e del palato.* Roma: Casa Editrice Luigi Pozzi, 1934, pp. 262-268.

Schoenborn D: Uber eine neue Methode der Staphylorraphie. *Archive Fuer Klinische Chirurgie* 19:527-531, 1876.

Schoenborn D: Vorstellung eines Falles vor Staphyloplastik. *Ver Deutsch Gest. Chirurgie* 15:57, 1886.

Schweiger J, Netsell R, and Sommerfeld R: Prosthetic management and speech improvement in individuals with dysarthria of the palate. *Journal of the American Dental Association* 80:1348-1353, 1970.

Selley WG: Dental and technical aids for the treatment of patients suffering from velopharyngeal disorders. In Ellis RE, and Flack FC (eds.): *Diagnosis and treatment of palato glossal malfunction.* London: College of Speech Therapists, 1979, pp. 53-61.

Semb G, and Shaw WC: Pharyngeal flap and facial growth. *Cleft Palate Journal* 27:217-224, 1990a.

Semb G, and Shaw WC: The influence of pharyngeal flap on facial growth. In Bardach J, and Morris HL (eds.): *Multidisciplinary management of cleft lip and palate.* Philadelphia: WB Saunders, 1990b, pp. 414-418.

Seyfer AE, Prohazka D, and Leahy E: The effectiveness of the superiorly based pharyngeal flap in relation to the type of palatal defect and timing of the operation. *Plastic and Reconstructive Surgery* 82:760-764, 1988.

Shprintzen RJ: The use of multiview videofluoroscopy and flexible fiberoptic nasopharyngoscopy as a predictor of success with pharyngeal flap surgery. In Ellis F, and Flack E (eds.): *Diagnosis and treatment of palato glossal malfunction.* London: College of Speech Therapists, 1979, pp. 6-14.

Shprintzen RJ: Pharyngeal flap surgery and the pediatric upper airway. *International Anesthesiology Clinics* 26:79-88, 1988.

Shprintzen RJ, Croft C, Berkman MD, and Rakoff S: Velopharyngeal insufficiency in the facio-auriculo-vertebral malformation complex. *Cleft Palate Journal* 17:132-143, 1980.

Shprintzen RJ, Lewin ML, Croft C, Daniller A, Argamaso R, Ship A, and Strauch B: A comprehensive study of pharyngeal flap surgery: tailor made flaps. *Cleft Palate Journal* 16:46-55, 1979.

Shprintzen RJ, McCall G, and Skolnick M: The effect of pharyngeal flap surgery on the movements of the lateral pharyngeal walls. *Plastic and Reconstructive Surgery* 4:570-573, 1980.

Shprintzen RJ, Singer L, Sidoti EJ, and Argamaso RV: Pharyngeal flap surgery: postoperative complications. *International Anesthesiology Clinics* 30:115-124, 1992.

Sirois M, Caouette-Laberge L, Spier S, Larocque Y, and Egerszegi EP: Sleep apnea following a pharyngeal flap: a feared complication. *Plastic and Reconstructive Surgery* 93:948-953, 1994.

Skolnick ML, and McCall G: Velopharyngeal competency and incompetence following pharyngeal flap surgery: a videofluoroscopic study in multiple projections. *Cleft Palate Journal* 9:1-12, 1972.

Skolnick ML, and McCall G: A radiographic technique for demonstrating the causes of persistent nasality in patients with pharyngeal flaps. *British Journal of Plastic Surgery* 26:12-15, 1973.

Skoog T: The pharyngeal flap operation for cleft palate. *British Journal of Plastic Surgery* 18:265-282, 1965.

Smith JK, and McCabe BF: Teflon injection in the nasopharynx to improve velopharyngeal closure. *Annals of Otology* 86:559-563, 1977.

Spratley M, Chenerey H, and Murdoch B: A different design of palatal lift appliance: review and case reports. *Australian Dental Journal* 33:491-495, 1988.

Stratoudakis AC, and Bambace C: Sphincter pharyngoplasty for correction of velopharyngeal incompetence. *Annals of Plastic Surgery* 12:243-248, 1985.

Sturim H, and Jacob C: Teflon pharyngoplasty. *Plastic and Reconstructive Surgery* 49:180-185, 1972.

Subtelny JD, and Pineda Nieto R: A longitudinal study of maxillary growth following pharyngeal flap surgery. *Cleft Palate Journal* 15:118-131, 1978.

Sullivan DE: Bilateral pharyngoplasty as an aid to velopharyngeal closure. *Plastic and Reconstructive Surgery* 27:31-39, 1961.

Thompson RPJ, Ferguson JW, and Barton M: The role of removable orthodontic appliances in the investigation and management of patients with hypernasal speech. *British Journal of Orthodontics* 12:70-77, 1985.

Thurston JB, Larson DL, Shanks JC, Bennett JE, and Parsons RW: Nasal obstruction as a complication of pharyngeal flap surgery. *Cleft Palate Journal* 17:148-154, 1980.

Tomes LA, Kuehn DP, and Peterson-Falzone SJ: Behavioral treatments of velopharyngeal impairment. In Bzoch KR (ed.): *Communicative disorders related to cleft lip and palate.* 4th ed. Austin: Pro-ed, 1997, pp. 529-562.

Trier WC: Pharyngeal flaps for the correction of velopharyngeal insufficiency. In Cohen M (ed.): *Mastery of plastic and reconstructive surgery.* Volume 1. Boston: Little, Brown, 1994, pp. 632-642.

Trigos I, Ysunza A, Gonzalez A, and Vazquez M: Surgical treatment of borderline velopharyngeal insufficiency using homologous cartilage implantation with videonasopharyngoscopic monitoring. *Cleft Palate Journal* 25:167-170, 1988.

Tudor C, and Selley W: A palatal training appliance and a visual aid for use in the treatment of hypernasal speech. *British Journal of Disorders of Communication* 9:117-122, 1974.

Valauri AJ: Cleft palate prosthetics. In Converse JM (ed.): *Reconstructive plastic surgery.* Volume 4. 2nd ed. Philadelphia: WB Saunders, 1977, pp. 2283-2295.

Van Demark DR, and Hardin MA: Longitudinal evaluation of articulation and velopharyngeal competence of patients with pharyngeal flaps. *Cleft Palate Journal* 22:163-172, 1985.

Walter JD: The design of prostheses used in the treatment of velopharyngeal insufficiency. *British Dental Journal* 151:338-342, 1981.

Ward PH, Goldman R, and Stoudt RJ: Teflon injection to improve velopharyngeal insufficiency. *Journal of Speech and Hearing Disorders* 31:267-273, 1966.

Ward PH, Stoudt RJ, and Goldman R: Improvement of velopharyngeal insufficiency by Teflon injection. *Transactions of the American Academy of Ophthalmology and Otolaryngology* 71:923-933, 1967.

Wedin S: Rehabilitation of speech in cases of palato-pharyngeal paresis with the aid of an obturator prosthesis. *British Journal of Communication Disorders* 7:117-130, 1972.

Weiss C: Success of an obturator reduction program. *Cleft Palate Journal* 8:291-297, 1971.

Weiss C, and Louis H: Toward a more objective approach to obturator reduction. *Cleft Palate Journal* 9:157-160, 1972.

Whitaker L, Randall P, Graham W, Hamilton R, and Winchester F: A prospective and randomized series comparing superiorly and inferiorly based posterior pharyngeal flaps. *Cleft Palate Journal* 9:304-311, 1972.

Witt PD, and D'Antonio LL: Velopharyngeal insufficiency and secondary palatal management: a new look at an old problem. *Clinics in Plastic Surgery* 20:707-721, 1993.

Witt PD, and Marsh JL: Advances in assessing outcome of surgical repair of cleft lip and palate. *Plastic and Reconstructive Surgery* 100:1907-1917, 1997.

Witt PD, D'Antonio LL, Zimmerman GJ, and Marsh JL: Sphincter pharyngoplasty: a preoperative and postoperative analysis of perceptual speech characteristics and endoscopic studies of velopharyngeal function. *Plastic and Reconstructive Surgery* 93:1154-1167, 1994.

Witt PD, Marsh JL, Grames, LM, and Muntz HR: Revision of the failed sphincter pharyngoplasty: an outcome assessment. *Plastic and Reconstructive Surgery* 96:129-138, 1995a.

Witt PD, Marsh JL, Grames LM, Muntz HR, and Gay WD: Management of the hypodynamic velopharynx. *Cleft Palate–Craniofacial Journal* 32:179-187, 1995b.

Witt PD, Rozelle AA, Marsh JL, Grames LM, Muntz HR, Gay WD, and Pilgram TK: Do palatal lift prostheses stimulate velopharyngeal neuromuscular activity? *Cleft Palate–Craniofacial Journal* 32:469-475, 1995c.

Witt PD, Marsh JL, Muntz HR, Grames LM, and Watchmaker GP: Acute obstructive sleep apnea as a complication of sphincter pharyngoplasty. *Cleft Palate–Craniofacial Journal* 33:183-189, 1996.

Witt PD, O'Daniel TG, Marsh JL, Grames LM, Muntz HR, and Pilgram TK: Surgical management of velopharyngeal dysfunction: outcome analysis of autogenous posterior pharyngeal wall augmentation. *Plastic and Reconstructive Surgery* 99:1287-1296, 1997.

Witzel MA, and Stringer DA: Methods of assessing velopharyngeal function. In Bardach J, and Morris HL (eds.): *Multidisciplinary management of cleft lip and palate.* Philadelphia: WB Saunders, 1990, pp. 763-776.

Wolford LM, Oelschlaeger M, and Deal R: Proplast as a pharyngeal wall implant to correct velopharyngeal insufficiency. *Cleft Palate Journal* 26:119-126, 1989.

Wong LP, and Weiss CE: A clinical assessment of obturator-wearing cleft palate patients. *Journal of Prosthetic Dentistry* 27:632-639, 1972.

Ysunza A, Garcia-Velasco M, Barcia-Garcia M, Haro R, and Valencia M: Obstructive sleep apnea secondary to surgery for velopharyngeal insufficiency. *Cleft Palate–Craniofacial Journal* 30:387-390, 1993.

Yules R, and Chase R: Pharyngeal flap surgery: a review of the literature. *Cleft Palate Journal* 6:303-308, 1969.

Yules RB, Chase RA, Blocksma R, and Lang BR: Secondary techniques for correction of palatopharyngeal incompetence. In Grabb WC, Rosenstein SW, and Bzoch KR (eds.): *Cleft lip and palate.* Philadelphia: WB Saunders, 1971, pp. 451-489.

Zwitman D: Velopharyngeal physiology after pharyngeal flap surgery as assessed by oral endoscopy. *Cleft Palate Journal* 19:36-39, 1982.

Chapter 14

Psychosocial and Educational Issues

When psychologists and other health care professionals first began to publish their concerns about patients with clefts and other facial differences, they were attempting to derive and organize information on a patient population that, for the most part, had not been studied from this perspective. The material they initially had to offer consisted of anecdotal reports, assessments of some broad aspects of development, ratings or reports of third-party reactions to facial disfigurement, observations of their own patients, and speculation about the meaning of those observations (Clifford 1967, 1969b, 1971, 1973; MacGregor, 1951; MacGregor et al., 1953; Richardson, 1971; Richardson et al., 1961; Richardson, Hastorf, and Dornbusch, 1964; Ruess, 1967; Tisza, Irwin, and Scheide, 1973). The effort these clinicians put into their task was admirable and often indefatigable. However, at least two factors led to subsequent problems in interpreting the information they derived. First, they often pooled subjects with cleft lip +/− palate (CL+/−P) and cleft palate only (CPO) because, at least in individual treatment centers, they did not have large patient populations to study. As you learned in Chapter 1, subjects with CPO are far more likely than subjects with CL+/−P to have other congenital anomalies or to fall into various syndromic categories. Some of the earlier studies on psychosocial concerns predated the knowledge of this important difference.[1]

The second factor that likely contributed to discrepancies in findings was the fact that investigators typically looked at just one or two aspects of psychosocial adjustment and behavior, e.g., Is IQ affected by a cleft? Do children with clefts do as well in school as children without clefts? Is there a "cleft palate personality"? Research designs in early studies often did not take into account the complex interactions among either the independent variables affecting their subjects or the dependent variables they were trying to measure. Endriga and Kapp-Simon (1999, p. 8) pointed to the importance of the development of research design in craniofacial research (in psychology) that included "multiple domains." For children with craniofacial anomalies (CFA), they described "domains of risk and protection" that include "variables related to child (e.g., cognition, severity of the [anomaly], temperament, and social competence), parent and family variables (e.g., psychological well-being, social support, marital satisfaction, and parenting style), and treatment variables (e.g., number and type of surgeries, therapeutic needs, and outcome of habilitation as it relates to factors such as speech, hearing and appearance)." The change in the rigor of research design found in recent publications and presentations should guide investigators well into the next decade.

It may give you a helpful perspective to know that, as of early 1999, although publications on various aspects of the psychosocial effects of clefts dated back at least four decades, nearly 40% of the pertinent articles, book chapters, and books on the topic were published *after* 1990. Like the areas of genetics and surgery, keeping abreast of new knowledge on psychosocial issues is an increasingly demanding task. In the mid-1990s, a Psychology Working Group on Craniofacial Conditions[2] was founded, bringing together leading researchers who published their first set of comprehensive, updated papers and reviews in 1997 (Berry et al., 1997; Broder, 1997; Kapp-Simon and McGuire, 1997; Pope and Speltz, 1997; Pope and Ward, 1997a; Richman, 1997). The recent Endriga and Kapp-Simon review (1999) addressed both clinical and research issues in "CFA" subjects, pooling the information from a large number of studies on cleft patients and those few available articles on other craniofacial birth defects.

[1]Even some of the more recent studies do not present evidence that their subjects were thoroughly examined to eliminate significant associated anomalies or syndromes, which may bring their results into question, especially when the studies included subjects with clefts limited to the secondary palate. See Chapters 2 and 8.

[2]Funded through the National Foundation for Facial Reconstruction.

Many reviews of the published information on the psychosocial impacts of clefts have appeared, each one covering most of the material that was available up to the date of that particular review (Clifford, 1973, 1979; Eder, 1995; Eliason, 1991; Endriga and Kapp-Simon, 1999; Lansdown, 1981; Lavigne and Wills, 1990; Madison, 1986; McWilliams, 1970, 1982; Richman and Eliason, 1982; Spriestersbach, 1973; Strauss and Broder, 1990; Tobiasen, 1990; Tobiasen and Speltz, 1996; Wirls, 1971). Some reviews focused particularly on research issues (Broder, 1997; Eliason, 1990; Pope and Speltz, 1997; Strauss and Broder, 1991; Tobiasen, 1984, 1993). If you develop an interest in particular aspects of psychosocial adjustment in patients with clefts and other craniofacial anomalies, you will find helpful references in the bibliographies of these articles.

In 1969, Clifford (1969a) recommended a *developmental* approach to psychosocial and educational concerns, that is, studying what is happening with the child and family at each developmental level or chronological age bracket. That approach has been adopted in current studies and reviews, although it took about 25 years for the change to occur (Eder, 1995; Eliason, 1991; Endriga and Kapp-Simon, 1999; Madison, 1984; Speltz et al., 1994b; Tobiasen, 1993; Tobiasen and Speltz, 1996). The developmental approach is a refreshing change from studies that asked broader questions (examples given above) across diverse age groups of patients. Coordinating topics of psychosocial concern with developmental stages or chronological age brackets yields the framework depicted in Table 14-1.

A NEW CHALLENGE: ANTICIPATION OF A CHILD WITH A CLEFT

From a chronological or developmental perspective, psychologists, social workers, family therapists and other psychosocial professionals *used* to focus first on how parents of newborn infants dealt with the shock of a child with a cleft. In the past two decades, however, there have been increasing numbers of about-to-be-parents who already know that their baby will have a cleft or other craniofacial anomaly. With specific regard to clefts, that foreknowledge (as of this writing) is usually limited to fetuses with cleft of

Table 14-1 **Psychosocial Concerns According to Developmental Stages of Patients**

Developmental Stage or Age Bracket	*Area of Concern*	*Specific Topics*
Prenatal	Adjustment to the impending birth of a child with a defect	
Birth, perinatal period	Adjustment to the birth of a child with a defect	Parent-infant bonding, feeding issues, reactions of other family members, dealing with reactions of others in the community; stress and financial demands of surgery*
Toddler years	Parent and family adjustment to multiple demands	Parents' attempts to protect the child from adverse reaction from extended family and community; child's normal attempt to assert self (before the realization of personal difference); stress of medical interventions
Preschool years (ages 3-6 years)	Self-concept; peer relationships; cognitive development	Unavoidable realization of facial difference for child and family; judgments by peers and teachers; interruptions from medical interventions; possible learning disabilities
Early school years (ages 6-10 years)	Self-concept, peer relationships, school adjustment, achievement	
Preteen years (ages 10-13 years)	Self-concept, peer relationships, school adjustment, achievement	Judgments by peers and teachers; interruptions caused by medical interventions; possible learning disabilities
Teens	Self-concept, peer relationships, school achievement	Final phases of physical management (e.g., orthodontics, surgery)
Adults	Social interactions, life partners, employment	

*Including the indirect costs of absences from work, travel, child care for siblings, housing, etc.

the lip +/– palate, in contrast to cleft palate only. Many of the multiple anomaly disorders such as Apert, Crouzon, and Pfeiffer syndromes, mandibulofacial dysostosis, and Nager syndromes are also visible on prenatal imaging. In addition, prenatal chromosome analysis or molecular genetic analysis can reveal the presence of many syndromes, although not the presence of cleft lip +/– palate alone. These advances in technology have forced cleft palate and craniofacial teams to push their professional expertise backward, chronologically, to aid about-to-be parents. This particular area of professional responsibility for counselors and their fellow team members was virtually unknown until recently, and thus we currently have no structured, systematic studies of the psychosocial impact on parents and families. It is likely that such studies will soon begin to appear in the literature and that clinicians will gain helpful information on how to assist families in handling this emotionally potent situation.

INFANTS AND THEIR PARENTS

The Initial Reaction

Clinicians have used a variety of approaches (structured interviews, questionnaires, anecdotal information) to learn about the feelings and fears of parents on the birth of a child with a cleft or other facial deformity. Many reports, including first-person accounts provided by parents, point to the importance of the baby being shown to the parents immediately after birth or as soon as possible (Clifford, 1973, 1979; Clifford and Crocker, 1971; Dar, Winter, and Tal, 1974; Gibbs, 1973; Lansdown, 1981; Rowe, 1983; Spriestersbach, 1973; Tisza and Gumpertz, 1962).[3] Delays in seeing the baby heighten anxiety, whereas being able to hold the infant and keep him nearby allows parents to realize that he is more like a normal child than not and that they can do normal things such as bathing, cuddling, and comforting (Gibbs, 1973; MacDonald, 1979; Rowe, 1983). The reported parental reactions to first learning of the baby's birth defect include disbelief, shock, anger, guilt, depression, resentment, grief, rage, frustration, fear, anxiety, protectiveness, and stigmatization (Barden et al., 1989; Benson and Gross, 1989; Brantley and Clifford, 1979; Carreto, 1981; Clifford, 1968, 1979; Clifford and Crocker, 1971; Drotar et al., 1975; Lansdown, 1981; Pope, 1999; Richman and Harper 1978a, 1978b; Slutsky, 1969; Spriestersbach, 1973; Stricker et al., 1979; Tisza and Gumpertz, 1962; Waechter, 1959).[4] Drotar et al. (1975) identified five successive stages of parental reaction to the birth of an infant with a congenital malformation (not exclusively clefts)—shock, denial, sadness and anger, adaptation, and reorganization—and reported that parents spent a variable amount of time in each of these stages.

New parents of a child with a cleft worry about how they will feed and care for the baby and about the baby's development, e.g., Will she have teeth? Will she talk OK? and perhaps the greatest fear, Is he going to be retarded? Embarrassment and fear of reaction of the public may lead some parents to try to conceal the infant (Bradbury and Hewison, 1984), and the parents themselves may withdraw from social contacts just at the time they are most in need of support from friends and relatives (Benson et al., 1991; Clifford, 1973, 1979; Pope, 1999). Pope (1999, p. 36) voiced the fear that "if parents are not able to make the emotional adjustment at this [neonatal] time, their unresolved feelings are likely to reappear and negatively influence their parenting." For parents of children with CL+/–P, compared with cleft palate only, the visibility of the lip defect can contribute to severity of their reaction (Natsume, Suzuki, and Kawai, 1987). However, some relatively recent data on parent-infant interaction indicate that this interaction may be adversely affected even when the cleft is "non-visible" (Endriga and Speltz, 1997). Several clinicians reported that the initial reactions of shock, anger, etc., dissipated fairly quickly in parents of cleft babies (Carreto, 1981; Clifford, 1968, 1979; Clifford and Crocker, 1971; Slutsky, 1969; Spriestersbach, 1973), a phenomenon that Clifford and Crocker (1971) attributed to the parents learning that the defect is "fixable." Subsequent investigations on this point have not yielded consistent results, possibly because of variation in such factors as severity of defect, family and social support, and how long after the birth the parents were interviewed. There has also been inconsistency in findings relative to effects of the birth on the marital relationship (Benson and Gross, 1989; Bradbury and Hewison, 1994; Clifford, 1968, 1969b, 1979; Clifford and Crocker, 1971; Speltz, Armsden, and Clarren, 1990).

Retrospectively, parents report that they wanted more information from the physician at the time of the birth, as well as more compassion and greater opportunity to discuss their fears (Strauss, Sharp, Lorch, and Kachalia, 1995). Early contact with other parents and with professionals, especially an interdisciplinary team, can aid in the adjustment of family (Clifford and Crocker, 1971). MacDonald (1979), a parent of a child with a cleft, stated, "Parents take their cues from professionals." That is, seeing the professionals smile at the baby, cuddle him, etc., can ease parental anxiety. Similarly, contact with other families who are raising a child with a cleft or other craniofacial anomaly can help build the parents' confidence and reduce the feeling of isolation (Benson et al., 1991; MacDonald, 1979). There are many local parent and patient groups that can serve as a source of information and support, and a few national groups as well.[5]

---

[3]Today, the idea of "protecting" parents by preventing them from immediately seeing their child with a craniofacial or other visible birth defect seems archaic, but there may well be communities where this practice is still considered to be in the best interest of the family.

[4]The studies cited here included some children with visible facial deformities other than clefts.

[5]To find these groups, contact the Cleft Palate Foundation, 1-800-24-CLEFT.

Dealing with Early Demands

Central to the parents' feelings of adequacy and competency is the ability to feed the infant comfortably and effectively. You read about some of the prosthetic approaches to this problem in Chapter 6. There is no question that most, but not all, babies with clefts exhibit early problems in weight gain and growth (Avedian and Ruberg, 1980; Ranalli and Mazaheri, 1975) unless there is early and effective intervention and that these problems add to parents' anxiety. Clinicians have always been concerned about these problems, but in recent years, investigators in psychology have also focused on the *interactive* physical and vocal cues exchanged between infant and mother at feeding times (Speltz et al., 1994a). In the latter study, infants with unrepaired clefts (CLP or CPO) were less likely than noncleft babies to smile or laugh during feeding and were rated lower in the "feeding cues" they gave their mothers. In other words, the negative influences on the baby and parents that become apparent in the baby's feeding and subsequent development may not be simply a function of the parent's difficulty in finding an effective means of feeding but may also stem in part from the baby. Speltz et al. (1994a) did a 12-month follow-up assessment on these same infants and found that they were exhibiting "normal patterns of feeding communication" and that maternal insensitivity did not influence the security of the mother-infant attachment.

In addition to managing the feeding and care of the infant, the reactions of friends and relatives and the general public, and possibly new marital stress, the parents face the demands of diagnostic evaluations (frequently requiring several visits with the team or individual practitioners) and the demands attendant on surgery. For the child with cleft lip and palate, there will be at least one operation in the first year of life, and more likely two. For the family the operations and the perioperative periods can be a time of conflict. In the early days and weeks of life, although the parents know that the baby is small and vulnerable, they often inquire about the possibility of immediate surgery to correct the visible defect (Eliason, 1991; Spriestersbach, 1973). When it is actually time for the lip surgery, parents typically are pleased that the defect is finally going to be "fixed," but because they will have had the child at home for 2 or 3 months before surgery, they may find that they are actually reluctant to see the appearance of the infant's face altered. It is not unusual for parents to admit a little sheepishly that they "don't really want to see his smile change." In addition, the hospitalization and operation can amplify feelings of guilt (e.g., "We did this to him."). Most hospitals now arrange for parents to sleep in the child's hospital room and to be the primary caregivers during hospitalization, which can help minimize the disruption in family life.

With specific regard to palate surgery, there are some additional sources of stress. The operative time is a little longer than the lapsed time for lip surgery, the infant is older and even more attached to the parents, and the immediate postoperative period typically involves the use of some form of arm restraints. In addition, the method of feeding will usually be different for a while. In total, the operative experience can amount to significant upset for both baby and parents. Tobiasen (1990) spoke of hospitalization as one of the "core stressors" for these families and one that recurs several times during the child's growing years. She also stated (1993, p. 623) that the "long-term invasive nature of treatment . . . may be extremely stressful and have adverse effects on [normal psychosocial] development."

There are some interesting data regarding effects of hospitalization in infancy on the subsequent development of the child. Schaffer and Callender (1959) were not looking at children with clefts but tried to study the psychological effects of hospitalization in children who had been through that experience between 3 and 51 weeks of age, with the length of that hospitalization being from 4 to 49 days. All the infants were less than 12 months old. The reactions seemed to fall into two distinct groups, based on whether the hospitalization occurred below or above the age of 7 months. Those older than 7 months who were hospitalized exhibited considerable upset when admitted to the hospital and a period of disturbance after returning home, with both reactions seeming to center around the need for the physical presence of the mother. In the group hospitalized under the age of 7 months, separation from the mother appeared to evoke "no observable disturbance," and instead there seemed to be an immediate adjustment to the new environment (that is, the hospital). On return to the home there was reportedly a "marked change of behavior [in most infants], but it was generally found to be of very brief duration." The authors suggested (p. 538), ". . . where there is a choice, hospitalization should be arranged to occur before the crucial age is reached." This study was perhaps the first to draw attention to the potential differential effects of hospitalization based on age of the infant.

Starr (1978a) looked at "hospitalization effects" on the behavior of preschoolers with cleft lip or palate. The children were aged 3 to 5 years and were compared with noncleft children on six behavior dimensions of a standardized behavioral checklist that was constructed to tap aggression, activity level, sociability, inhibition, sleep disturbance, and somatization.[6] Starr found no significant differences between the children with clefts and those without clefts. At the time, 20+ years ago, the author felt that his findings should be comforting to parents of children with clefts. However, he assumed that the lack of significant differences meant that hospitalization (from 1 month to 5½ years) was the only factor influencing his

[6]"Somatization" refers to turning psychological stresses into self-perceived physical symptoms or self-perceived differences in body parts or organs.

results because this was essentially the only factor he was examining.

Today, hospitalization does not mean as much isolation from parents as it once did because of changes in policies of patient and parent management, but the potential for disruption of family life and parent-child attachments is nevertheless of concern.

Parent-Infant Bonding

Problems in early parent-infant bonding have been studied from several different aspects. Clifford (1969a) had parents of babies with clefts, all under the age of 2 years at the time of the study, rate perceived severity of the child's medical condition, activity level, and general attractiveness. In this study, all types of clefts were combined (CLO [cleft lip only], CPO, CLP). Clifford found that the higher the rating of severity of the defect, the more likely the infant was to be perceived by the parents as active-irritable and as less pleasant in personality characteristics. Rubin (1975) reported that mothers of infants with clefts showed a delay in touching their babies. Field and Vega-Lahr (1984) found that mothers of infants with cleft lip and palate in the 3- to 6-month age range were less interactive with their babies than were mothers in a comparison group; that is, they were less playful, less responsive when the baby initiated a new behavior, and less facially expressive. The babies were also less facially expressive, showing less smiling and looking at their mothers less than noncleft babies did.[7] Field and Vega-Lahr (1984) conjectured that the mothers they studied may have felt inadequate, causing an adverse effect on parent-child bonding. A later report on a diverse group of five infants in the same age range, all with different types of craniofacial anomalies (Barden et al., 1989) yielded results that were essentially consistent with those of Field and Vega-Lahr (1984). Two studies by Wasserman (Wasserman and Allen, 1985; Wasserman, Allen, and Solomon, 1986) also yielded similar results. However, each of these studies included children who were syndromic, a factor that could obviously influence results. Some subsequent studies on attachment in later infancy (e.g., 9 to 12 months) found that babies with craniofacial anomalies were at no greater risk for insecure attachment than were babies without such anomalies (Hoeksma and Koomen, 1991; Wasserman, Lennon, Allen, and Shilansky, 1987).

Endriga and Speltz (1997) observed mother-infant dyads when the infants with clefts (CLP or CPO) were 3 months old. Interestingly, the mothers of the CPO babies appeared less involved in en face interaction than the mothers of the CLP infants. However, the authors did not find significant differences between the mother-infant pairs in the combined cleft groups and pairs in which the infants were noncleft. They concluded that there was little evidence to suggest that "anomalous facial appearance" had a significant influence on the quality of early mother-infant interaction. They conjectured that the age of 3 months may be too late to detect such differences. Perhaps the observation made by Clifford and Crocker (1971) that parents work through the initial crises relatively quickly means that the age of 3 months is in fact too late to pick up differences in parent-infant interaction.

Speltz, Armsden, and Clarren (1990) looked at maternal functioning during the late infancy and toddler periods (ages 1 to 3 years, average age 20 months). The babies had CLP, CPO, or isolated synostosis of the sagittal suture of the cranium. The data consisted of the mothers' self-reports of psychological and emotional status and of the quality of their relationships with spouses and others plus direct observation of mother-infant interactions. The mothers reported higher levels of stress, lower evaluations of their own competence, and a higher degree of marital conflict than mothers in a comparison group did. However, the observational measures showed no group differences in maternal response to the children or in the behavior and responsiveness of the children themselves. Thus, the mothers perceived themselves as stressed and inadequate, even when direct observations of their behavior with the babies did not verify these perceptions. Speltz, Armsden, and Clarren (1990) also observed that the presence of facial disfigurement in their CLP subgroup was not associated with uniquely higher levels of maternal stress or problems in parenting competence and marital interaction.

In summary, there are many obvious threats to parent-infant bonding, and they may not be as simple as was once assumed. Much of the research by Tobiasen (Tobiasen, 1984, 1987; Tobiasen and Hiebert, 1993a, 1993b, 1994; Tobiasen et al., 1987) focused on the adverse impact of abnormal facial appearance on early parent-child relationships as well as subsequent development of the child in the toddler, preschool, and school years. However, the research of Speltz and coworkers (Speltz, Armsden, and Clarren, 1990; Speltz, Galbreath, and Greenberg, 1995; Speltz et al., 1994b) did not validate facial appearance as the predominant factor in parent-infant attachment. Speltz et al. (1994b, p. 66) did state, "There is preliminary evidence for the existence of early difficulties in mother-infant interaction, including compromised maternal responsiveness and lack of clarity in the infant's communication of positive emotion and feeding cues. Such problems may lead to higher-than-average rates of insecure attachment . . . although this has yet to be investigated and should be a priority for future infancy research."

Infant Development

Several early studies on cognitive and other types of development in babies with clefts signaled an increased risk for developmental delay, but in many of these studies the

[7] Speltz, Galbreath, and Greenberg (1995) conjectured that infants with craniofacial anomalies may not be able to produce normal facial expressions that would serve as cues for their parents and that this might interfere with parent-infant communication. Endriga and Kapp-Simon (1999) and Pope (1999) echoed the same thought. The only actual data on the ability of children with clefts to produce facial expressions were derived in the 1993 study of Krueckeberg, Kapp-Simon, and Ribordy on preschoolers, discussed later in this chapter.

types of clefts were combined and syndromic involvement may not have been entirely eliminated, especially when babies with CPO were not separated from those with CL+/−P. It is thus somewhat ironic that many of the more recent studies (and reviews of the literature) on infant development have combined babies with clefts with babies exhibiting other craniofacial anomalies.

Starr et al. (1977) assessed development in 75 children with clefts (24 CPO, 31 CLP, 20 CLO). The measure used was the Bayley Scales of Infant Development (Bayley, 1969), an instrument still in wide use more than 30 years later. They had no noncleft controls, but simply compared the scores to the test norms, and presented cross-sectional and longitudinal data (6, 12, 18, and 24 months of age). In both the cross-sectional and longitudinal data, the performance of the CLP children was not significantly different from the norms for the test, but the scores for the cleft palate only group were significantly different. The authors expressed some surprise that the performance of the infants with CPO was so different from that for infants with CL+/−P. The knowledge that infants with cleft palate only are much more likely than infants with cleft lip +/− palate to have associated anomalies or syndromic involvement had been in the literature for nearly 30 years when this study was published (e.g., Fogh-Andersen, 1942) but was still relatively unrecognized in the United States. Starr et al. (1977) also reported that their findings across the five dimensions of responsiveness to mother, object orientation, imaginative play, activity, and reactivity levels were suggestive of greater passivity or a greater tendency to avoid sensorimotor stimuli in the children with clefts compared with noncleft children.

Fox, Lynch, and Brookshire (1978) also found evidence of developmental delay in children less than 3 years old with a variety of clefts (UCLP, BCLP, CPO). The subjects ranged in age from late infancy to toddlerhood, averaging 17.7 months of age, and were matched with a control group. The data were primarily language-based, consisting of the Denver Developmental Screening Scale (Frankenburg and Dodds, 1969), the REEL scale (Receptive-Expressive Emergent Language) (Bzoch and League, 1971), and the Birth-to-Three Scale (Bangs and Garrett, 1973). The authors found it was possible to group 79% of the subjects accurately (cleft versus control groups) solely on the basis of developmental data. This study became one of the "wake-up" calls to developmental concerns in very young children with clefts, even children without associated anomalies or syndromes.[8] Long and Dalston (1982) demonstrated delays in the development of gestural language in 12-month old children with cleft lip and palate, a finding that was surprising at that time because all the previous studies on language had focused primarily on oral expressive language, in which negative effects of the cleft palate were expected. Delays in nonoral language development were less easily explained. Subsequent studies have also demonstrated delays or deficiencies in cognitive and language development. Neiman and Savage (1997) studied infants and toddlers at four age levels: 5 months, 13 months, 25 months, and 36 months. With use of the Kent Infant Development Scale (Reuter and Bickett, 1985) and the Minnesota Child Development Inventory (Ireton and Thwing, 1977), both caregiver reports, Nieman and Savage found evidence of "at risk" or delayed development in the motor, self-help, and cognitive domains in 5-month old children, especially when the cleft involved the palate. Interestingly, even the children with CLO exhibited depressed full-scale and motor developmental quotients, a finding that the authors suggested may have been due to factors attendant to lip surgery (arm restraints, lip adhesion as a first procedure [see Chapter 4], posturing of the caregiver, etc.). The authors also postulated that early feeding difficulties may interrupt opportunities for infant participation in "preintentional" communication, meaning nonverbal and vocal behaviors such as body posture, facial expression, limb extension, hand gestures, directed gaze, gaze eversion, crying, cooing, and babbling. At 13 months the children were within normal limits in all developmental domains except for those with CPO, who were "at risk" in the motor domain. The authors concluded (p. 224), "Developmental measures indirectly reflect the success with which the infant interacts with his or her environment to manage the effects of the congenital malformation and/or recovery from surgery. Conversely, these results document the 'at-risk' nature of 5-month old infants according to cleft types and specific domains, and underscore the need for developmental measures in craniofacial team assessments." Performance of the children in this study essentially worsened in the toddler period, as discussed in the next section.

A recent study of linguistic and cognitive skills in toddlers (Broen et al., 1998) used the mental scales of the Bayley Scales of Infant Development at the age of 24 months plus administration of the Minnesota Child Development Inventory at the age of 30 months, together with various linguistic measures. The children had either complete cleft lip and palate or cleft palate only. The authors reported that their subjects ". . . although well within the normal range, performed significantly below the children in the control group on the Bayley, some subscales of the MCDI, and the number of words acquired by the age of 24 months." Broen et al. (1998, p. 676) stated that the differences in results were in the verbal versus the nonverbal test, but they were also careful to consider both the status of velopharyngeal function and the hearing status of their subjects. When intergroup differences in these variables were added into the analysis, the significant differences on the Bayley and the MCDI scales were essentially erased. The authors' approach to their data in this study could have served as a model for earlier investigators and certainly highlighted the traps investigators can fall into when attempting to assess development at this early age.

[8]However, the grouping of children with CPO with other types of clefts is always suspect.

The extent to which development can be reasonably assessed in any baby or toddler depends on many factors, and in infants with clefts there is a high likelihood of other structural anomalies or other threats to development. In fact, given all the potential threats to communication development in children with craniofacial anomalies, it is something of a miracle that so many of them emerge from their growing and treatment years with normal communication skills and learning abilities. However, recent studies on learning problems in school-aged children with clefts, cited in a later portion of this chapter, have reminded us once again of the importance of early and ongoing assessment and intervention.

TODDLERS AND THEIR PARENTS

The toddler years see children (with or without clefts) start to assert themselves and develop their own personalities. The child and the parents are caught up in an independence-dependence struggle: the basic necessities of life (including affection, comfort, and security) must be provided by the parents, but toddlers want to do many things for themselves, and the parents would like a little freedom of their own. Parents have their own conflicts: they do not want to smother the child, but they do want to protect him or her. How they balance these needs will have an important effect on the child's socialization and learning.

As background, it should be noted that the toddler years are not typically a time of surgical intervention, but some of the articles or reviews (e.g., Pope, 1999) relevant to development in the toddlers have cited "hospitalization" as a possible source of stress in parent and child and thus a possible cause of developmental differences. Some toddlers with clefts may have late palatal surgery because of either failure of the first repair or a delay in repair due to medical problems. Myringotomies may be required on a repeated basis in some toddlers, but this surgery does not require hospitalization or isolation from parents. Of course, ongoing ear disease and hearing loss can always be a source of differences in development.

As in the studies of infants, studies of toddlers in the past two decades or so have focused on parent behavior as well as that of the child and have often combined children with a variety of types of craniofacial anomalies, not just clefts alone. In a series of studies, Wasserman and coauthors (Wasserman and Allen, 1985; Wasserman, Allen, and Linares, 1988; Wasserman, Allen, and Solomon, 1985, 1986) looked at various aspects of toddler development and parent-toddler relationships. Each of these studies included a few children with clefts (CLO, CLP, CPO) as well as children with more complex craniofacial anomalies, and all were combined into the "CFA" (craniofacial anomaly) group. Wasserman and Allen (1985) reported that mothers of "handicapped" toddlers exhibited a tendency to withdraw from their children. Furthermore, although the children's Bayley scores had not differed from those of healthy children when they were evaluated at the age of 1 year, children of mothers who tended to ignore them had lower concurrent 2-year IQ scores and an average 30-point drop between the two evaluations. The study of Wasserman, Allen, and Solomon of 1985 was a longitudinal study of children with "physical handicap" (which also included some children with limb anomalies) who were videotaped with their mothers at the ages of 9, 12, 18, and 24 months. These children performed more poorly on measures of social initiative, focused play, language production, and a measure of intelligence quotient used at the age of 2 years. They showed increased distractibility, decreased compliance, and more reluctance to separate from their mothers than did children who were not physically handicapped. Their mothers showed more initiating behaviors and were seen as less responsive than control mothers; interestingly, they were more likely both to encourage *and* to ignore their toddlers. The authors conjectured that some of the developmental deficits observed in toddlers with physical handicap might be affected "or even induced" by parenting patterns, a suggestion that seemed to be verified in their subsequent report of 1986. The latter study (Wasserman, Allen, and Solomon, 1986) used the same group of toddlers (at age 2 years) with "physical disabilities" plus a group of toddlers who had been premature; they found that mothers of children in both groups used less effective strategies in managing their children, although the children themselves were just as compliant in performing an assigned task as children in the control group.

Wasserman, Allen, and Linares (1988) later expanded the group of children with clefts to look at maternal interaction and language development in what they termed "children with and without speech-related anomalies." However, their group of toddlers "without" speech-related anomalies was not well chosen because it included Goldenhar syndrome, VATER association, ear tags, arthrogryposis, and so on. In addition, the group with "speech-related anomalies" included children with cleft lip (for whom speech should not be an issue) and children with cleft palate only, increasing the likelihood of associated anomalies or syndromes. The children with the "speech-related" anomalies showed significantly poorer performance than controls on standardized tests of intelligence and language. The average in this group was more than 10 points below that in the children with non-speech-related anomalies and more than 20 points below that in a group of controls. Similar differences were found in "verbal ability." In fact, the "verbal ability quotient" in these three groups paralleled the reported IQs. The mothers of the children with speech-related anomalies showed more physical teaching activity and initiating behaviors than did mothers in either of the other two groups. The authors concluded (p. 319) that maternal interactive behavior "is not global in its response to child disability; rather it varies with the particular pattern of child disabilities. . . ." However, the design of the study was questionable at best.

Allen, Wasserman, and Seidman (1990, p. 328), commenting on studies of toddlers, stated ". . . the second year may be a particularly difficult time for the families of nonretarded disabled/disfigured children [citing Starr et al., 1977; Wasserman and Allen, 1985; Wasserman, Allen, and Solomon, 1985]. At 2 years, children exhibited a range of problems including distractibility and failure to keep pace with developmental milestones such as language development. In the Wasserman studies, mothers reacted to this pattern by increasing their activity level in dyadic interaction compared to mothers of nondisabled toddlers, as though they were attempting to compensate for their children's problems. . . . In addition, most mothers of children with facial anomalies evidence a degree of burnout and withdrawal from their youngsters . . . children of these mothers performed increasingly poorly on standardized tests across their second year." Allen, Wasserman, and Seidman (1990) studied parent-child interaction in 3-year-old children with craniofacial anomalies and observed that these interactions during free play and teaching times were similar to those of controls. However, there was a tendency for an action-dominant, controlling parental style in the mothers of children with craniofacial anomalies.

The previously cited study by Speltz, Armsden, and Clarren (1990) underscored the effects of a variety of sources of stress on the comfort and sense of self-competence in mothers of toddlers with craniofacial anomalies. These mothers reported higher levels of stress, a lower sense of competence, and higher levels of marital conflict than did mothers in a comparison group, although direct observation of their behavior did not verify these perceptions. Speltz, Armsden, and Clarren (1990) stated that parental reaction to the atypical appearance of the child may be more dependent on such variables as maternal psychological status and marital functioning than on the nature of the disfigurement itself. In a follow-up study on these children at ages 5 to 7 years (Speltz et al., 1993) the authors found a relationship between the maternal interaction variables that had been observed in the same mother-child dyads when the children were toddlers and the child's later self-perception: the self-perception scores were higher for children whose mothers had placed less emphasis on correct performance and were less directive during play times.

Kapp-Simon and Krueckeberg (1995) found that children with clefts exhibited delays at the age of 25 months as measured on the Bayley Scales of Infant Development, which is a global measure of development without specific domains. In contrast, the 25-month-old toddlers in the Neiman and Savage study (1997) cited earlier showed developmental quotients in all domains of the Kent Infant Developmental Scales and the Minnesota Child Development Inventory consistent with a normative group. However, the 36-month-old toddlers in this cross-sectional study demonstrated significantly lower developmental performance in fine motor, gross motor, and expressive language domains. Of all the developmental domains, the cognitive and language domains seemed to be more strongly influenced by "environmental effects." In the study of Allen, Wasserman, and Seidman (1990), 3-year-old children with a variety of types of craniofacial anomalies were administered an intelligence test (Stanford-Binet)[9] and a preschool language scale. The authors reported that the children's performance on the intelligence and language tests was related to socioeconomic scale but not to "medical risk." They also observed that the children with craniofacial anomalies were more socially reticent and compliant than their peers.

The studies on early language development in infants and toddlers provoke a question of the chicken-egg variety: "which came first?" Did structurally based delays in phonologic development cause delays in language development that then led to broader delays in development than could be measured on standardized tests of language and phonologic development? Or are there inherent developmental delays that are reflected in language measures, among other domains? Recent studies on school-age children have shown that concerns regarding very early cognitive and language development in children with clefts may not only be justified but sadly overlooked in previous estimates of intellectual function of children with clefts. (See the section on school-age children below.)

There are obvious conflicts in the data on toddlers with clefts (and other craniofacial anomalies) and their parents and in the conclusions that have been drawn. It is difficult to control all independent variables in any clinical investigation, and at this age there are rather "muddy" variables such as adequacy of previous surgical intervention in minimizing either facial disfigurement or speech defect, persistent ear disease despite myringotomies and tubes, and adjustment of parents to what can still be a self-perceived sense of inadequacy. Pope (1999) conjectured that ongoing medical attention gives the message (to the toddler) that he is not competent and that the world is too dangerous. However, she had no data verifying that medical interventions were frequent during the toddler period. She warned that craniofacial team members should be alert for signs of developmental and psychosocial disturbance in toddlers, a warning that is well taken.

THE PRESCHOOL YEARS

In the age range of roughly 4 to 6 years, children with clefts and their families face some new challenges. Many children start to perceive their own facial differences during this period. The first experience with a school situation may mean the first time the child is confronted with questions, querying looks, and teasing from other children. Some secondary surgery may be done to improve appearance, specifically lip and nose revisions (nasoseptal reconstruction is typically deferred until age 6 years to minimize interference with growth of this portion of the face—see Chapter 4). The necessity of ongoing evaluations and treatment may interfere with the child's socialization and adaptation to his new school environment. Not surprisingly, in a study of 20 children ages 4 through 7 years with

[9]See the note in the following section on preschool children regarding the use of language-based tests on children with craniofacial anomalies.

a variety of types of congenital facial anomalies, Fisk et al. (1985) found "increasing emotional indicators" in those children who had had more or later operations. They found that "surgical decisions," rather than degree of deformity, affected the child's value judgment, identification, and friendship preference.

In the literature the earliest age at which researchers have attempted to measure intelligence in children with clefts has generally been in the preschool years. (The subjects of intelligence and school achievement are discussed in greater detail in the section on school-age children.) Richman and Eliason (1982) warned that intellectual assessments during this period should be interpreted with caution, especially when highly verbal measures are used. That is, problems in what most authors in the psychology literature term "expressive language" (but which may actually be articulation or phonologic problems) may interfere with accurate assessment of intelligence. They suggested that early IQ level as measured on the Stanford-Binet test, for example, may not be a good predictor of later intellectual functioning. A study by Musgrave, McWilliams, and Matthews (1975) in which the measurement instrument was the Stanford-Binet Form L-M may have been proof of this point: the authors reported some very interesting findings regarding IQ distribution in 19 children with CPO (in this case, clefts of the soft palate only) who were followed longitudinally from the preschool years through age 10 years. In the preschool years, children tested at low average, with 70% falling below the normal range. But by 10 years of age they tested in the high-average range, with about half the group a little above the population mean and ranging into the superior areas. Two thirds of the children at the time of the initial testing, and all but one at the time of final assessment, had hearing levels no greater than 20 dB in the better ear. Nevertheless, it is possible that early problems in speech or hearing may have affected the underestimation of intelligence in the preschoolers. Not surprisingly, subsequent studies of preschoolers verified deficits in expressive and receptive language (Eliason, 1990; Eliason and Richman, 1990; Nation, 1970) that could easily affect the accuracy of attempted intelligence measures. Nearly a quarter of a century after the study of Musgrave, McWilliams, and Matthews (1975), Endriga and Kapp-Simon (1999) concluded that cognitive development and achievement in preschoolers with clefts and other craniofacial anomalies was "understudied," meaning there is a paucity of actual data except for the studies of language.

The behavior and social skills of preschoolers have been examined in a few studies. Schneiderman and Auer (1984) obtained behavioral ratings from parents and teachers for a group of children with cleft lip and palate ranging in age from preschool up through the ninth grade. The measure was the Behavior Problem Checklist (Quay and Peterson, 1979). The number of behavior problems as perceived by both parents and teachers increased significantly between the preschool years and the elementary school years. Conduct problems, personality problems, and "socialized delinquency" problems were all judged to increase in severity as the child aged. Krueckeberg, Kapp-Simon, and Ribordy (1993) investigated social knowledge, social skills, and cognitive and physical competence as perceived by parents and teachers in 3- to 6-year-old children with various types of craniofacial anomalies compared with a control group. The craniofacial anomaly group included some children with CLO, some with CPO, and some with CLP; about 70% had visible facial disfigurement. The study included parent and teacher questionnaires to rate perceived physical competence, cognitive competence, peer acceptance, and maternal acceptance; facial encoding and decoding tasks (for which the children tried to produce specific facial expressions and also decode expressions in pictures); a "social knowledge" interview of the child; and a social skills behavioral rating completed by "significant adults" in the child's life. Interestingly, in the facial encoding and decoding tasks, the control children and the craniofacial anomaly children performed equally well (see footnote 9). In only two areas were the children with craniofacial anomalies rated lower than the control children: attractiveness and friendliness. On the self-perception measures, it was a surprise to the investigators that the boys with craniofacial anomalies fell in the average range for self-perception, whereas the girls rated themselves *above* average. The authors conjectured that the demands on these children may be less during the preschool years than at other times. They may not yet realize they are different or may not yet have had negative social experiences that can lead to problems in self-esteem. Krueckeberg, Kapp-Simon, and Ribordy (1993, p. 480) concluded, "It is disconcerting that craniofacial anomaly children were rated as less attractive and that they responded to hypothetical social situations in a less friendly manner, especially since friendliness is a predictive factor for social skill. Perhaps children with CFA start out with similar levels of social skills, but encounter problems in continuing to develop their skills while handling the numerous stressors that accompany a craniofacial anomaly (e.g., stigmatizing reactions to their facial appearance and stressful medical procedures)." Their suggestion was verified in a follow-up study on a small group of those children 3 years later (Krueckeberg and Kapp-Simon, 1997) in which 31% received global behavior problem scores in the clinical range as rated by either teacher or parent report. Speltz et al. (1993) found similar results at ages 5 to 7 years: about 18% of these children obtained "clinically significant scores" on the basis of both parent and teacher reports. Girls with craniofacial anomalies received higher scores for externalizing or "acting-out" behavior, on the basis of parent reports, than either boys with craniofacial anomalies or control children. This gender-specific finding was generally the reverse of what had been found in other studies of behavior in children with craniofacial anomaly, but may have been an artifact due to the small sample size of girls.

In a companion study to their investigation of social skills in preschoolers, Krueckeberg and Kapp-Simon (1993) also looked at the effect of parental factors on those skills. They found no differences between the craniofacial anomaly and control groups (same children as in the previously discussed study of Krueckeberg, Kapp-Simon, and Ribordy [1993]) on measures of parenting stress, parenting style, or social network characteristics. The parents of children with visible defects did find their social support networks to be more helpful, but the authors pointed out that the sample was biased because all the families were receiving regular consultation from a psychosocial support staff, beginning with their first clinic visit to an interdisciplinary team. In the parents who did see themselves as stressed during the preschool years, that rating was significantly correlated with parent, teacher, and self-reports of poorer social competence. Thus, as pointed out by Krueckeberg and Kapp-Simon (1993) there seems to be an interactive effect between children's social skills and parental stress: parents feel more stressed when their children have difficulty in reacting to social challenges, but at the same time how the parent views his or her child's social skills is greatly influenced by how stressed [the parent] is feeling.

Obviously the areas of self-concept, behavior, and social skills are intricately tied together in children with craniofacial anomalies. The finding by Fisk et al. (1985) that "later" surgery in the 4- to 7-year age range produced more emotional problems coincides with the conclusion of Krueckeberg, Kapp-Simon, and Ribordy (1993) that the preschool years may be a time relatively free of emotional stress. That is, the children in the study of Fisk et al. (1985) evidenced greater emotional problems when their surgery stretched into the early school years as opposed to preschool. Whereas Endriga and Kapp-Simon (1999) stated that self-concept is a difficult construct to measure in the preschool ages, Fisk et al. (1985) felt that in the age range of 4 to 7 years the facial anomalies affected "the ways in which the child represents himself to self and to others." Eliason (1991) concluded that during the preschool years, a child's self-image and feelings about self are derived primarily from the parents' attitudes and behaviors. As the child's interaction with the world expands in the school years, the effects on self-image, socialization, school adjustment, and academic achievement become much more complex.

SCHOOL-AGE YEARS

From the first through the eighth grades the child with a cleft or other craniofacial anomaly—and his family—will face challenges in self-concept and self-esteem, peer judgments and relationships, conflicts with parents, school adjustment and achievement, much like children who do *not* have physical anomalies but amplified by several factors attendant to the cleft. It is difficult to deal with each of these issues separately because they are so interdependent: the youngster's own feelings about how he or she looks and functions is inevitably tied to how the parents and other family members view him or her. The parents' comfort is in part determined by how these children feel about themselves, how they relate to other children, and how they do in school. The child's ability to make friends is a measure of social skills but is also dependent on those skills, and how comfortable the child feels is in part dependent on how comfortable the parents are. All these concerns are interdependent at nearly any age level in the school years.

Intelligence, Learning Disabilities, School Achievement

Most of the historical studies on "IQ" in individuals with clefts were carried out on children in the "middle" ages of childhood (e.g., 9 to 12 years old) and teenagers, and in many of these studies the results were not sorted by type of cleft, nor were associated anomalies always ruled out. Ruess (1967) summarized data from several early studies (each without delineation of type of cleft or elimination of associated defects) from several countries, including the United States, and concluded that there was some evidence that children with clefts have a mean IQ between 2 and 6 points below the statistical population mean.[10] Estes and Morris (1970) reported that a larger proportion of cleft palate subjects aged 9 to nearly 16 years fell into the lower end of the normal IQ distribution compared with the normative data for the Stanford-Binet and the Wechsler Intelligence Scale for Children (WISC) and also found that scores were lower for the CPO subjects than for children with CL+/−P. Their subjects did better on the performance portions of the WISC than the verbal portions, something that had previously been noted by Goodstein (1961) and by Morris (1962a). Subsequent studies on intelligence in children with clefts generally indicated (1) mean IQ scores either equivalent to or a couple of points below those in the general population (Richman, 1976, 1978a, 1978b, 1980; Richman and Harper, 1978b; Ruess, 1965, 1967; Smith and McWilliams, 1966)[11] and (2) more discrepancy between cleft and noncleft children on verbal portions of intelligence tests than on performance sections, although not consistently across all studies (Eliason, 1991; Lamb, Wilson, and Leeper, 1973; Richman, 1980; Richman and Eliason, 1982).

McWilliams and Matthews (1979) reported some interesting data that underscored the differences between cleft diagnostic groups on tests of intelligence. In their subject pool of 226 children (mean age 10 years), the verbal, performance, and full-scale IQs on the WISC varied in a

---

[10]Two studies from Europe (Cervenka and Drabkova, 1965; Gabka and Weber, 1984) offered similar results but did not specify the age of the subjects at the time of testing. The former study did report that roughly one fourth of their patients with BCLP had IQs falling below 68, whereas none of the subjects in the other cleft groups fell this low. However, these authors also did not specify the test or whether the test included verbal as well as performance sections. Gabka and Weber (1984) stated their subjects "showed weaker results but still within the norm region" on the intelligence test they used.

[11]The Richman studies of 1976 and 1978 did *not* show a significant difference in mean full-scale IQ between CLP and CPO subjects, nor did the earlier study of Lamb, Wilson, and Leeper (1973).

consistent direction depending on whether the subjects had UCLP or CPO, with or without other anomalies. The patients with other anomalies included some with complex syndromes that we now recognize as predisposing toward lower intellectual development (e.g., Apert syndrome, otopalatodigital syndrome). The children with UCLP without other anomalies did best (mean verbal IQ 104.9, performance 104.25, full scale 105.05), CPO without other anomalies ranked next (verbal 101.28, performance 97.32, full scale 99.49), UCLP with other anomalies next (verbal IQ 95.2, performance 95.93, full scale 94.94), and CPO with other anomalies last (verbal IQ 90.55, performance 92.40, full scale 91.00). Note that all these mean scores fell within the normal range; only a few of these differences were statistically significant, but they did show a persistent drift downward depending on the specific diagnostic group. Interestingly, scores on the Vineland Social Maturity Scale on each of these four groups of subjects followed the same pattern. We do not find these data remarkable today, but 20 years ago this study was a significant milestone.

Richman's 1980 study identified two subgroups of children within those who showed lower verbal than performance IQs. The first subgroup seemed to have a general language disability, whereas the second showed a relatively high level of verbal mediation ability despite their lower verbal IQ scores. These children had only a verbal expression problem and performed significantly better than the first group on tasks requiring categorization and associated reasoning. Richman stated (p. 455), "It may be that the slightly depressed intellectual functioning, and in particular depressed verbal skills, frequently identified in groups of cleft palate children, is based on group mean IQ scores influenced by sub-groups of . . . children with language deficits. These language deficits may not have a common etiology. . . ." Subsequent studies continued to identify language problems in children with clefts that could certainly affect measures of IQ (Kommers and Sullivan, 1979; Richman and Eliason, 1993; Richman, Eliason, and Lindgren, 1988), with CPO children being more likely to show these deficits than CLP children (Clifford, 1979; Richman and Eliason, 1982; Tobiasen, 1990).[12]

Older studies of intelligence and of school achievement in children with clefts, as well as in noncleft children, did not distinguish specific learning disabilities from overall intelligence or achievement. This began to change with the studies cited above, which identified specific language problems. Recent studies have revealed much more about learning disabilities in children with craniofacial defects. Endriga and Kapp-Simon (1999) concluded that although nonsyndromic children with craniofacial anomalies are at a slightly higher risk for mental retardation (4% to 6%) in comparison to the general population (2%), learning disabilities occur in 30% to 40% (compared with 15% to 20% of the general population) on the basis of data presented by Broder, Richman, and Matheson (1998), Richman (1978a, 1980), Richman and Eliason (1984), Richman and Millard (1992), and Richman, Eliason, and Lindgren (1988). Reading disabilities out of proportion to children's full-scale IQs were documented by Richman and Eliason (1984) and Richman, Eliason, and Lindgren (1988). The data of Broder, Richman, and Matheson (1998) were particularly jarring: in 168 children ranging in age from 6 through 18 years, all with average intellectual function, 46% were learning disabled, 47% were functioning below grade level, and 27% had repeated at least one grade. Males with CPO had a significantly higher rate of learning disabilities than either males or females with CLP or females with CLP.[13]

From the time of entry into primary school, classroom achievement in children with clefts may be affected by much more than just "native" intelligence or learning disabilities. The complex interactions are conceptualized in Fig. 14-1. Richman (1976) reported that children with clefts demonstrated significantly lower scores on standardized achievement tests than noncleft controls did, even when the two groups were matched for IQ. Brantley and Clifford (1979) also reported lower parental expectations for achievement in children with clefts. Richman (1978b) looked at teachers' perceptions of ability in children with clefts aged 9 to 14 years, dividing the children into one group with minimal facial disfigurement and one with significant disfigurement. The two groups did not actually differ on intellectual, behavior, or achievement data. The teachers rated the ability of the first group more accurately than they did the group with significant disfigurement: for the latter group, the teachers tended to underestimate the ability of the brighter children and overestimate the ability of less bright children. Richman (1978a) also investigated

[12]In his 1971 review, Wirls stated that intellectual ability was the only area of psychosocial research in which differences had consistently been found between cleft and noncleft subjects (up to that time). However, he was prescient in pointing out the variables of severity of defect, hearing loss, social maturation, and speech problems as confounding the results of both intellectual and personality assessments.

[13]Similar gender-by-sex differences were reported by Lamb, Wilson, and Leeper (1973) and would be predicted on the basis of more significant or severe defects occurring in the less-often-affected sex for the type of cleft: males are more apt to have UCLP than females, etc. (see Chapter 1). In a study of the relationship between "clinical findings" (major malformations and neurologic dysfunction) and school achievement in children with clefts, Gall et al. (1972) expressed surprise that the highest prevalence of poor school performance and of "frank mental retardation" was in boys with CPO. They thought the youngsters with visible cleft lip would be doing more poorly because they would be subject to "labeling." They did report that the highest proportion of children with multiple malformations was in boys with CPO and the lowest in girls with CLP. This study reflects the naiveté in many early studies in not recognizing (1) that individuals with CPO are known to be more apt to have additional malformations than those with CLP and (2) the likelihood of additional physical and functional findings is higher in individuals of the less frequently affected sex (boys with CPO, girls with CLP).

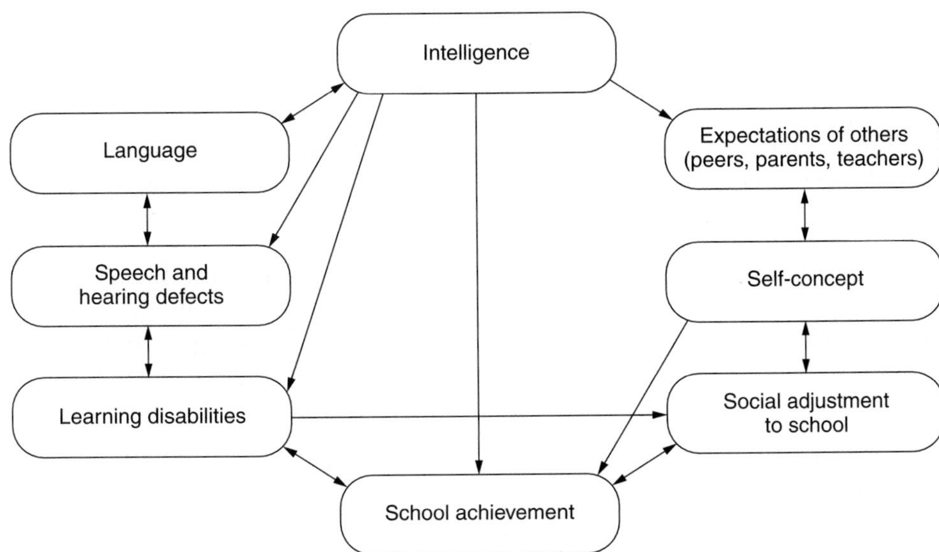

Figure 14-1 Theoretical interactions among variables affecting school achievement.

parents' and teachers' ratings of behavior of 7- to 12-year-old children and found that teachers rated the children as significantly more inhibited in the classroom than the parents observed at home. Richman (1978a) suggested that differential expectations at home and at school may contribute to different perceptions. The teachers expected more at school and when they did not see it they felt the children were inhibited; the parents may not have expected as much from their children in terms of school performance and thus did not rate them as inhibited. Both these studies (Richman 1978a, 1978b) pointed to the possible influence of expectations on behavior and achievement. Mitchell, Lott, and Pannbacker (1984) mailed questionnaires about children with clefts to classroom teachers, special education teachers, and speech-language pathologists, asking about academic problems and adjustment and also asking for suggestions regarding the need for in-service training about clefts. The answers really consisted primarily of speculation because 87% of the teachers and 85% of the special educators had had *no* experience with clefts. The special educators thought that children with clefts had lower academic potential, whereas classroom teachers and speech-language pathologists thought they had the same potential as their peers. Very few of the respondents, except for classroom teachers, though that children with clefts were as equally well adjusted as their peers. The value of this study is obviously limited because so few of the respondents had any experience with clefts, but it does speak to the possible effect of expectation. Tobiasen (1984, 1987) suggested that achievement may be affected by what others, including peers, expect of these children. Broder and Strauss (1989) echoed the same concern.

In their 1982 review of their own data and the published data of other authors on psychological characteristics of children with clefts, Richman and Eliason concluded the following with regard to school achievement: (1) as a group, children with clefts tend to achieve below expectations based on their intellectual skills, (2) teachers tend to underestimate the intellectual ability of average and above-average children with more facial disfigurement, (3) children with clefts are frequently perceived as being more inhibited in the classroom, (4) a general verbal or language deficiency in some children may result in significant academic failure, and (5) parents may have lower expectations for the cleft child, resulting in lower academic aspirations. In their reviews, McWilliams (1982), Tobiasen (1990), and Endriga and Kapp-Simon (1999) emphasized many of these same points. Probably the most significant new findings with regard to school achievement that have emerged in recent years were those of Broder, Richman, and Matheson (1998), reviewed above. Certainly those findings brought to a halt any complacency clinicians had had that children with clefts were essentially normal by the time they reached the preadolescent or adolescent years.

Self-Concept

Systematic study of self-concept in children with clefts began with the 1979 work of Kapp on children in the 11- to 13-year age group, although later studies extended "backward" into the preschool years (Krueckeberg, Kapp-Simon, and Ribordy, 1993) and early primary school years (Kapp-Simon, 1986). As pointed out by Endriga and Kapp-Simon in 1999, self-concept is a difficult entity to measure in the preschool years, but in the study of Krueckeberg, Kapp-Simon, and Ribordy (1993) on 3- to 6-year-old children with several types of craniofacial anomalies, all scores were generally in the average range. The authors were surprised that on the Pictorial Scale of Perceived Competence and Social Acceptance for Young Children (Harter and Pike, 1984), the little girls yielded higher self-concept scores higher than either the boys with craniofacial anomalies or control subjects, which the authors conjectured may have been due to "the characteristics of the developmental period the children [were] in

(p. 479)" because other studies on non-cleft preschool children had also shown that youngsters in this age group tended to overrate themselves highly. The thought was that this may have reflected a defensive or self-preservation strategy, something that was not assumed to be unique to children with craniofacial anomalies. In the follow-up study 3 years later (Krueckeberg and Kapp-Simon, 1997), a more positive social acceptance at age 9 years was correlated with the preschooler's ability to produce a recognizable facial expression and also with the preschooler's friendliness in a structured play interview (see the notes on this study in the section on preschoolers).

Eder (1995) also looked at self-concept in the early school-age years, using puppets to learn what 5-year-old children with craniofacial anomalies (not just clefts) were thinking about their own well-being, self-control, and social acceptance. In comparison to control subjects the children with craniofacial anomalies were feeling more alienated by others, more aggressive, and more scared, mad, and upset. However, they were like their peers without craniofacial anomalies in terms of how they liked themselves and felt about working hard, being leaders, and having friends. Eder (1995) reported that the mothers of these children were consistent with their own progeny, viewing them as more aggressive and emotionally upset although they did not perceive the same sense of alienation. In an earlier study, Speltz et al. (1993) used the same puppet strategy with 5- to 7-year-old children. This was a follow-up on the infants and toddlers that they had studied in 1990. From maternal ratings of behavior, Speltz et al. (1993) concluded that children with craniofacial anomalies have at least twice the risk of behavior problems at school entry, although in their sample relative deficits in behavioral adjustment were found only for girls. The authors also reported that behavior problems risk could be predicted by clinic observations of mother-child interactions during late infancy, but they found no significant differences between CFA children and comparison groups.

Kapp-Simon's 1986 study of children in the 5- to 9-year-old age group used the Primary Self Concept Inventory (PSCI) of Muller and Leonetti (1974). The children had a mixture of clefts: some had CLO; most had CLP; and some had CPO (thus, both visible and invisible defects). The children had a significantly lower global self-concept. They perceived themselves as less socially adept and more frequently sad and angry than did their noncleft peers. Kapp-Simon (1986) conjectured that the poor self-concept of these children could be related to concerns in multiple areas—speech, appearance, parental expectations, or a combination of all of these. Broder and Strauss (1989) used the same self-concept scale as Kapp-Simon (1986) in their study of 7-year-old children with a mixture of CLO, CLP, and CPO. They found that the children with visible defects (CLO or CLP) had the lowest self-concept scores and recommended that future research in this area should consider each cleft type as a distinct and discrete group, a recommendation that regrettably has not been followed in most studies.

In Kapp's first examination of self-concept in children with clefts (1979), she looked at children aged 11 to 13 years with a mixture of visible and invisible clefts. The sample was also heterogeneous with regard to speech, hearing, and physical appearance. Both boys and girls in this age group had lower global self-concept scores than noncleft subjects did and reported a significantly greater dissatisfaction with appearance. In addition, the girls in this early adolescent age group reported greater unhappiness and dissatisfaction, less success in school, and more anxiety. Kapp (1979) conjectured girls may be more affected by the stigma of the cleft because of the importance of physical attractiveness in our society. Subsequent investigations have generally been in agreement with Kapp's data regarding dissatisfaction and anxiety about facial appearance being greater in girls than in boys, although there has been some variation from study to study.

Several studies examined self-concept in more than one age group of children. Leonard et al. (1991) looked at one group of 8- to 11-year-old children and another group from 12 to 18 years. The subjects were again a mix of CLO, CLP, and CPO. They were also rated for presence or absence of hypernasality in speech. However, in the total group of subjects, visibility of the defects and/or presence or absence of hypernasality apparently had little effect on self concept as measured on the Piers-Harris scale (Piers, 1969): 98% of the children had average or above-average self-concept scores. There was an interaction between age and gender, in that adolescent girls had a more negative self-concept than the younger girls but the adolescent boys had a more positive self-concept than the younger boys. In her commentary on this article, Broder (1991) pointed out that the "physical appearance" dimension of the Piers-Harris scale does not necessarily address specific areas that might be of concern to this patient population (e.g., mouth, nose) but rather consists of a more global appearance rating. Jones (1984) used the same scale in his study of CLP children over the very broad age range of 8 to 18 years. He reported that these children, regardless of sex, had significantly lower global self-concept scores than noncleft subjects did, but he did not break down the results by ages. He also found that males with clefts felt less popular than their noncleft peers, and that females expressed significantly more anxiety than noncleft peers. Jones (1984) also had the parents of his subjects complete a questionnaire about the child's relationship with the family and peers and about progress in school. The parents reported more negative responses than a control group regarding the teasing their children were experiencing because of facial appearance and the effect the child's facial appearance had on school progress (as they perceived it).

Broder, Smith, and Strauss (1994) looked at three groups of children ages 5 to 9 years, 10 to 13 years, and 14 to 18 years. They kept their data separate for visible defects

(CLO or CLP) and invisible defects (CPO). The measurement tool was a standardized interview, and the study primarily emphasized satisfaction with appearance (discussed later in this chapter) but also addressed accomplishment of psychosocial tasks. Differences in results across age groups were examined for the four areas of satisfaction with appearance, self-perception of popularity, self-perception of inability to solve hard problems, and self-perception of social independence. The three independent variables were age group, sex, and visibility versus invisibility of the cleft defect. Satisfaction with facial appearance was lower in the 5- to 9-year-old girls with visible defects than in girls with invisible defects or in the control group; interestingly, this satisfaction decreased significantly with age in the latter two groups, despite the absence of a visible cleft. With regard to popularity, the subjects with clefts (visible or invisible) indicated that they had more friends than did subjects in the control group, and subjects with visible defects yielded self-ratings of popularity that tended to increase with age. The authors viewed both these findings with skepticism because they were contrary to a substantial amount of prior data—derived by direct observation, peer ratings, and teacher reports—demonstrating that children with clefts are more socially isolated and unaccepted by peers (Kapp-Simon and Simon, 1991; Richman and Harper, 1978a; Schneiderman and Harding, 1984; Sigelman, Miller, and Whitworth, 1986). Broder, Smith, and Strauss (1994) felt the high self-rating of popularity could reflect denial, a higher need for acceptance, or both. Self-ratings of the ability to solve hard problems were significantly lower in children with CPO and higher in this group in the youngest age bracket. The authors pointed out that this difference by cleft type probably reflected the higher prevalence of learning and speech problems in this cleft group (Richman, Eliason, and Lindgren, 1988).[14] "Social independence" was assessed by the children's expression of a preference for playing by themselves or playing with others; both cleft groups had a higher percentage of children preferring to play with others than found in the control group, with the difference more marked in the girls than in the boys. Broder, Smith, and Strauss (1994) pointed out that the children may have been overcompensating because of their experience of low peer acceptance. Their interpretation of their results with regard to popularity and social independence brings to mind a statement made by Wirls in 1971 (p. 127): "[The child with a cleft might be] forced by the circumstances of his physical disability to learn coping behavior and to develop as a part of his self-concept a view of himself as successful in mastering difficult and painful situations." This comment about "enhanced self-esteem" coincided with the results of Broder, Smith, and Strauss (1994) a quarter of a century later.

Two relatively recent studies on self-concept in the preadolescent to early adolescent years used subjects with a variety of craniofacial anomalies (Kapp-Simon, Simon, and Kristovich, 1992; Pope and Ward, 1997a, 1997b). Kapp-Simon, Simon and Kristovich (1992) used a self-perception scale, a personality inventory for children, and a behavior problem checklist. They found that measures in each of the areas of self-perception, social skills, and inhibition were "within the normal range" for their rather heterogeneous group of young adolescents (mean age 12.3 years). Pope and Ward (1997b) used a variety of measures to assess "self-perceived facial appearance and psychosocial adjustment" and reported that the feelings of their young adolescents with regard to facial appearance were positively correlated with measures of global self-worth, self-perceived social acceptance, and number of same-sex close friends. Not unexpectedly, feelings of self-worth were inversely correlated with loneliness and parent-rated social problems. Dissatisfaction with facial appearance was associated with peer relationship problems and low global self-esteem, but not with other aspects of self-concept or other adjustment problems. Also, as one would expect, when the children were more dissatisfied with their facial appearance, their parents were concerned about their children's peer relationships and increased their support and advice. Overall, the authors reported that only social problems were associated with concerns about facial appearance, not other measures of psychosocial adjustment problems. They also pointed out that their results were consistent with Kapp's 1979 findings on the same age group. Brantley and Clifford (1979) looked at three age groups from the ages of 10 to 18 years, but their published study did not identify the types of clefts in the study population. They looked at cognitive, self-concept, and body image measures in normal, cleft palate, and obese teenagers, and reported that the subjects with clefts had self-reported no pervasive feelings of body distortion. The teenagers with clefts showed their sensitivity to what their parents had been through as revealed in a "When I Was Born" probe, but they maintained high self-esteem. Similar to the 1971 observation of Wirls (cited earlier), Brantley and Clifford (1979, p. 182) stated, "Perhaps heightened self-esteem arises after they [children with clefts] have managed to cope successfully with the experience of having had clefts." However, the authors also wanted to alert future clinicians and researchers to potential problems in teenagers: "Only in the area of self-concept, particularly with regard to perceived familial acceptance and enhanced self-esteem, does the cleft palate adolescent appear to be different" (p. 182).

Richman and Eliason (1982) synthesized pertinent information on self-concept that had been published up to the time of their review. They concluded that children with clefts were generally within a normal range on self-concept measures but did show situational concerns specific to facial appearance, most likely to become apparent in female

[14]Which in turn probably reflects the higher likelihood of associated anomalies and syndromes.

adolescents. Most of the studies published since the time of this review have fit this pattern.

Several studies have focused upon patient and family satisfaction with the patient's facial appearance and have used this information to make some inferences about self-concept. In the school children interviewed by Broder, Smith, and Strauss (1994), children with CLP were less likely to report being "very pleased" with their appearance compared with CPO children (40% versus 90%). The girls in both the Kapp (1979) and Leonard et al. (1991) studies were more likely than the boys to report dissatisfaction with appearance and less happiness.

Broder, Smith, and Strauss (1992) reported that 54% of children (ages 5 to 18 years) with CLO, CLP, or CPO were very pleased with their appearance and 62% were very pleased with their speech. There were no age differences in satisfaction with appearance. The parents of the girls expressed more concern about their daughters' appearance, whereas the parents of the boys were more concerned about speech. The boys themselves were just as concerned about their looks as the girls. Because previous authors had reported more concern about appearance in girls with clefts than in boys (Berscheid and Gangsted, 1982; Kapp, 1979; Kapp-Simon, 1986), the authors wondered (p. 266) if this lack of difference might reflect "a more current cultural norm or trend, which emphasizes the importance of facial appearance regardless of gender." In a slightly later study on an expanded group of patients in the same age range, Broder, Smith, and Strauss (1994) reported that only a low percentage of teenage girls were "very pleased" with their appearance, which the authors felt may have reflected the increased social pressure for attractiveness at this age although they acknowledged that not all the teenagers had completed all their surgeries at the time of the last interview. (About half the children in this study had visible clefts.)

Tobiasen's research (Tobiasen, 1984; 1987; 1990; 1993; Tobiasen and Heibert, 1984, 1988, 1993a, 1993b; 1994; Tobiasen and Speltz, 1996; Tobiasen, Hiebert, and Boraz, 1991) placed primary emphasis on facial appearance and its effect on self-esteem and social competence. From her own work and that of others, Tobiasen (1993) concluded that self-ratings of severity of cleft impairment—not peer ratings—strongly predicted psychosocial adjustment in several areas, including global self-esteem, mood, and social competence. She also concluded (p. 630) ". . . it is unclear how the individual differences in self-perception of appearance develop and if they remain stable over time or if they can be altered. . . ." To the extent that physical treatment affects facial appearance and that changes in facial appearance do or do not alter self-concept, a large amount of helpful data should become available within the next several years as the American Cleft Palate–Craniofacial Association pursues a nationwide (federally funded) study on treatment outcomes.

In summary, it seems clear that there are many factors potentially affecting self-concept and self-esteem in children with clefts and other craniofacial anomalies during the school-age years. Standardized tests and interviews tend to yield scores indicating lowered self-esteem, although this is not entirely consistent across studies and may be influenced by age, gender, severity of defect, parental attitudes, and so on. Pope (1999) made an excellent point to clinicians, namely, that it is important to be sensitive about what is communicated to the child about appearance because it will influence self-concept.

Personality, Behavior, Social Relationships[15]

Psychologists and other clinicians in the field of facial clefts long ago discarded the notion that there was such an entity as a "cleft palate personality" (Clifford, 1973, 1979; Corah and Corah, 1963; Goodstein 1960, 1968; Harper and Richman, 1978; McWilliams, 1982; Richman and Harper, 1979; Simonds and Heimburger, 1978; Spriestersbach, 1973; Wirls, 1971; Wirls and Plotkin, 1971). Actually, given the diversity of individuals who have clefts and the many influences upon their lives and personalities, it is a mystery why anyone would have proposed in the first place that there was a specific personality type associated with clefts. In addition, no one has found evidence of an increased occurrence of personality disorders or psychopathology in this population (Endriga and Kapp-Simon, 1999; Madison, 1986; McWilliams, 1982; Richman and Eliason, 1982; Simonds and Heimburger, 1978; Strauss and Broder, 1991; Tobiasen, 1984, 1990; Wirls, 1971; Wirls and Plotkin, 1971).[16]

Similarly, many of the studies published through the 1970s and early 1980s also concluded that there was no evidence of significant behavioral or social maladjustment in individuals with clefts (Jones, 1984; Lansdown, 1981; Madison, 1986; McWilliams, 1982; Richman and Eliason, 1982; Richman and Harper, 1978b, 1979; Tobiasen, 1984). However, there are *specific* areas of behavior, adjustment, and socialization that require attention, especially when clinicians try to minimize or even prevent the development of problems.

Many behavioral studies on school-age children with clefts have reported that these children tend to be more inhibited than their noncleft peers, based on parent or teacher ratings, self-reports, or direct observation (Harper and Richman, 1978; Harper, Richman, and Snider, 1980; Richman, 1976, 1978b, 1983; Richman and Harper, 1978b, 1979; Tobiasen and Hiebert, 1984). Although inhibition of impulse is something we expect children to gradually develop as they mature, children with clefts seem to show greater inhibition (sometimes equated with

[15]In the literature the topic of "school adjustment" is sometimes treated as being synonymous with "school achievement." This discussion will include material on "school adjustment" as it pertains to social relationships rather than to academic achievement.

[16]An important exception is velocardiofacial syndrome, in which there is a high likelihood of significant psychopathology, as mentioned in Chapter 3 (Carlson et al., 1997; Karayiorgou et al., 1992; Papolos et al., 1996; Pulver et al., 1994; Shprintzen et al., 1992).

shyness, social withdrawal, etc.) than considered normal for chronological age. Clinicians and researchers have attributed the increase in inhibition to an unconscious attempt by the child to avoid calling attention to himself or to avoid situations that give rise to negative responses from others. As Richman and Eliason (1982) pointed out, this may be a positive adaptive response rather than a sign of maladjustment. In a study on children between the ages of 4 and 13 years with various types of both visible and invisible birth defects, including cleft lip and palate, Heller et al. (1985) reported that 12% of the children with clefts were maladjusted, primarily boys who were described as "uncommunicative." The authors also reported that increasing amounts of maladjustment were found as age increased in all their subject groups and that in all cases those children experiencing embarrassment associated with their condition appeared to be at greatest risk, especially the children with clefts. Their data showed a strong relationship between maladjustment in the children and a lack of understanding of the medical aspects of CLP and an inverse relationship between maladjustment and the education and social status of the mothers.

Tobiasen and coworkers (Tobiasen and Hiebert, 1984; Tobiasen et al., 1987) examined parents' perceptions of their children's conduct. The children were all males, ranging in age from 2 to 12 years and were sorted into four groups: UCLP, UCLP with associated malformations, CPO, and CPO with associated malformations. The parents were asked to rate whether the children "never, sometimes, or usually" had any of the following problems in school: not following instructions, talking out of turn, slow learning, short attention span, not finishing work, not getting along with other children. The authors found notable variability in *which* behaviors the parents considered to be a problem and also found that parents tended to be more tolerant of socially inappropriate behavior than parents of children without craniofacial anomalies. Not surprisingly, the boys with associated malformations, whether they had UCLP or CPO, were rated as having more serious school or conduct problems in comparison with the boys with isolated clefts.

When the child with a cleft or other craniofacial anomaly begins school, one of the most potent determinants of adjustment, behavior, and ability to develop appropriate social relationships will be how the child handles teasing. All children are teased about something, and as Pope (1999) pointed out, the reasons for which they are continually teased are mainly related to the way in which they respond. Several studies have contained parent reports or perceptions that their children with craniofacial anomalies suffered teasing (Jones, 1984; Noar, 1991; Turner et al., 1997). Pope (1999) emphasized the role that parents play in preparing the child for these experiences: even before the child's school entry, the parents will likely have developed a "family story" about the cleft to tell to new acquaintances, and this gives the child a better chance to handle the situation naturally. A good example of this was the story told by Rowe (1983), who had prepared her little boy for school with the advice, ". . . if they ask you silly questions, give them silly answers." When he was asked at the beginning of a new school year what had happened to his lip, he answered that on the Saturday before school started he fell out of a helicopter and then when he hit the ground he was attacked by a lion. The child reported to his mother with delight that his questioner (another little boy) had believed him, adding, "He must be stupid if he believes that."

Looking at how the conduct, behavior, and socialization of children with a craniofacial anomaly may change over time, we find some evidence of an "age" effect. In the previously cited Schneiderman and Auer study (1984) of parents' and teachers' perceptions of the behavior of CLP children from preschool up through ninth grade, boys were judged to exhibit significantly more behavior problems during the elementary and junior high school years, compared with the preschool years. They were also judged to have more "social delinquency" problems than girls during the junior high years. Richman (1997) collected longitudinal data on behavior, facial disfigurement, and speech defectiveness, looking for interaction among these variables in 65 children with CPO or CLP at the ages of 6, 9, and 12 years. He was also looking at effects of gender and IQ. At 6 years of age, there were no significant relationships among speech ratings, facial disfigurement, and behavior, but there was a significant effect of gender, in that boys were more likely than girls to "act out." At ages 9 and 12 years, the combination of gender and IQ did affect behavior: boys with lower IQs were likely to act out, and girls with higher IQs tended to show more inhibition of behavior. Richman (1997) concluded that by the age 6 years, speech and facial appearance variables may not have yet produced lasting traits and that the "acting out" of boys this age is probably true of noncleft children as well. He found a significant effect of speech ratings, but not facial ratings, on internalization (inhibition)[17] at age 9 years and a significant effect of facial ratings, but not speech, on internalization at age 12 years.[18] Richman (1997) observed that the influence of cleft-related conditions on behavior at one age may not necessarily apply at another age for the same child and that many of the behavioral concerns may be transitory states amenable to change with intervention. Richman and Millard (1992, 1997) reported longitudinal data on behavior in 44 children from the ages of 4 to 12 years. They found that boys internalized (showed inhibition of impulse) at all of these ages, but there was an age effect for externalizing or acting-out behaviors, with more of such behavior at the ages of 6 to 7 years and less of it at ages 11 to 12 years. Girls showed rather normal scores for internalizing (inhibition) at ages 4 to 6 years but higher

[17]Psychologists call behavior that is inhibited "internalized" and aggressive, acting-out behavior "externalized" or "externalization."

[18]Perhaps this "flip-flop" is a product of approaching adolescence and its preoccupation with appearance.

than normal scores above that age. Externalizing behaviors were higher than normal in girls by the ages of 11 to 12 years, but they were also registering higher on internalizing behaviors, suggesting a frustration-aggression dynamic. Levels of conduct problems in boys fluctuated with age. Among their other conclusions, the authors (Richman and Millard, 1992, 1997) reported that their attempts to relate speech, hearing, or facial disfigurement to a prediction of behavior or achievement by age 9 years did not work. However, the changes they saw by age 12 years were potentially important for patient management. Kapp-Simon and Dawson (1998), studying children with various craniofacial anomalies between the ages of 4 and 18 years, found that boys showed more acting-out behavior than girls only in the age range of 10 to 13 years; in all other age groups, it was the girls who were exhibiting more of such behavior. Endriga and Kapp-Simon (1999) pointed out that when children have significant behavior or emotional problems, high scores on both internalizing (inhibited behavior) and externalizing (acting-out behavior) scales are not uncommon. They also pointed out that research on this topic suggests that children who show both inhibition and acting-out behaviors are demonstrating the consequences of their frustration at not being able to achieve their goals.

Some of the behavioral problems in children with clefts may be related to how they are being accepted by peers, particularly to the extent that such acceptance is based on facial appearance. Richardson (1970) compared the social preferences of children for photographs of other children with no disability, crutches and leg brace, wheel chair, arm amputation, obesity, and repaired cleft lip. The children with obesity and those with cleft lip were least preferred. Richardson also found that teenagers and adults were even harsher in their judgments than younger children. Clifford and Walster (1973) handed fifth-grade teachers identical report cards to which photos were attached and found that attractive children were rated as being more popular, more intelligent, and more likely to be academically successful. Schneiderman and Harding (1984) found that children in the second, third, and fourth grades rated color slides of children with cleft lip more negatively than slides of noncleft faces, and they rated slides of bilateral clefts more negatively than unilateral clefts. The ratings were in a forced-choice format, pairing good/bad adjectives (interesting/boring, friendly/mean, happy/sad, etc.). Interestingly, the older children (around age 10 years) tended to rate the slides of children with clefts less harshly than the younger judges, although this was not constant. Adults also rated slides of children with clefts as less socially acceptable in an earlier study by Glass et al. (1981).[19] Tobiasen (1987) used judges of both sexes and ranging in age from 8 to 16 years to judge either uncorrected or photographically corrected pictures of children with clefts. She found no effect for age or sex of the rater; that is, older raters were just as harsh as younger ones, and males and females did not differ. The pictures of children with clefts were rated as less popular, friendly, and smart and a less likely choice as a friend. Amount of facial deformity was judged more severely in pictures of females as opposed to males, an observation that fits other reports that facial appearance is more worrisome to girls with clefts than to boys up to a certain age level, although it may become of equal concern to both sexes in the teenage years as a natural consequence of being an adolescent (Broder, Smith, Strauss, 1992).[20]

Assessment of social development of children with clefts is unavoidably tied to assessment of personality and the general category of adjustment and should also be referenced to what we know about social skills in physically normal children.[21] Again, the literature points not so much to general deficits as to situational or age-specific concerns. Children with clefts are in fact at risk for problems in the development of age-appropriate social skills, something that is pluripotential both in etiology and in effects on other aspects of their lives. Many studies have illustrated or underscored these differences, but clinicians and researchers do see most such findings as situational or potentially changeable with professional intervention, rather than unavoidable (Richman and Millard, 1997.) Tobiasen and Hiebert (1984) conjectured that the parents in their study may have fostered feelings in their sons of being less able to perform in a socially appropriate manner and concluded (p. 84) that the child with a cleft ". . . may have substantively different social skills learning experiences than a child without a cleft defect." Pertinent to this point were the findings of Campis, DeMaso, and Twente (1995), who found that, in 6- to 12-year-old children with a variety of craniofacial anomalies, maternal adjustment and maternal perceptions of mother-child relationships were more potent predictors of the children's emotional adjustment than either severity of their medical condition or the amount of maternal social support. In other words, how the mothers felt and how they saw their relationship with their child had a direct effect on the child's adjustment.

In summary, the data to date on psychosocial and educational concerns during the school-age years seem to indicate that children with clefts:

1. Are not apt to be significantly different from their peers in terms of personality measures or occurrence of psychopathology

[19]Shaw (1981) demonstrated that even mild dental anomalies, without any cleft, negatively influenced ratings that 11- to 13-year-old children gave to facial photographs.

[20]There have been several studies on the relationship between judgments of facial appearance and judgments of speech in individuals with clefts (Falk and McGlone, 1976; Glass and Starr, 1979; Podol and Salvia, 1976; Sinko and Hedrick, 1982).

[21]A point that speech-language pathologists, as well as other healthcare givers, repeatedly lose track of. Children are difficult (they don't come with manuals), and teenagers are worse, etc. However, most clinicians and researchers providing information on psychosocial problems in clefts have been careful to compare their findings to those in noncleft individuals.

2. May be more apt to exhibit behavioral problems, with this difference to some extent dependent on age and gender
3. May have some personality characteristics that differentiate them from noncleft peers, although the results seem to depend on sex, age, treatment success, and the particular independent variables chosen by investigators
4. Are subject to teasing and other forms of abuse from peers and need assistance in learning how to handle this
5. Are prone to difficulties in academic achievement, particularly in reading and other areas linked to language competencies

A CLOSER LOOK AT ADOLESCENTS

Probably anyone who has raised children could, in retrospect, identify at least two particularly battle-torn periods in that process: toddlerhood and adolescence. The teenage years see a resurgence of the need for autonomy in the child, and typically a resurgence of anxiety on the part of the parents. As the youngster goes through this final stage toward becoming a grown-up, earlier parent-child patterns of interaction and parenting styles will most likely still have some residual effects. "Support without smothering" is a difficult assignment for parents. The teenager still needs support and nurturing but also needs independence and self-confidence. For a youngster with a cleft or other craniofacial anomaly, and for the parents, it may be even more difficult to shake off old patterns.

Richman and Harper (1978a) examined how adolescent boys with clefts perceived the parenting behavior of their mothers in comparison to the way control subjects and boys with cerebral palsy perceived their mothers. The boys with clefts saw their mothers as exerting greater intrusiveness and encouraging less independent development to an extent not found in either the control group or the group with cerebral palsy. The authors concluded that the boys may have become less accepting of their mothers' fostering of dependence as they moved into adolescence, viewing this maternal behavior as restrictive and intrusive rather than nurturing. Parenthetically, it is interesting to ponder why this was true in boys with clefts and not in the boys with cerebral palsy.

Kapp-Simon (1995) pointed out that the normal developmental tasks of adolescents include individuation from family, development of a sense of personal identity, and establishment of satisfactory peer relationships. All these are potentially difficult for a teenager coping with a cleft or other craniofacial anomalies. Kapp-Simon (1995) made specific suggestions for helping the teen handle teasing, drawn from her social skills training program (Kapp-Simon and Simon, 1991) in which hypothetical situations are presented to the youngster for "rehearsing" responses that are direct, honest, and unlikely to stimulate further teasing. (See the section of this chapter devoted to prevention and intervention.)

Kapp-Simon (1995) also pointed out that, in addition to other challenges, teenagers with craniofacial anomalies are challenged by the medical decision making they must make in cooperation with their parents and caregivers. The teenager will often volunteer, "I'm satisfied with the way I look" as a way of avoiding another hospitalization or other interruption in his or her busy life and is likely to be met with a dug-in response from the parents (e.g., "We need to follow the doctor's recommendations and do what's best for you") (Kapp-Simon, 1995). Actually, studies on just how much older children and teenagers are taught or told about their condition and the required treatment have pointed out a disappointing failure of care providers (and parents) to share information and treatment decisions with youngsters. Walesky-Rainbow and Morris (1978) reported that children between the ages of 8 and 19 years had less than adequate information about the general impact of a cleft, the cause of clefts, the rationale for cleft management, and future management of their problem. Things may not have changed all that much in the more than 22 years since that study. When Paynter, Edmonson, and Jordan (1991) assessed the accuracy of information reported by parents and children who had been evaluated by a cleft palate team, the children's responses were accurate only 67% of the time, and the parents' responses 80.6% of the time. The authors warned clinicians not to overestimate what children and families will store and process of the information given to them by the team. Pannbacker and Scheuerle (1993) found that only 57% of parents were satisfied with their involvement in team treatment decisions, which means that only a little more than half of them felt they were part of the decision process, and, by inference, far too many treatment decisions are made without adequate input from the patient and family. Turner et al. (1997) reported that almost one fourth of 15-year-old children with clefts felt they had been excluded from treatment decisions.

Bernstein and Kapp (1981) wrote an article about potential problems in teenagers with clefts that consisted basically of "arm-chair philosophy" rather than data but did offer some interesting perspectives. They felt that the social and emotional problems associated with a cleft stemmed from multiple sources (speech and hearing problems, parents' feelings of guilt and anxiety, protracted contact with physicians, and the visible scars) and that these factors retarded the development of a satisfactory self-image and the process of individualization. On the other hand, they expressed the opinion that continuing medical care such as later corrective surgery, regular evaluations, speech therapy, and psychotherapy could help "relieve the adolescent's misery." These authors also suggested that surgical procedures during adolescence might alter facial expressions, thus further affecting and social communications; however, this was pure conjecture without data. (Kapp-Simon subsequently went on to gather large amounts of data related to the questions and points she and Bernstein had raised.) Canady (1995), a plastic surgeon, cautioned his colleagues about making too many automatic assumptions about the effects of plastic surgery on the emotional well-being of teenagers, urging among other things systematic psychological assessment and availability of counseling.[22]

Strauss, Broder and Helms (1988) examined satisfaction with appearance and with speech in teenagers with CLO, CLP, or CPO. About 60% were very pleased with their facial appearance, and about 60% were pleased with the way they talked. About 9% were very disappointed with their looks, and a total of 28% rated themselves as not understandable or only moderately understandable. In the patients with clefts of the lip, approximately 36% (and 44% of their parents) were less than "very pleased" with appearance. The authors warned fellow clinicians (p. 341), "This study discredits the assumption that time and treatment uniformly result in the patient's being 'out of the woods.' "

Endriga and Kapp-Simon (1999) summarized the published information on psychosocial issues in teenagers with craniofacial anomalies. Global self-concept seems to fall within the normal range (Leonard et al., 1991; Starr, 1978b). They stated that the literature indicated nonpathological elevations in inhibition and social introversion. Some subsets of teens (e.g., older adolescent girls) may be less well adjusted, perhaps owing to continued anxiety about facial appearance and its effect on social relationships. Adolescent girls do report more feelings of being unpopular, anxious, unhappy, and dissatisfied with their appearance (Broder, Smith, and Strauss, 1994; Kapp, 1979; Leonard et al., 1991). The work of Harper and Richman (1978) and Richman (1983) revealed dissatisfaction with educational and social functioning, self-doubt, and discomfort in interpersonal relationships. Tobiasen and Hiebert (1993a) found that teens whose self-ratings of facial impairment were less severe than peer ratings of that impairment had better self-esteem and psychosocial adjustment, as common sense would predict. However, Richman, Holmes, and Eliason (1985) found that teens who were well adjusted by parent report rated their own facial appearance in a manner similar to their teachers' ratings but reported levels of social inhibition that were consistent with the perceptions of their parents. By contrast, teens who were poorly adjusted rated their own appearance higher than their teachers did and underestimated their own levels of inhibition. The authors conjectured that, in the teens who were less realistic in their self-perceptions, the denial of facial disfigurement was a defense mechanism that resulted in greater social withdrawal.[23]

Endriga and Kapp-Simon (1999) felt that the learning capacities of adolescents with craniofacial anomalies had not been well studied, although many studies of intelligence in individuals with craniofacial anomalies contained teenagers within their samples. They concluded that what data were available did make it seem likely that these teenagers show a pattern of poorer academic achievement, similar to that found in school-age children.

Kapp-Simon and McGuire (1997) offered some interesting data derived from observations of the behavior of teenagers with craniofacial anomalies in a natural, daily occurring situation—their school cafeteria. Observers recorded subject initiations (of contacts with peers), responses, peer initiations and responses, conversation events, and nondirected comments. The teens with craniofacial anomalies behaved differently from their peers. They were often at the periphery of the group, acting more like observers than participants. They were not approached as often as their peers, and they often made nondirected comments. Their nonaffected peers initiated more contact and responded more frequently to peer initiation. The authors summarized their findings as indicative of "decreased social contact," consistent with previous studies indicating social isolation and a need for intervention.

All these problems in teenagers with clefts or other craniofacial anomalies tell us that, as put by Strauss, Broder, and Helms (1988), these youngsters are not necessarily "out of the woods" as a natural consequence of maturation or physical treatment (orthodontics, surgery) by the time they are on the brink of adult life. Current work focuses on what the youngsters perceive, how they react, and what professionals and families can do to minimize conflicts and, perhaps, to alter or escape old parent-child interaction problems laid down when the child was much younger. Pope and Ward (1997a) found greater social competence in teenagers if the parents worried less about their child's friendships but at the same time actively encouraged the child's efforts to engage with peers. In the 1992 study of Kapp-Simon et al. on children aged 10 to 16 years, the two best predictors of adjustment were social skills and athletic competence. Both of these reports raise the question of interactive effects. In the study of Kapp-Simon, Simon, and Kristovich (1992), were social skills better because the teenagers were better "adjusted," or vice versa? In the Pope and Ward (1997a) report, were the teenagers more competent in their social relationships because the parents were giving them more freedom, or were the parents giving them more freedom because they perceived their children as more socially competent? Both studies highlight the potential for professionals to intervene and provide a better psychosocial outcome for teenagers if that intervention is timely.

ADULTS

The majority of studies and surveys on adults with CL+/−P that focused on various aspects of "success" in life (e.g.,

[22]Such services are mandated by the American Cleft Palate–Craniofacial Association, both in their "Parameters for Evaluation and Treatment" document (1993) and in the "Standards of Team Care" document (1998), and are a part of the care provided by most teams but not by most surgeons working outside team settings.

[23]One is also tempted to wonder whether the poorly adjusted group was poorly adjusted, at least in part, because their facial appearance was worse than that of the better-adjusted group.

educational level, employment, marriage) were published several decades ago. Because of the time of their publication, most of them did not recognize the important difference between CPO and CL+/−P in assessing life outcomes. Although these studies are still widely cited, it is only reasonable to assume that some of the information they contain is outdated either by advances in treatment or by societal changes in general. By comparison, there are very few recent studies on the status of adults.

One parameter that has been used to assess adult status is the level of education achieved. Demb and Ruess (1967) reported that the high school dropout rate for individuals with clefts was 25% compared with 42% for their siblings. This was at a time when the national average was 30%. The authors hypothesized that family patterns rather than the presence of a cleft formed the primary basis for whether a youngster would complete high school. The higher dropout rate for their siblings was unexplained but invites speculation that parents were putting more emphasis on school for their youngsters with clefts or that the attention those youngsters were getting within the family may have stimulated rebellion in their siblings. In a study that examined several aspects of function in adults with clefts, Clifford, Crocker, and Pope (1972) analyzed their results for differences among cleft types (CLO, CPO, CLP) and between sexes rather than in comparison to a control group; they found no significant differences in educational level either among cleft types or between sexes. McWilliams and Paradise (1973) found a similar dropout rate (23%) for individuals with clefts but, in contrast to the findings of Demb and Ruess (1967), only a 13% rate for their siblings. In the latter study, when the upper end of the educational scale was evaluated, subjects with clefts attended college and graduated from college with the same frequency as their siblings. Both the cleft subjects and their siblings achieved a significantly higher level of education than did either their fathers or their mothers, although the cleft subjects dropped out of school more often. Family differences accounted for some of these findings: in families that did not have a pattern of continuing education, a significantly larger number of cleft patients dropped out of high school in comparison to their siblings, but this was not true in families that did have a pattern of continuing education. Thus, the authors felt the presence of a cleft was more influential in families where there was already a pattern of not stressing education than in families who did.

A Finnish study (Lahti, Rintala, and Soivio, 1974) looked at school attendance (meaning highest grade level achieved) and military service as indices of educational level and reported lower percentages of individuals with clefts, as compared to noncleft individuals, in the higher ranks either for grade level achieved or level of military service. A study published in the same year in the United States (Peter and Chinsky, 1974b) examined educational level by cleft type, but the results were essentially nonsignificant. The dropout rate was 25% for individuals with CLP and 27% for CPO, compared with 31% for random control subjects and 25% for their siblings. The percentage of individuals who completed college was 14% for all three groups. Peter and Chinsky (1974a) also reported that their cleft subjects tended to marry persons with equal or higher educational attainment only slightly less frequently than did their siblings or random controls and that type of cleft did not substantially affect the choice of mate in terms of educational attainment.[24] A relatively recent study from Norway (Ramstad, Ottem, and Shaw, 1995) also reported few differences between adults with clefts and control subjects with regard to educational attainment.

Peter, Chinsky, and Fisher (1975a) looked at occupational levels of adults with clefts. They found no significant differences between cleft palate subjects and control subjects based on the U.S. census socioeconomic scales, nor were there significant differences between cleft types. However, the cleft adults did have significantly lower incomes than control subjects, leading the authors (p. 199) to conclude that adults with clefts "experience some limitation in their ability to secure vocational and economic rewards from society." McWilliams and Paradise (1973) found no significant differences between the occupational levels of their cleft subjects and those of either their fathers or their nearest-age siblings, although both the cleft subjects and their siblings had achieved higher levels of education than their parents, a finding that may be consistent with the conclusion of Peter, Chinsky, and Fisher (1975a). Similarly, Ramstad, Ottem, and Shaw (1995) reported few differences between adults with clefts and control subjects with respect to employment but also that incomes tended to be lower among married men and single women with clefts than among controls. In the study of Clifford, Crocker, and Pope (1972), there were no significant differences among cleft types for the number of jobs held, but men with clefts had had more jobs than women with clefts had. Overall, the subjects' satisfaction with their employment was high.

The social adjustment of adults with clefts has been assessed by looking at their patterns of interaction with others, dating and marriage, and their self-reported satisfaction with appearance and treatment on the assumption that that satisfaction influences (and is influenced by) social relationships. Clifford, Crocker, and Pope (1972) reported that 21 of their 98 subjects were unmarried, but they did not specify the ages of the subjects so there may have been a time-dependent factor. McWilliams and Paradise (1973), Peter and Chinsky (1974a), and Ramstad, Ottem, and Shaw (1995) all reported that individuals with clefts marry

[24]A 1971 study in England on "speech and intelligence in adult cleft-palate patients" (Lovius, 1971) reported no significant differences between the intelligence of cleft subjects (actually age 14 years and up) and that of a small group of control subjects matched for age and chosen because they had "spent long periods in hospital" as children. The cleft subjects were a mixture of repaired, prosthetically treated, and untreated individuals; the speech data were naive; and there was no evidence that the intelligence assessment tool was administered by a qualified psychologist.

later and less frequently; in the Peter and Chinsky study (1974a), the percentages of adults who were unmarried were about the same for CPO and CLP. Peter and Chinsky (1974a) also reported that there were childless couples among adults with clefts and fewer children per marriage. Interestingly, childless couples who eventually divorced were found 35% more frequently among adults with CLP as opposed to CPO.

Peter, Chinsky, and Fisher (1975b) looked at other aspects of social integration in adults with clefts in comparison to their siblings and a large group of controls: family interdependence, geographic mobility, home activities, initial social contacts, friendship patterns, neighbor integration, and voluntary associations. They found a reliance on extended family for mutual aid and social activities. The cleft adults participated less frequently in voluntary associations and relied on just a few one-to-one friendships. Their social activities tended to be that of "informal visiting patterns." Of all the cleft subjects, males with CPO tended to be the least well socially integrated. (This is reminiscent of the 1985 finding of Heller et al. of the likelihood of maladjustment in "uncommunicative" boys.) The authors offered the interpretation that society might be more supportive of persons whose physical problems are visible in that social norms require differential behavior toward this group. On the other hand, perhaps CLP subjects encounter greater rejection from society and adopt more aggressive behavior to compensate for the threats of rejection, whereas CPO subjects may experience less rejection but conversely are less able to cope with it when it does occur.

Richman and Harper (1980) compared personality profiles of a group of young adults with cleft lip and palate and another group with orthopedic problems, just as they had studied persons with similar physical problems as teenagers (Harper and Richman, 1978). All the subjects had normal intelligence. The young adults with clefts seemed to show less self-doubt and worry over interpersonal relations than had previously been identified in adolescents with clefts. No psychopathology was found.

In telephone interviews touching upon various aspects of function in adults with CLO, CLP, or CPO, Heller, Tidmarsh, and Pless (1981) reported finding evidence of psychosocial maladjustment in from 10% to 30% of subjects, depending on the criteria used. Their questions focused on educational achievement, work performance, and social integration. Unfortunately, they did not differentiate their results by cleft type. Their telephone respondents expressed a high rate of persistent dissatisfaction with appearance, hearing, speech, teeth, and social life.

Several other studies have also examined satisfaction with appearance and treatment results in adults with clefts. In the study of Clifford, Crocker, and Pope (1972), the subjects expressed a high degree of satisfaction with their treatment and overall appearance, with the lowest points of satisfaction being their teeth and their speech. However, as the authors pointed out, all the subjects were "volunteers" and were thus more likely to be those who had made the most satisfactory life adjustments. (The fact that only 4% were dissatisfied with their appearance could also reflect either denial or the need that most of us have to believe that we have had the best medical care available.) The authors also queried their subjects on the perceived influence of the cleft on their lives; the mean scores on this measure fell in the range of low influence, which again may have reflected some degree of bias or a need to present themselves as doing well in life despite adverse circumstances. Noar's 1991 study on young adults (age range 16 to 25 years) also indicated general satisfaction with treatment and overall facial appearance but specific aspects of dissatisfaction with regard to speech and the appearance of the nose, lip, profile, and teeth. These subjects, like those of Clifford, Crocker, and Pope (1972), did not feel they had been significantly handicapped socially or emotionally by their clefts. Starr (1982) assessed self-perceived physical attractiveness and self-esteem by mail-in standardized questionnaires and reported (not surprisingly) that the more attractive a person rated himself, the higher the self-esteem. He found no difference between CPO and CLP individuals on their responses to the questions in either self-esteem or perceived attractiveness. However, he had no control subjects.

From his review of the psychosocial literature, Clifford (1979) concluded that individuals with clefts, as adults, assume reasonable positions in society and do not appear to be remarkably different from others. The data that have been derived in the intervening 20 years continue to support this conclusion. No consistent, significant differences between adults with clefts and control subjects have emerged in studies of educational levels, employment, or social integration. With regard to the social status of adults with clefts, Clifford (1979, p. 48) stated "It is clear . . . that the drastic effects on heterosexual relationships put forth by Bryt (1953) for patients with craniofacial anomalies do not apply to subjects with cleft palate." However, specific areas of concern remain (e.g., appearance and society's reaction to facial differences). Also, it must again be pointed out that most of the information discussed in this section is quite dated. Updated studies on adults, reflecting the results of current standards of practice, are certainly needed.

PREVENTION AND INTERVENTION

As the amount of information on psychosocial and educational concerns for patients with clefts and other craniofacial anomalies has ballooned over the past few decades, clinicians have increasingly advocated preventive and therapeutic strategies in the effort to minimize the prevalence and severity of problems. Approaching this area of care chronologically,[25] intervention by the team

[25]For the time being, we have little to offer parents-to-be of fetuses who are already known to have a craniofacial anomaly, other than support from the team and contact with other families if they so desire.

psychologist or other mental health professional is urged from the earliest contact, regardless of the age of the patient. Endriga and Speltz (1997) urged that visits with the team for regular rechecks of weight gain in infants include information exchange between parents and the team. These authors also emphasized the importance of intake screening (again, regardless of age) and availability of intervention for all patients. Drotar et al. (1975) urged early "crisis counseling" for new parents. In their study of preschoolers, Krueckeberg, Kapp-Simon, and Ribordy (1993) stated that the challenge for professionals was to identify the strengths children possess and to nurture those skills as the children face a variety of challenges in the process of maturation. Broder and Strauss (1989) also urged routine psychosocial screening by teams and preventive psychosocial intervention to help these children develop their potential and to improve behavioral adjustment. Tobiasen (1990) strongly urged that at least one psychological assessment be completed for every child with a cleft before entrance into school and repeated every 2 to 3 years thereafter. She also recommended that older children and their parents should routinely be offered consultations with a psychologist before and after each major surgery.[26] In 1991, Strauss and Broder pointed to the efforts made by mental health workers to develop support groups for families, provide nursing and feeding instructions, dispense literature to enlighten family members and school personnel about cleft conditions, assess patients and family systems, and provide counseling to patients and their families. However, they were pleading for outcome data (p. 152): "We believe that these efforts [of the mental health workers] reduce stress, increase awareness, decrease fear of the unknown, improve self-concept, and promote positive communication and family stability, yet no published data exist that verify these beliefs." Although the literature tells us that most individuals with clefts seem to do very well in various aspects of adjustment and development, as Pope (1999, p. 38) put it, ". . . it can be critical for families to have some assistance in navigating the stressors associated with living with a CFA." Pope and Ward (1997a) emphasized the need for appropriate referrals and intervention for children with craniofacial anomalies in the preadolescent years. The disturbing findings of Broder, Richman, and Matheson (1998) with regard to school achievement, together with the information they reviewed about other aspects of development and adjustment in children with clefts, spurred the authors to recommend early screening and continuing psychological assessment for children with clefts. Other professionals who urged that psychological treatment be regularly made available for children with craniofacial anomalies and their families were Bennett and Stanton (1993), Bjornsson and Agustsdottir (1987), Broder and Richman (1987), and Heller, Tidmarsh, and Pless (1981). The sequential studies of Speltz, Armsden, and Clarren (1990) and Speltz et al. (1993) pointed to the possibility of forestalling or minimizing behavior problems in 5- to 7-year-old children by intervening when certain mother-child interactions are observed during late infancy. Richman's 1997 findings on the interaction among various "cleft-related" conditions" and behavior between the ages of 6 and 9 years led him to observe than many of the behavioral worries may be amenable to change with intervention. Kapp-Simon and Simon (1991) devised a hands-on social skills training program for teenagers with craniofacial anomalies, designed to teach them how to handle difficult social situations, deal with pesky peers, and maintain a healthy and balanced attitude as they mature through these difficult years. Another social interaction training program for individuals with facial disfigurement was published by Robinson, Rumsey, and Partridge in 1986.

The push for preventive measures and intervention with regard to psychosocial problems in individuals with clefts comes into toe-to-toe opposition with the 1990s' push for minimizing costs of care by reducing that care to the lowest possible level. When psychologists and other mental health care professionals first had an opportunity to examine and counsel these patients and their families in the 1950s, 1960s, and 1970s, many craniofacial teams were funded by federal grants that supported the interdisciplinary approach to treatment. Sadly, that is no longer the case. As we leave the 1900s, we know more than we have ever known about these needs and have fewer resources to meet them than our predecessors had in previous decades.

[26]Clifford (1973) and Lefebvre and Barclay (1982) warned about the dangers of unrealistic preoperative expectations and unilateral decisions about surgery.

REFERENCES

Allen R, Wasserman GA, and Seidman S: Children with congenital anomalies: the preschool period. *Journal of Pediatric Psychology* 15:327-345, 1990.

Avedian L, and Ruberg RL: Impaired weight gain in cleft palate infants. *Cleft Palate Journal* 17:24-26, 1980.

Bangs TE, and Garrett SB: *Birth to three scale (experimental edition).* Houston: Speech and Hearing Institute, 1973.

Barden C, Ford M, Jensen AG, Rogers-Salyer M, and Salyer KE: Effects of craniofacial deformity in infancy on the quality of mother-infant interactions. *Child Development* 60:819-824, 1989.

Bayley N: *Bayley scales of infant development.* San Antonio (TX): Psychological Corporation, 1969.

Bennett ME, and Stanton ML: Psychotherapy for persons with craniofacial deformities: can we treat without theory? *Cleft Palate–Craniofacial Journal* 30:406-410, 1993.

Benson BA, and Gross AM: The effect of a congenitally handicapped child on the marital dyad: a review of the literature. *Clinical Psychology Review* 9:747-458, 1989.

Benson BA, Gross AM, Messer SM, Kellum G, and Passmore LA: Social support networks among families of children with craniofacial anomalies. *Health Psychology* 10:252-258, 1991.

Bernstein NR, and Kapp KA: Adolescents with cleft palate: body-image and psychosocial problems. *Psychosomatics* 22:697-701, 1981.

Berry LA, Witt PD, Marsh JL, Pilgram TK, and Eder RA: Personality attributions based on speech samples of children with repaired cleft palates. *Cleft Palate–Craniofacial Journal* 34:385-389, 1997.

Berscheid E, and Gangested S: Social-psychological implications of facial physical attractiveness. *Clinics in Surgery* 9:198-202, 1982.

Bjornsson A, and Agustsdottir S: A psychosocial study of Icelandic individuals with cleft lip or cleft lip and palate. *Cleft Palate Journal* 24:152-156, 1987.

Bradbury ET, and Hewison J: Early parental adjustment to visible congenital disfigurement. *Child Care, Health and Development* 20:251-266, 1984.

Brantley H, and Clifford E: Cognitive, self-concept, and body image measures of normal, cleft palate, and obese patients. *Cleft Palate Journal* 16:177-182, 1979.

Broder HL: Commentary on Leonard et al., 1991. *Cleft Palate–Craniofacial Journal* 28:353, 1991.

Broder HL: Psychological research of children with craniofacial anomalies: review, critique, and implications for the future. *Cleft Palate–Craniofacial Journal* 34:402-404, 1997.

Broder HL, and Richman LC: An examination of mental health services offered by cleft/craniofacial teams. *Cleft Palate Journal* 24:158-162, 1987.

Broder HL, and Strauss RP: Self-concept of early primary school age children with visible or invisible defects. *Cleft Palate Journal* 26:114-117, 1989.

Broder HL, Richman LC, and Matheson PB: Learning disability, school achievement, and grade retention among children with cleft: a two-center study. *Cleft Palate–Craniofacial Journal* 35:127-131, 1998.

Broder HL, Smith FB, and Strauss RP: Habilitation of patients with clefts: parent and child ratings of satisfaction with appearance and speech. *Cleft Palate–Craniofacial Journal* 29:262-267, 1992.

Broder HL, Smith FB, and Strauss RP: Effects of visible and invisible orofacial defects on self-perception and adjustment across developmental eras and gender. *Cleft Palate–Craniofacial Journal* 31:429-436, 1994.

Broen PA, Devers MC, Doyle SS, Prouty JM, and Moller KT: Acquisition of linguistic and cognitive skills by children with cleft palate. *Journal of Speech, Language, and Hearing Research* 41:676-687, 1998.

Bzoch KR, and League R: *Assessing language skills in infancy.* Gainesville (FL): Tree of Life Press, 1971.

Campis LB, DeMaso DR, and Twente AW: The role of maternal factors in the adaptation of children with craniofacial disfigurement. *Cleft Palate–Craniofacial Journal* 32:55-61, 1995.

Canady JW: Emotional effects of plastic surgery on the adolescent with a cleft. *Cleft Palate–Craniofacial Journal* 32:120-124, 1996.

Carlson C, Papolos D, Pandita RK, Faedda GL, Veit S, Goldberg R, Shprintzen RJ, Kucherlapati R, and Morrow B: Molecular analysis of velo-cardio-facial syndrome patients with psychiatric disorders. *American Journal of Human Genetics* 60:851-859, 1997.

Carreto V: Maternal responses to an infant with cleft lip and palate: a review of the literature. *Maternal-Child Nursing Journal* 10:197-206, 1981.

Cervenka J, and Drabkova H: The intelligence quotient in cleft lip and palate. *Acta Chirurugiae Plasticae* 7:58-61, 1965.

Clifford E: Connotative meaning of concepts related to cleft lip and palate. *Cleft Palate Journal* 4:165-173, 1967.

Clifford E: The impact of symptom on the child: comparative studies of clinical populations. *Journal of School Health* 38:342-350, 1968.

Clifford E: Parental ratings of cleft palate infants. *Cleft Palate Journal* 6:235-244, 1969a.

Clifford E: The impact of symptom: a preliminary comparison of cleft-lip-palate and asthmatic children. *Cleft Palate Journal* 6:221-227, 1969b.

Clifford E: Cleft palate and the person: psychologic studies of its impact. *Southern Medical Journal* 64:1516-1520, 1971.

Clifford E: Psychosocial aspects of orofacial anomalies: speculations in search of data. *Asha Report #8: Orofacial anomalies: clinical and research implications: proceedings of the conference.* Washington (DC): American Speech and Hearing Association, 1973, pp. 2-29.

Clifford E: Psychological aspects of cleft lip and palate. In Bzoch KR (ed.): *Communicative disorders related to cleft lip and palate.* 2nd ed. Boston: Little, Brown, 1979, pp. 37-51.

Clifford E, and Crocker EC: Maternal responses: the birth of a normal child as compared to the birth of a child with a cleft. *Cleft Palate Journal* 8:298-306, 1971.

Clifford E, Crocker EC, and Pope BA: Psychological findings in the adulthood of 98 cleft lip–palate children. *Plastic and Reconstructive Surgery* 50:234-237, 1972.

Clifford MM, and Walster E: Research note: the effect of physical attractiveness on teacher expectations. *Sociology in Education* 46:248-258, 1973.

Corah NL, and Corah PS: A study of body image in children with cleft palate and cleft lip. *Journal of Genetic Psychology* 103:133-173, 1963.

Dar H, Winter S, and Tal Y: Families of children with cleft lips and palates: concerns and counseling. *Developmental Medicine and Child Neurology* 16:513-517, 1974.

Demb N, and Reuss A: High school drop-out rate for cleft palate patients. *Cleft Palate Journal* 4:327-333, 1967.

Drotar D, Baskiewisz A, Irvin H, Kennell J, and Claus M: The adaptation of parents to the birth of an infant with a congenital malformation: a hypothetical model. *Pediatrics* 56:710-717, 1975.

Eder RA: Individual differences in young children's self-concepts: implications for children with cleft lip and palate. In Eder RA (ed.): *Developmental perspectives on craniofacial problems.* New York: Springer-Verlag, 1995, pp. 141-157.

Eliason MJ: Neuropsychological perspectives of cleft lip and palate. In Bardach J, and Morris HL (eds.): *Multidisciplinary management of cleft lip and palate.* Philadelphia: WB Saunders, 1990, pp. 825-830.

Eliason MJ: Cleft lip and palate: developmental effects. *Journal of Pediatric Nursing* 5:107-113, 1991.

Eliason MJ, and Richman LC: Language development in preschoolers with clefts. *Developmental Neuropsychology* 6:173-182, 1990.

Endriga MC, and Kapp-Simon KA: Psychological issues in craniofacial care: state of the art. *Cleft Palate–Craniofacial Journal* 36:3-11, 1999.

Endriga MC, and Speltz ML: Face-to-face interaction between infants with orofacial clefts and their mothers. *Journal of Pediatric Psychology* 22:439-453, 1997.

Estes RE, and Morris HL: Relationships among intelligence, speech proficiency, and hearing sensitivity in children with cleft palates. *Cleft Palate Journal* 7:763-773, 1970.

Falk ML, and McGlone EL: Social response to acoustic and visual characteristics of oral cleft. *Cleft Palate Journal* 13:181-183, 1976.

Field TM, and Vega-Lahr N: Early interactions between infants with craniofacial anomalies and their mothers. *Infant Behavior and Development* 7:527-530, 1984.

Fisk SB, Pearl RM, Schulman GI, and Wong H: Congenital facial anomalies among 4- through 7-year-olds: psychological effects and surgical decisions. *Annals of Plastic Surgery* 14:37-42, 1985.

Fogh-Andersen P: *Inheritance of harelip and cleft palate.* Copenhagen: Munksgaard, 1942.

Fox D, Lynch J, and Brookshire B: Selected developmental factors of cleft palate children between two and thirty-three months of age. *Cleft Palate Journal* 15:239-245, 1978.

Frankenburg WK, and Dodds JB: *Denver developmental screening test.* Mead Johnson Laboratories, 1969.

Gabka K, and Weber B: Intelligence studies in patients with cleft lip, jaw and palate. *Stomatologie der DDR* 34:257-265, 1984.

Gall JC, Hayward JR, Harper ML, and Garn SM: Studies of dysmorphogenesis in children with oral clefts. I: Relationship between clinical findings and school performance. *Cleft Palate Journal* 9:324-334, 1972.

Gibbs JM: Cleft palate babies: one mother's experience. *Nursing Care* 7:19-23, 1973.

Glass L, and Starr CD: A study of relationships between judgments of speech and appearance of patients with orofacial clefts. *Cleft Palate Journal* 16:436-440, 1979.

Glass L, Starr CD, Stewart, RE, and Hodge SE: Identikit model II—a model tool for judging cosmetic appearance. *Cleft Palate Journal* 18:147-151, 1981.

Goodstein LD: Personality test differences in parents of children with cleft palates. *Journal of Speech and Hearing Research* 3:39-43, 1960.

Goodstein LD: Intellectual impairment in children with cleft palates. *Journal of Speech and Hearing Research* 4:287-294, 1961.

Goodstein LD: Psychosocial aspects. In Spriestersbach DC, and Sherman D (eds.): *Cleft palate and communication.* New York: Academic Press, 1968, pp. 201-224.

Harper D, and Richman LC: Personality profiles of physically impaired adolescents. *Journal of Clinical Psychology* 34:636-642, 1978.

Harper D, Richman LC, and Snider B: School adjustment and degree of physical impairment. *Journal of Pediatric Psychology* 5:377-383, 1980.

Harter S, and Pike R: The pictorial scale of perceived competence and social acceptance for young children. *Child Development* 55:1969-1982, 1984.

Heller A, Tidmarsh W, and Pless IB: The psychosocial functioning of young adults born with cleft lip or palate. *Clinical Pediatrics* 20:459-465, 1981.

Heller A, Rafman S, Zvagulis I, and Pless IB: Birth defects and psychosocial adjustment. *Archives of Adolescent and Pediatric Medicine* 139:257-263, 1985.

Hoeksma JB, and Koomen H: *Development of early mother-child interaction and attachment.* Amsterdam: Pro Lingua, 1991.

Ireton H, and Thwing E: *Minnesota infant development inventory.* Minneapolis: Behavior Science Systems, 1977.

Jones JE: Self-concept and parental evaluation of peer relationships in cleft lip and palate children. *Pediatric Dentistry* 6:132-138, 1984.

Kapp KA: Self concept of the cleft lip and/or palate children. *Cleft Palate Journal* 16:171-176, 1979.

Kapp-Simon KA: Self-concept of primary-school-age children with cleft lip, cleft palate, or both. *Cleft Palate Journal* 23:24-27, 1986.

Kapp-Simon KA: Psychological interventions for the adolescent with cleft lip and palate. *Cleft Palate–Craniofacial Journal* 32:104-108, 1995.

Kapp-Simon KA, and Dawson P: Behavior adjustment and competence of children with craniofacial conditions. Proceedings of the American Cleft Palate–Craniofacial Association, Baltimore, MD, April 1998.

Kapp-Simon KA, and Krueckeberg SM: Mental development in infants with cleft lip and/or palate. Proceedings of the American Cleft Palate–Craniofacial Association, Tampa, FL, April 1995.

Kapp-Simon KA, and McGuire DE: Observed social interaction patterns in adolescents with and without craniofacial conditions. *Cleft Palate–Craniofacial Journal* 34:380-384, 1997.

Kapp-Simon KA, and Simon D: *Meeting the challenge: a social skills training program for adolescents with special needs.* Chicago: University of Illinois, 1991.

Kapp-Simon KA, Simon DJ, and Kristovich S: Self-perception, social skills, adjustment, and inhibition in young adolescents with craniofacial anomalies. *Cleft Palate Journal* 29:340-345, 1992.

Karayiogou M, Morris MA, Morrow B, Shprintzen RJ, Goldberg RB, Borrow J, Gos A, Nestadt G, Wolyniec PS, Lasseter VK, Eisen W, Childs B, Kazazian HH, Kucherlapata R, Antonariakis SE, Pulver AD, and Housman DE: Schizophrenia susceptibility associated with interstitial deletions of chromosome 22z11. *Proceedings of the National Academy of Sciences of the United States of America* 92:7612-7616, 1992.

Kommers MS, and Sullivan MD: Written language skills of children with cleft plate. *Cleft Palate Journal* 16:81-85, 1979.

Krueckeberg SM, and Kapp-Simon KA: Effect of parental factors on social skills of preschool children with craniofacial anomalies. *Cleft Palate–Craniofacial Journal* 30:490-496, 1993.

Krueckeberg SM, and Kapp-Simon KA: Longitudinal follow-up of social skills in children with and without craniofacial anomalies. Proceedings of the American Cleft Palate–Craniofacial Association, New Orleans, April 1997.

Krueckeberg SM, Kapp-Simon KA, and Ribordy SC: Social skills of preschoolers with and without craniofacial anomalies. *Cleft Palate–Craniofacial Journal* 30:475-481, 1993.

Lahti A, Rintala A, and Soivio AL: Educational level of patients with cleft lip and palate. *Cleft Palate Journal* 11:36-40, 1974.

Lamb MM, Wilson FB, and Leeper HA: The intellectual function of cleft palate children compared on the basis of cleft type and sex. *Cleft Palate Journal* 10:367-377, 1973.

Lansdown R: Cleft lip and palate: a prediction of psychological disfigurement? *British Journal of Orthodontics* 8:83-88, 1981.

Lavigne JV, and Wills KE: Psychological aspects of clefting. In Kernahan D, and Rosenstein S (eds.): *Cleft lip and palate: a system of management.* Baltimore: Williams & Wilkins, 1990, pp. 37-46.

Lefebvre A, and Barclay S: Psychosocial impact of craniofacial deformities before and after reconstructive surgery. *Canadian Journal of Psychiatry* 27:579-584, 1982.

Leonard BJ, Brust JD, Abrahams G, and Sielaff B: Self-concept of children and adolescents with cleft lip and/or palate. *Cleft Palate–Craniofacial Journal* 28:347-353, 1991.

Long NV, and Dalston RM: Gestural communication in twelve-month-old cleft lip and palate children. *Cleft Palate Journal* 19:57-61, 1982.

Lovius BBJ: Speech and intelligence in adult cleft-palate patients. *The Dental Practitioner* 21:290-293, 1971.

MacDonald S: Parental needs and professional responses: a parental perspective. *Cleft Palate Journal* 16:188-192, 1979.

MacGregor FC: Some psychosocial problems associated with facial deformities. *American Sociological Review* 16:629-638, 1951.

MacGregor FC, Abel TM, Bryt A, Lauer E, and Weissman S: *Facial deformities and plastic surgery: a psychosocial study.* Springfield (IL): CC Thomas, 1953.

Madison L: Psychologic aspects of cleft lip and palate. *Ear, Nose, and Throat Journal* 65:337-341, 1986.

McWilliams BJ: Psychosocial development and modification. *Asha Report #5: Speech and the dentofacial complex: the state of the art.* Washington (DC): American Speech and Hearing Association, 1970, pp. 165-187.

McWilliams BJ: Social and psychological problems associated with cleft palate. *Clinics in Plastic Surgery: Symposium on Social and Psychological Considerations in Plastic Surgery* 9:317-326, 1982.

McWilliams BJ, and Matthews HP: A comparison of intelligence and social maturity in children with unilateral complete clefts and those with isolated cleft palates. *Cleft Palate Journal* 16:363-372, 1979.

McWilliams BJ, and Paradise JL: Educational, occupational, and marital status of cleft palate adults. *Cleft Palate Journal* 10:223-229, 1973.

Mitchell CK, Lott R, and Pannbacker M: Perceptions about cleft palate held by school personnel: suggestions for in service training development. *Cleft Palate Journal* 21:308-312, 1984.

Morris HL: Communication skills of children with cleft lips and palates. *Journal of Speech and Hearing Research* 5:79-90, 1962.

Muller DB, and Leonetti R: *Primary self-concept inventory test manual.* Austin (TX): Learning Concepts, 1974.

Musgrave R, McWilliams BJ, and Matthews J: A review of two different surgical procedures for the repair of clefts of the soft palate only. *Cleft Palate Journal* 12:281-290, 1975.

Natsume N, Suzuki T, and Kawai T: Maternal reactions to the birth of a child with cleft lip and/or palate. *Plastic and Reconstructive Surgery* 79:1003-1004, 1987.

Nation JE: Vocabulary comprehension and use of speech in preschool cleft palate and normal children. *Cleft Palate Journal* 7:639-644, 1970.

Neiman GS, and Savage HE: Development of infants and toddlers with clefts from birth to three years of age. *Cleft Palate–Craniofacial Journal* 34:219-225, 1997.

Noar JH: Questionnaire survey of attitudes and concerns of patients with cleft lip and palate and their parents. *Cleft Palate–Craniofacial Journal* 28:279-284, 1991.

Pannbacker MP, and Scheuerle J: Parents' attitudes toward family involvement in cleft palate treatment. *Cleft Palate–Craniofacial Journal* 30:87-89, 1993.

Papolos DF, Faedda GL, Veit S, Goldberg R, Morrow B, Kucherlapati R, and Shprintzen RJ: Bipolar spectrum disorders in patients diagnosed with velo-cardio-facial syndrome: does a hemizygous deletion of chromosome 22q11 result in bipolar affective disorder? *American Journal of Psychiatry* 153:1541-1547, 1996.

Paynter ET, Edmonson TW, and Jordan WJ: Accuracy of information reported by parents and children evaluated by a cleft palate team. *Cleft Palate–Craniofacial Journal* 28:329-337, 1991.
Peter JP, and Chinsky RR: Sociological aspects of cleft palate adults. I. Marriage. *Cleft Palate Journal* 11:295-309, 1974a.
Peter JP, and Chinsky RR: Sociological aspects of cleft palate adults. II. Education. *Cleft Palate Journal* 12:443-449, 1974b.
Peter JP, Chinsky RR, and Fisher MJ: Sociological aspects of cleft palate adults. III. Vocational and economic aspects. *Cleft Palate Journal* 12:193-199, 1975a.
Peter JP, Chinsky RR, and Fisher MJ: Sociological aspects of cleft palate adults. IV. Social integration. *Cleft Palate Journal* 12:301-310, 1975b.
Piers EV: *Manual for the Piers-Harris children's self-concept scale.* Nashville (TN): Counselor Recordings and Tests, 1969.
Podol J, and Salvia J: Effects of visibility of a prepalatal cleft on the evaluation of speech. *Cleft Palate Journal* 13:361-366, 1976.
Pope AW: Points of risk and opportunity for parents of children with craniofacial conditions. *Cleft Palate–Craniofacial Journal* 36:36-39, 1999.
Pope AW, and Speltz ML: Research on psychosocial issues of children with craniofacial anomalies: progress and challenges. *Cleft Palate–Craniofacial Journal* 34:371-373, 1997.
Pope AW, and Ward J: Factors associated with peer social competence in preadolescents with craniofacial anomalies. *Journal of Pediatric Psychology* 22:455-470, 1997a.
Pope AW, and Ward J: Self-perceived facial appearance and psychosocial adjustment in preadolescents with craniofacial anomalies. *Cleft Palate–Craniofacial Journal* 34:396-401, 1997b.
Pulver AE, Nestadt G, Goldberg R, Shprintzen RJ, Lamacz M, Wolyniec PS, Morrow B, Karayiorgou M, Antonarakis SE, Housman D, and Kucherlapati F: Psychotic illness in patients diagnosed with velo-cardio-facial syndrome and their relatives. *Journal of Nervous and Mental Disorders* 182:476-478, 1994.
Quay HC, and Peterson DR: *Behavior problem checklist.* Champaign (IL): University of Illinois, 1979.
Ramstad T, Ottem E, and Shaw WC: Psychosocial adjustment in Norwegian adults who had undergone standardised treatment of complete cleft lip and palate. *Scandinavian Journal of Plastic and Reconstructive and Hand Surgery* 29:251-257, 1995.
Ranalli DN, and Mazaheri M: Height-weight growth of cleft children, birth to six years. *Cleft Palate Journal* 12:400-404, 1975.
Reuter J, and Bickett L: *The Kent infant developmental scale manual.* 2nd ed. Kent (OH): Kent Developmental Metrics, 1985.
Richardson SA: Age and sex differences in values toward handicaps. *Journal of Health and Social Behavior* 11:207-214, 1970.
Richardson SA: Handicap, appearance, and stigma. *Social Science and Medicine* 5:621-626, 1971.
Richardson SA, Hastorf AH, and Dornbusch SM: Effects of physical disability on a child's description of himself. *Child Development* 35:893-907, 1964.
Richardson SA, Goodman N, Hastorf A, and Dornbusch S: Cultural uniformity in reaction to physical disabilities. *American Sociological Review* 26:241-247, 1961.
Richman LC: Behavior and achievement of cleft palate children. *Cleft Palate Journal* 13:4-10, 1976.
Richman LC: Parents and teachers: differing views of behavior of cleft palate children. *Cleft Palate Journal* 15:360-364, 1978a.
Richman LC: The effects of facial disfigurement on teachers' perception of ability in cleft palate children. *Cleft Palate Journal* 15:155-160, 1978b.
Richman LC: Cognitive patterns and learning disabilities in cleft palate children with verbal deficits. *Journal of Speech and Hearing Research* 23:447-456, 1980.
Richman LC: Self-reported social, speech, and facial concerns and personality adjustment of adolescents with cleft lip and palate. *Cleft Palate Journal* 20:108-112, 1983.
Richman LC: Facial and speech relationships to behavior of children with clefts across three age levels. *Cleft Palate–Craniofacial Journal* 34:390-395, 1997.
Richman LC, and Eliason MJ: Type of reading disability related to cleft type and neuropsychological patterns. *Cleft Palate Journal* 21:1-6, 1984.
Richman LC, and Eliason MJ: Psychological characteristics of children with cleft lip and palate: intellectual, achievement, behavioral, and personality variables. *Cleft Palate Journal* 19:249-257, 1982.
Richman LC, and Eliason MJ: Communication disorders of children. In Walker CE, and Roberts MC (eds.): *Handbook of clinical child psychology* (revised). New York: John Wiley, 1993, pp. 697-722.
Richman LC, and Harper DC: Observable stigmata and perceived maternal behavior. *Cleft Palate Journal* 15:215-219, 1978a.
Richman LC, and Harper DC: School adjustment of children with observable disabilities. *Journal of Abnormal Child Psychology* 6:11-18, 1978b.
Richman LC, and Harper DC: Self identified personality patterns of children with facial or orthopedic disfigurement. *Cleft Palate Journal* 16:257-261, 1979.
Richman LC, and Harper DC: Personality profiles of physically impaired young adults. *Journal of Clinical Psychology* 36:668-671, 1980.
Richman LC, and Millard TL: Neuropsychological aspects of language/learning based reading disorder in children with cleft. Presented before the American Cleft Palate–Craniofacial Association, Portland, OR, May 1992.
Richman LC, and Millard TL: Cleft lip and palate: longitudinal behavior and relationships of cleft conditions to behavior and achievement. *Journal of Pediatric Psychology* 22:487-494, 1997.
Richman LC, Eliason MJ, and Lindgren SC: Reading disability in children with clefts. *Cleft Palate Journal* 25:21-25, 1988.
Richman LC, Holmes CS, and Eliason MJ: Adolescents with cleft lip and palate: self-perceptions of appearance and behavior related to personality adjustment. *Cleft Palate Journal* 22:93-96, 1985.
Robinson E, Rumsey N, and Partridge J: An evaluation of the impact of social interaction skills training for facially disfigured people. *British Journal of Plastic Surgery* 49:281-289, 1986.
Rowe C: Why has he got a funny nose, Mum? *Nursing Mirror* 156:356-359, 1983.
Rubin R: Maternal tasks in pregnancy. *Maternal-Child Nursing Journal* 4:143-153, 1975.
Ruess A: A comparative study of cleft palate children and their siblings. *Journal of Clinical Psychology* 21:354-360, 1965.
Ruess A: Convergent psychosocial factors in the cleft palate clinic. In Lencione R (ed.): *Cleft palate habilitation: proceedings of the fifth annual symposium on cleft palate habilitation.* Syracuse: Syracuse University, 1967, pp. 53-70.
Schaffer HR, and Callender WM: Psychologic effects of hospitalization in infancy. *Pediatrics* 24:528-539, 1959.
Schneiderman CR, and Auer KE: The behavior of the child with cleft lip and palate as perceived by parents and teachers. *Cleft Palate Journal* 21:224-228, 1984.
Schneiderman CR, and Harding JB: Social ratings of children with cleft lip by school peers. *Cleft Palate Journal* 21:219-223, 1984.
Shaw W: The influence of children's dentofacial appearance on their social attractiveness as judged by peers and lay adults. *American Journal of Orthodontics and Dentofacial Orthopedics* 79:399-415, 1981.
Shprintzen RJ, Goldberg R, Golding-Kushner KJ, and Marion R: Late-onset psychoses in velo-cardio-facial syndrome. *American Journal of Medical Genetics* 42:141-142, 1992.
Sigelman CK, Miller TE, and Whitworth LA: The early stigmatizing reactions to physical differences. *Journal of Applied Developmental Psychology* 7:17-23, 1986.
Simonds JF, and Heimburger RE: Psychiatric evaluation of youth with cleft lip–palate matched with a control group. *Cleft Palate Journal* 15:195-201, 1978.

Sinko GR, and Hedrick DL: The interrelationships between ratings of speech and facial acceptability in persons with cleft palate. *Journal of Speech and Hearing Research* 25:402-407, 1982.

Slutsky H: Maternal reaction and adjustment to birth and care of cleft palate child. *Cleft Palate Journal* 6:425-429, 1969.

Smith RM, and McWilliams BJ: Creative thinking abilities of cleft palate children. *Cleft Palate Journal* 3:275-283, 1966.

Speltz ML, Armsden GC, and Clarren SS: Effects of craniofacial birth defects on maternal functioning postinfancy. *Journal of Pediatric Psychology* 15:177-195, 1990.

Speltz ML, Galbreath H, and Greenberg MT: A developmental framework for psychosocial research on young children with craniofacial anomalies. In Eder RA (ed.): *Craniofacial anomalies: psychological perspectives.* New York: Springer-Verlag, 1995, pp. 258-286.

Speltz ML, Morton K, Goodell EW, and Clarren SK: Psychological functioning of children with craniofacial anomalies and their mothers: follow-up from late infancy to school entry. *Cleft Palate–Craniofacial Journal* 30:482-489, 1993.

Speltz ML, Goodell EW, Endriga MC, and Clarren SK: Feeding interactions of infants with unrepaired cleft lip and/or palate. *Infant Behavior and Development* 17:131-140, 1994a.

Speltz ML, Greenberg MT, Endriga MC, and Galbreath H: Developmental approach to the psychology of craniofacial anomalies. *Cleft Palate–Craniofacial Journal* 31:61-67, 1994b.

Spriestersbach DC: *Psychological aspects of the cleft palate problem.* Volumes 1 and 2. Iowa City: University of Iowa Press, 1973.

Starr P: Hospitalization effects upon behavior of pre-schoolers with cleft lip and/or palate: a pilot study. *Cleft Palate Journal* 15:182-185, 1978a.

Starr P: Self-esteem and behavioral functioning of teen-agers with oral-facial clefts. *Rehabilitation Literature* 93:233-235, 1978b.

Starr P: Physical attractiveness and self-esteem ratings of young adults with cleft lip and/or palate. *Psychological Reports* 50:467-470, 1982.

Starr P, Chinsky R, Canter H, and Meier J: Mental, motor, and social behavior of infants with cleft lip and/or cleft palate. *Cleft Palate Journal* 14:140-147, 1977.

Strauss RP, and Broder HL: Psychological and sociocultural aspects of cleft lip and palate. In Bardach J, and Morris HL (eds.): *Multidisciplinary treatment of cleft lip and palate.* Philadelphia: WB Saunders, 1990, pp. 831-837.

Strauss RP, and Broder HL: Directions and issues in psychosocial research and methods as applied to cleft lip and palate and craniofacial anomalies. *Cleft Palate–Craniofacial Journal* 28:150-156, 1991.

Strauss RP, Broder HL, and Helms RW: Perceptions of appearance and speech by adolescent patients with cleft lip and palate and by their parents. *Cleft Palate–Craniofacial Journal* 25:335-342, 1988.

Strauss RP, Sharp MC, Lorch SC, and Kachalia B: Physicians and the communication of "bad news": parent experiences of being informed of their child's cleft lip and/or palate. *Pediatrics* 96:82-89, 1995.

Stricker G, Clifford E, Cohen L, Giddon D, Meskin L, and Evans C: Psychosocial aspects of craniofacial disfigurement. *American Journal of Orthodontics* 76:410-422, 1979.

Tisza VB, and Gumpertz E: The parents' reaction to the birth and early care of children with cleft palate. *Pediatrics* 30:86-90, 1962.

Tisza VB, Irwin E, and Scheide E: Children with oral-facial clefts: a study of the psychological development of handicapped children. *Journal of the American Academy of Child Psychiatry* 12:292-313, 1973.

Tobiasen JM: Psychosocial correlates of congenital facial clefts: a conceptualization and model. *Cleft Palate Journal* 21:131-139, 1984.

Tobiasen JM: Social judgments of facial deformity. *Cleft Palate Journal* 24:323-327, 1987.

Tobiasen JM: Psychosocial adjustment to cleft lip and palate. In Bardach J, and Morris HL (eds.): *Multidisciplinary management of cleft lip and palate.* Philadelphia: WB Saunders, 1990, pp. 820-825.

Tobiasen JM: Clefting and psychosocial judgment: influence of facial aesthetics. *Advances in Management of Cleft Lip and Palate: Clinics in Plastic Surgery* 20:623-631, 1993.

Tobiasen JM, and Hiebert JM: Parents' tolerance for the conduct problems of the child with cleft lip and palate. *Cleft Palate Journal* 21:82-85, 1984.

Tobiasen JM, and Hiebert JM: Reliability of aesthetic judgments of cleft impairment. *Cleft Palate Journal* 25:313-316, 1988.

Tobiasen JM, and Hiebert JM: Clefting and psychosocial adjustment. *Clinics in Plastic Surgery: Advances in Management of Cleft Lip and Palate* 20:623-631, 1993a.

Tobiasen JM, and Hiebert JM: Combined effects of severity of cleft impairment and facial attractiveness on social perception: an experimental study. *Cleft Palate–Craniofacial Journal* 30:82-86, 1993b.

Tobiasen JM, and Hiebert JM: Facial impairment scales for clefts. *Plastic and Reconstructive Surgery* 93:31-41, 1994.

Tobiasen JM, and Speltz ML: Cleft palate: a psychosocial developmental perspective. In Berkowitz S (ed.): *Cleft lip and palate: perspectives in management.* Volume II: *An introduction to other craniofacial anomalies.* San Diego: Singular, 1996, pp. 15-23.

Tobiasen JM, Hiebert JM, and Boraz RA: Development of scales of severity of facial cleft impairment. *Cleft Palate–Craniofacial Journal* 28:419-424, 1991.

Tobiasen JM, Levy J, Carpenter MA, and Hiebert JM: Type of facial cleft, associated congenital malformations, and parents' ratings of school and conduct problems. *Cleft Palate Journal* 24:209-215, 1987.

Turner SR, Thomas PWN, Dowell T, Rumsey N, and Sandy JR: Psychological outcomes amongst cleft patients and their families. *British Journal of Plastic Surgery* 50:1-9, 1997.

Waechter E: Concerns of parents related to the birth of a child with a cleft of the lip and palate with implications for nurses [thesis]. Chicago: University of Chicago, 1959.

Walesky-Rainbow PA, and Morris HL: An assessment of informative-counseling procedures for cleft palate children. *Cleft Palate Journal* 15:20-29, 1978.

Wasserman GA, and Allen R: Maternal withdrawal from handicapped infants. *Journal of Child Psychology and Psychiatry* 26:381-387, 1985.

Wasserman GA, Allen R, and Solomon CR: At-risk toddlers and their mothers: the special case of physical handicap. *Child Development* 56:82-85, 1985.

Wasserman GA, Allen R, and Solomon CR: Limit setting in mothers of toddlers with physical anomalies. *Rehabilitation Literature* 47:290-294, 1986.

Wasserman GA, Allen R, and Linares LO: Maternal interaction and language development in children with and without speech-related anomalies. *Journal of Communication Disorders* 21:319-331, 1988.

Wasserman GA, Lennon MC, Allen R, and Shilansky M: Contributors to attachment in normal and physically handicapped infants. *Journal of the American Academy of Child and Adolescent Psychiatry* 26:9-15, 1987.

Wirls CJ: Psychosocial aspects of cleft lip and palate. In Grabb W, Rosenstein W, and Bzoch KR (eds.): *Cleft lip and palate: surgical, dental, and speech aspects.* Boston: Little, Brown, 1971, pp. 119-129.

Wirls CJ, and Plotkin RR: A comparison of children with cleft palate and their siblings on projective test personality factors. *Cleft Palate Journal* 8:399-407, 1971.

SUPPLEMENTARY READING LIST

The following articles contain psychosocial information about craniofacial anomalies other than, or in addition to, cleft lip and palate.

Allen R, Wasserman GA, and Seidman S: Children with congenital anomalies: the preschool period. *Journal of Pediatric Psychology* 15:327-345, 1990.

Arndt EM, Travis F, Lefebvre A, and Munro IR: Psychosocial adjustment of 20 patients with Treacher Collins syndrome before and after reconstructive surgery. *British Journal of Plastic Surgery* 40:605-609, 1987.

Barden RC, Ford ME, Jensen AG, Rogers-Salyer M, and Salyer KE: Effects of craniofacial deformity in infancy on the quality of mother-infant interactions. *Child Development* 60:819-824, 1989.

Barden RC, Ford ME, Wilhelm W, Rogers-Salyer M, and Salyer KE: Emotional and behavioral reactions to facially deformed patients before and after craniofacial surgery. *Plastic and Reconstructive Surgery* 82:409-418, 1988.

Barden RC, Ford ME, Wilhelm W, Rogers-Salyer M, and Salyer KE: The physical attractiveness of facially deformed patients before and after craniofacial surgery. *Plastic and Reconstructive Surgery* 82:229-235, 1988.

Beder OE, and Weinstein F: Explorations of the coping of adolescents with orofacial anomalies using the Cornel Medical Index. *Journal of Prosthetic Dentistry* 43:565-570, 1980.

Bennett ME, and Stanton ML: Psychotherapy for persons with craniofacial deformities: can we treat without therapy? *Cleft Palate–Craniofacial Journal* 30:406-410, 1993.

Benson BA, and Gross AM: The effect of a congenitally handicapped child on the marital dyad: a review of the literature. *Clinical Psychology Review* 9:747-458, 1989.

Benson BA, Gross AM, Messer SM, Kellum G, and Passmore LA: Social support networks among families of children with craniofacial anomalies. *Health Psychology* 10:252-258, 1991.

Berscheid E, and Gangested S: Social-psychological implications of facial physical attractiveness. *Clinics in Surgery* 9:198-202, 1982.

Bjornsson A, and Agustsdottir S: A psychosocial study of Icelandic individuals with cleft lip or cleft lip and palate. *Cleft Palate Journal* 24:152-156, 1987.

Bradbury ET, and Hewison J: Early parental adjustment to visible congenital disfigurement. *Child Care, Health and Development* 20:251-266, 1984.

Broder HL, and Richman LC: An examination of mental health services offered by cleft/craniofacial teams. *Cleft Palate Journal* 24:158-162, 1987.

Broder HL, and Strauss RP: Self-concept of early primary school age children with visible or invisible defects. *Cleft Palate Journal* 26:114-118, 1989.

Broder HL: Psychological research of children with craniofacial anomalies: review, critique, and implications for the future. *Cleft Palate–Craniofacial Journal* 34:402-404, 1997.

Broder HL, Smith FB, and Strauss RP: Effects of visible and invisible orofacial defects on self-perception and adjustment across developmental eras and gender. *Cleft Palate–Craniofacial Journal* 31:429-436, 1994.

Broder HL, and Strauss RP: Self-concept of early primary school age children with visible or invisible defects. *Cleft Palate Journal* 26:114-117, 1989.

Campis LB, DeMaso DR, and Twente AW: The role of maternal factors in the adaptation of children with craniofacial disfigurement. *Cleft Palate–Craniofacial Journal* 32:55-61, 1995.

Carlson C, Papolos D, Pandita RK, Faedda GL, Veit S, Goldberg R, Shprintzen RJ, Kucherlapati R, and Morrow B: Molecular analysis of velo-cardio-facial syndrome patients with psychiatric disorders. *American Journal of Human Genetics* 60:851-859, 1997.

Charkins H: *Children with facial difference: a parents' guide.* Bethesda (MD): Woodbine, 1996.

Chibbaro PD: Living with craniofacial microsomia: support for the patient and family. *Cleft Palate–Craniofacial Journal* 36:40-42, 1999.

Clifford E, Cohen N, and Swanson D: Psychologic aspects of craniofacial anomalies. In Converse J, McCarthy J, and Wood-Smith D (eds.): *Symposium on diagnosis and treatment of craniofacial anomalies.* St. Louis: Mosby, 1979, pp. 117-127.

Clifford E: Psychosocial aspects of orofacial anomalies: speculations in search of data. *Asha Report #8: Orofacial anomalies: clinical and research implications.* Washington (DC): American Speech and Hearing Association, 1973, pp. 2-29.

Dion KK, Berscheid E, and Walster E: What is beautiful is good. *Journal of Personality and Social Psychology* 24:285-290, 1972.

Drotar D, Baskiewisz A, Irvin H, Kennell J, and Claus M: The adaptation of parents to the birth of an infant with a congenital malformation: a hypothetical model. *Pediatrics* 56:710-717, 1975.

Eder RA (ed.): *Developmental perspectives on craniofacial problems.* New York: Springer-Verlag, 1995.

Endriga MC, and Kapp-Simon KA: Psychological issues in craniofacial care: state of the art. *Cleft Palate–Craniofacial Journal* 36:3-11, 1999.

Field TM, and Vega-Lahr N: Early interactions between infants with craniofacial anomalies and their mothers. *Infant Behavior and Development* 7:527-530, 1984.

Fisk SB, Pearl RM, Schulman GI, and Wong H: Congenital facial anomalies among 4- through 7-year-olds: psychological effects and surgical decisions. *Annals of Plastic Surgery* 14:37-42, 1985.

Hanus SA, Bernstein NR, and Kapp KA: Immigrants into society. *Clinical Pediatrics* 20:37-41, 1981.

Harper D, and Richman LC: Personality profiles of physically impaired adolescents. *Journal of Clinical Psychology* 34:636-642, 1978.

Harper D, Richman LC, and Snider B: School adjustment and degree of physical impairment. *Journal of Pediatric Psychology* 5:377-383, 1980.

Heller A, Rafman S, Zvagulis I, and Pless IB: Birth defects and psychosocial adjustment. *Archives of Adolescent and Pediatric Medicine* 139:257-263, 1985.

Hoeksma JB, and Koomen H: *Development of early mother-child interaction and attachment.* Amsterdam: Pro Lingua, 1991.

Horowitz F: Design factors in the assessment of intelligence. *Annals of Otology, Rhinology, and Laryngology* 88:64-73, 1979.

Kapp-Simon KA, and Simon D: *Meeting the challenge: a social skills training program for adolescents with special needs.* Chicago: University of Illinois, 1991.

Kapp-Simon K: Mental development and learning disorders in children with single suture craniosynostosis. *Cleft Palate–Craniofacial Journal* 35:197-203, 1998.

Kapp-Simon KA, Figueroa AA, Jocher C, and Schafer M: Longitudinal assessment of mental development in infants with nonsyndromic craniosynostosis with and without cranial release and reconstruction. *Plastic and Reconstructive Surgery* 92:831-839, 1993.

Kapp-Simon KA, Simon DJ, and Kristovich S: Self-perception, social skills, adjustment, and inhibition in young adolescents with craniofacial anomalies. *Cleft Palate Journal* 29:340-345, 1992.

Krueckeberg SM, and Kapp-Simon KA: Effect of parental factors on social skills of preschool children with craniofacial anomalies. *Cleft Palate–Craniofacial Journal* 30:490-496, 1993.

Krueckeberg SM, Kapp-Simon KA, and Ribordy SC: Social skills of preschoolers with and without craniofacial anomalies. *Cleft Palate–Craniofacial Journal* 30:475-481, 1993.

Lansdown R, and Polak L: A study of the psychological effects of facial deformity in children. *Child Care, Health and Development* 1:85-91, 1975.

Lazarus RS: Psychological stress and coping process. New York: McGraw-Hill, 1966.

Lefebvre A, and Barclay S: Psychosocial impact of craniofacial deformities before and after reconstructive surgery. *Canadian Journal of Psychiatry* 27:579-584, 1982.

MacGregor FC: Facial disfigurement: problems and management of social interactions and implications for mental health. *Aesthetic Plastic Surgery* 14:249-257, 1990.

MacGregor FC: Some psychosocial problems associated with facial deformities. *American Sociological Review* 16:629-638, 1951.

MacGregor FC, Abel TM, Bryt A, Lauer E, and Weissman S: *Facial deformities and plastic surgery: a psychosocial study.* Springfield (IL): CC Thomas, 1953.

Maris CL, Endriga MC, Omnell ML, and Speltz ML: Psychological adjustment in twin pairs with and without hemifacial microsomia. *Cleft Palate–Craniofacial Journal* 36:43-50, 1999.

McWilliams BJ: Psychosocial development and modification. *Asha Report #5: Speech and the dentofacial complex: the state of the art.* Washington (DC): American Speech and Hearing Association, 1970, pp. 165-187.

Moss EM, Batshaw ML, Solot CB, Gerdes M, McDonald-McGinn DM, Driscoll DA, Emanuel BS, Zackai EH, and Wang PP: Psychoeducational profile of the 22q11.2 microdeletion: a complex pattern. *Pediatrics* 134:193-198, 1999.

Padwa BL, Evans CA, and Pillemer FC: Psychosocial adjustment in children with hemifacial microsomia and other craniofacial deformities. *Cleft Palate–Craniofacial Journal* 28:354-359, 1991.

Palkes HS, Marsh JL, and Talent BK: Pediatric craniofacial surgery and parental attitudes. *Cleft Palate Journal* 23:137-143, 1986.

Papolos DF, Faedda GL, Veit S, Goldberg R, Morrow B, Kucherlapati R, and Shprintzen RJ: Bipolar spectrum disorders in patients diagnosed with velo-cardio-facial syndrome: does a hemizygous deletion of chromosome 22q11 result in bipolar affective disorder? *American Journal of Psychiatry* 153:1541-1547, 1996.

Pertschuk MJ, and Whitaker LA: Psychosocial adjustment and craniofacial malformations in childhood. *Plastic and Reconstructive Surgery* 75:177-181, 1985.

Pertschuk MJ, and Whitaker LA: Psychosocial considerations in craniofacial deformities. *Clinics in Plastic Surgery* 14:163-168, 1987.

Pertschuk MJ, and Whitaker LA: Psychosocial outcome of craniofacial surgery in children. *Plastic and Reconstructive Surgery* 82:741-746, 1988.

Phillips J, and Whitaker LA: The social effects of craniofacial deformity and its correction. *Cleft Palate Journal* 16:7-15, 1979.

Pillemer FB, and Cook CV: The psychosocial adjustment of pediatric craniofacial patients after surgery. *Cleft Palate Journal* 26:201-207, 1989.

Pope AW: Points of risk and opportunity for parents of children with craniofacial conditions. *Cleft Palate–Craniofacial Journal* 36:36-39, 1999.

Pope AW, and Speltz ML: Research on psychosocial issues of children with craniofacial anomalies: progress and challenges. *Cleft Palate–Craniofacial Journal* 34:371-373, 1997.

Pope AW, and Ward J: Factors associated with peer social competence in preadolescents with craniofacial anomalies. *Journal of Pediatric Psychology* 22:455-470, 1997a.

Pope AW, and Ward J: Self-perceived facial appearance and psychosocial adjustment in preadolescents with craniofacial anomalies. *Cleft Palate–Craniofacial Journal* 34:396-401, 1997b.

Pulver AE, Nestadt G, Goldberg R, Shprintzen RJ, Lamacz M, Wolyniec PS, Morrow B, Karayiorgou M, Antonarakis SE, Housman D, and Kucherlapati F: Psychotic illness in patients diagnosed with velo-cardio-facial syndrome and their relatives. *Journal of Nervous and Mental Disorders* 182:476-478, 1994.

Richardson SA: Age and sex differences in values toward handicaps. *Journal of Health and Social Behavior* 11:207-214, 1970.

Richardson SA: Handicap, appearance, and stigma. *Social Science and Medicine* 5:621-626, 1971.

Richardson SA, Hastorf AH, and Dornbusch SM: Effects of physical disability on a child's description of himself. *Child Development* 35:893-907, 1964.

Richardson SA, Goodman N, Hastorf A, and Dornbusch S: Cultural uniformity in reaction to physical disabilities. *American Sociological Review* 26:241-247, 1961.

Richman LC: The effects of facial disfigurement on teachers' perception of ability in cleft palate children. *Cleft Palate Journal* 15:155-160, 1978.

Richman LC, and Harper D: School adjustment of children with observable disabilities. *Journal of Abnormal Child Psychology* 6:11-18, 1978.

Richman LC, and Harper D: Self identified personality patterns of children with facial or orthopedic disfigurement. *Cleft Palate Journal* 16:257-261, 1979.

Richman LC, and Harper D: Personality profiles of physically impaired young adults. *Journal of Clinical Psychology* 36:668, 1980.

Robinson E, Rumsey N, and Partridge J: An evaluation of the impact of social interaction skills training for facially disfigured people. *British Journal of Plastic Surgery* 49:281-289, 1986.

Schwartz AH, and Landwirth J: Birth defects and the psychological development of the child: some implications for management. *Connecticut Medicine* 32:457-464, 1968.

Shprintzen RJ, Goldberg R, Golding-Kushner KJ, and Marion R: Late-onset psychoses in velo-cardio-facial syndrome. *American Journal of Medical Genetics* 42:141-142, 1992.

Sigelman CK, Miller TE, and Whitworth LA: The early stigmatizing reactions to physical differences. *Journal of Applied Developmental Psychology* 7:17-23, 1986.

Speltz ML, Armsden GC, and Clarren SS: Effects of craniofacial birth defects on maternal functioning postinfancy. *Journal of Pediatric Psychology* 15:177-195, 1990.

Speltz ML, Galbreath H, and Greenberg MT: A developmental framework for psychosocial research on young children with craniofacial anomalies. In Eder RA (ed.): *Craniofacial anomalies: psychological perspectives.* New York: Springer-Verlag, 1995, pp. 258-286.

Speltz ML, Endriga MC, and Mouradian WE: Presurgical and postsurgical mental and psychomotor development of infants with sagittal synostosis. *Cleft Palate–Craniofacial Journal* 34:374-379, 1997.

Speltz ML, Morton K, Goodell EW, and Clarren SK: Psychological functioning of children with craniofacial anomalies and their mothers: follow-up from late infancy to school entry. *Cleft Palate–Craniofacial Journal* 30:482-489, 1993.

Speltz ML, Greenberg MT, Endriga MC, and Galbreath H: Developmental approach to the psychology of craniofacial anomalies. *Cleft Palate–Craniofacial Journal* 31:61-67, 1994.

Strauss RP, and Broder HL: Directions and issues in psychosocial research and methods as applied to cleft lip and palate and craniofacial anomalies. *Cleft Palate–Craniofacial Journal* 28:150-156, 1991.

Stricker G, Clifford E, Cohen L, Giddon D, Meskin L, and Evans C: Psychosocial aspects of craniofacial disfigurement. *American Journal of Orthodontics* 76:410-422, 1979.

Wasserman GA, Allen R, and Solomon CR: At-risk toddlers and their mothers: the special case of physical handicap. *Child Development* 56:82-85, 1985.

Wasserman GA, Allen R, and Linares LO: Maternal interaction and language development in children with and without speech-related anomalies. *Journal of Communication Disorders* 21:319-331, 1988.

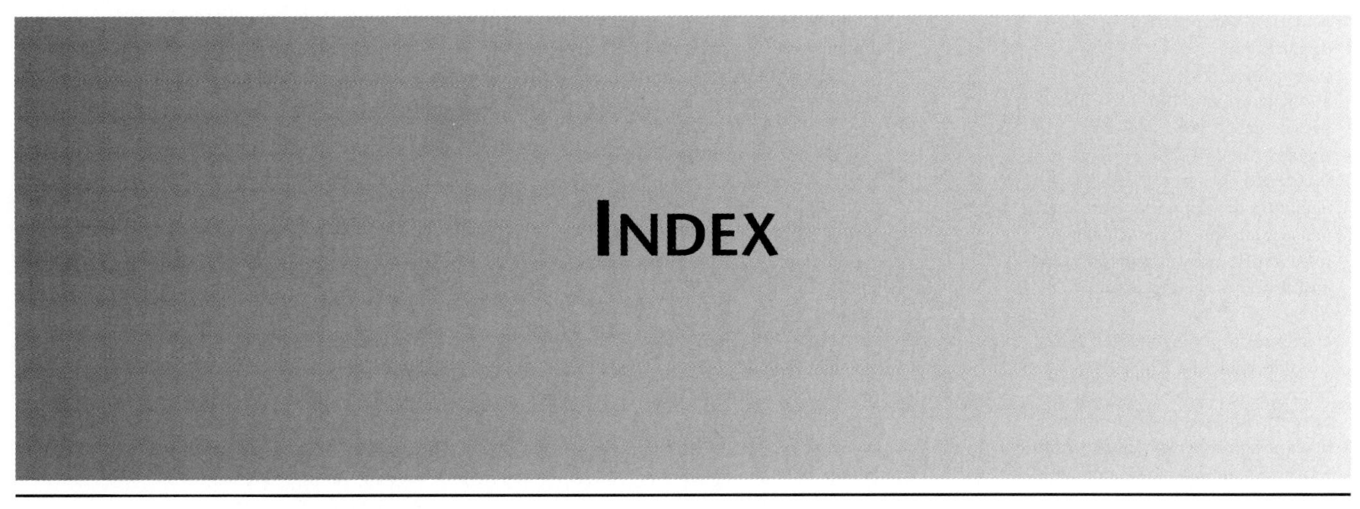

INDEX

b indicates box; *f*, figure; n, footnote; *t*, table.

W

Z